Genetic Disorders of
Human Sexual Development

OXFORD MONOGRAPHS ON MEDICAL GENETICS

General Editors

Arno G. Motulsky   Martin Bobrow   Peter S. Harper   Charles Scriver

Former Editors

J. A. Fraser Roberts   C. O. Carter

OXFORD MONOGRAPHS ON MEDICAL GENETICS NO. 38

Genetic Disorders of Human Sexual Development

LEONARD PINSKY, M.D.
Professor and Chair of Human Genetics
Professor of Medicine and Pediatrics
McGill University

ROBERT P. ERICKSON, M.D.
Professor of Pediatrics and Molecular and Cellular Biology
The University of Arizona Health Sciences Center

R. NEIL SCHIMKE, M.D.
Professor of Medicine and Pediatrics
The University of Kansas Medical Center

New York   Oxford
OXFORD UNIVERSITY PRESS
1999

Oxford University Press

Oxford   New York
Athens   Auckland   Bangkok   Bogotá   Buenos Aires   Calcutta
Cape Town   Chennai   Dar es Salaam   Delhi   Florence   Hong Kong   Istanbul
Karachi   Kuala Lumpur   Madrid   Melbourne   Mexico City   Mumbai
Nairobi   Paris   São Paulo   Singapore   Taipei   Tokyo   Toronto   Warsaw

and associated companies in
Berlin   Ibadan

Copyright © 1999 by Oxford University Press, Inc.

Published by Oxford University Press, Inc.
198 Madison Avenue, New York, New York 10016

Library of Congress Cataloging-in-Publication Data
Pinsky, Leonard.
Genetic disorders of human sexual development /
Leonard Pinsky, Robert P. Erickson, R. Neil Schimke.
p. cm.—(Oxford monographs on medical genetics; no. 38)
Includes bibliographical references and index.
ISBN 0-19-510907-4
1. Sexual disorders—Genetic aspects.   2. Sexual differentiation disorders—Genetic aspects.
3. Developmental disorders—Genetic aspects.   4. Sex chromosome abnormalities.
5. Generative organs—Abnormalities—Genetic aspects.
I. Erickson, Robert P., 1939– .   II. Schimke, R. Neil, 1935– .
III. Title.   IV. Series.
[DNLM: 1. Gonadal Disorders—genetics.   2. Sex Chromosome Abnormalities—genetics.
3. Sex Chromosomes—genetics.   4. Sex Maturation—genetics.   5. Genetics, Biochemical.
WK 900 P658g   1999]   RC881.5.P55   1999   616.6'9042—dc21
DNLM/DLC   for Library of Congress   98-42996

9 8 7 6 5 4 3 2 1

Printed in the United States of America
on acid-free paper

To Merrille, Susan, Todd, Karen, and Gina
for having tolerated a lot of
inattention over nearly 40 years.
L. P.

To the memory of
Tracy Lynn Erickson,
1969–1997
R. P. E.

To my grandchildren
Chad, Tony, Heather, Cora, and Conner
R. N. S.

Preface

We are three clinical geneticists who share a long and abiding interest in disorders of human sexual development. We have joined as coauthors because each of us has felt the need for a single, practical, everyday source of information that can provide up-to-date understanding and guidance in the delineation, diagnosis, and management of these disorders. There are, of course, encyclopedic volumes that deal in more or less depth with diverse forms of sexual maldevelopment, as one among many other categories of human maldevelopment. And there are textbooks of endocrinology that deal comprehensively with common forms of sexual maldevelopment, and cursorily with less common forms, but they do so in stereotypical textbook fashion, with little or no space for inquiry, integration, speculation, or the authors' own clinical experience. We have integrated genetically whenever possible, questioned frequently, speculated liberally (even across species barriers), and shared our personal experiences to their professional limits. As geneticists, we have treasured the value of the rare case that makes a disproportionate contribution to knowledge, but we have not overlooked the cross-sectional predictions that are meaningful to individuals, even if they have been derived from the longitudinal analysis of groups.

The powerful tools of molecular genetics have produced an avalanche of new information about the factors that carry out normal sexual development, about the genes that encode these factors, and about the mutations that impair them structurally, numerically, or functionally. Quite simply, we know a lot more now than we did 20 years ago about the structure and function of the sex chromosomes, about the identity, distribution, and role of the sex-*determining* genes, and about the hormonal substances (endocrine, paracrine, or autocrine) that mediate the processes of sex *differentiation*. It is safe to say that knowledge about normal and abnormal sexual development has passed from the stage of pure description to the first stage of biochemical-molecular understanding. The next two decades will likely bring us close to a full understanding of normal and abnormal sexual development. That does not necessarily mean that we will often be able to prevent or reverse sexual maldevelopment, but it does mean at least that explanation and choice will often be available to help people and families deal with the perceived or actual burdens of sexual maldevelopment.

We have designed this book to deal with basic facts as well as emerging information at the frontier of knowledge. Therefore, our book should be as readily useful to the senior medical student assigned to a case as to the gynecologist, urologist, endocrinologist, or clinical geneticist–dysmorphologist who is ultimately responsible for the person who is each case.

We have not tried to be exhaustive. For instance, we have not catalogued every chromosome abnormality that may inhibit normal sexual development, nor have we identified every nonchromosomal syndrome of multiple congenital anomalies that may include sexual maldevelopment. At the same time, just as we have not disregarded the value of the important rare case, we have tried hard to increase the reader's accessibility to established syndromal forms of sexual maldevelopment in males and/or females. To approach this goal we have classified these syndromes in several ways: alphabetically according to their common names, according to anomalies in single nonreproductive organs, in groups that have an underlying systemic or metabolic basis, and by reference to appropriate syndromes in those sections of the book that deal with specific nonsyndromal forms of sexual maldevelopment.

Above all, we have sought to compile a modern, *genetic* overview of human sexual maldevelopment as we approach the new millennium. We believe we have provided a solid framework upon which the reader can add personal experience or published information as these become available.

We feel privileged that Oxford University Press has chosen us to add a key volume to the series of Oxford Monographs on Medical Genetics, and we hope to be involved in the preparation of subsequent editions as these become mandated by the inevitable accrual of knowledge about human sexual maldevelopment.

Montreal, Quebec   L. P.
Tucson, Arizona   R. P. E.
Kansas City, Kansas   R. N. S.

Acknowledgments

It is a pleasure to acknowledge my formidable first mentors: F. Clarke Fraser, who inspired my interest in developmental genetics; Angelo M. DiGeorge who promoted the pursuit of endocrine genetics; and Robert S. Krooth, who promoted the power of cultured somatic cells to solve problems in human organismal genetics. Bradley N. White allowed me to float through his laboratory during a sabbatical year in order to immerse myself in human genomics. The influence of each of them is embodied in what became a career-long research program: the use of genital skin fibroblasts (and their nucleic acids) to identify and characterize mutant androgen receptors responsible for the extremely diverse phenotypes of androgen resistance. Alexandra Costa and Elpida Artemiou searched the literature databases for me, and from these searches all three of us learned a lot. Rhona Rosenzweig's endless devotion to the book kept me going whenever the task seemed daunting. Linda Van Inwegen generated an imaginative jacket illustration at the last minute. Thankfully, Charles Annis kept a watchful eye over our editorial indiscretions. The gentle persistence of Jeffrey House was indispensable.

L. P.

I want to thank my early mentors in genetics, Tahir Rizki, Leonard and Leonore Herzenberg, and Salome G. Waelsch for recruiting me to the field. My interest in human sexual differentiation was initially stimulated by Charles J. Epstein. Bryan Hall helped my understanding of the dysmorphological aspects, and Peter N. Goodfellow allowed me to participate in his early work on the molecular aspects. Workers in my laboratory who contributed to our research in normal and abnormal sexual differentiation include Asangla Ao, Stan R. Blecher, Timothy R. Boyer, Majed Dasouki, Mitchell M. Drumm, Edward J. Durbin, Penelope Graves, Linda M. Kalikin, Marisol L. Lopez, John R. D. Stalvey, Vera C. Verga, Michal Witt, and Theresa A. Zwingman. I appreciate how much they have taught me. I would like to thank Drs. Nabeel Affara, Christopher Cunniff, Malcom Ferguson-Smith, and Randall

Heidenreich for comments on various portions of the manuscript. I would also like to thank Ms. Carole Meyer for the typing of the manuscript and, above all, my wife Sandra, the value of whose support cannot be adequately expressed.

R. P. E.

I am indebted to Robert Manning who stimulated my interest in genetics, Elizabeth (Tibby) Russell who was kind enough to underwrite a stay at the Jackson Laboratory early in my career and helped me gain an appreciation of mouse genetics, and, of course, Victor McKusick who helped me put it all together and who has remained an inspiration over these many years. I would also like to thank my secretaries, Melissa Thomas and Mary Lynch, who put up with the correspondence and the often times confusing drafts and redrafts of various portions of the manuscript. I would also like to apologize to my wife, Loretta, for my occasional testy personality while the manuscript was in progress.

R. N. S.

Contents

III Gonadal Maldevelopment

IV Sexual Maldevelopment

V Genetic Forms of Gamete Failure

I

NORMAL GONADAL AND SEXUAL DEVELOPMENT

1

The Embryology of Normal Gonadal and Genital Development

The genetic sex of the embryo is established at fertilization. Although the developmental events that subsequently occur in sex differentiation have long been known, the precise genetic, biochemical, endocrine, and molecular mechanisms have been only partially elucidated (Schafer, 1995). The evaluation of patients with chromosome anomalies, with mendelian traits, and with multifactorial conditions that involve absent, incomplete, or inadequate gonadal development and genital ambiguity has been invaluable in our effort to unravel the complexities of human sex differentiation. Similarly, studies in other mammals, particularly mice, have offered considerable insight into the various mechanisms involved.

A brief review of normal gonadal and genital development is provided in this chapter as groundwork for a fuller understanding of the nature and timing of anomalous sexual differentiation. The genetic factors known to be responsible for the various events will be briefly mentioned and elaborated upon in later chapters.

DEVELOPMENT OF THE GONADS

The Indifferent Gonad.   Gonadal development is first apparent during the fifth week of gestation as a thickened area of coelomic or mesodermal epithelium on the medioventral border of the urogenital ridge (Moore, 1988). Further proliferation of this epithelium and its underlying mesenchyme produces a bulge on the medial side of the mesonephros, the gonadal ridge. Shortly thereafter, epithelial projections, called primary sex cords, grow into the mesenchyme, thereby defining two arbitrary zones, an outer cortex and the inner medulla.

Primordial germ cells are large, spherical cells recognizable during the fourth week in the yolk sac wall near the origin of the allantois. These cells increase mitotically and migrate toward the gonadal ridge through the dorsal mesentery of the hindgut (Byskov, 1956). By the sixth week, they enter the gonadal ridge and are incorporated into the primary sex cords. Before the sixth week of gestation, gonadal tissue of either sex is indistinguishable. Without germ cells, the gonadal ridge in the female remains undeveloped, whereas in males, testis development continues (Grumbach and Conte, 1992). Germ cells number more than 500,000 by 8 weeks (Baker and Eastwood, 1983). Those that fail to reach the gonad at the time of sex differentiation usually degenerate but occasionally may persist and develop later into extragonadal germ cell tumors.

There is a close spatial relationship between the gonad and kidney anlagen in the urogenital ridge and the developing adrenal at this stage, and it is likely that specific genes affect the ontogeny of two or more of these organs simultaneously. For example, heterozygous mutations in the so-called Wilms tumor gene-1 (WT-1) in man, located on the short arm of chromosome 11 (11p13), lead to a range of developmental abnormalities in the kidney and gonad (Hastie, 1994). In mice, null homozygotes for the analogous gene Wt-1 fail to develop either kidneys or gonads (Kriedberg et al., 1993). Another gene in mice, Sf-1 (steroidogenic factor 1), one alternative splice product of the gene Ftz-F1, codes for a nuclear receptor that not only regulates the steroid hydroxylase enzyme system but appears to be essential for adrenal and gonadal development in general (Parker and Schimmer, 1997). A similar gene in man has been mapped to 9q33 (Taketo et al., 1995). Homing and survival of germ cells in mice require the Sf-1 gene, along with the c-kit protooncogene and its ligand, which are the products of the W and S1 loci, respectively (Wylie and Heasma, 1993).

There is a distinct temporal difference in gonadal differentiation between the sexes. Under the influence of testis-determining genes, testis organization begins between the sixth and seventh week. In contrast, the ovary does not emerge from the indifferent state until about 12 weeks.

Testis.   Testicular differentiation is evident in the male embryo by the end of the seventh week (Gustafson and Donahoe, 1994). By this time, the primitive sex cords, now termed seminiferous or testicular cords, have condensed and extended into the center or medulla of the developing gonad, where they anastomose and branch to form the rete testis. Contact of the seminiferous cords with the surface epithelium is broken by development of a thick fibrous capsule, the tunica albuginea. The seminiferous cords are separated by mesenchyme that will later give rise to interstitial or Leydig cells. In addition to primitive germ cells, the seminiferous cords contain Sertoli cells derived from the surface epithelium. The previous mitotic proliferation of germ cells is now suppressed, and shortly thereafter, müllerian regression occurs. Both these phenomena are likely mediated by the Sertoli cells. It is thought that Sertoli cells elaborate a meiosis-preventing substance that arrests germ cell maturation at the primitive spermatogonia stage. An alternative explanation is that inhibition of germ cell meiosis occurs because of the physical separation of the spermatogonia from the rete testis, which possibly secretes a meiosis-inducing substance. Sertoli cells do secrete Müllerian-inhibiting substance (MIS), also termed müllerian-inhibiting factor (MIF) or anti-müllerian hormone (AMH) (Josso et al., 1993). This substance is a glycoprotein with structural similarity to transforming growth factor beta (TGF-β). Its gene is on the short arm of chromosome 19. MIS has a paracrine function: it diffuses to the paired müllerian duct primordia and causes their dissolution, probably by apoptosis. The expression of MIS is controlled by SRY (sex-determining regions on the Y chromosome), through one or more intermediary steps (Haqq et al., 1994). The Sertoli cells also produce inhibin, and an androgen-binding protein, and probably play an as yet undefined role in testicular descent.

Leydig cells are detected in the testis by 60 days gestation, and they rapidly proliferate during the third and fourth months, possibly under the influence of MIS (Behringer et al., 1994). Testosterone synthesis by the Leydig cells begins at about 9 weeks, perhaps stimulated by placenta-derived chorionic gonadotropin (hCG), although this is controversial (Word et al., 1989), and later by fetal pituitary luteinizing hormone (LH). Testosterone and its reduced metabolite, dihydrotestosterone, regulate male internal and external differentiation. Peak fetal serum concentration of testosterone occurs at roughly 16 weeks gestation and thereafter declines to a level similar to that seen in a prepubescent male. The glycoprotein hormones hCG and LH also are necessary for intrauterine growth of the penis and scrotum, and for testicular descent, although the precise role of each hormone is uncertain.

At birth, the seminiferous cords are populated by early spermatogonia, which are quiescent until late in the prepubescent period when proliferation gives rise to primary spermatocytes. The cords become canalized to become seminiferous tubules. Meiosis begins at puberty, with the process ultimately leading to the production of mature spermatozoa. Unlike the germ cell attrition that occurs in the ovary, male germinal epithelium continues to be active throughout life.

In addition to SRY, genes on the Y chromosome, on the X chromosome, and on autosomes are necessary for development, differentiation, and maturation of the testis (Schafer, 1995). The various effects of these genes are discussed in later chapters.

Ovary. Without the concerted action of a set of testis-determining genes, the undifferentiated gonad will inherently develop as an ovary, as long as surviving germ cells are present. As indicated earlier, the indifferent stage of ovarian development persists until about 12 weeks of gestational life. The germ cells proliferate and become recognizable as oogonia, perhaps under the influence of a meiosis-inducing substance elaborated by the rete ovarii. No oogonia form after birth. By the twelfth week of gestation, the transition of oogonia into oocytes is evident, and this phase of differentiation marks the true beginning of the ovary. By 16 weeks, the cortical cords begin to break up into clusters of primordial follicles. Follicle formation is maximal between 20 and 25 weeks under the influence of fetal follicle-stimulating hormone (FSH), with a peak population of 6 to 7 million, in various stages of differentiation and degeneration, by 7 months *in utero*. Thereafter, the number diminishes and the oocytes that survive are arrested in prophase of the first meiotic division (diplotene). They remain in this state until ovulation. At ovulation, the first polar body is extruded, but the second polar body is not lost until the ovum is penetrated by a spermatozoan. The fetal ovary has the ability to synthesize estradiol, but there is no evidence that fetal estradiol is of developmental significance.

The granulosa cell of the ovary is homologous to the Sertoli cell, and the theca cell is derived from the same mesenchymal elements as the Leydig cell. Neither cell type is known to contribute for certain to female ovarian or genital development, although MIS secreted by granulosa cells has been suggested to exert an antimeiotic effect on oocytes (Lee and Donahoe, 1993).

Genes on both X chromosomes are essential for ovarian maintenance, as evidenced by the accelerated follicular atresia seen in women with monosomy X. Autosomal genes are also important in ovarian development and maintenance, for a number of autosomal inherited forms of 46,XX gonadal dysgenesis exist (Chapter 15).

DEVELOPMENT OF THE GENITAL DUCTS

Early Stages.   Male and female embryos each have two pairs of genital ducts (Figure 1–1). The mesonephric or wolffian ducts drain the mesonephric kidney, and elements of this duct become essential parts of the male reproductive system. Except for a few vestigial remnants, the mesonephric ducts in females largely disappear. In contrast, the paramesonephric (müllerian) ducts are an integral part of the female reproductive system. These ducts are derived from an invagination of the coelomic epithelium lateral to each mesonephros. The paramesonephric system in males degenerates with the exception of a terminal remnant attached to each testis, the appendix testis. By the third month, respective male and female internal development is complete.

Male Duct.   In a number of pioneering studies, Jost (1953, 1972) and Jost and colleagues (1973) demonstrated the importance of paracrine and endocrine secretions of the testis in directing genital development. Secretion of MIS by the Sertoli cells is local and unilateral: if one testis is absent, an ipsilateral oviduct will develop. Testosterone from the Leydig cell acts locally and directly to stabilize the wolffian duct, probably by a concentration effect, and also as a blood-borne hormone on male external genital primordia. Because wolffian duct tissue lacks the enzyme 5 α-reductase, it is testosterone and not the reduced metabolite dihydrotestosterone that binds to the cytosolic androgen receptor to induce male internal genital development.

Under the influence of testosterone, elements of the degenerating mesonephric ducts persist. The tubules nearest the testis become the efferent ductules and con-

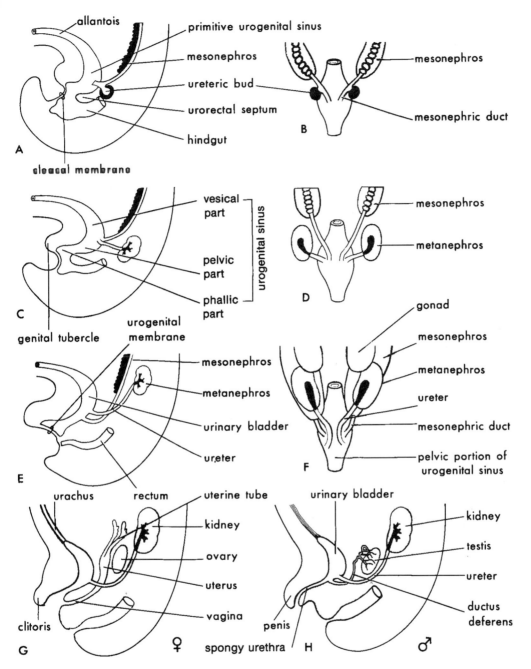

FIGURE 1–1. Diagrams showing: (1) division of the cloaca into the urogenital sinus and rectum, (2) absorption of the mesonephric ducts, (3) development of the urinary bladder, urethra, and urachus, and (4) changes in the location of the ureters. *A,* Lateral view of the caudal half of a five-week embryo. *B, D,* and *F,* Dorsal views. *C, E, G,* and *H,* Lateral views. The stages shown in *G* and *H* are reached by the twelfth week. (Reproduced from Moore KL and Persaud TVN, 1993. *The Developing Human: Clinically Oriented Embryology,* 5th ed., Philadelphia, Saunders, with permission.)

7

nect the seminiferous tubules via the rete testis to the main portion of the persistent wolffian duct, which becomes the epididymal duct. The more distal wolffian duct acquires a smooth muscle coat and becomes the vas deferens. Seminal vesicles are lateral outgrowths of each wolffian duct. That portion of the wolffian duct between the duct of the seminal vesicles and the urethra is the definitive ejaculatory duct.

As mentioned earlier, MIS facilitates müllerian duct degeneration. Males with absent, deficient, or structurally abnormal MIS or similar defects in the MIS receptor have various degrees of persistence of the müllerian system (Chapter 9). Similarly, males with Leydig cell hypoplasia, abnormalities in testosterone biosynthesis, and androgen receptor defects have rudimentary or hypoplastic wolffian derivatives with external genital feminization or ambiguity (Chapter 11).

Female Duct. Female internal duct development is an autonomous phenomenon. In the absence of a gonad or a functional testis, and hence MIS, the cranial ends of the paired müllerian ducts become the fallopian tubes. Remnants of the cranial ends of the müllerian ducts not utilized in development of the infundibulum of the fallopian tubes may persist as a small appendage known as the hydatid of Morgagni. Distally, the ducts cross the midline anterior to the degenerating wolffian ducts and fuse to form the uterovaginal primordium. This fusion process brings together two peritoneal folds that become the broad ligaments.

Elements of the wolffian ducts may persist in females. The cranial end may be represented by a structure called the appendix vesiculosa. Nearer the ovary, blind tubular components and duct, together called the epoophoron, which are analogous to the efferent ductules and epididymal duct in the male, may be found within the broad ligament. Close to the uterus, wolffian remnants may be detected as rudimentary tubules termed paroophoron. Still other parts of the wolffian system, corresponding to the male vas deferens and ejaculatory duct, may persist as Gartner's duct or as Gartner's duct cysts between layers of the broad ligament.

Despite the essential involution of the wolffian duct in the female, some interaction or codependence of this system and the müllerian duct must exist. The evidence for this is that agenesis or aplasia of the mature (metanephronic) kidney, which arises from an outbud of the wolffian duct, is often accompanied by uterine and fallopian tube anomalies with or without vaginal agenesis. This association is discussed further in Chapter 7.

DEVELOPMENT OF THE EXTERNAL GENITALIA

Indifferent Stage. The external genital primordia of both sexes are indistinguishable until after the eighth week of gestation, and it is not until the twelfth week that the sexes can be fully differentiated. During the fourth week, a genital tubercle develops at the anterior end of the cloacal membrane in both sexes. Posterior to the tubercle and on the medial aspect of the membrane, urethral folds develop, and laterally, labioscrotal folds become apparent. As the urorectal septum proliferates and descends to intersect with the cloacal membrane in the sixth week, it induces eventual breakdown of the membrane, thereby dividing the cloaca into an anterior segment, the urogenital sinus, and a posterior cavity, the eventual rectum and anus (O'Rahilly, 1977; Escobar et al., 1987).

Male External Genitalia. In the presence of an intact testis with normal steroidogenic capacity, normal 5α-reductase activity in the external genital anlagen, and functional androgen receptors, male external development proceeds. The major, if not the sole, determining factor in male external differentiation is dihydrotesterone. Under the influence of this hormone, the genital tubercle develops into a glans penis, the urethral folds elongate and fuse in the midline to form the cavernous urethra and corpus spongiosum, and the labioscrotal folds fuse and move posteriorly to become the definitive scrotum. The line of fusion of the labioscrotal folds is the midline raphae, which dorsally contributes to the ventral epidermis of the penis. Penile length increases at about 0.7 mm per week from roughly 10 weeks to term, a rate of increase almost four times that of the clitoris. The prostate gland and the bulbourethral (Cowper's) glands are outgrowths of the urogenital sinus, and their development is also controlled by dihydrotestosterone.

Female External Genitalia. The caudal ends of the paired müllerian ducts fuse in the midline to form a urovaginal primordium that projects into the urogenital sinus. This urovaginal projection probably represents the müllerian contribution to the vagina, although the issue is controversial (Cunha, 1975). It does appear, however, that interaction between the terminal fused müllerian ducts and the urogenital sinus is necessary for normal development and canalization of the vagina. The vesicovaginal septum proliferates, forcing the vaginal orifice posteriorly and creating separate openings to the urethra and vagina. The urogenital sinus in females is essentially obliterated, although Skene's paraurethral glands and the vestibular glands of Bartholin remain as homologues of the prostate and Cowper's glands in the male.

The genital tubercle enlarges to form the clitoris. The urethral folds essentially remain open to become the labia minora, the posterior segment fusing as the frenulum. Both the extreme anterior and posterior parts of the labioscrotal folds fuse to become the mons pubis and the posterior labial commissure, respectively. The large midportion remainder of the labioscrotal folds remain unfused, eventually forming two large skin folds, the labia majora.

REFERENCES

Baker T G, Eastwood J (1983). Origin and differentiation of germ cells in man. *Bibl Anat* 24: 67–76.

Behringer R R, Finegold M J, Cate R L (1994). Müllerian-inhibiting substance function during mammalian sexual development. *Cell* 79:415–425.

Byskov A G (1986). Differentiation of mammalian embryonic gonad. *Physiol Rev* 66:71–117.

Cunha G R (1975). The dual origin of vaginal epithelium. *Am J Anat* 143:357–392.

Escobar L F, Weaver D D, Bixler D, et al. (1987). Urorectal malformation sequence. *Am J Dis Child* 141:1021–1024.

Grumbach M M, Conte F A (1992). Disorders of sex differentiation. In *Williams Textbook of Endocrinology*. Wilson J D, Foster D W (eds.), 8th ed. Philadelphia, W B Saunders, pp 853–951.

Gustafson M L, Donahoe P K (1994). Male sex determination: current concepts of male sexual differentiation. *Annu Rev Med* 45:5-505–524.

Haqq C M, King C-Y, Ukijama E, et al. (1994). Molecular basis of mammalian sexual determination: activation of Müllerian inhibiting substance gene expression by SRY. *Science* 266:1454–1500.

Hastie N D (1994). The genetics of Wilms' tumor—a case of disrupted development. *Annu Rev Genet* 28:523–558.

Josso N, Lamarre I, Picard J-Y, et al. (1993). Anti-Müllerian hormone in early human development. *Early Human Dev* 33:91–99.

Jost A (1953). Studies on sex differentiation in mammals. *Recent Prog Horm Res* 8:379–418.

Jost A (1972). A new look at the mechanism controling sex differentiation in mammals. *Johns Hopkins Med J* 130:38–53.

Jost A, Vigier B, Drepin J, et al. (1973). Studies on sex differentiation in mammals. *Recent Prog Horm Res* 29:1–41.

Kriedberg J A, Sariola H, Loring J M, et al. (1993). WT-1 is required for early kidney development. *Cell* 74:679–691.

Lee M M, Donahoe P K (1993). Müllerian inhibiting substance: a gonadal hormone with multiple functions. *Endocr Rev* 14:152.

Moore C C D, Grumbach M M (1992). Sex determination and gonadogenesis: a transcription cascade of sex chromosome and autosome genes. *Semin Perinatal* 16:266–278.

Moore K L (1988). *The Developing Human; Clinically Oriented Embryology*, ed. 4, Philadelphia, W B Sanders, pp 262–275.

O'Rahilly R (1977). The development of the vagina in the human. *Birth Defects* 13:123.

Parker K L, Schimmer B P (1997). Steroidogenic factor 1: a key determinant of endocrine development and function. *Endocr Rev* 18:361–377.

Schafer A J (1995). Sex determination and its pathology in man. *Adv Genet* 33:275–329.

Taketo M, Parker K L, Howard T A, et al. (1995). Homologs of drosophila Fuski-Tarazo factor 1 map to mouse chromosome 2 and human chromosome 9q33. *Genomics* 25:565–567.

Word R A, George F W, Wilson J D, et al. (1989). Testosterone synthesis and adenylate cyclase activity in the early fetal testis appear to be independent of human chorionic gonadotropin control. *J Clin Endocrinol Metab* 69:204–208.

Wylie C C, Heasma J (1993). Migration, proliferation and potency of primordial germ cells. *Semin Devel Biol* 4:161–170.

2

Sex Chromosome and Autosome Contributions to Normal Gonadal Development

Research on the genetics of sexual determination and differentiation has resulted in many recent advances. These include the cloning of the testis-determining factor (*SRY*), identification of candidate downstream genes for its action, and localization of genes whose role in sexual differentiation is not fully understood. This chapter attempts to review the current status of this fast moving field without ignoring the unanswered questions.

Sex Chromosomes

THE Y CHROMOSOME IS MALE-DETERMINING

"Classical" Human Cytogenetic Discoveries. It has been known since 1923 that humans have X and Y chromosomes (Painter, 1923). However, nothing was known about their respective roles in mammalian sex determination until 1959, when the

crucial contribution of the Y chromosome became clear. In that year, Welshons and Russell (1959) demonstrated that XO mice are female; Jacobs and Strong (1959) discovered that a male with Klinefelter syndrome had a 47,XXY karyotype; and Ford and colleagues (1959) reported that a woman with Turner syndrome had a 45,XO chromosomal constitution. Together, these observations demonstrated that a mammalian embryo develops as a male in the presence of a Y chromosome and as a female in the absence of a Y chromosome. Additionally, they indicated that this Y-chromosome action was independent of the number of X chromosomes.

Definition of Testis-determining Factor (TDF).   Along with Jost's illuminating experiments on the central role of the testes in mediating primary sex differentiation (see Chapters 1 and 3), the aforementioned cytogenetic evidence was interpreted to indicate that the Y chromosome possessed a gene or genes, the presence or absence of which determined the destiny of the bipotential gonad as a testis or ovary, respectively. It was also assumed that gonadal hormones would control the development of the dimorphic secondary sexual characteristics. In humans, the hypothetical Y-chromosomal gene was named *TDF* (testis-determining factor); in mice, it was named *Tdy* (testis-determining gene on the Y). Many patients with translocations and/or deletions involving the Y chromosome were studied in an effort to localize *TDF* on the Y chromosome. Most of the evidence could be interpreted in terms of localization to the short arm of the Y chromosome (Yp) (Davis, 1981).

The introduction of molecular genetics during the 1980s brought finer localization, but during the two preceding decades a large number of genes and sequences were studied as candidates for the elusive *TDF*. One such candidate was the Y-linked histocompatibility antigen (H-Y). It was originally detected by skin grafting between the two sexes within inbred strains of mice; later, a putative serological equivalent was found. The observation that antibodies raised in inbred female mice that received transplants of male skin reacted with XY cells of a variety of species led to the proposal that the H-Y antigen was the product of *TDF* (Wachtel, et al., 1975). This hypothesis was excluded by the finding of XX, sex-reversed (*Sxr*) male mice that did not express H-Y (McLaren, et al., 1984) and XY human females who were H-Y positive (Simpson, et al., 1987). We now know that a transplantation H-Y antigen is encoded by *SMCY*, which maps to the long arm of the human Y chromosome (Yq), not Yp (Wang, et al., 1995). Another *TDF* candidate was the repetitive sequence *Bkm* ("Banded krait minor") originally isolated from the snake *Bungarus fasciatus* (Jones and Singh, 1981) and found only in the sex chromosomes of many vertebrates. This hypothesis was rejected because in the human these sequences are not concentrated on Yp (Kiel-Metzger et al., 1985).

SRY IS TDF

Finer Localization of TDF.   The discovery that 46,XX males usually have translocations of Yp to one of their Xps was a major breakthrough (see Chromosome Mutations, 46,XX Males with *SRY* in Chapter 6 for further details) in the ability to map *TDF* on the Y chromosome (Evans et al., 1979; Magenis et al., 1982). The X

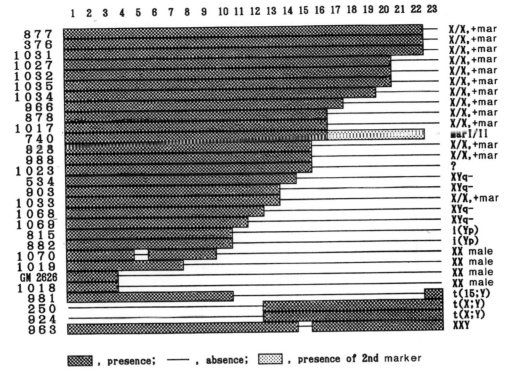

FIGURE 2–1. Example of a deletion map of the Y chromosome using 23 probes in 29 patients. Numbers for probes are indicated at the top, sample numbers on the left, and simplified karyotype designations on the right. Because there are two kinds of aberrant Y chromsomes in sample 740, the presence of fainter hybridizing sequences are indicated by a faint bar (from Nakahori et al., *Genomics* 9:765–769, 1991; by permission).

and Y are seen to pair at meiosis and this configuration is called the sex bivalent. This pairing is in a homologous segment located at the terminus of their short arms. Because of the high rate of genetic exchange between the X and Y chromosomes in this region, genes located in this region appear to be neither X-linked or Y-linked. Thus, this portion of the sex chromosomes is called "pseudoautosomal." The occurrence of crossovers centromeric to the pseudoautosomal region can result in the transfer of *TDF* to the X chromosome. These translocations involved an illegitimate recombination during paternal meiosis due to crossing-over between unpaired segments (Gueallaen et al., 1984; Stalvey et al., 1989). Molecular analyses of the different fragments of Y chromosome present in these patients permitted the construction of a deletion map with seven intervals: the first three covered all of Yp, the fourth corresponded to the centromeric region, and the remaining three represented the long arm, Yq (Vergnaud, et al., 1986). This map demonstrated that the terminal region of Yp (interval 1) was essential for testicular differentiation. Finer maps soon followed (Nakahori et al., 1991; Figure 2–1).

Page and colleagues (1987) subsequently subdivided Yp into 13 intervals. The interval 1A2, containing 140 kb, was found in a XX male who retained only 300 kilobases (kb) of Y chromosome, but not in a woman whose karyotype was

46X,−X,+t(Y;22). The Y;22 translocation retained only 160 kb of Y chromosome. The authors concluded that the interval 1A2 contained an essential part or all of *TDF* and they used different subclones from this region to search for evolutionarily conserved sequences from Y chromosomes of various mammals. One of the subclones identified a unique-sequence DNA in all males, but not in females, among those mammals studied. This subclone hybridized with another fragment of DNA present in both sexes. The nucleotide sequence of this clone revealed an open reading frame for a protein of 404 amino acids containing 13 zinc fingers, a domain common among transcription-regulating factors. The putative protein coded for by this clone was proposed as the product of *TDF*. It was suggested that this protein regulated the transcription of other genes in the pathway leading to testis differentiation. They named this gene *ZFY* (zinc *finger* gene on Y chromosome), and its X chromosome homologue *ZFX*. Notably, Page and colleagues (1987) mentioned that one of their XX males did not have *ZFY*. The finding of more such patients (Palmer et al., 1989; Verga and Erickson, 1989) suggested that *ZFY* could not be *TDF*.

Identification and Characterization of SRY *and* Sry *and Demonstration of Their Role in Sex Determination: Discovery and Confirmation by Mutational Analysis.*   The resumed search for *TDF* was targeted on 35 kb of DNA between the proximal limit of the pseudoautosomal region of the Y chromosome (i.e., the region that has homology to a corresponding segment of the X) and the breakpoint in XX, *ZFY⁻* negative males. The subclones generated from this target were hybridized with DNA from males of various mammals. One subclone detected sex-specific sequences in multiple mammals (Sinclair et al., 1990). Lower hybridization stringency exposed additional autosomal bands shared by males and females. These bands represent homologous sequences, some of which are involved in sex differentiation (see below).

The nucleotide sequence of this subclone encoded a protein containing a segment of 80 amino acids homologous to the mating-type protein of the *mat-3M* gene in *Schizosaccharomyces pombe* and to a conserved 80-amino-acid, DNA-binding motif present in the HMG1 and HMG2 (*high mobility group*) proteins (Sinclair et al., 1990) and in other transcription-regulating proteins (Jantzen et al., 1990). Northern analyses of a variety of tissues disclosed a transcript of 1.1 kb only in the testis. This gene, designated *SRY* (sex-determining region, Y chromosome) was suggested to be *TDF* (Sinclair et al., 1990).

Soon thereafter mutations in the *SRY* gene were found in some cases of XY, pure gonadal dysgenesis (Berta et al., 1990; Jäger et al., 1990; Hawkins et al., 1992; Affara et al., 1993). Subsequent studies disclosed that 46,XY females with mutations in *SRY* have streak gonads composed of ovarian-like stroma; in contrast, patients without *SRY* mutations have gonads composed of undifferentiated stroma with either seminiferous tubules or a *rete* structure (Vilain et al., 1993; see Alterations in *SRY* causing Gonadal Dysgenesis in Chapter 5 for fuller discussion). This difference indicates that in the presence of functional *SRY*, testicular formation begins but is halted, whereas in its absence, no evidence for an onset of testicular formation is found. The female patient originally described as having a simple Y;22 translocation

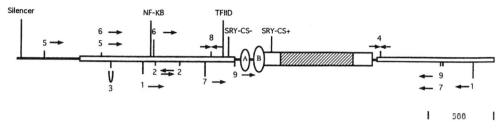

FIGURE 2–2. Diagrammatic illustration of various features on the flanking sequences of the human *SRY* gene. The *SRY* gene is represented by the large box. The shaded area indicates the coding region of the gene. Two ovals, A and B, indicate the location of the GC-rich core promoter and 40 nucleotides of 5' untranslated region of the *SRY* gene. The A + T contents are 71% and 66% for the upstream and downstream AT-rich blocks, respectively. The human *SRY* gene has 46% G + C content. The sequences homologous to the silencer of the MHC class I gene, immunoglobulin κB, and the binding site for TFID are identified. Two binding sites, SRY-CS+ and SRY-CS−, for the HMG domain of the SRY protein are present in both the plus and minus strands, respectively, as indicated. Several examples of repeats are identified by numbers: 1 and 2 = complementary inverted repeats; 3 = hairpin loop; 4 and 8 = direct inverted repeats; 5 and 6 = tandem repeats; and 7 and 9 = imperfect inverted repeats. The arrows indicate the orientations of the respective repeats (from Su H and Lau Y C, *Am J Hum Genet* 52:24–38, 1993; by permission).

(Page et al., 1987) was subsequently shown to have an additional deletion of interval 1A, which included the *SRY* gene (Page et al., 1990).

Identification and Characterization of SRY *and* Sry *and Demonstration of their Role in Sex Determination: Confirmation by Transgenesis.*　The mouse *Sry* gene was cloned at the same time as *SRY* (Gubbay et al., 1990). Partial deletion of the gene in XY female mice corroborated the finding of *SRY* mutations in XY human females (Lovell-Badge and Robertson, 1990). Mice transgenic for a 14-kb fragment containing *Sry* showed 40,XX sex-reversal—that is, mice otherwise destined to be female had a normal male appearance, although they were sterile (Koopman et al., 1991). Testes of these mice were histologically similar to those of human XX males. However, sex reversal did not always occur, even with a particular transgenic insertion. This incomplete penetrance seems unrelated to variation in the number of *Sry* transgenes. It may, however, be related to the influence of genetic background on *Sry* transgene expression (Hacker et al., 1995). Such variability has also been known in families in which some individuals with *SRY* mutations show XY gonadal dysgenesis while others are normal males who can transmit the mutated *SRY* (see Chapter 6). It will be of interest to determine whether or not variations in genetic background are also the explanation for this variable expression of mutations in *SRY*. In this context, it is relevant to point out that *SRY* did not cause sex reversal in transgenic mice.

SRY AS A TRANSCRIPTIONAL (TRANSACTING) FACTOR

Physical Chemistry of SRY *Compared to Other HMG Proteins.*　The *SRY* gene has a simple structure containing only one exon and no introns (Figure 2–2). The five-prime flanking sequence does not contain TATA or CCAT boxes, is rich in GC doublets, and contains two tandem Sp1 recognition sites (Sp1 is a zinc finger transcription factor, its target sequence is found in many promoters and enhancers), a sequence known to potentiate transcription (Vilain et al., 1992). The region transcribed consists of 841 base pairs, producing a protein of 204 amino acids with a molecular weight of 23.9 kDa. The gonadal ridge transcript has been defined for *Sry* (Hacker et al., 1995; Jeske et al., 1995). The HMG box is located centrally, at amino acids 57–137 of the protein (Su and Lau, 1993). Almost all the *SRY* mutations in XY females have occurred in the HMG box (see Chapter 5).

Two types of proteins contain HMG boxes: canonical and generalized. In the canonical group, 50% of residues are conserved, the HMG box is a major portion of the protein, the proteins are abundant, and they localize to the nucleus. They are thought to have a role in chromatin structure. The generalized group is very diverse and less abundant. The HMG box is a small portion of the protein and its strongly conserved portion consists of only eight residues. Of these, two are invariably prolines, two are positively charged amino acids, and four are aromatic residues. The HMG boxes of SRY and Sry correspond to generalized HMG boxes (Bianchi et al., 1992). The SRY HMG box binds to synthetic DNA fragments of the sequence AA-CAAAG (Nasrin et al., 1991); however, it also binds to cruciform DNA structures independently of their sequence (Ferrari et al., 1992). This ambivalence of DNA binding is apparently resolved by structural studies showing that the consensus sequence and the cruciform structure adopt a similar conformation in solution (King and Weiss, 1993). It has been suggested that the union of SRY with linear DNA induces a bend of about 80°, similar to that encountered in cruciform DNA. Other HMG proteins bind with great affinity to DNA cruciform structures. Because these other HMG proteins are much more abundant than SRY in the nucleus, it is likely that SRY favors DNA binding dependent on sequence (Ferrari et al., 1992). Notably, the sequence AACAAAG has been identified at positions −3 to +4 relative to the site of transcription initiation of the SRY gene, suggesting a possible autoregulatory role (Vilain et al., 1992). The resolution of the solution structure of the SRY-octamer DNA complex indicates that a concave surface, made of multiple amino acids, binds to the minor grove, inducing a large conformational change in the DNA (Werner et al., 1995). The solution structure also aids the interpretation of the mutations in *SRY*. Several mutations showing variable penetrance cause defects that would be expected to destabilize the protein, presumably leading to more rapid degradation; other mutations in the HMG box alter the conformation of DNA-contact sites in a way that precludes the usual deformation of the DNA (Werner et al., 1995).

Other Classes of SRY *Mutations.*   One would also expect to find promoter mutations affecting the expression of *SRY*; the analysis of 2 kb 5' to *SRY* in 52 patients disclosed one candidate promoter mutation (Kwok et al., 1996). To date, the controlling elements of *SRY* have not been elucidated although, as already mentioned, there is a consensus SRY binding element at the *SRY* transcription site. Mutations that presumably cause their effect by altering *SRY* expression include a deletion of 25 to 52 kb of DNA starting 1.7 kb upstream of the gene (McElreavey et al., 1992) and a deletion 2–3 kb 3' to the coding sequence mutation (McElreavey et al., 1996).

These deletions are deleterious either by removing controlling elements or by a position effect.

The Search for Genes Directly Regulated by SRY   Given that SRY can bind and alter the conformation of DNA, there has been great interest in identifying genes whose expression is directly regulated by the binding of SRY. This search has focused on genes expressed after SRY is expressed in the gonadal ridge (see next section). We will discuss other genes potentially involved in sex determination below, but they (SF1, SOX9, WT1) are initially expressed prior to this time. However, the finding that SRY is transcribed in the preimplantation embryo (see below) indicates that SRY could be involved in their regulation as well. One study demonstrated that the HMG box of SRY recognizes, in a specific manner and with great affinity, the promoter elements of the genes for müllerian inhibitory substance (MIS; discussed in a later section) and aromatase P450, suggesting that the SRY protein controls masculine development by regulating these target genes (Haqq et al., 1993). More recently, it has been shown that despite this high affinity binding, a direct interaction of SRY protein with the promoter is not essential for the regulation of MIS seen in cells cotransfected with the MIS promoter driving a recorder gene, and SRY (Haqq et al., 1994). The MIS promoter was activated in a cell line from urogenital ridges when SRY was transfected into the cell line. However, mutations in the SRY binding site found upstream of MIS did not inhibit the effect. Thus, the authors postulate an indirect interaction with SRY and an intermediate gene whose product stimulates the MIS promoter. They tested one candidate protein (SF1) and found negative results, although others have shown that SF1 can regulate MIS expression (Shen et al., 1994). Activation of Fos-related antigen 1 promoter constructs that contain potential SRY binding sites was shown in cotransfection experiments with SRY in Chinese hamster ovary (CHO) K1 cells but mutational analysis to show that the effect is a direct one has not been done (Cohen et al., 1994). It has also been proposed that the HMG domain of SRY binds to regulatory DNA sequences and represses a hypothetical gene Z, considered to be a negative regulator of male sex determination (McElreavey et al., 1993). This gene is postulated to be in a region of Xp21 that, when duplicated, results in 46,XY females (see below). Recent results are compatible with this notion and suggest that it is the increased amount of the duplicated gene's (DAX1) product that inhibits testis differentiation (see below). Finally, the knockout of Desert hedgehog (a homologue of the Drosophila hedgehog genes) results in complete absence of sperm due to the absence of its expression in pre-Sertoli cells (Bitgood et al., 1996), suggesting that it could be an early target of SRY.

WHEN DOES SRY (SRY) WORK?

Gonadal Ridge and Preimplantation Embryo Expression.   Studies on expression of Sry have focused on presumptive Sertoli cells in the gonadal ridge at the time of gonadal differentiation, that is, 11.5 days (Koopman et al., 1990). These authors examined embryos carrying a a mutated allele (W^e) at the W (Dominant spotting) locus, which causes abnormal germ cell migration, at 7.5 days post-coitus, and at later times, and found no expression until 11.5 days (Koopman et al., 1990). When such studies were extended to day 1.5 to 4.5 (i.e., the preimplantation embryo), abundant evidence for transcription of *Sry* and *Zfy* was found from two-cell to blastocyst stages (Zwingman et al., 1993). Quantitation disclosed that there are approximately 40 to 100 copies per cell in a male blastocyst (Cao et al., 1995). As in adult testes (Capel et al., 1993; Zwingman et al., 1994), both circular, nontranslated, and linear, potentially translatable, *Sry* RNAs are found (Boyer and Erickson, 1993). The functional importance of circular transcripts of *Sry* is unclear; they are not made by *SRY*. The difference is explained by the finding that *Sry* is located in the middle of a large inverted repeat whereas *SRY* is not.

Sry and *Zfy* and their human homologues are closely linked in the sex-determining region of mouse and human Y chromosomes, respectively. Recently, another gene, *Smcy*, which determines a Y-histocompatibility antigen (see below), has been cloned from this region of the mouse chromosome; it is also abundantly transcribed in the mouse and primate preimplantation embryos (Agulnik et al., 1994; Kent-First et al., 1996). The findings of early transcription of sex-determining region genes have been confirmed in the human preimplantation embryo (Ao et al., 1994; Fiddler et al., 1995). *SRY*, *ZFY*, and *ZFX* (zinc finger X) transcripts have been found shortly after fertilization; *ZFX* transcripts were found in the oocyte.

The aforementioned sex-determining region genes have only been shown to be transcribed. However, it is now well established that the male-specific antigen (MSA, serological H-Y) is detectable on preimplantation mouse embryos (Krco et al., 1976; Epstein et al., 1980). These results have, somewhat variably, been extended to bovine (White et al., 1987a), ovine (White et al., 1987b), porcine (White et al., 1987c), and equine (Wood et al., 1988) embryos. Some of the variability is related to the titer of antisera (Piedrahita and Anderson, 1985). In all cases, half the embryos are reactive and, when karyotypes have been performed, only Y-bearing embryos are antigen-positive. This gene product cannot be the sex-determining factor, but its expression shows one early translational difference between male and female embryos. The evidence that *Smcy*, which is transcribed abundantly in the preimplantation embryo, is a gene for a histocompatibility-Y antigen (Scott et al., 1995) shows that it (and another H-Y antigen; Greenfield et al., 1996) is translated. We conclude that at least one of the three sex-determining region genes abundantly transcribed in the preimplantation embryo (*Smcy*) is likely to be translated and all three may be (the experiments have not, to our knowledge, been performed). Such translation could be essential for sex determination.

It is possible that the first candidate gene for *TDF*, *ZFY*, is an important player. The potential role of *ZFY* in sexual differentiation is supported by studies of its expression. Initial Northern analyses of *ZFY* expression detected it in all Y-chromosome-positive cell lines studied (T-cell leukemia, neuroblastoma, fibroblast, and lymphoblastoid lines; Schneider-Gadicke et al., 1989). Palmer and colleagues (1990) used RT-PCR to demonstrate expression of *ZFY* in fetal brain and adult liver as well as testis. Lau and Chan (1989) found *ZFY* to be expressed as major 3 kb and minor 5.7 kb transcripts in testes and found the minor transcript in a variety of somatic cells (although only data from tumor lines were presented). Affara and colleagues (1989) found the apparently same minor transcript in fetal testis. Some authors also studied the expression of the closely homologous, X-linked copy, *ZFX*.

ZFX was expressed in all the tissues in which they had found ZFY to be expressed and also in adult testes by Schneider-Gadicke and colleagues (1989). Palmer and colleagues (1989) found ZFX to be expressed in all adult or fetal tissues studied and Lau and Chan (1989) added ovary to the list. ZFX was well expressed from the inactivated X (Schneider-Gadicke et al., 1989; Palmer et al., 1990). The knockout of Zfx leads to decreased viability, growth deficiency, and reduced numbers of germ cells in homozygous deficient females and hemizygous deficient males (Luoh et al., 1997). Male fertility was apparently normal, despite decreased numbers of sperm, therefore, Zfx might be implicated in preventing some features of Turner syndrome (see Genomic Mutations, Turner Syndrome, in Chapter 6) but not sexual development; ZFY/Zfy may still have such a role.

Zfy is represented by Zfy-1 and Zfy-2 in mice. They are closely linked and structurally similar (Mahaffey et al., 1997). They have undergone unequal crossover in the Sxr^a fragment to create the Sxr^b fragment which thus has only one copy of a hybrid Zfy but still is male determining because Sry remains intact (Simpson and Page, 1991). Zfy-1 and Zfy-2 are both expressed in adult testes: cDNA for each was found in testes but not in other tissues, including brain, heart, kidney, liver, lung, and spleen, as detected by Northern analyses (Mardon and Page, 1989). Southern analysis of RT-PCR products suggested that low levels of Zfy are expressed in a variety of fetal tissues (Nagamine et al., 1990. Zfy expression appears at pachytene during spermatogenesis (Nagamine et al., 1990) but increases postmeiotically (Kalikin et al., 1989); preferential expression of Zfy-2 (Nagamine et al., 1990) and Zfy-1 (Kalikin et al., 1989) has been suggested, As in human tissue, Zfx was found to be expressed in all mouse tissues studied (Mardon and Page, 1989). Mice differ from humans (see Genomic/Chromosomal Disorders in Chapter 7) in having an autosomal processed (intronless) copy of Zfx, Zfa, which is expressed in testes at a time that the 8 kb Zfx transcript is less readily detected by Northern analysis (Ashworth et al., 1990). The differences in modes of X-inactivation (Ashworth et al., 1991; Adler et al., 1991) and the possible need for a Zfx-like protein during spermatogenesis when the X is inactivated are the presumed explanation. Thus, studies in mice also suggest an important role of Zfy and/or cognate genes.

Zfy is also expressed in secondary sexual organs in the mouse, specifically in the epididymis (Mastrangelo et al., 1994). In this study, Northern blotting and RT-PCR were used to examine gene transcription of Zfy in the testis and epididymis of XX, Sxr^a pseudomales (one hybrid Zfy copy) as compared to XY littermates. Contrary to results reported by other researchers, both methods detected Zfy transcription, not only in the normal testis but also in the pseudomale testis. Northern blotting failed to demonstrate Zfy transcription in normal or pseudomale epididymis. However, RT-PCR studies demonstrated Zfy transcription in the normal epididymis. These data suggest a role for Zfy gene function in the development of the epididymis. Further work is needed to see if ZFY has a similar role in the human epididymis.

More Rapid Growth of Y-bearing Preimplantation Embryos.   Embryos that blastulate early *in vitro* are predominantly male (Tsunoda et al., 1985). The simplest explanation is that the difference is caused by a "growth factor" on the Y chromosome. Alternatively, the female-imprinted X of a male embryo might promote rapid growth that could be inhibited by the simultaneous presence of a male-imprinted X in a female embryo. (Imprinting is the term used to describe epigenetic differences in gene expression that depend on the parent-of-origin of the gene.) The evidence for early X-chromosome imprinting and its effects on X-linked gene expression and on survival of androgenones, gynogenones, and parthenogenones has recently been reviewed (Latham, 1996). Burgoyne (1993) has resolved these alternatives for crosses involving Y chromosomes from the CDI and MFI inbred strains, showing linkage of the growth factor Y effect to these Y chromosomes in blastocysts. An apparent exception was found to the growth factor Y effect at the blastocyst stage when the Y chromosome from the RIII inbred strain did not show more rapid embryonic development on a MFI background (Burgoyne, 1993).

The growth factor Y effect is not the result of preferential survival of male versus female embryos after transfer to pseudopregnant females (Zwingman et al., 1993), and it persists to mid-gestation (Scott and Holsen, 1977; Seller and Perkins-Cole, 1987). This effect is also seen in *bovidae* (Avery, 1992; Xu et al., 1992) and in humans. In human in vitro fertilization (IVF) programs, the number of blastomeres at the time of embryo transfer partially predicts the sex of the offspring (Pergament et al., 1994). Differing rates of fertilization by X-and Y-bearing sperm are unlikely to be involved, because the studies in *bovidae* and humans involved *in vitro* fertilization.

The differences in growth rates are reflected in differences in metabolic activity. Male bovine morulae and expanded blastocysts (cultured) have a higher total glucose consumption than do their female counterparts, which show higher pentose-phosphate pathway activity (Tiffin et al., 1991). Higher uptakes of glucose and pyruvate, and production of lactate, were also found for human male embryos at this stage (Ray et al., 1995).

In contrast to the apparently Y-determined blastocyst effect, Thornhill and Burgoyne (1993) reported that a maternally imprinted X chromosome accelerates the development of the 10.5-day mouse embryo. These data were contrasted to previous data in which 40,XO embryos with a paternal X were delayed compared with XX sibs (Burgoyne et al., 1983). Thus, Thornhill and Burgoyne suggest that a paternally imprinted X delays development in either XX or XO embryos (Thornhill and Burgoyne, 1993). However, others have not found differences in development between XX and XO embryos (Omoe and Endo, 1993). It now seems likely that both a Y- and an X-imprinting effect are involved—the former early and the latter later (Burgoyne et al., 1995).

Mittwoch demonstrated that at the earliest time male and female gonads can be distinguished, the testis is already larger in rats (Mittwoch et al., 1969) and humans (Mittwoch and Mahadevaiah, 1980). In contrast, Mittwoch found that in birds, the ovary (i.e., the gonad of the heterogametic sex) was faster growing than the testis (Mittwoch, 1971). Thus, one could hypothesize that manipulations slowing growth could cause XY sex reversal. In this light, it is provocative that Cattanach and colleagues (1995) have found ovarian development in mouse XY embryos in the presence of any one of a number of autosomal deletions that slow growth of the embryo. Additionally, mouse knockouts for the *Polycomb* homologue, *M33*, show male-to-female sex reversal with delayed gonadal growth (Katoh-Fukui, et al. 1998).

The theory that heterogametic sex chromosomes regulate sex determination by causing more rapid growth of the fetal gonad suffered from the lack of evident mechanisms by which to relate the growth rate of a gonad to the quality of its differentiation. The expression of sex-determining region genes in the preimplantation embryo may provide a molecular mechanism for this relation. The case of a "true hermaphrodite" with a somatic mutation in *SRY* is illustrative (Braun et al., 1993). This individual had ambiguous genitalia, and the histology of the one gonad studied demonstrated oocyte-like cells disseminated among Sertoli cells and spermatogonia (however, immature testis can have many such cells); no Leydig cells were seen (Braun et al., 1993). One interpretation of this case is that normal *SRY* expression in the embryo before gonadal differentiation permitted faster somatic and gonadal growth, thereby allowing the degree of testicular differentiation seen despite detection of only mutant *SRY* in the one "ovotestis." Presumably, some androgen production occurred in the other gonad (or had previously in the sectioned gonad) to explain the degree of masculinization.

The Y-bearing preimplantation embryo probably does not always develop more rapidly. As mentioned, Burgoyne did not detect growth factor Y in the *RIII* inbred strain of mice (Burgoyne, 1993). He has also shown that *Sry* cannot be the responsible gene, because *Sry*-negative XY fetuses are larger than their XX siblings at day 10.5, yet do not develop as males (Burgoyne, 1993). The contention that XX, *Sxr* fetuses are the same overall size as their sibs at day 10.5 (Burgoyne, 1993), yet develop as males (the *Sxr* fragment includes *Sry*), may simply be overlooking a difference in the gonadal size at this time. These apparent discrepancies would be resolved if more rapid growth of the Y-bearing embryo is required for successful sex determination, but that it does not have to always include the preimplantation stage.

THE ROLES OF THE X CHROMOSOME IN GONADAL DEVELOPMENT

Is the Major Role of SRY *to Inactivate a X-chromosomal Locus?*   The marked species variation in the amino acid sequence of *SRY* outside its conserved HMG box presents some problems for understanding of *SRY* function. Dubin and Ostrer (1994) have shown that both human/mouse *SRY/Sry* are transactivators in transfected cultured cells, but the finding may be misleading because the "transactivating" domain is not found in some rodents (Tucker and Lundigram, 1993). Alternatively, as mentioned earlier, it has been proposed that *SRY* represses (negatively regulates) a hypothetical gene, Z, that is itself a negative regulator of male sex determination (McElreavey et al., 1993). This model has been further developed by Jimenez and colleagues (1996). *DAX1* is a good candidate for this target gene (see below) but, as already discussed, it seems unlikely that this is the sole role for *SRY*. *SOX3*, a highly conserved X-linked member of the *SRY*-related, HMG-box gene family, which is also found on the X in marsupials (Stevanovic et al., 1993; Foster and Marshall-Graves, 1994) is not a good alternative candidate. Although it is the *Sox* gene most closely related to *Sry* (and its probable ancestral homologue), it is predominantly expressed in the developing nervous system (Collignon et al., 1996).

Xp21 Duplications in 46,XY Females (see Chapter 5). A number of 46,XY individuals with sex reversal have partial duplications of the Xp and an intact *SRY* gene. They usually have normal female external and internal genitalia with partial gonadal dysgenesis (Bardoni et al., 1994). Bernstein and colleagues (1980) presented two cases and concluded that "testis-determining genes of the Y chromosome may be suppressed by regulatory elements of the X." Other reports focused on the fact that the duplicated Xp region includes *ZFX* (Scherer et al., 1989); but if this was the cause of the sex reversal, subjects with a 46,XXY karyotype should not develop testes, because *ZFX* escapes inactivation; that is, whatever the locus (or loci), it should be X-inactivated or XXY would not develop as males under this hypothesis. It is of interest that some XXY triploids have shown sexual ambiguity (Graham et al., 1989); however, lack of X-inactivation may be the cause (Petit el al., 1992).

Ogata and coworkers (1992, 1994) further defined the critical region for Xp duplication with sex reversal, and Bardoni and colleagues (1994) narrowed it to a 160-kb span. They hypothesized a single gene in the region and named it *DSS* (*d*osage *s*ensitive *s*ex reversal). This region includes *DAX1* (*d*osage sensitive sex reversal—*a*drenal hypopolasia congenita gene on the X chromosome gene *1*), a gene whose defects cause adrenal hypoplasia congenita (Muscatelli et al., 1994; Zanaria et al., 1994). *DAX1* is a candidate for *DSS*. However, if *DAX1* is *DSS*, it indicates that *DSS* is not necessary for male differentiation, because absence of *DAX1* function does not impair male, or female (Yu et al., 1998) development. *DAX1* is an orphan member of the nuclear hormone receptor family, meaning that its ligand is unknown. *DAX1* is related to *SF1*, which is involved in gonad development (see below). Capel (1995) has argued that *DAX1* may be involved in the fetal response to maternal hormones in such a manner that an increased dosage of *DAX1* would override the *SRY* signal for testis development. This hypothesis is supported by the fact that *DAX1* is normally down-regulated in the developing testis while its expression persists in the developing ovary (Swain et al., 1996), and overexpression in Dax1 transgenics delays testicular development and can result in sex reversal in the presence of weak-functioning (hypomorphic) *Sry* (Swain, et al, 1998). *DAX1* is autosomal in marsupials, suggesting that its X location is not critical for its potential role in sexual differentiation (Pask et al., 1997).

Another class of genes found within the *DSS* critical region has been named *DAM* (DSS/AHC [adrenal hypoplasia congenita] critical interval genes belonging to the *MAGE* [melanoma antigen] superfamily). Five *DAM* genes are clustered within 50 kb of *DSS*. (Dabovic et al., 1995). Two of these are expressed in adult testes and are highly similar to the MAGE family of tumor-associated antigens and mouse necedin. Their potential role in sex reversal is yet to be determined. The possible role of *DAM* genes can be tested by creating transgenic mice with increased copies of the mouse homologous genes.

Male Pseudohermaphroditism in the X-linked α-thalassemia and Mental Retardation Syndrome. Weatherall and colleagues (1981) noted the concurrence of α-thalassemia and mental retardation but the X-linkage and distinctive dysmorphology were delimited by Wilkie and colleagues *et al* (1990, 1991). The syndrome has been named "ATR-X" and includes microcephaly, short stature, tented upper lip, everted lower lip, anteverted nostrils, epicanthal folds and/or hypertelorism, and macrostomia (see Chapter 5). Male pseudohermaphroditism is an occasional feature and dysgenetic testis has been described (McPherson et al., 1995). One of the original defining cases was a 46,XY female, but most cases have merely had cryptorchidism or hypospadias. Recently, McPherson and colleagues (1995) reported a family in which three out of four XY individuals were raised as females, and Reardon and colleagues (1995) reported two similar sibs in another family. In the first family, the hematological abnormalities were mild, consistent with the hypothesis that the ATR-X gene encodes a transacting factor involved in many developmental processes (hematologic, CNS, facies, etc.) and that different mutations could differentially affect its function. This hypothesis was confirmed by the cloning of *XH2*, a member of the helicase superfamily that includes transcriptional factors, and the demonstration that it is mutated in the ATR-X syndrome (Gibbons et al., 1995). It is possible that some mutations might affect one developmental role more than another. Alternatively, the presence of a paternal uncle with bladder exstrophy in the pedigree studied by Reardon and colleagues (1995) might suggest that modifying genes are the major determinant of the varying presence of pseudohermaphroditism.

The Role of the X Chromosome in Ovarian Development. Clear-cut testicular development occurs in the absence of germ cells; this is not true of ovarian development. Normal oocytes require two X chromosomes and supporting cells differentiate as pre-follicle or pre-granulosa cells under the influence of oocytes. By the time of birth, the development of oocytes is essentially complete with entry into meiosis and arrest at the diplotene stages. Both X's are active before this process commences (Mangia et al., 1975). The oocytes then influence the development of follicles that are dependent on the continued presence of germ cells (Yost and Magre, 1989). Although the differentiation of supporting Sertoli cells does not require germ cells, their maintenance usually requires them. Morphological abnormalities in Sertoli cells occur in the absence of germ cells in Klinefelter syndrome (Chemes et al., 1977) and in XX, *Sxr* mice (Chung, 1974).

It has been hypothesized that there is a critical region at Xq1-Xq27 that must be intact on both X chromosomes for normal ovarian development to occur (Sarto et al., 1973; Summitt et al., 1978). Women with translocation breakpoints in this region usually have primary amenorrhea, but oligomenorrhea and early menopause also occur (Kaiser et al., 1984; Krauss et al., 1987). There are exceptions to this "rule" (Barnabei et al., 1981; Madan et al., 1981; Wegner et al., 1982; Markovic et al., 1985; Rivera et al., 1986). The effects on reproductive phenotype of Xq26-Xqter deletions have been more variable but have usually included oligomenorrhea or early menopause (Trunca et al., 1984). In order to explain the variability of both the effects and the location of deletions, it has been hypothesized that there are multiple X genes involved in female fertility and that there is an inverse relationship between the number of them (in two copies) and the duration of fertility—that is, the life span of oocytes (Fitzgerald et al., 1984).

Autosomal Chromosomes

SEX DETERMINATION INVOLVES A CASCADE OF GENE EXPRESSION

Testis Differentiation without SRY.   XX true hermaphroditism without apparent Y chromosomal sequences has been known for some time (Ramsay et al., 1988). Such cases occur at a frequency of one in several thousand among Bantu-speaking blacks, and these patients usually show some degree of sexual ambiguity with ovo-testis. Recently, it has been shown that these patients do not have *SRY* or uniparental disomy of the X (Spurdle et al., 1995), unlike the true hermaphrodite (Braun et al., 1993) discussed above. Thus, they achieve a major degree of testis differentiation in the absence of *SRY*, a result paralleled by recent findings in voles. Voles include species in which no Y chromosome can be resolved cytogenetically. Recently, it has been shown that two of these species do not contain *Sry* (Just et al., 1995), but the authors were able to detect *Sry* in a closely related species. Thus, the problem was not one of detecting distantly related *Sry* sequences. It is apparent that in these two species of voles, male sex is determined without *Sry*. The obvious hypothesis is that a gene downstream of *Sry* has mutated so as to become *Sry*-independent or that a gene normally suppressing the pathway (e.g., *DSS*) is altered. The presence and location of Y chromosomal sequences thought to be important for spermatogenesis—for example, *AZF* (*AZoospermia* Factor, see Azoospermia and Yq Alterations in Chapter 5—have yet to be determined in these species of vole.

Abundance of 46,XY Females.   The population frequency of 46,XY females is not accurately known; however, it is clear that this disorder is not exceedingly rare and that its etiology is heterogenous. Interestingly, deletion of Yp (i.e., the reciprocal of the translocation typically found in 46,XX males) is not a common finding. Most 46,XY females have had an intact Y chromosome and only 10% to 20% of them have mutations in *SRY* (Hawkins et al., 1992). It is clear that mutations in a number of different genes that contribute to the testis differentiation cascade can result in individuals with female external appearances, (e.g., Smith-Lemli-Opitz or campto-melic dysplasia). These disorders will be discussed further in other chapters. It is also interesting to consider the mode of ascertainment of 46,XY females. Frequently, they are found unexpectedly when a karyotype is performed for the purpose of investigating delayed development or dysmorphism. Occasionally, they are discovered accidentally. We recently had an illustrative case: a postmortem was performed on a 9-year-old girl dead of sepsis. The pathologist noted streak gonads and obtained a karyotype that was 46,XY. One would expect a number of 46,XY females to be discovered from karyotypes performed for primary amenorrhea. However, at least in our experience, most cases have been discovered from karyotypes performed by pediatric geneticists, not endocrinologists.

SOME AUTOSOMAL GENES ALREADY IMPLICATED

Wilms Tumor 1.   The association between the Wilms tumor 1 (*WT1*) gene and testis development was recognized from investigations into the Denys-Drash syndrome (see Chapter 7 for further description) and the WAGR syndrome, which consists of Wilms tumor, aniridia, genitourinary anomalies, and mental retardation. The latter syndrome is caused by deletions of 11p13 and hemizygosity in this region. Further, the deletions suggested that there was a tumor suppressor in this region related to Wilms tumor (for review, see Van Heyningen and Hastie, 1992). In Denys-Drash syndrome, there is a complex nephropathy and sexual ambiguity. Patients with the WAGR syndrome may have undescended testes and hypospadias, whereas male patients with Denys-Drash syndrome may have female or ambiguous external genitalia with dysgenic gonads. When the WT1 gene was cloned, it was found to code a DNA-binding, zinc-finger transcription factor with multiple isoforms due to alternative splicing. Expression studies show that high levels of WT1 are expressed in the developing kidney, especially in glomeruli and mesangial cells that are involved in the above-mentioned nephropathy. High levels were also found in the indifferent gonads, in Sertoli cells, and in granulosa cells. It has been suggested that the WT1 gene is involved in mesenchymal-epithelial interactions (Van Heyningen and Hastie, 1992); for example, between Sertoli cells and Leydig cells. Such interactions are crucial in both the developing kidney and gonad. Analysis of the defects of kidney development in WT-1 knockout mice strongly support the notion that WT-1 is involved in the mesenchyme-to-epithelial transition (Sainio et al., 1997). It is probable that defects in these interactions disrupt testicular development so that Leydig cell function and testosterone production are inadequate. This could explain the pseudohermaphroditism sometimes seen in Denys-Drash syndrome. *Emx*2 (the mouse homologue of the *Drosophila* head gap gene *empty spiracles, ems*) is also involved in the early development of the urogenital tract; knockouts lack kidneys, gonads, ureters, and genital tracts (Miyamoto et al., 1997).

SOX9.   Camptomelic dysplasia is a skeletal dysplasia in which camptomelia (i.e., bowing of the long bones, especially the legs,) is a prominent feature (see Autosomal Single-Gene Disorders in Chapter 7 for fuller description). Actually camptomelia is not an essential feature of the condition, but the hypoplastic scapulae, non-mineralized thoracic pedicles, and vertically narrow iliac bones are sufficient for the diagnosis (Hall and Spranger, 1980). Importantly, 46,XY sex reversal frequently occurs; up to two thirds of 46,XY patients with camptomelic dysplasia are phenotypically female. The gonads may have an ovarian appearance with primary follicles (Mansour et al., 1995). Thus, it was hypothesized that the locus for camptomelic dysplasia encodes an autosomal testis differentiation gene.

Translocation breakpoints in patients suggested a gene at 17q24-25 and the mouse homology map suggested *SOX9*, a gene expressed in developing cartilage, as a candidate (Wright et al., 1995). This gene is a member of a family of *SOX* (SRY-type HMG box) genes. Many others have been identified since the discovery of *SRY*. It has been reported that *SOX9* is also expressed in mouse fetal genital ridges and early gonads (Wright et al., 1995); its expression pattern closely parallels the development of Sertoli cells (da Silva et al., 1996). Mutation analysis of *SOX9* has revealed various mutations in several patients (Foster et al., 1994). Little is known about the function of *SOX9* in gonadal development, but it might be regulated by *SRY* in mammals and even substitute for it in birds (da Silva et al., 1996).

Steroidogenic Factor-1.   Steroidogenic factor-1 (SF-1; homologous to the *Drosophila* gene *Fushi tarazu* 1 factor and sometimes referred to as *Ftz F1*) is an orphan nuclear receptor that has been shown to be a key regulator of steroidogenic en- zymes in adrenocortical cells (Lala et al., 1992). Developmental studies demon- strated that it is expressed in the urogenital ridge at embryonic day 9 to 9.5 in the mouse. This is an early stage of organogenesis of the developing gonads, prior to the time of expression of *Sry* (Ikeda et al., 1994). The embryonic stem cell "knock- out" of *Sf-1* resulted in mice that died 8 days after birth (Luo et al., 1994). The knockout mice lacked adrenal glands and gonads and had a resulting deficiency in corticosterone that was the likely cause of death. More recent expression studies (Hatano et al., 1994; Shen et al., 1994) have demonstrated a sexually dimorphic expression pattern of *Sf-1* with persistence in males and a discontinuation of ex- pression of females, which was hypothesized to link the expression of *Sry* to that of the *MIS*. SF1 was shown to regulate MIS *in vitro* (Shen et al., 1994) and *in vivo* (Giulli et al., 1997), but another *in vitro* study could not demonstrate that SF-1 could mediate between *SRY* and *MIS* (Haqq et al., 1994; see above). Dramatic co- stimulation of the MIS promoter by WT-1 (isoforms lacking lys-thr-ser between the third and fourth zinc finger [-KTS]; see Chapter 7) with SF-1 has been demonstrated (Nachtigal et al., 1998) and can be antagonized by Dax1; transcription of the Leydig insulin-like gene is also mediated (Zimmerman et al., 1998). Although no patients have yet been described with disease entities known to be caused by mutations in SF-1, one might predict a phenotype associated with predominantly female ap- pearance and severe neonatal problems due to lack of steroid hormones. SF-1 maps to 9q33 (Taketo et al., 1995), a region not yet associated with problems of sexual differentiation.

A Possible Sex Differentiation Gene on 9p.   Across the years, a number of cases of XY sex-reversal associated with monosomy 9p have been reported (Jotterand and Juillard, 1976; Fryns et al., 1986; Crocker et al., 1988). However, these patients had translocations with various partial trisomies (3p, 7q, 13q), so the relative pathoge- nicity of monosomy 9p and their trisomies could not be distinguished. Recently, a case of *de novo* deletion 9p in a 46,XY individual with female development, but dysplastic gonads, indicated that monosomy 9p alone can be responsible for 46,XY sex reversal (Bennett et al., 1993). Thus, testicular development had commenced as in other cases in which *SRY* was normal (*SRY* showed a normal sequence in this case). Other cases of monosomy 9p have consisted of sexual ambiguity without dysplastic gonads (Huret et al., 1988). Thus, it is possible that modifying genes or the loss of sufficient material for general fetal growth retardation is also required for failure of gonadal development. Similar findings with ring chromosome 9 sug- gest that the phenotype of sex reversal may be caused by deficiencies of one of the chromosome termini (i.e., 9p) (Metaxotou and Kalpini-Mavrou, 1977). One report of a male with underdeveloped genitalia suggested a location distal to D9S168 for the gene involved in sex differentiation (Ogata et al., 1997), and another (Veitia et al., 1998) located it more distally, beyond D9S1813. More recently, two other studies have situated the gene even more telomerically, beyond marker D9S1770, with the smallest region of overlap spanning 9p24-pter (Flejter et al., 1998; Guioli et al., 1998). The recent discovery that the mammalian orthologue of a gene involved in sex determination in *C. elegans* and *Drosphila* (*DMT1*) maps to this region provides a strong candidate for the gene involved (Raymond et al., 1998).

It is of interest that an autosomal homologue of ZFY was mapped to 9p22-pter by *in situ* hybridization (Affara et al., 1989). The role of an autosomal copy of ZFY in humans (studies in mice are not helpful because *Zfa* is located on mouse chromosome 10 in a region homologous to human 10q and 6q but not to 9p) is not known. A contribution of ZFY to masculine sexual differentiation is possible because SRY^+, ZFY^- individuals have some degree of sexual ambiguity (Palmer et al., 1989).

A Possible Sex Differentiation Gene on 10q.   Deletions of 10q have been associated with male sexual maldevelopment (Wulfsberg et al., 1989). All males have had undescended testes; two thirds have had micropenis, and one third have had frank sexual ambiguity (Wulfsberg et al., 1989). Recently, one 46,XY $10q^-$ patient had female external genitalia and another had an intersex phenotype; the first patient had no detectable gonads, the second had a testis with a "normal distribution of germ Sertoli and Leydig cells" (Wilkie et al., 1993). These patients have had deletions from 10q26-qter. These deletions are close to a potential candidate gene, PAX 2, which maps to 10q25. PAX 2 is a member of the family of paired box genes. These genes were cloned on the basis of sequence homology to genes involved in *Drosophila* segmentation. Interestingly, heterozygous expression of half-normal levels of their respective proteins are frequently involved in developmental defects: PAX 3 with Waardenburg syndrome in humans and *Splotch* in mice; PAX 6 with *Aniridia* in humans and small eyes in mice (Hastie, 1991): PAX 2, like *Hox* 4E, is expressed in mesodermal structures, including the developing urogenital tract (Nornes et al., 1990; Fickenscher et al., 1993). PAX 2 is required for the epithelial conversion of mesenchyme found in renal development (Rothenpieler and Dressler, 1993). Overexpression (Dressler et al., 1993) and underexpression (Keller et al., 1984) lead to renal anomalies in mice; there are retinal defects as well in the *Pax*-2 deletion mice. A frameshift mutation of exon 5 of PAX 2 was associated with optic nerve colobomas, renal hypoplasia, and vesicoureteral reflux (Sanyanusin et al., 1995). Other mutations (or possibly deletions on some genetic backgrounds) could be associated with genital anomalies, for Fickensher and colleagues (1993) reported high levels of *Pax* 2 transcripts in male and female genital tracts.

Conclusions

As seen in Figure 2–3, the data reviewed in this chapter suggest that multiple genes are involved in the sex-determination pathway. This is not surprising in that the usual major player, SRY, is not essential for male development in some humans and two species of voles. One interesting feature of the postulated interactions of the currently identified "players" (and, certainly, more are to come) is the degree to which they may be involved in more than one stage of sexual determination/ differentiation. SOX9 is actively transcribed prior to the appearance of a distinguishable testis; later, its transcription may be stimulated by SRY and be essential for Sertoli cell development. SF1 seems to be essential for development of intermediate mesoderm as gonadal ridge and preadrenal; later, it is expressed in Sertoli

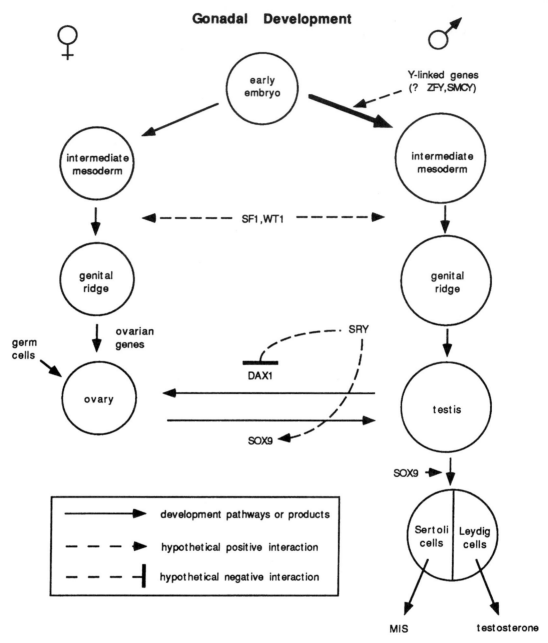

FIGURE 2–3. Postulated scheme of genetic and developmental interactions involved in sex determination and sex differentiation of the gonad. Note larger size of gonad structure on the right side (male). See concluding section of Chapter 2 for fuller discussion.

cells and has been postulated to play a role in the induction of *MIS* expression (although a specific *in vitro* test of this relationship was negative). *ZFY* is transcribed in the early embryo, in the developing epididymis, and later during spermatogenesis. *ZFY* shares aspects of the structure of known, zinc-finger transacting factors, thus it is likely to have target genes that are yet to be identified.

Another aspect of Figure 2–3 is the indication of the vulnerability of males in sexual determination. Thus, events, genetic or environmental, that slow early embryonic growth may cause XY sex reversal. A double dosage of *DAX1*, or a deficiency of *SOX9*, can also have this effect. Although more frequently seen experimentally than clinically, transformation of ovary to testes can also occur. For instance, ovaries transplanted under the adult kidney capsule may develop testicular structures; *SOX9* expression occurs concomitantly (da Silva et al., 1996). Finally, it is important to point out that a number of genes must be specifically involved in ovarian development. We have indicated possible locations for the actions of some of them (including some influence from germ cells that seem essential for ovarian development), but much remains to be learned.

REFERENCES

Adler D A, Bressler S L, Chapman V M, Page D C, Disteche C M (1991). Inactivation of the *Zfx* gene on the mouse X chromosome. *Proc Natl Acad Sci USA* 88:4592–4595. 1991.

Affara N A, Chalmers I J, Ferguson-Smith M A (1993). Analysis of *SRY* in 22 sex-reversed XY females identifies four new point mutations in the conserved DNA binding domain. *Hum Mol Genet* 2:785–789.

Affara N A, Chambers D, O'Brien J, Habeegu S S M, Kalaitsidaki M, Bishop C E Ferguson-Smith M A (1989) Evidence for distinguishable transcripts of the putative testis determining gene (*ZFY*) and mapping of homologous cDNA sequences to chromosomes X,Y, and 9. *Nucleic Acids Res* 17:2987–2999.

Agulnik A L, Mitchell M J, Lema J L, Woods D R, Bishop C E (1994). A mouse Y chromosome gene encoded by a region essential for spermatogenesis and expression of male-specific minor histocompatibility antigens. *Hum Mol Genet* 3:873–878.

Ao A, Erickson R P, Winston R M L, Handyside A H (1994). Transcription of paternal Y-linked genes in the human zygote as early as the pronucleate stage. *Zygote* 2:281–287.

Ashworth A, Rastan S, Lovell-Badge R, Kay G (1991). X-chromosome inactivation may explain the difference in viability of XO humans and mice. *Nature* 351:406–408.

Ashworth A, Skene B, Swift S, Lovell-Badge R (1990). Zfa is an expressed retroposon derived from an alternative transcript of the *Zfx* gene. *EMBO J* 9:1529–1534.

Avery B, Jorgensen C B, Madison V, Greve T (1992). Morphological development and sex of bovine *in vitro* fertilized embryos. *Mol Reprod Dev* 32:265–270.

Bardoni B, Zanaria E, Guioli S, Floridia G, Worley K C, Tonini G, Ferrante E, Chiumello G, MCabe E R B, Fraccaro M, Zuffardi O, Camerino G (1994). A dosage sensitive locus at chromosome Xp21 is involved in male to female sex reversal. *Nat Genet* 7:497–501.

Barnabei V M, Wyandt H E, Kelly T E (1981). A possible exception to the critical region hypothesis. *Am J Hum Genet* 33:61–66.

Bennett C P, Docherty Z, Robb S A, Ramani P, Hawkins J R, Grant D (1993). Deletion 9p and sex reversal. *J Med Genet* 30:518–520.

Bernstein R, Jenkins T, Dawson B, Wagner J, Dewald G, Koo G C, Wachtel S S (1980). Female phenotype and multiple abnormalities in sibs with a Y chromosome and partial X chromosome duplication: H-Y antigen and Xg blood group findings. *J Med Genet* 17:291–300.

Berta P, Hawkins J R, Sinclair A H, Taylor A, Griffiths B L, Goodfellow P N, Fellous M (1990). Genetic evidence equating *SRY* and the testis-determining factor. *Nature* 348:448–450.

Bianchi M E, Falciola L, Ferrari S, Lilley D M J (1992). The DNA binding site of HMG1 protein is composed of two similar segments (HMG boxes), both of which have counterparts in other eukaryotic regulatory proteins. *EMBO J* 11:1055–1063.

Bitgood M J, Shen L, McMahon A P (1996). Sertoli cell signaling by Desert hedgehog regulates the male germline. *Curr Biol* 6:298–304.

Boyer T, Erickson R P (1993) Detection of circular and linear transcripts of *Sry* in preimplantation mouse embryos: differences in requirement for reverse transcriptase. *Biochem Biophys Res Commun* 198:492–496.

Braun A, Kammerer S, Cleve H, Löhrs U, Schwarz H-P, Kuhnle U (1993). True hermaphroditism in a 46,XY individual, caused by a postzygotic somatic point mutation in the male gonadal sex-determining locus (*SRY*): molecular genetics and histological findings in a sporadic case. *Am J Hum Genet* 52:578–585.

Burgoyne P S (1993). A Y-chromosomal effect on blastocyst cell number in mice. *Development* 117:341–345.

Burgoyne P S, Tam P P L, Evans E P (1983). Retarded development of XO conceptuses during early pregnancy in the mouse. *J Reprod Fertil* 68:387–393.

Burgoyne P S, Thornhill A R, Kalmus Boudrean S, Darling S M, Bishop C E, Evans E P (1995). The genetic basis of XX-XY differences present before gonadal sex differentiation in the mouse. *Phil Trans R Soc Lond B* 350:253–261.

Cao Q P, Gaudette M F, Robinson D H, Crain W R (1995). Expression of the mouse testis-determining gene *Sry* in male preimplantation embryos. *Mol Reprod Dev* 40:196–204.

Capel B (1995). New bedfellows in the mammalian sex-determination affair. *Trends Genet* 11: 161–163.

Capel T, Swain A, Nicolis S, Hacker A, Walter M, Koopman P, Goodfellow P, Lovell-Badge R. (1993) Circular transcripts of the testis-determining gene *Sry* in adult mouse testis. *Cell* 73:1019–1030.

Cattanach B M, Rasberry C, Beechey C V. (1995). XY sex reversal associated with autosomal deletions. *Mouse Genome* 93:426.

Chemes H E, Dym M, Fawcett D W, Javadpour N, Sherins R J (1977). Patho-physiological observations of Sertoli cells in patients with germinal aplasia or severe germ cell depletion: ultrastructural findings and hormone levels. *Biol Reprod* 17:108–123.

Chung K W (1974). A morphological and histochemical study of Sertoli cells in normal and XX, sex-reversed mice. *Am J Anat* 139:369–375.

Cohen D R, Sinclair A H, McGovern J D (1994) *SRY* protein enhances transcription of Fos-related antigen 1 promoter constructs. *Proc Natl Acad Sci USA* 91:4372–4376.

Collignon J, Sockanathan S, Hacker A, Cohen-Tannoudji M, Norris D, Rastan S, Stevanovic M, Goodfellow P-N, Lovell-Badge R (1996). A comparison of the properties of *Sox-3* with *Sry* and two-related genes, *Sox-1* and *Sox-2*. *Development* 122:509–520.

Crocker M, Coghill S B, Cortinho R (1988). An unbalanced autosomal translocation (7;9) associated with feminization. *Clin Genet* 34:70–73.

Dabovic B, Zanaria E, Bardoni B, Lisa A, Bordignon C, Russo V, Matessi C, Traversari C, Camerino G (1995). A family of rapidly evolving genes from the sex reversal critical region of Xp21. *Mammal Genome* 6:571–580.

da Silva S M, Hacker A, Harley V, Goodfellow P, Swain A, Lovell-Badge R (1996). *SOX9* expression during gonadal development implies a conserved role for the gene in testis differentiation in mammals and birds. *Nat Genet* 14:62–68.

Davis R M (1981). Localization of male determining factors in man: a thorough review of structural anomalies of the Y chromosome. *J Med Genet* 18:161–195.

Dressler G R, Wilkinson J E, Rothenpieler U W, Patterson L T, Williams-Simons L, Westphal H (1993). Deregulation of *Pax-2* expression in transgenic mice generates severe kidney abnormalities. *Nature* 362:65–67.

Dubin R A, Ostrer H (1994). *Sry* is a transcriptional activator. *Mol Endocrinol* 8:1182–1192.

Epstein C J, Smith S, Davis B (1980). Expression of H-Y antigen on preimplantation mouse embryos. *Tissue Antigens* 15:63–67.

Evans H S, Buckton K E, Spowart G, Carothers A D (1979). Heteromorphic X chromosomes in 46,XX males: evidence for the involvement of X-Y interchange. *Hum Genet* 49:11–31.

Ferrari S, Harley V R, Pontiggia A, Goodfellow P N, Lovell-Badge R, Bianchi M E (1992). *SRY* like HMG1, recognizes sharp angles in DNA. *EMBO J* 11:4497–4506.

Fickenscher H R, Chalepakis G, Gruss P (1993). Murine Pax-2 protein is a sequence-specific *trans*-activator with expression in the genital system. *DNA Cell Biol* 12:381–391.

Fiddler M, Abdel-Rahman B, Rappolee D A, Pergament E (1995). Expression of *SRY* transcripts in preimplantation human embryos. *Am J Med Genet* 55:80–84.

Fitzgerald P H, Donald R A, McCormick P (1984). Reduced fertility in women with X chromosome abnormality. *Clin Genet* 25:301–309.

Flejter W L, Fergestad J, Gorski J, Varvill T, Chandrasekharappa S (1998). A gene involved in XY sex reversal is located on chromosome 9, distal to marker D9S1779. *Am J Hum Genet* 63:794–802.

Ford C E, Jones K W (1959). A sex chromosome anomaly in a case of gonadal dysgenesis (Turner's syndrome). *Lancet* 1:711–713.

Foster J W, Dominguez-Steglich M A, Guioli S, Kwok C, Weller P A, Stevanovic M, Weissenbach J, Mansour S, Young I D, Goodfellow P N, Brook J D, Schafer A J (1994). Campomelic dysplasia and autosomal sex reversal caused by mutations in an *SRY*-related gene. *Nature* 374:525–530.

Foster J W, Marshall-Graves J A (1994). An *SRY*-related sequence on the marsupial X chromosome: implications for the evolution of the mammalian testis-determining gene. *Proc Natl Acad Sci USA* 91:1927–1931.

Fryns J P, Kleczkowska A, Casaer P, Van Den Berghe H (1986). Double autosomal chromosomal aberration (3p trisomy/9p monosomy) and sex-reversal. *Ann Genet* 29:49–52.

Gibbons R J, Picketts D J, Villard L, Higgs D R (1995). Mutations in a putative global transcriptional regulator cause X-linked mental retardation with α-thalassemia (ATR-X syndrome). *Cell* 80:837–845.

Giuili G, Shen W-H, Ingraham H A (1997). The nuclear receptor SF-1 mediates sexually dimorphic expression of müllerian inhibiting substance, *in vivo*. *Development* 124:1799–1807.

Graham J M Jr, Rawnsley A F, Simmons G M, Wurster-Hills D H, Park J P, Parin-Padilla M, Crow H C (1989). Triploidy: pregnancy complications and clinical findings in seven cases. *Prenatal Diagnosis* 9:409–419.

Greenfield A, Scott D, Pennisi D, Ehrmann I, Ellis P, Cooper L, Simpson E, Koopman P (1996). An H-YD[b] epitope is encoded by a novel mouse Y chromosome gene. *Nat Genet* 14:474–478.

Gubbay J, Collignon J, Koopman P, Capel B, Economou A, Münsterberg A, Vivian N, Goodfellow P, Lovell-Badge R (1990). A gene mapping to the sex-determining region of the mouse Y chromosome is a member of a novel family of embryonically expressed genes. *Nature* 346:245–250.

Gueallaen G, Casanova M, Bishop C, Geldwerth D, Andre G, Fellous M, Weissenboch J (1984). Human XX males with Y single-copy DNA fragments. *Nature* 307:172–173.

Guioli S, Schmitt K, Critcher R, Bouzyk M, Spurr N K, Ogata T, Hoo J J, Pinsky L, Gimelli G, Pasztor L, Goodfellow P N (1998). Molecular analysis of 9p deletions associated with XY sex reversal: refining the localization of a sex-determining gene to the tip of the chromosome. *Am J Hum Genet* 63:905–908.

Hacker A, Capel B, Goodfellow P, Lovell-Badge R (1995). Expression of *Sry*, the mouse sex-determining region gene. *Development* 121:1603–1614.

Hall B D, Spranger J W (1980). Campomelic dysplasia. *Am J Dis Child* 134:285–289.

Haqq C M, King C-Y, Donahoe P K, Weiss M A (1993). *SRY* recognizes conserved DNA sites in sex-specific promoters. *Proc Natl Acad Sci USA* 90:1097–1101.

Haqq C M, King, C-Y, Ukiyama E, Falsafi S, Haqq T N, Donahoe P K, Weiss M A. Molecular basis of mammalian sexual determination: activation of Müllerian inhibiting substance gene expression by *SRY*. *Science* 266:1494–1500. 1994.

Hastie N D 1991. *Pax* in our time. *Current Biol* 1:342–344.

Hatano O, Takayama K, Imai T, Waterman M R, Takakusu A, Omura T, Morohashi K-I (1994). Sex-dependent expression of a transcription factor, Ad4BP, regulating steroidogenic P-450 genes in the gonads during prenatal and postnatal rat development. *Development* 20:2787–2797.

Hawkins J R, Taylor A, Goodfellow P N, Migeon C J, Smith K D, Berkovitz G D. Evidence for increased prevalence of *SRY* mutations in XY females with complete rather than partial gonadal dysgenesis. *Am J Hum Genet* 51:979–984. 1992.

Huret J L, Leonard C, Forestier B, Rethore M O, Lejeune J (1988). Eleven new cases of del(9p) and features from 80 cases. *J Med Genet* 25:741–749.

Ikeda Y, Shen W-H, Ingraham H A, Parker K L (1994). Developmental expression of mouse steroidogenic factor 1, an essential regulator of the steroid hydroxylases. *Mol Endocrinol* 8:654–662.

Jacobs P A, Strong J A (1959). A case of human intersexuality having a possible XXY sex-determining mechanism. *Nature* 183:302–303.

Jäger R J, Anvret M, Hall K, Scherer G (1990). A human XY female with a frame shift mutation in the candidate testis-determining gene *SRY*. *Nature* 348:452–454.

Jantzen H-M, Admon A, Bell S P, Tjian R (1990). Nucleolar transcription factor hUBf contains a DNA-binding motif with homology to HMG proteins. *Nature* 344:830–836.

Jeske Y W A, Bowles J, Greenfield A, Koopman P (1995). Expression of a linear *Sry* transcript in the mouse genital ridge. *Nat Genet* 10:480–482.

Jimenez R, Sanchez A, Burgos M, de la Guardia R D (1996) Puzzling out the genetics of mammalian sex determination. *Trends Genet* 12:164–166.

Jones K W, Singh L (1981). Conserved repeated DNA sequences in vertebrate sex chromosomes. *Hum Genet* 58:46–53.

Jotterand M, Juillard E (1976). A new case of trisomy for the distal part of 13q due to maternal translocation, (9;13) (p21; q21). *Hum Genet* 33:213–222.

Just W, Rau W, Vogel W, Akhverdian M, Fredga K, Marshall-Graves J A, Lyapunova E (1995). Absence of *Sry* in species of the vole *Ellobius*. *Nat Genet* 11:117–118.

Kaiser P, Harprecht W, Steuernagel P, Daume E (1984). Long arm deletions of the X chromosome and their symptoms: a new case (bp q24) and a short review of the literature. *Clin Genet* 26:433–439.

Kalikin L M, Fujimoto H, Witt M P, Verge V, Erickson R P (1989). A genomic clone of *Zfy-1* from a Y[DOM] strain detects post-meiotic gene expression of *Zfy* in testes. *Biochem Biophys Res Commun* 165:1286–1291.

Katoh-Fukui Y, Tsuchiya R, Shiroishi T, Nakahara Y, Hashimoto N, Noguchi K, Higashinakagawa T (1998). Male-to-female sex reversal in *M33* mutant mice. *Nature* 393:688–692.

Keller S A, Jones J M, Boyle A, Barrow L L, Killen P D, Green D G, Kapousta N V, Hitchcock P F, Swank R T, Meisler M H (1994). Kidney and retinal defects *(Krd)*, a transgene-induced mutation with a deletion of mouse chromosome 19 that includes the *Pax2* locus. *Genomics* 23:309–320.

Kent-First M G, Maffitt M, Maallem A, Brisco P, Shultz J, Ekenburg S, Agulnik A I, Agulnik I, Shramm D, Bavister B, Abdul-Mawgood A, VandeBerg J (1996). Gene sequence and evolutionary conservation of human *SMCY*. *Nat Genet* 14:128–129.

Kiel-Metzger K, Warren G, Wilson G N, Erickson R P (1985). Evidence that the human Y chromosome does not contain clustered DNA sequences (Bkm) associated with heterogametic sex determination in other vertebrates. *N Engl J Med* 313:242–245.

King C-Y, Weiss M A (1993). The *SRY* high-mobility-group box recognizes DNA by partial intercalation in the minor grove: a topological mechanism of sequence specificity. *Proc Natl Acad Sci USA* 90:11990–11994.

Koopman P, Gubbay J, Vivian N, Goodfellow P, Lovell-Badge R (1991). Male development of chromosomally female mice transgenic for *Sry*. *Nature* 351:117–121.

Koopman P, Münsterberg A, Capel B, Vivian N, Lovell-Badge R (1990) Expression of a candidate sex-determining gene during mouse testis differentiation. *Nature* 348:450–452.

Krauss C M, Turksoy R N, Atkins L, McLaughlin C, Brown L G, Page D C (1987). Familial premature ovarian failure due to an interstitial deletion of the long arm of the X chromosome. *N Engl J Med* 317:125–131.

Krco C J, Goldberg E H (1976) Detection of H-Y (male) antigen in 8-cell mouse embryos. *Science* 193:1134–1135.

Kwok C, Tyler-Smith C, Mendonca B B, Hughes I, Berkovitz G D, Goodfellow P N, Hawkins J R (1996). Mutation analysis of the 2 kb 5' to *SRY* in XY females and Y intersex subjects. *J Med Genet* 33:465–468.

Lala D S, Rice D A, Parker K L (1992) Steroidogenic factor 1, a key regulator of steroidogenic enzyme expression, is the mouse homolog of fushi tarazu factor 1. *Mol Endocrinol* 6:1249–1258.

Latham K E (1996). X chromosome imprinting and inactivation in the early embryo. *Trends Genet* 12:134–138.

Lau Y-F, Chan K (1989). The putative testis-determining factor and related genes are expressed as discrete-size transcripts in adult gonadal and somatic tissues. *Am J Hum Genet* 45:942–952.

Lovell-Badge R, Robertson E (1990). XY female mice resulting from a heritable mutation in the primary testis-determining-gene, *Tdy*. *Development* 109:635–646.

Luo X, Ikeda Y, Parker K L (1994). A cell-specific nuclear receptor is essential for adrenal and gonadal development and sexual differentiation. *Cell* 77:481–490.

Luoh S-W, Bain P A, Polakiewicz R D, Goodheart M L, Gardner H, Jaenisch R, Page D C (1997). *Zfx* mutation results in small animal size and reduced germ cell number in male and female mice. *Development* 124:2275–2284.

Madan K, Hompes P G A, Schoemaker J, Ford C E (1981). X-autosome translocation with a breakpoint in Xq22 in a fertile woman and her 47,XXX infertile daughter. *Hum Genet* 59:290–296.

Magenis R E, Webb M J, McKean R S, Tomar D, Allen L J, Kammer H, VanDyke D L, Lourien E (1982). Translocation (X: Y) (p 22.33; p 11.2) in XX males: etiology of male phenotype. *Hum Genet* 62:271–276.

Mahaffey C L, Bayleran J K, Yeh G Y, Lee T C, Page D C, Simpson E M (1997). Intron/exon structure confirms that mouse *Zfy* 1 and *Zfy* 2 are members of the *ZFY* gene family. *Genomics* 41:123–127.

Mangia F, Albo-Halsbach G, Epstein C J (1975). X-chromosome expression during oogenesis in the mouse. *Dev Biol* 45:366–368.

Mansour S, Hall C M, Pembrey M E, Young I D (1995). A clinical and genetic study of compomelic dysplasia. *J Med Genet* 32:415–420.

Mardon G, Page D C (1989). The sex-determining region of the mouse Y chromosome encodes a protein with a highly acidic domain and 13 zinc fingers. *Cell* 56:765–770.

Markovic V D, Cox D W, Wilkinson J (1985). X; 14 translocation an exception to the critical region hypothesis on the human X chromosome. *Am J Med Genet* 20:87–96.

Mastrangelo P, Zwingman T, Erickson R P, Blecher S R (1994). *Zfy* is transcribed in the normal mouse epididymis and in the XX*Sxr* "sex reversed" testis. *Dev Genet* 15:129–138.

McElreavey K, Vilain E, Abbas N, Costa J M, Souleyreau N, Kucheria K, Boucekkine C, Thibaud E, Brauner R, Flamant F, Fellous M (1992). XY sex reversal associated with a deletion 5' to the *SRY* "HMG box" in the testis-determining region. *Proc Natl Acad Sci USA* 89:11016–11020.

McElreavey K, Vilain E, Abbas N, Herskowitz I, Fellous M (1993). A regulatory cascade hypothesis for mammalian sex determination: *SRY* represses a negative regulator of male development. *Proc Natl Acad Sci USA* 90:3368–3372.

McElreavey K, Vilain E, Barbaux S, Fuqua J S, Fechner P Y, Souleyreau N, Doco-Fenzy M, Gabriel R, Quereux C, Fellous M, Berkovitz G D (1996). Loss of sequences 3' to the testis-determining gene, *SRY*, including the Y pseudoautosomal boundary associated with partial testicular determination. *Proc Natl Acad Sci USA* 93:8590–8594.

McLaren A, Simpson E, Tomonari K, Chandler P, Hogg H (1984). Male sexual differentiation in mice lacking H-Y antigen. *Nature* 312:552–555.

McPherson E W, Clemens M M, Gibbons R J, Higgs D R (1995). X-linked α-thalassemia/mental retardation (ATR-X) syndrome: a new kindred with severe genital anomalies and mild hematologic expression. *Am J Med Genet* 55:302–306.

Metaxotou C, Kalpini-Mavrou A (1977). Ring chromosome 9: 46,XY,r(9) in a male with ambiguous external genitalia. *Hum Genet* 37:351–354.

Mittwoch U (1971). Sex determination in birds and mammals. *Nature* 231:432–434.

Mittwoch U, Delhanty J D A, Beck F (1969). Growth of differentiating testes and ovaries. *Nature* 224:323–325.

Mittwoch U, Mahadevaiah S (1980). Additional growth—a link between mammalian testes, avian ovaries, gonadal asymmetry in hermaphrodites and the expression of H-Y antigen. *Growth* 44:287–300.

Miyamoto N, Yoshida M, Kuratani S, Matsuo I, Aizawa S (1997). Defects of urogenital development in mice lacking *Emx2*. *Development* 124:1653–1664.

Muscatelli F, Strom T M, Walker A P, Zanaria E, Récan D, Meindl A, Bardoni B, Guioli S, Zehetner G, Rabl W, Schwarz H P, Kaplan J-C, Camerino G, Meitinger T, Monaco A P (1994). Mutations in the *DAX-1* gene give rise to both X-linked adrenal hypoplasia congenita and hypogonadotropic hypogonadism. *Nature* 372:672–676.

Nachtigal M W, Hirokawa Y, Enyeart-VanHouten D L, Flanagan J N, Hammer G D, Ingraham H A (1998). Wilms' tumor 1 and Dax-1 modulate the orphan nuclear receptor SF-1 in sex-specific gene expression. *Cell* 93:445–454.

Nagamine C M, Chan K, Hake L E, Lau Y-FC (1990). The two candidate testis-determining Y genes (*Zfy-1* and *Zfy-2*) are differentially expressed in fetal and adult mouse tissues. *Genes Dev* 4:63–74.

Nakahori Y, Tamua T, Nagafuchi S, Fujieda K, Minowada S, Fukutani K, Fuse H, Hayashi K, Kuroki Y, Fukushima Y, Agematsu K, Kuno T, Kaneko S, Yamada K, Kitagawa T, Nonomura M, Fukuda S, Kusano M, Onigata S, Hibi I, Nakagome Y (1991). Molecular cloning and mapping of 10 new probes on the human Y chromosome. *Genomics* 9:765–769.

Nasrin N, Buggs C, Kong X F, Carnazza J, Goebl M, Alexander-Bridges, M (1991). DNA-binding properties of the product of the testis-determining gene and a related protein. *Nature* 354:317–320.

Nornes H O, Dressler G R, Knapik E W, Deutsch U, Gruss P (1990). Spatially and temporally restricted expression of *Pax* 2 during murine neurogenesis. *Development* 109:797–809.

Ogata T, Hawkins J R, Taylor A, Matsuo N, Hata J, Goodfellow P N (1992). Sex reversal in a child with a 46,X,Yp+ karyotype: support for the existence of a gene(s), located in distal Xp, involved in testis formation. *J Med Genet* 29:226–230.

Ogata T, Matsuo N (1994). Testis determining gene(s) on the X chromosome short arm: chromosomal localisation and possible role in testis determination. *J Med Genet* 31:349–350.

Ogata T, Muroya K, Matsuo N, Hata J, Fukushima Y, Suzuki Y (1997). Impaired male sex development in an infant with molecularly defined partial 9p monosomy: implication for a testis forming gene(s) on 9p. *J Med Genet* 34:331–334.

Omoe K, Endo A (1993). Growth and development of 39, X mouse embryos at mid-gestation. *Cytogenet Cell Genet* 63:50–53.

Page D C, Mosher R, Simpson E M, Fisher E M C, Mardon G, Pollack J, McGillivray B, de la Chapelle A, Brown L G (1987). The sex-determining region or the human Y chromosome encodes a finger protein. *Cell* 51:1091–1104.

Page D C, Fisher E M C, McGillivray B, Brown L G (1990). Additional deletion in sex-determining region of human Y chromosome resolves paradox of X,t (Y;22) female. *Nature* 346:279–281.

Painter T S. Mammalian spermatogenesis: *J Exp Zool* 137:291. 1923.

Palmer M S, Sinclair A H, Berta P, Ellis N A, Goodfellow P N, Abbas N E, Fellous M (1989). Genetic evidence that *ZFY* is not the testis-determining factor. *Nature* 342:937–939.

Palmer M S, Berta P, Sinclair A H, Pym B, Goodfellow P N (1990). Comparison of human *ZFY* and *ZFX* transcripts. *Proc Natl Acad Sci USA* 87:1681–1685.

Pask A, Toder R, Wilcox S A, Camerino G, Marshall-Graves J A. (1997). The candidate sex-reversing *DAX1* gene is autosomal in marsupials: implications for the evolution of sex determination in mammals. *Genomics* 41:422–426.

Pergament E, Fiddler M, Cho N, Johnson D, Holmgren W (1994). Sexual differentiation and preimplantation cell growth. *Human Reprod* 9:1730–1732.

Petit P, Moerman P H, Fryns J P (1992). Full 69,XXY triploidy and sex-reversal: a further example of true hermaphrodism associated with multiple malformations. *Clin Genet* 41: 175–177.

Piedrahita J A, Anderson G B (1985). Investigation of sperm cytotoxicity as an indicator of ability of antisera to detect male-specific antigen on preimplantation mouse embryos. *J Reprod Fertil* 74:637–644.

Ramsay M, Berstein R, Zwane E, Page D C, Jenkins T (1988). XX true hermaphroditism in southern African blacks: an enigma of primary sexual differentiation. *Am J Hum Genet* 43:4–13.

Ray P F, Conaghan J, Winston R M L, Handyside A H (1995). Increased number of cells and metabolic activity in male human preimplantation embryos following *in vitro* fertilization. *J Reprod Fertil* 104:165–171.

Raymond C S, Shamu C E, Shen M M, Seifert K J, Hirsch B, Hodgkin J, Zarkower D (1998). Evidence for evolutionary conservation of sex-determining genes. *Nature* 391:691–695.

Reardon W, Gibbons R J, Winter R M, Baraitser M (1995). Male pseudohermphroditism in sibs with the α-thalassemia/mental retardation (ATR-X) syndrome. *Am J Med Genet* 55: 285–287.

Rivera H, Enríquez-Guerra M A, Rolón A, Jiménez-Sáinz M E, Núñez-González L, Cantú J M (1986). Whole-arm t (X;17) (Xp17q^{q}17p) and gonadal dysgenesis: a further exception to the critical region hypothesis. *Clin Genet* 29:425–428.

Rothenpieler U W, Dressler G R (1993). *Pax-2* is required for mesenchyme-to-epithelium conversion during kidney development. *Development* 119:711–720.

Sainio K, Hellstedt P, Kreidberg J A, Saxen L, Sariola H (1997). Differential regulation of two sets of mesonephric tubules by WT-1. *Development* 124:1293–1299.

Sanyanusin P, Schimmenti L A, McNoe L A, Ward T A, Pierpont M E M, Sullivan M J, Dobyns W B, Eccles M R (1995). Mutation of the *PAX2* gene in a family with optic nerve colobomas, renal anomalies and vesicoureteral reflux. *Nat Genet* 9:358–363.

Sarto G E, Therman E, Patau K (1973). X inactivation in man: a woman with t(Xq−;12q+). *Am J Hum Genet* 25:262–270.

Scherer G, Schempp W, Baccichetti C, Lenzini E, Bricarelli F D, Carbone L D L, Wolf U (1989). Duplication of an Xp segment that includes the ZFX locus causes sex inversion in man. *Hum Genet* 81:291–294.

Schneider-Gadicke A, Beer-Romero P, Brown L G, Nussbaum, R, Page DXC (1989). *ZFX* has a gene structure similar to *ZFY*, the putative human sex determinant, and escapes X inactivation. *Cell* 57:1247–1258.

Scott D M, Ehrmann I E, Ellis P S, Bishop C E, Agulnik A I, Simpson E, Mitchell M J (1995). Identification of a mouse male specific transplantation antigen, H-Y. *Nature* 376:695–698.

Scott W J, Holsen J F (1977). Weight differences in rat embryos prior to sexual differentiation. *J Embryol Morphol* 40:259–263.

Seller M J, Perkins-Cole K J (1987). Sex differences in mouse embryonic development at neurulation. *J Reprod Fertil* 79:159–161.

Shen W-H, Moore C C D, Ikeda Y, Parker K L, Ingraham H A (1994). Nuclear receptor steroidogenic factor 1 regulates the Müllerian inhibiting substance gene: a link to the sex determination pathway. *Cell* 77:651–661.

Simpson E, Chandler P, Goulmy E, Disteche C M, Ferguson-Smith M A, Page D C (1987). Separation of the genetic loci for the H-Y antigen and for testis determination on human Y chromosome. *Nature* 326:876–878.

Simpson E M, Page D C (1991). An interstitial deletion in mouse Y chromosomal DNA created a transcribed *Zfy* fusion gene. *Genomics* 11:601–608.

Sinclair A H, Berta P, Palmer M S, Hawkins J R, Griffiths B L, Smith M J, Foster J W, Frischauf

A-M, Lovell-Badge R, Goodfellow P N (1990). A gene from the human sex-determining region encodes a protein with homology to a conserved DNA-binding motif. *Nature* 346: 240–244.

Spurdle A B, Shankman S, Ramsay M (1995). XX true hermaphroditism in southern African blacks: exclusion of SRY sequences and uniparental disomy of the X chromosome. *Am J Med Genet* 55:53–56.

Stalvey J R D, Durbin E J, Erickson R P (1989). Sex vesicle "entrapment": translocation or nonhomologous recombination of misaligned Yp and Xp as alternative mechanisms for abnormal inheritance of the sex-determining region. *Am J Med Genet* 32:564–572.

Stevanovic M, Lovell-Badge R, Collignon J, Goodfellow P N (1993). *SOX3* is an X-linked gene related to *SRY*. *Hum Mol Genet* 2:2013–2018.

Su H, Lau Y C (1993). Identification of the transcriptional unit, structural organization, and promoter sequence of the human sex-determining region Y(*SRY*) gene, using a reverse genetic approach. *Am J Hum Genet* 52:24–38.

Summitt R L, Tipton R E, Wilroy R S Jr., Martens P R, Phelan J P (1978). X-autosome translocations: a review. *Birth Defects* 14:219–247.

Swain A, Narvaez V, Burgoyne P, Camerino G, Lovell-Badge R, (1998). *Dax1* antagonizes *Sry* action in mammalian sex determination. *Nature* 391:761–767.

Swain A, Zanaria E, Hacker A, Lovell-Badge R, Camerino G (1996). Mouse *Dax1* expression is consistent with a role in sex determination as well as in adrenal and hypothalamus function. *Nat Genet* 12:404–409.

Taketo M, Parker K L, Howard T A, Tsukiyama T, Wong M, Niwa O, Morton C C, Miron P M, Seldin M F (1995). Homologs of Drosophila Fushi-Tarazu factor 1 map to mouse chromosome 2 and human chromosome 9q33. *Genomics* 25:565–567.

Thornhill A R, Burgoyne P S (1993). A paternally imprinted X chromosome retards the development of the early mouse embryo. *Development* 118:171–174.

Tiffin G J, Rieger D, Betteridge K J, Yadar B R, King W A (1991). Glucose and glutamine metabolism in pre-attachment cattle embryos in relation to sex and stage of development. *J Reprod Fertil* 93:125–132.

Trunca C, Therman E, Rosenwaks Z (1984). The phenotypic effects of small, distal Xq deletions. *Hum Genet* 68:87–89.

Tsunoda Y, Tokunaga T, Sugie T (1985). Altered sex ratio of live young after transfer of fast- and slow-developing mouse embryos. *Gamete Res* 12:301–304.

Tucker P K, Lundigan B L (1993). Rapid evolution of the sex determining locus in Old World mice and rats. *Nature* 364:715–717.

Van Heyningen V, Hastie N D. (1992). Wilms' tumor: reconciling genetics and biology. *Trends Genet* 8:16–21.

Veitia R A, Nunes M, Quintana-Murci L, Rappaport R, Thibaud E, Jaubert F, Fellous M, McElreavey K, Gonçalves J, Silva M, Rodrigues J C, Caspurro M, Boieiro F, Marques R, Lavinha J (1998). Swyer syndrome and 46,XY partial gonadal dysgenesis associated with 9p deletions in the absence of monosomy-9p syndrome. *Am J Hum Genet* 63:901–905.

Verga V, Erickson R P (1989). An extended long-range restriction map of the human sex-determining region on Yp, including *ZFY*, finds marked homology on XP and no detectable Y sequences in an XX male. *Am J Hum Genet* 44:756–765.

Vergnaud G, Page D C, Simmler M C, Brown L, Rouyer F, Noel B, Botstein D, de la Chapelle A, Weissenbach J (1986). A deletion map of the human Y chromosome based on DNA hybridization. *Am J Hum Genet* 38:109–124.

Vilain E, Fellous M, McElreavey K (1992). Characterization and sequence of the 5' flanking region of the human testis-determining factor *SRY*. *Methods Mol Cell Biol* 3:128–134.

Vilain E, Jaubert F, Fellous M, McElreavey K. Pathology of 46,XY pure gonadal dysgenesis: absence of testis differentiation associated with mutation in the testis-determining factor. *Differentiation* 52:151–159.

Wachtel S S, Ohno S, Koo G C, Boyse E A (1975). Possible role for H-Y antigen in the primary determination of sex. *Nature* 257:235–236.

Wang W, Meadows L R, den Haan J M M, Sherman N E, Chen Y, Blokland E, Shabanowitz J, Agulnik A I, Hendrickson R C, Bishop C E, Hunt D F, Goulmy E, Engelhard V H (1995). Human H-Y: a male-specific histocompatibility antigen derived from the *SMCY* protein. *Science* 269:1588–1590.

Weatherall D J, Higgs D R, Bunch C, Old J M, Hunt D M, Pressley L, Clegg J B, Bethlenfalvay N C, Sjolin S, Koler R D, Magenis E, Francis J L, Bebbington D (1981). Hemoglobin H disease and mental retardation: a new syndrome or a remarkable coincidence? *N Engl J Med* 305:607–612.

Wegner R D (1982). Translocation t(X;1) and the "critical region hypothesis." *Hum Genet* 61: 79.

Welshons W J, Russell L B (1959). The Y-chromosome as the bearer of male-determining factors in the mouse. *Proc Natl Acad Sci USA* 45:560–566.

Werner M H, Huth J R, Gronenborn A V, Clore G M (1995). Molecular basis of human 46,XY sex reversal revealed from the three-dimensional solution structure of the human *SRY*-DNA complex. *Cell* 81:705–714.

White K L, Anderson G B, BonDurant R H (1987a). Expression of a male-specific factor on various stages of preimplantation bovine embryos. *Biol Reprod* 37:867–873,

White K L, Anderson G B, Pashen R L, BonDurant R H (1987b). Delection of histo-compatibility-Y (H-Y) antigen: identification of sex of preimplantation ovine embryos. *J Reprod Immunol* 10:27–32.

White K L, Anderson G B, Berger T J, BonDurant R H, Pashen R L (1987c). Identification of a male-specific histocompatibility protein on preimplantation porcine embryos. *Gamete Res* 17:107–113.

Wilkie A O, Zeitlin H C, Lindenbaum R H, Buckle V J, Fischel-Ghodsian N, Chui D H, Gardner-Medwin D, MacGillivray M H, Weatherall D J, Higgs D R (1990). Clinical features and molecular analysis of the alpha-thalassemia/mental retardation syndromes. II. Cases without detectable abnormality of the alpha globin gene complex. *Am J Hum Genet* 46:1127–1140.

Wilkie A O, Gibbons R J, Higgs D R, Pembrey M E (1991). X-linked alpha-thalassemia/mental retardation: spectrum of clinical features in three related males. *J Med Genet* 28:738–741.

Wilkie A O, Campbell F M, Daubeney P, Grant D B, Daniels R J, Mullarkey M, Affara N A, Fitchett M, Huson S M (1993). Complete and partial XY sex reversal associated with terminal deletion of 10q: report of 2 cases and literature review. *Am J Med Genet* 46:597–600.

Wood T G, White K L, Thompson Jr D L, Garza Jr F (1988). Evaluation of the expression of a male-specific antigen on cells of equine blastocysts. *J Reprod Immunol* 14:1–8.

Wright E, Hargrave M R, Christiansen J, Cooper L, Kun J, Evans T, Gangadharan U, Greenfield A, Koopman P (1995). The *Sry*-related gene *SOX9* is expressed during chondrogenesis in mouse embryos. *Nat Genet* 9:15–20.

Wulfsberg E A, Weaver R P, Cunniff C M, Jones M C, Lyons Jones K (1989). Chromosome 10qter deletion syndrome: a review and report of three new cases. *Am J Med Genet* 32: 364–367.

Xu K P, Yadav B R, King W A, Betteridge K J (1992). Sex-related differences in developmental rates of bovine embryos produced and cultured *in vitro*. *Mol Reprod Dev* 31:229–234.

Yost A, Magre S (1989). Control mechanisms of testicular differentiation. *Phil Trans R Soc B* 323:35–61.

Yu R N, Ito M, Saunders T L, Camper S A, Jameson J L (1998). Role of *Ahch* in gonadal development and gametogenesis. *Nat Genet* 20:353–357.

Zanaria E, Muscatelli F, Bardoni B, Strom T M, Guioli S, Guo W, Lalli E, Moser C, Walker A P, McCabe E R B, Meitinger T, Monaco A P, Sassone-Corsi P, Camerino G (1994). An unusual member of the nuclear hormone receptor superfamily responsible for X-linked adrenal hypoplasia congenita. *Nature* 372:635–641.

Zimmerman S, Schwärzler A, Buth S, Engel W, Adham I M (1998). Transcription of the

Leydig insulin-like gene is mediated by Steroidogenic Factor-1. *Mol Endocrinol* 12:706–713.

Zwingman T, Erickson R P, Boyer T, Ao A (1993). Transcription of the sex determining region genes *Sry* and *Zfy* in the mouse preimplantation embryo. *Proc Natl Acad Sci USA* 90:814–817.

Zwingman T, Fujimoto H, Lai L-W, Boyer T, Ao A, Stalvey J R D, Blecher S R, Erickson R P (1994). Transcription of circular and noncircular forms of *Sry* in mouse testes. *Mol Reprod Dev* 37:370–381.

3

Introductory Biochemistry and Endocrinology of Sexual Development

Sexual development can be said to begin after the gonads have been determined to become testes or ovaries. It is usually divided into two levels: *primary*, referring to internal and external genital morphogenesis that is testis-dependent in males, but testis-independent in females, and *secondary*, referring to pubertal growth and maturation of the respective reproductive axes enabling reproduction. But there is reason to recognize a *tertiary* level: the emotional and interpersonal aspects of sexual development, including gender identity and role, and homosexual or heterosexual orientation.

PRIMARY SEXUAL DEVELOPMENT

Because internal and external genital morphogenesis is constitutively female (it occurs even in the physical or functional absence of embryonic gonads), ovaries obviously do not contribute substantively to primary sexual development in females. It is important to appreciate, however, that the large amount of androgen made by the fetal female adrenal glands is sufficient to masculinize the external genitalia of

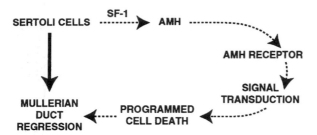

FIGURE 3–1. Sertoli cells are ultimately responsible for müllerian duct regression (solid arrow). A series of steps in this process is indicated by dashed arrows.

female fetuses if there is insufficient placental aromatase activity to convert the adrenal androgen to estrogen. The consequences of aromatase deficiency are discussed in Chapter 13. It is not clear whether, and to what extent, the placentally derived estrogen is competitively anti-androgenic, or whether it serves simply to "drain" what would otherwise be a large masculinizing pool of androgen.

To override the constitutivity of female primary sexual development, normal male internal and external genital morphogenesis requires the active intervention of a very large number of chronologically integrated factors. Thus, to accomplish müllerian duct regression, the organism needs Sertoli cells; the factor(s), such as steroidogenesis factor-1 (SF-1), that regulates the synthesis and secretion of anti-müllerian hormone (AMH) by these cells; the AMH receptor on the surface of cells that are targets of AMH action; and the cascade of intracellular signaling molecules that culminates in müllerian duct regression by apoptosis (Fig. 3–1).

SF-1, a multipotent transcriptional regulator of steroid organogenesis and hormonogenesis, is discussed later in this chapter. AMH, a member of the transforming growth factor–β (TGF-β) superfamily, and the AMH receptor, a serine/threonine protein kinase with a single transmembrane domain, are described in Chapter 9, which contains descriptions of their mutations and the consequences thereof.

The requirements for wolffian duct differentiation are at least as numerous as those for müllerian duct regression (Fig. 3–2). They include Leydig cells; the steroid acute regulatory (StAR) protein that is responsible for cholesterol transport into Leydig cell mitochondria in order to start the process of steroid biosynthesis; the

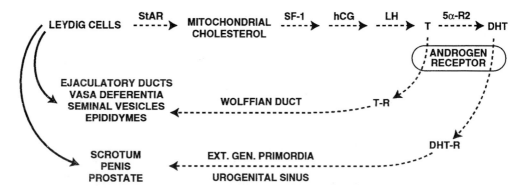

FIGURE 3–2. Leydig cells are ultimately responsible for internal and external genital masculinization (solid arrows). A set of steps in these processes is indicated by dashed arrows.

factors, such as SF-1 and, perhaps, DAX-1 (see below), that regulate the expression of enzymes that catalyze certain steps in the sequential biosynthesis of testosterone (T); the androgen receptor (AR), a typical nuclear receptor, within cells of the wolffian duct; and, undoubtedly, a host of unknown genes (some targets of T action; many others not) whose interacting products underlie the morphogenesis of wolffian duct–derived structures. In other words, normal sexual morphogenesis, both internal and external, must depend on morphogens having nothing directly to do with sex hormones, whether in the male or female. This is why sexual dysmorphogenesis so often accompanies nonsexual anomalies in a multitude of malformation syndromes that have very diverse etiologies. Furthermore, some individuals with completely female external genitalia—because of AR or Leydig cell defects—nevertheless have epididymes and vasa deferentia. Thus, other "factors" may sometimes fulfill the role of T in these aspects of wolffian duct differentiation; alternatively, even small amounts of androgenic activity may be adequate, in a paracrine fashion, for some aspects of wolffian duct differentiation (Erickson, 1997). The consequences of mutation causing underactivity of the StAR protein and, in various forms, of Leydig cells are both recorded in Chapter 13; those resulting from deficient or defective AR activity are presented in Chapter 14. Prostate and external genital morphogenesis are one level more complicated than internal genital morphogenesis, because their primordia must develop *a sufficient amount* of 5α-reductase, type 2 (5α-R2) activity, *at the right time*, in order that enough precursor T is converted to 5α-dihydrotestosterone (DHT). This androgenic hormone acts on the AR in an autocrine and/or paracrine fashion to induce differentiation of the prostate, penis, and scrotum. 5α-R2 deficiency is discussed in Chapter 13.

SECONDARY SEXUAL DEVELOPMENT

Human chorionic gonadotropin (hCG) maintains Leydig cell testosterone biosynthesis in embryonic life, but the initiation of that process may be autogenous (Word et al., 1989). Luteinizing hormone (LH) stimulates the resumption of Leydig cell testosterone biosynthesis in late fetal and neonatal life, and at male puberty (Fig. 3–3). At female puberty, LH also induces ovulation, formation of the corpus luteum, and ovarian steroid secretion by acting on both theca and granulosa cells. Follicle-stimulating hormone (FSH) stimulates ovarian follicular growth and, together with LH, promotes ovarian estrogen synthesis by acting on granulosa cells; it also supports spermatogenesis by acting on Sertoli cells, and Sertoli cells, in turn, produce a factor that stimulates Leydig cell steroidogenesis (Boujrad et al., 1995). LH and FSH are made in the anterior pituitary by basophilic cells called gonadotrophs (or gonadotropes). These cells differentiate under the control of a pituitary transcription factor, PROP1 (see Chapter 17). LH and FSH are dimeric glycoproteins; they share a common α subunit coupled to different β subunits. LH and CG β subunits are so similar that they share the same receptor. FSH has its own receptor. Both receptors are of the 7-transmembrane helix type coupled to G proteins. At puberty, the pulsatile release of gonadotropin-releasing hormone (GnRH; also known as LHRH), a decapeptide produced by the hypothalamus, stimulates the pulsatile secretion of LH primarily, and of FSH as well (Shupnik, 1996). LH secretion in the male is subject to negative feedback by androgen primarily, and by estrogen. The androgen inhibits at both the hypothalamic and pituitary levels; the estrogen only

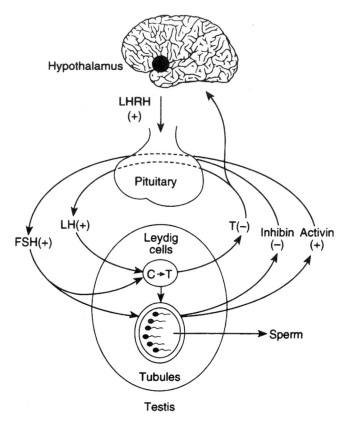

FIGURE 3–3. A simplified scheme of the regulatory relations among various secretions of the hypothalamic-pituitary-testis axis. An ovary version of this scheme is given in the text. C → T, cholesterol → testosterone biosynthesis. (Reproduced from Griffin, J E and Ojida S R (eds), 1996. *Textbook of Endocrine Physiology*, 3rd ed., New York, Oxford University Press, p. 211.)

at the hypothalamic. GnRH pulse frequency and amplitude have differential regulatory effects on the genes that encode the β subunits of LH and FSH. For example, frequency alteration can favor LH or FSH synthesis. Likewise, gonadal steroid feedback has a greater negative effect on LH, and gonadal peptides either increase FSH release (activin) or decrease it (inhibin; follistatin), but do not affect LH. Inhibin is a protein containing an α subunit and one or another of two homologous β subunits that resemble a subunit of TGF-β. Activin is a homodimer of β subunits (Mayo, 1994). Follistatin, an unrelated peptide, nullifies activin by binding to it. Mutations of activin, inhibin, or follistatin have not yet been discovered. Mutations of LH, FSH, GnRH, and the GnRH receptor are discussed in Chapter 10; those of the LH receptor, the post-LH receptor cascade, and the FSH receptor are covered in Chapter 11.

STEROIDOGENIC FACTOR (SF-1)

SF-1 is a universal regulator of *development* and *function* of the hypothalamic-pituitary-gonadal axis. Structurally, it is a member of the nuclear receptor super-family; thus, it is closely related to the steroid receptors and similar transcriptional regulatory proteins. Like them, it has a ligand-binding domain (but no known ligand; hence "orphan"), and a DNA-binding domain built around typical zinc fingers. Its gene maps to human chromosome 9q33.

SF-1 was originally recognized as a cell-specific protein that retarded the mobility (in gel shift assays) of promoter elements in the 5'-flanking regions of the genes for various cytochrome P450 steroid hydroxylases, enzymes responsible for certain steps in steroidogenesis (Lala et al., 1995). Later, SF-1 was discovered to also regulate the genes encoding gonadotropin subunits (Halvorson et al., 1996) and the müllerian-inhibiting substance (Shen et al., 1994). Thus, SF-1 was initially considered to be a global transcriptional regulator (directly or indirectly) of hormones involved in primary and secondary sexual differentiation (Parker and Schimmer, 1996). After the SF-1 gene was cloned, *in situ* hybridization permitted detection of its mRNA transcripts in the earliest gonadal and adrenal primordia, well before the onset of steroidogenesis. This implied that SF-1 was involved in the genesis of these organs, not just in their mature functions. Interestingly, SF-1 expression is inhibited in fetal ovaries, but continues to be expressed in fetal Sertoli and Leydig cells as well as in the Leydig cells of mature testes. Importantly, SF-1 transcripts are also detected in portions of the hypothalamus related to GnRH neurons, and in the anterior pituitary gland itself. The implications of the foregoing observations were affirmed when SF-1 knockout mice were found to lack adrenal glands, gonads, LH and FSH, and the ventromedial hypothalamic (VMH) nucleus. These observations proved the omnipotent influence of SF-1 on development of the hypothalamic-pituitary-gonad axis but raised other questions. For instance, SF-1 knockout mice respond to exogenous GnRH by release of LH and FSH, yet their own GnRH neurons do have GnRH (Parker and Schimmer, 1996). Apparently, what they lack is a signal from the VMH to release their GnRH.

The following basic aspects of SF-1 need to be resolved: (1) what controls SF-1 expression, positively in most places of the developing human, but negatively in the ovary during female sexual differentiation; (2) how many (and which?) genes are targets of SF-1 action, particularly the one(s) whose product(s) prevents the programmed cell death that is responsible for regression of the adrenal glands and gonads in SF-1 knockout mice; (3) what is the ligand(s) for SF-1?; (4) is it modified post-translationally, such as by phosphorylation; and (5) does it interact with other transcriptional regulatory factors, either directly at the protein-protein level or, in some measure indirectly, through the mediation of regulatory sequences of nucleotides? There are no known disorders due to natural SF-1 mutations. However, a minority of subjects with apparently autosomal recessive congenital adrenal hypoplasia (Chapter 10) may be candidates for such mutations, as may individuals with different forms of apparent delay in testis differentiation (Fuqua et al., 1996) and/or maturation (Meyer et al., 1978).

DAX-1

DAX-1 shares many properties with SF-1 (Ikeda et al., 1996). Its gene was originally identified by positional cloning as the one responsible for X-linked congenital adrenal hypoplasia (Chapter 10) associated with hypogonadotropic hypogonadism (Zanaria et al., 1994). The name *DAX-1* is derived from its localization within the *d*osage-sensitive sex reversal locus and the *AHC* (adrenal hypoplasia congenita) locus on the X chromosome. The DAX-1 gene consists of two exons separated by a 3.4 kb intron. Like SF-1, DAX-1 is also an orphan nuclear receptor. It has a typical ligand-binding domain, but it does not have a typical zinc-finger DNA-binding domain. Instead, its amino-terminal portion contains a novel domain in which several repeats of two putative zinc-finger structures are found. Strikingly, DAX-1 and SF-1 are expressed in essentially the same places: the adrenal glands, the gonads, the hypothalamus, and the pituitary gland. This suggests that DAX-1 and SF-1 are interacting transregulatory proteins that collaborate to share control of various target genes.

It is striking to behold that particular transcriptional regulatory factors (DAX-1; SF-1; see above and below) have been conserved to serve the multiple purposes of adrenogenesis, gonadogenesis, and male (and probably female) sexual steroidogenesis. Such evolutionatory conservatism has evidently served as a successful strategy in the management of a biological process as fundamental as reproduction.

STEROID BIOSYNTHESIS

Biosynthetic sequences leading to the production of sex steroids are shown in Figure 3–4. The first committed step in the pathway, the conversion by side chain cleavage (SCC) of c27 cholesterol to c21 pregnenolone, is catalyzed by a cytochrome P450 mixed-function oxidase (CYP11A) that resides on the inner *mitochondrial* membrane. Cytochromes P450 are enzymes that increase the water solubility of hydrophobic substrates by the process of hydroxylation. Transport of cholesterol to the residence of this enzyme is necessary for normal enzyme activity. Deficient transport leads to congenital lipoid adrenal hypoplasia (Chapter 13).

The next two steps in the Δ^5 pathway (double bond between c5 and c6) are catalyzed by a bifunctional P450 enzyme (CYP17) that is bound to *microsomes*: they are 17α-hydroxylation of pregnenolone to 17-OHpregnenolone, and cleavage between c17 and c20 of 17-OHpreg to produce a c19 product, dehydroepiandrosterone (DHEA). Some DHEA, particularly in the adrenal cortex, becomes sulfated (not shown). Each Δ^5 precursor can be converted to its 3-keto-Δ^4 product by a non-P450 enzyme, 3β-hydroxysteroid dehydrogenase (HSD)/$\Delta^5 \rightarrow \Delta^4$ isomerase. Androstenedione can be released from the adrenal cortex or ovary and converted to testosterone (T) peripherally. This is the major androgen source in females. In the testis, some DHEA may be converted to T through another intermediate, Δ^5-androstenediol (not shown). The main products in the testis, T and androstenedione, can be peripherally aromatized to estradiol or estrone, respectively. Just as important, T can be reduced peripherally to 5α-dihydrotestosterone by steroid 5α-reductase, types 1 or 2.

In the ovary, the main products are estradiol and estrone because of indigenous aromatase activity. The enzyme responsible for the catalytic conversion of c19 (androgenic) steroids to c18 estrogens (P450arom) belongs to the cytochrome P450 superfamily of heme proteins. It is one member of a two-component complex (the other component is NADPH-cytochrome P450 reductase) that resides in the endoplasmic reticulum of certain cells (and organs): granulosa (ovary), Leydig (testis), syncytiotrophoblast (placenta), fibroblasts (adipose and skin), and certain portions

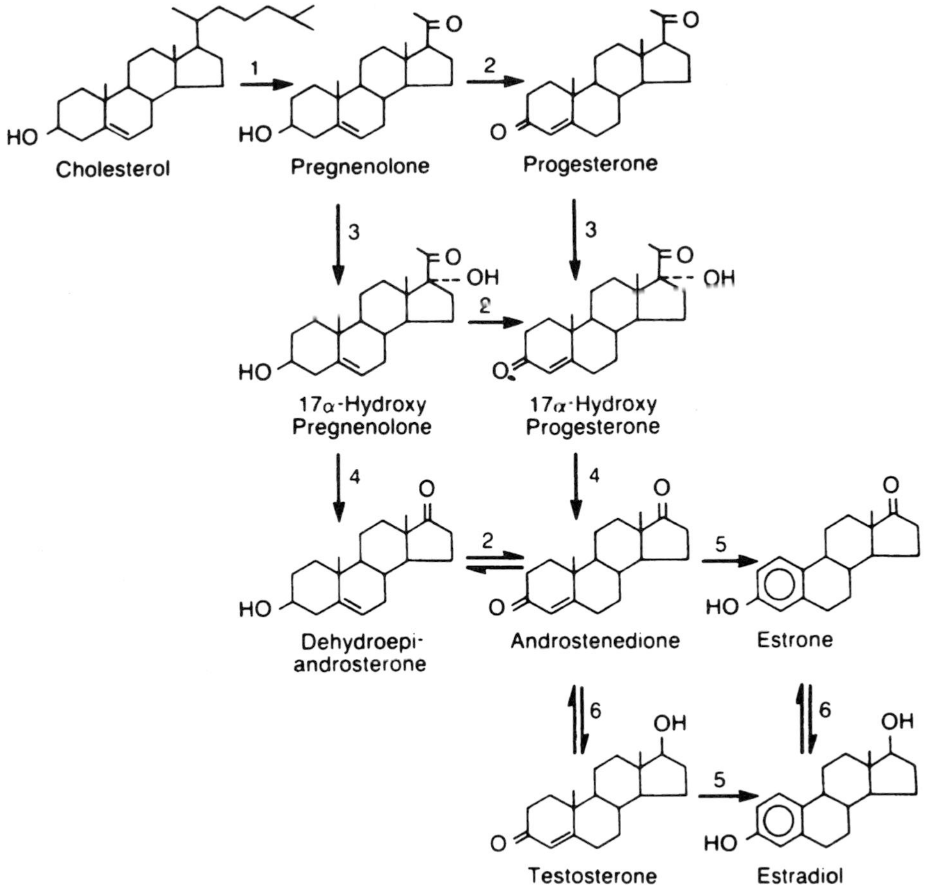

FIGURE 3–4. The biosynthesis of sex steroids. (1) cholesterol side-chain cleavage enzyme complex; (2) 3β-hydroxysteroid dehydrogenase; (3) 17α-hydroxylase; (4) 17,20-lyase; (5) aromatase; (6) 17β-hydroxysteroid dehydrogenase. (Reproduced from Griffin J E and Ojida S R (eds), 1996. *Textbook of Endocrine Physiology*, 3rd ed., New York, Oxford University Press.)

of brain (Simpson et al., 1994). Organs vary in the nature of their predominant C_{19} substrates and, therefore, in their principal estrogenic products. For example, the ovary converts testosterone (T) to 17β-estradiol (E_2) primarily, adipose synthesizes estrone (E_1) from Δ^4-androstenedione, and placenta makes estriol (E_3) from 16α-hydroxyandrostenedione that is ultimately derived from dehydroepiandrosterone sulfate (DHEAS) made in the fetal and maternal adrenal glands. Mutations that increase or decrease aromatase activity are described in Chapter 13.

The biosynthesis of aldosterone and cortisol in the adrenal cortex (Fig. 3–5) depends on the precursors, progesterone and 17-OH progesterone. It is apparent from Figure 3–5 that accumulation of these precursors, and their progenitors, due to deficiency of 21-hydroxylase (CYP21) or 11β-hydroxylase (CYP11B1) will be diverted to the synthesis and release of DHEA and/or androstenedione. Each of these weak androgens is convertible peripherally to T. Excess T is harmful because it masculinizes females and virilizes males. In Chapter 13, genetic defects of sex ste-

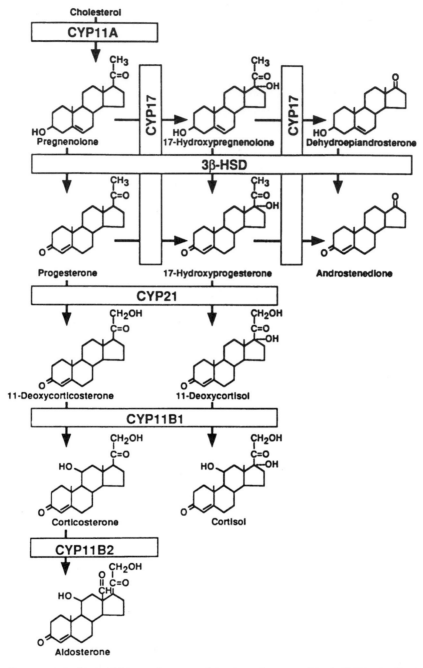

FIGURE 3–5. Steroid biosynthesis in the adrenal cortex. (Top) CYP11A, CYP17, and 3β-HSD, the enzymes shared by adrenocorticosteroid and sex steroid biosynthesis. (Bottom) CYP21, CYP11B1, and CYP11B2, the enzymes devoted to adrenocorticosteroid synthesis. The catalytic activities of the three shared enzymes, of CYP21, and of CYP11B1 are defined in the text; those of CYP11B2 are not considered in this volume. (Reproduced from Donohoue P A, Parker K, Migeon C J (1995) Congenital adrenal hyperplasia. Scriver C R, Beaudet A L, Sly W S, Valle D (eds). *Metabolic and Molecular Bases of Inherited Disease*, 7th ed., New York, McGraw-Hill, pp. 2929–2966.)

roidogenesis are considered in three sections: in combination with defects of adrenocortical steroidogenesis and, apart from them, as defects in androgenesis and estrogenesis, or as defects in estrogenesis alone.

REFERENCES

Boujrad N, Ogwuegbu O, Garnier M, Lee C-H, Martin B M, Papadopoulos V (1995). Identification of a stimulator of steroid hormone synthesis isolated from testis. *Science* 268: 1609–1612.

Erickson K P (1997). Does sex determination start at conception? *Bioessays* 19:1027–1031.

Fuqua J S, Sher E S, Perlman E J, Urban M D, Ghahreman M, Pelletier J, Migeon C J, Brown T R, Berkovitz G D (1996). Abnormal gonadal differentiation in two subjects with ambiguous genitalia, Müllerian structures, and normal testes: evidence for a defect in gonadal ridge development. *Hum Genet* 97:506–511.

Halvorson L M, Kaiser U B, Chin W W (1996). Stimulation of luteinizing hormone beta gene promoter activity by the orphan nuclear receptor, steroidogenic factor-1. *J Biol Chem* 271: 6645–6650.

Ikeda Y, Swain A, Weber T J, Hentges K E, Zanaria E, Lalli E, Tamai T, Sassone-Corsi P, Lovell-Badge R, Camerino G, Parker K L (1996). Steroidogenic factor 1 and Dax-1 colocalize in multiple cell lineages: potential links in endocrine development. *Mol Endocrinol* 10:1261–1272.

Lala D S, Ikeda Y, Luo X, Baity I. A, Meade J C, Parker K L (1994). A cell-specific nuclear receptor regulates the steroid hydroxylases. *Steroids* 60:10–14. 1995.

Mayo K E. Inhibin and activin: molecular aspects of regulation and function. *Trends Endocrinol Metab* 5:407–415.

Meyer W J, Keenan B S, De Lacerda L, Park I J, Jones H E, Migeon C J (1978). Familial male pseudohermaphroditism with normal Leydig cell function at puberty. *J Clin Endocrinol Metab* 46:593–603.

Parker K L, Schimmer B P (1996). The roles of the nuclear receptor steroidogenic factor 1 in endocrine differentiation and development. *Trends Endocrinol Metab* 7:203–207.

Shen W-H, Moore C C D, Ikeda Y, Parker K L, Ingraham H A (1994). Nuclear receptor steroidogenic factor 1 regulates the Müllerian inhibiting substance gene: a link to the sex determination cascade. *Cell* 77:651–661.

Shupnik M A (1996). Gonadotropin gene modulation by steroids and gonadotropin-releasing hormone. *Biol Reprod* 54:279–286.

Simpson E R, Mahendroo M S, Means G D, Kilgore M W, Hinshelwood M M, Graham-Lorence S, Amarneh B, Ito Y, Fisher C R, Michael M D, Mendelson C R, Bulun S E (1994). Aromatase cytochrome P450, the enzyme responsible for estrogen biosynthesis. *Endocr Rev* 15:342–355.

Word R A, George F W, Wildon J D, Carr B R (1989). Testosterone synthesis and adenylate cylase activity in the early human fetal testis appear to be independent of human chorionic gonadotropin control. *J Clin Endocrinol Metab* 69:204–208.

Zanaria E, Muscatelli F, Bardoni B, Strom T M, Guioli S, Guo W, Lalli E, Moser C, Walker A P, McCabe E R B, Meltinger T, Monaco A P, Sassone-Corsi P, Camerino C (1994). An unusual member of the nuclear hormone receptor superfamily responsible for X-linked adrenal hypoplasia congenita. *Nature* 372:635–641.

II

CLINICAL APPROACH

4

The Clinical Approach to Genetic Abnormalities of Gonadal and Sexual Development

The assessment of genital ambiguity in the newborn is a psychosocial emergency (Grumbach and Conte, 1992). Appropriate gender assignment is critical because all surgical, hormonal, and psychological therapy must be in concert and appropriate for the decision, and early and usually repeated reinforcement of the decision will be required. The ultimate goal is a sexually functional and, if possible, fertile individual.

DIAGNOSIS

Precisely what constitutes genital ambiguity is sometimes difficult to define. For example, clitoral enlargement may be a manifestation of virilization in a female with an adrenogenital (AG) syndrome variant, an isolated anomaly, or part of a complex syndrome of known or unknown genesis. However, it may also be due to incomplete virilization in a male with any number of disorders of chromosomal, biochemical, or molecular etiology.

Similarly, bilateral undescended testes with a normal-appearing phallus and phallic urethra may be caused by gonadal agenesis or nonspecific cryptorchidism or could be the result of extreme intrauterine androgenization of a female, perhaps secondary to 21-hydroxylase deficiency or a maternal ovarian tumor. In general, it is best to err on the side of too much rather than too little suspicion about the genital state, and to be thorough rather than superficial in the approach to management. To adopt a wait-and-see attitude may have profound later consequences for the infant and his or her family.

History. Paramount to any decision regarding gender assignment is a good maternal and gestational history, including any history of other relatives in whom there were problems in sex assignment. If the child has other nongenital abnormalities, it is important to inquire whether any of these were present in any relative as well, for some syndromes may be so variable that only a portion of affected individuals have genital anomalies, or if they do, they may be less severe or have been historically minimized.

A maternal drug history is also important. As noted elsewhere in this volume (Chapter 17) certain drugs may nonspecifically interfere with both internal and external genital development in both sexes. Others may affect only external features, as would be the case with androgen ingestion by the mother of an otherwise normal female fetus. Although contemporary oral contraceptives have progestins that are not appreciably androgenic, older preparations contained progesterone derivatives of considerably more androgenic potency and a missed pill or two, followed by resumption of cyclic therapy, could easily obscure early pregnancy. Anti-androgens such as spironolactone commonly used in women for treatment of hirsutism and acne could, in sufficient doses, interfere with male external genital development.

The mother herself should be examined for signs of virilization and/or hirsutism. A maternal ovarian or adrenal androgen-secreting tumor could have profound effects on the developing female fetus (Verhoevern et al., 1973). A luteoma of pregnancy, defined as a benign hCG-dependent ovarian tumor, can cause maternal virilization and, in roughly two thirds of cases, signs of virilization in the newborn female. The evidence of excess androgen production in the mother disappears rapidly after delivery, but the condition may be recurrent (Thomas et al., 1972). Although uncommon, undetected, and hence untreated, maternal non-salt-losing adrenogenital syndrome can contribute sufficient transplacental androgens to virilize a female fetus, who would be at least a heterozygote. Rare causes such as isolated placental aromatase deficiency might be considered if maternal serum estrogen levels were low during pregnancy (Chapter 13).

Physical Examination. The initial physical examination of the newborn by the attending pediatrician or family physician is of critical importance because that individual should either initiate appropriate studies or seek the assistance of a pediatric endocrinologist and perhaps, if warranted, a clinical geneticist. Sufficiently detailed investigation should be carried out in the newborn period to avoid any uncertainty about gender assignment. Absent or grossly abnormal genitalia are unlikely to be overlooked by even a casual observer. However, more subtle abnormalities are also of importance, such as slight clitoral enlargement, labial pigmentation, and inguinal masses or hernias in otherwise normal females. Either unilateral or bilateral cryptorchidism, hypospadias, particularly if second-or third-degree and accompanied by cryptorchidism, micropenis, or unusually small testes are cause for concern in apparent males. If other congenital anomalies are evident, more careful evaluation is necessary because some of these may be immediately life-threatening. A careful rectal examination may provide palpable evidence of a uterus.

Clinical evidence of metabolic derangement, such as tachypnea or excessive urine output, may be indicative of systemic acidosis and warrants more detailed study of plasma electrolytes and acid-base balance.

Laboratory Evaluation. In order to understand the pathophysiology of genital ambiguity better, a peripheral blood karyotype is mandatory, and sufficient metaphases should be examined to exclude mosaicism; one hundred is generally accepted as desirable. Because the process takes a few days to complete, it is one of the first tests to be ordered. If the karyotype is 46,XX, it is imperative that steroid studies be done to exclude the various virilizing forms of the AG syndrome (female pseudohermaphroditism), because the salt-losing forms of this syndrome are lethal if not promptly recognized and treated with hydrocortisone and fluids (Chapter 13). Obviously, if an inguinal or labial gonad is palpated, it raises the possibility of true hermaphroditism, for the majority of those patients are 46,XX (Chapter 6). Most other forms of female pseudohermaphroditism require no immediate therapy, but sonographic evaluation of the urinary tract and lumbosacral spine x-rays are appropriate.

A 46,XY karyotype with genital ambiguity creates a different kind of dilemma (male pseudohermaphroditism), for the various conditions that can produce this clinical picture are numerous and are discussed at length elsewhere in this volume. In some instances, the genitalia are so clearly male or female that sex assignment is simple, regardless of the presence of a Y chromosome. However, in most such infants, more detailed studies will be required. For example, plasma levels of 17-hydroxyprogesterone, DHEA, androstenedione, testosterone, and dihydrotestosterone may provide evidence of a biosynthetic block or end-organ unresponsiveness. If the values are at all equivocal, both ACTH and hCG stimulation tests can be performed. As an aside, penile growth after stimulation with hCG may be a prognostically useful indicator of target tissue responsiveness to androgens in later life. Pelvic ultrasound and/or MRI should be done to assess the internal genitourinary structures. Depending on the nature of the anomaly, injection of radiocontrast dye into the urethra or apparent vagina may aid in delineation of the functional internal anatomy. If there is still a question, laparotomy with gonadal biopsy should be undertaken. Generally, if surgery is deemed necessary, the ambiguity is so significant as to preclude male gender assignment, and definitive internal reconstruction may be considered at this time.

Additional efforts to establish an etiology may require molecular studies of the X and Y chromosomes, even if they appear morphologically intact. If the extragenital features are sufficiently suggestive, the possible presence of other known molecular lesions, such as that associated with camptomelic dysplasia (Chapter 7), can be pursued.

Sex Assignment

As soon as the various studies have been completed, gender assignment should be made, and there should be no question in the minds of the physician, nurses, ancillary personnel, and especially the parents and immediate family, including grandparents, as to the sex-of-rearing. Insofar as possible, this should be done before the infant leaves the newborn nursery. Ambiguous names should be avoided. The infant should be under the care of a physician who understands the developmental potential of the genitalia and is well versed on the need and timing of hormone replacement therapy.

SEX REASSIGNMENT

In a series of studies spanning decades, Money and colleagues (1955, 1984) have shown that change in sex-of-rearing is possible and can probably be done without harm up to 18 months of age. More controversial is change later (i.e., up to 30 months of age). If such delay is unavoidable because of failure of early diagnosis, parental confusion, or misguided advice, sex change can be considered, but only after intensive conversation with the immediate family, and only when adequate provision for close follow-up of the patient and the family is possible. Thereafter, any gender modification is fraught with probably irreparable psychological harm.

It is true, however, that in certain cultures, maleness, even grossly equivocal maleness, is considered to be of such importance that the parents insist on male reconstructive surgery, no matter how inadequate the result. The dramatic change in phenotype in males with 5 alpha-reductase deficiency (Chapter 13) at the time of puberty and the gender change at that time is quite acceptable in some areas of the world.

Later in life, the patient may decide that he or she has been reared in the wrong sex and desire change. If the anatomy is appropriate, surgical reconstruction may be considered, but only after detailed psychological evaluation has been performed and legal experts have been consulted.

THERAPY

Any treatment modality must be practical and functional, and accomplished within anatomical constraints. It is not sexist to acknowledge that it is generally easier to do surgical reconstruction as a female than a male in a situation where there is gross ambiguity. Although the majority of patients with genital ambiguity will be infertile, in certain instances—such as virilized females who have the AG syndrome(s)—early surgery increases the chances for later fertility and procreation because the internal genitalia are perfectly normal. In general, and when overall health permits, genital surgery should be accomplished as soon as feasible, preferably before the child is a year old.

Most authorities advocate clitoral recession rather than clitorectomy as a first step in restoration of female anatomy. Whether vaginoplasty per se is accomplished early or later is controversial. When the procedure is done in early childhood, it is likely that the introitus and/or vault will become stenosed, requiring reoperation when function is desired. With surgery in adolescence, various molds can be used by the individual to enlarge the vagina (Costa et al., 1997). In genetic males reared as females, many would opt for vaginal reconstruction at adolescence when sexual relations commence. However, if a shallow vagina already exists, the use of molds early on will cause some degree of vaginal enlargement, and may facilitate later surgery. The type and timing of surgery may depend on the precise anatomy (Powell et al., 1995). Clearly, in potentially fertile individuals with female pseudohermaphroditism, establishing continuity between the vagina and uterus is mandatory.

There are well-established procedures to deal with male hypospadias. A child in whom male gender assignment has been decided on, who has a small phallus with or without hypospadias, may respond to a depot preparation of testosterone, usually at a dose of 50 mg monthly for 3 to 4 months. If enlargement does occur, it augurs well for later and greater response to male hormones at adolescence. This short course dose of testosterone will not alter bone age appreciably. Moreover, penile enlargement may improve operative results from hypospadias repair, simply by providing more tissue. For this same reason, circumcision should be avoided. If the gonads are absent or are surgically removed, prosthetic testes can be used to enlarge the scrotum. Adult-sized prostheses can then be placed at adolescence.

Internal genital surgery should be consistent with external sex—for example, removal of uterus and fallopian tubes in someone reared as a male. Early gonadectomy is controversial, but most feel that the procedure should be accomplished when reconstruction is done. If, for whatever reason, definitive surgery is put off until later in childhood, the gonads should be examined yearly at least by ultrasound and, if necessary, by MRI to monitor for gonadal malignancy. The incidence of malignancy varies from condition to condition, but in general if the individual harbors a Y cell line, the gonad should be considered a potential dysgenetic testis, an organ that will likely not be adequately functional, and one in which the risk of malignant degeneration is significant. By the same token, early orchidopexy should be accomplished for cryptorchid testes, both for the purpose of facilitating fertility and to place gonads where they can be easily examined, because it is known that the incidence of testicular cancer, although lower than in persistently cryptorchid testes, is still higher than in normal gonads. Current recommendations are for orchiopexy by one year of age (Kass et al., 1996). Unfortunately, even with early orchiopexy, fertility is still reduced (Lee et al., 1996).

In both sexes and in almost all instances, hormone replacement therapy will be essential, not only for sexual function and external appearance but to prevent osteoporosis (Vered et al., 1997). Mention has been made earlier about the use of long-acting testosterone esters in situations in which there is microphallus, generally considered to be a phallus, less than 2.5 cm in extended length. Some advocate periodic use of this hormone (e.g., 2 to 3 months every 1 to 2 years until adolescence) in such individuals, because there is some evidence that good early growth portends a better sexually functional penis later. At adolescence, larger and more frequent doses of testosterone will be necessary in patients with absent or non-functional gonads. Currently available oral preparations are usually avoided because of potential hepatotoxicity. The role of transdermal testosterone remains to be defined.

Phenotypic females with absent or dysgenetic ovaries, who have an intact uterus and vagina, should be treated with cyclic oral estrogen and progesterone. However, if menses are not considered appropriate, as might be the case for hygienic reasons in severely retarded females, daily low-dose combined oral estrogen-progesterone preparations may be more useful, mainly to avoid the structural and cardiovascular complications of estrogen deficiency. In the absence of a uterus, progestins are unnecessary, and daily oral estrogens are generally used, although transdermal preparations may be substituted if compliance is a problem.

Patients whose gonadal hormone deficiency is of pituitary origin should, for practical purposes, be treated as if they have end-organ deficiency, for replacement of pituitary hormone analogues is complex and requires injection therapy. In selected circumstances, combinations of hCG and human menopausal gonadotropin (hMG) can be used to induce ovulation preparatory to natural or *in vitro* fertilization. Combined therapy is rarely successful for sustained germ cell maturation in affected males. If the hypogonadotropic hypogonadism is hypothalamic in origin, which it is most commonly, GnRH agonists have been used successfully in both sexes to induce pituitary FSH and LH secretion. This therapy is more likely to be effective if the hypogonadotropism is only partial.

Specific replacement therapy with cortisol or synthetic derivatives is essential for patients with the more severe varieties of the AG syndrome(s). Supplementation with a synthetic mineralocorticoid may be useful as well. The theoretical basis for this form of therapy is discussed elsewhere in this volume (Chapter 13). For more explicit details, the reader should consult a comprehensive textbook of endocrinology.

COUNSELING

A frank discussion of the embryology of the internal and external genitalia in lay terms often helps the family to understand how variations from the norm occur. It should include the concept of a normal double set of internal sex organs in early fetal life, and the later events that trigger expansion or regression of the various components of the dual anlage that are necessary for complete internal and external sex differentiation.

Whenever the etiology of the anomaly is known, the discussion can be expanded to clarify precisely where things went wrong. If the lesion is recognizably genetic, appropriate recurrence risk factors can be stated as well as possibilities for early diagnosis, *in utero* therapy, alternative family planning, and so forth.

The most important aspect of a counseling session is to emphasize that there should be no uncertainty in gender assignment, such that the growing child and his or her parents have no doubt about the correctness of the sex assignment.

REFERENCES

Costa E M F, Mendonca B B, Inácio Metal (1997). Management of ambiguous genitalia in pseudohermaphroditism: new perspectives on vaginal dilation. *Fertil Steril* 67:229–232.

Grumbach M M, Conte F A (1992). Disorders of sex differentiation, in Wilson J D, Foster D W (eds) *Williams Textbook of Endocrinology*, 8th ed. W B Saunders Co., Philadelphia, pp 853–951.

Kass E, Kogan S J, Manley C, et al (1996). Timing of elective surgery on the genitalia of male children with particular reference to the risks, benefits, and psychological effects of surgery and anesthesia. *Pediatrics* 97:590–594.

Lee P A, O'Leary L A, Songer N J, et al (1996). Paternity after unilateral cryptorchidism: a controlled study. *Pediatrics* 98:676–679.

Money J, Hampson J C, Hampson J L (1955). Hermaphroditism: recommendations concerning assignment of sex, change of sex, and psychologic management. *Johns Hopkins Med J* 97: 284–295.

Money J, Schwartz M, Lewis V G (1984). Adult erotosexual status and fetal hormonal masculinization and demasculinization: 46, XX congenital virilizing adrenal hyperplasia and 46, XY androgen insensitivity compared. *Psychoneuroendocrinology* 9:405–414.

Powell D M, Newman K D, Randolph J (1995) A proposed classification of vaginal anomalies and their surgical correction. *J Pediatr Surg* 30:271–275.

Shozu M, Akasofu K, Takenori T, et al (1991). A new cause of female pseudohermaphroditism: placental aromatase deficiency *J Clin Endocrinol Metab* 72:560–566.

Thomas E, Mestman J H, Henneman C, et al. (1992). Bilateral luteomas of pregnancy with virilization: a case report. *Obstet Gynecol* 39:577–584.

Vered I, Kaiserman I, Vered Sela B, et al (1997). Cross genotype sex hormone treatment in two cases of hypogonadal osteoporosis. *J Clin Endocrinol Metab* 82:576–578.

Verhoeven A T M, Mastboom J L, Van Leusden H A I M, et al. (1973) Virilization in pregnancy coexisting with an (ovarian) mucinous cystadenoma: a case report and review of virilizing ovarian tumors in pregnancy. *Obstet Gynecol Surg* 28:597–622.

III

GONADAL MALDEVELOPMENT

5

Y Chromosome Aberrations

This chapter covers gonadal maldevelopment caused by Y chromosome aberrations. We begin with a comprehensive treatment of *SRY* mutations because more is known about this testis-determining gene than any other. This is followed by a brief discussion of a rare combination: 46,XX males who are infertile and *ZFY*-negative but apparently *SRY*-positive. This combination implies that *ZFY* has a role, perhaps facultative, in achieving fully normal testis development. Finally, we deal with Yq alterations that impair spermatogenesis. Strictly speaking, the affected individuals have defective gametogenesis rather than defective testis differentiation; hence, they could also have been discussed as one form of "gamete failure" in Part V.

ALTERATIONS IN *SRY* CAUSING GONADAL DYSGENESIS

A number of causes for the occurrence of 46,XY females are described in this book (see Chapter 2 for an introduction). Such patients fall into the category of gonadal dysgenesis because they have streak gonads. Patients with streak gonads who did not have Turner syndrome were initially described by Swyer (1995), hence the appellation Swyer syndrome. However, the condition is clinically (Berkovitz et al., 1991) and genetically (see Chapters 6 and 7) heterogenous. Another designation proposed by Hoffenberg and Jackson (1957) that fits most of these patients is that of pure gonadal dysgenesis. The causal heterogeneity of patients with pure gonadal dysgenesis can be seen in the variety of their chromosomal constitutions. Among 40 patients classified as having pure gonadal dysgenesis, nine were 46,XY; 21 were 46,XX; two were 45,X/46,XX; three were 45,X/46,XY; and five had structural abnormalities of the X chromosome (Hamerton, 1971). Given the role of *SRY* in testicular development, as described in Chapter 2, mutations in *SRY* are one cause of such maldevelopment and these are reviewed here.

Clinical and Imaging Presentation.   Most cases are ascertained because of pubertal delay or primary amenorrhea. Some patients are found because of very mild manifestations of sexual ambiguity (e.g., slight clitoromegaly) (Schmitt-Ney et al., 1995); in many patients, external genitalia are infantile (e.g., Lida et al., 1994). Ultrasound examination reveals an absence of ovaries or, more often, streak gonads. The fallopian tubes and uterus are frequently described as normal or small. Gonadoblastoma is sometimes disclosed by the ultrasound examination because the presence of a Y chromosome in an intra-abdominal gonad greatly increases the risk of gonadoblastoma (see below). Some patients are found as prepubertal siblings of an older affected patient. One patient presented as premature ovarian failure (Brown, et al, 1998). Finally, as discussed previously, gonadal dysgenesis may be one finding in patients with multiple birth defects.

Laboratory Features.   Basal serum levels of follicle-simulating hormone and luteinizing hormone are usually elevated, and estrogen and androgen levels are low.

Genotyping.   A large number of *SRY* mutations have been found in these patients. These are presented in Table 5–1. Some of the mutations are compatible with the phenotype of a fertile male who can transmit the mutation to multiple XY daughters (Vilain et al., 1992; Jäger, et al, 1992), whereas other transmitted mutations seem to be the result of paternal mosaicism, including the germ line (Schmitt-Ney et al., 1995), or are indeterminate for the two possibilities (Berta et al., 1990; Hawkins et al., 1992a). Somatic mosaicism for a *SRY* mutation resulted in true hermaphroditism in one case (Braun et al., 1993; discussed in Chapter 2). As can be seen from Table 5–1, most of the point mutations are in the DNA-binding domain,—the HMG box (which also encodes a nuclear localization signal [Poulat et al., 1995]; see Chapter 2 for a discussion of the biochemistry of *SRY*). Many of the protein products of these mutated *SRY* genes have decreased DNA-binding activity (Harley and Goodfellow, 1994). Like other disorders discussed in this book (e.g. camptomelic dysplasia) (see Chapter 7), position effects also seem to occur. Thus, a deletion that has its distal termination at least 1.8 kb upstream of the *SRY* coding sequence was associated with XY sex reversal (McElreavey et al., 1992a) and a deletion 2–3 kb 3' to the coding sequence was associated with partial gonadal dysgenesis (McElreavey et al., 1996).

TABLE 5–1. Summary of *SRY* Mutations and Their Phenotypes

Mutation	Phenotype	Reference(s)
1. In HMG Box		
a. nonsense		
70 trp	XY female	Hawkins et al., 1992a; Graves et al., 1999
92 lys	XY female	Müller et al., 1992
93 gln	XY female	McElreavey et al., 1992a
107 trp	XY female	Lida et al., 1994
127 tyr	XY female	McElreavey et al., 1992b
b. missense		
60 val > leu	Fertile male + XY female	Vilain et al., 1992
62 arg > gly	XY female	Affara et al., 1993
64 met > ile	Fertile male + XY female	Berta et al., 1990
68 ile > thr	XY female	Berta et al., 1990
78 met > thr	XY female	Affara et al., 1993
90 ile > met	XY female	Hawkins et al., 1992a
91 ser > gly	XY female	Schmitt-Ney et al., 1995
95 gly > arg	XY female	Hawkins et al., 1992a
106 lys > isoleu	XY female	Hawkins et al., 1992b
109 phe > ser	XY female	Jäger et al., 1990
112 ala > thr	XY female	Zeng et al., 1993
125 pro > leu	XY female	Schmitt-Ney et al., 1995
127 tyr > cys	XY female	Poulat et al., 1994
133 arg > trp	XY female	Affara et al., 1993; Veitia et al., 1997
Mosaic 44 leu > cys	True hermaphrodite	Braun et al., 1993
c. frameshift		
108 (1 bp deletion)	XY female	Hawkins et al., 1992b
122 (4 bp deletion)	XY female	Jäger et al., 1990
2. Other Coding Region		
2 gln > stop	XY female with some ovarian function	Brown et al., 1998
12 tyr > stop	XY female	Veitia et al., 1997
162 leu > stop	XY female	Tajima et al., 1994
3. Possible Control Regions		
1 out of 49 studied for 2kb 5'	fertile male + XY female	Kwok et al., 1996
4. More Distant		
≤ 1.8 kb upstream to ≥ 30 kb upstream	XY female	McElreavey et al., 1992a
2–3 kb downstream	XY female	McElreavey et al., 1996

Management.   For most of the XY females who are found from a workup for amenorrhea, genetic counseling about the cause and possible treatment of their infertility will be the major need. As in Turner syndrome, oocyte donation and hormone replacement can lead to successful pregnancies (Frydman et al., 1988; Sauer et al., 1989; Bianco et al., 1992; Kan et al., 1997). In addition, because the Y-chromosomal gene responsible for the high risk of malignancy in Y-containing gonadal cells maintained at 37°C maps to Yq (Tsuchiya et al., 1995), surgical removal of the streak gonads is indicated. As the mutations have sometimes been familial, either due to variable penetrance or mosaicism, a careful search for other affected members of the family is indicated.

Discussion.   Because there are many causes of 46,XY sex reversal, some guidelines as to when it is useful to search for mutations in *SRY* would be useful. Hawkins and colleagues (1992b) first suggested that the prevalence of *SRY* mutations in XY females with complete gonadal dysgenesis is greater than in those with partial gonadal dysgenesis. This observation was extended by Fellous's group (Vilain et al., 1993), who pointed out that the streak gonads of patients with *SRY* mutations show no evidence of beginning testicular differentiation—that is, no *rete*, which would be indicative of early, partial testicular development. Rather, exclusively ovarian-like stroma was seen in these cases. In contrast, patients with streak gonads that contained either tubules or a *rete* structure did not have a mutated *SRY* gene. This suggests that many cases of 46,XY gonadal dysgenesis that started out on the male differentiation pathway in the presence of a normal *SRY* were diverted from it because of other genetic or environmental causes. However, in the absence of a functional *SRY*, this differentiation pathway did not even start. In our experience, female dysmorphic patients in whom 46,XY sex reversal is a chance finding have not had *SRY* mutations (Graves et al., 1999). Such patients are likely to have alterations in the sex differentiation pathway related to the causes of the dysmorphism.

REFERENCES

Affara N A, Chalmers I J, Ferguson-Smith M A (1993). Analysis of the *SRY* gene in 22 sex-reversed XY females identifies four new point mutations in the conserved DNA binding domain. *Hum Mol Genet* 2:785–789.

Berkovitz G D, Fechner P Y, Zacur H W, Rock J A, Snyder H M, Migeon C F, Perlman E J (1991). Clinical and pathologic spectrum of 46,XY gonadal dysgenesis: its relevance to the understanding of sex differentiation *Medicine* 70:375–383.

Berta P, Hawkins J R, Sinclair A H, Taylor A, Griffiths B L, Goodfellow P N, Fellous M (1990). Genetic evidence equating *SRY* and the testis-determining factor. *Nature* 348:448–450.

Bianco S, Agrifoglio V, Mannino F, Cefalu E, Cittalini E (1992). Successful pregnancy in a pure gonadal dysgenesis with karyotype 46,XY patient (Swyer's syndrome) following oocyte donation and hormonal therapy. *Acta Eur Fertil* 23:37–38.

Braun A, Kammerer S, Cleve H, Lohrs U, Schwarz H-P, Kuhnle U (1993). True hermaphroditism in a 46,XY individual, caused by a postzygotic somatic point mutation in the male gonadal sex-determining locus (*SRY*): molecular genetics and histological findings in a sporadic case. *Am J Hum Genet* 52:578–585.

Brown S, Yu C C, Lanzano P, Heller D, Thomas L, Warburton D, Kitajewski J, Stadtmauer L (1998). A *de novo* mutation (Gln2stop) at the 5' end of the SRY gene leads to sex reversal with partial ovarian function. *Am J Hum Genet* 62:189–192.

Frydman R, Parneix I, Fries N, Testart J, Raymond J P, Bouchard P (1998). Pregnancy in 46 XY patient. *Fertil Steril* 50:813–814.

Graves P E, Erickson R P, Lopez M L, Mendez J P, Kofman-Alfaro S, Davis D, Speer I E (1999). Letter to the Editor: Ascertainment and mutation of SRY in nine patients. *Am J Med Genet*, in press.

Hamerton J H (1971). In *Human Cytogenetics*, Vol. 2, Clinical Cytogenetics, Academic Press, New York.

Harley V R, Goodfellow P N (1994). The biochemical role of *SRY* in sex determination. *Mol Reprod Dev* 39:184–193.

Hawkins J R, Taylor A, Berta P, Levilliers J, Van der Auwera B, Goodfellow P N (1992a). Mutational analysis of *SRY*: nonsense and missense mutations in XY sex reversal. *Hum Genet* 88:471–475.

Hawkins J R, Taylor A, Goodfellow P N, Migeon C J, Smith K D, Berkovitz G D (1992b). Evidence for increased prevalence of *SRY* mutations in XY females with complete rather than partial gonadal dysgenesis. *Am J Hum Genet* 51:979–984.

Hoffenberg R, Jackson W P U (1957). Gonadal dysgenesis: modern concepts. *Br Med J* 2:1457–1462.

Jäger R J, Anvret M, Hall K. Scherer G (1990). A human XY female with a frame shift mutation in the candidate testis-determining gene *SRY*. *Nature* 348:452–454.

Jäger R J, Harley V R, Pfeiffer R A, Goodfellow P N, Scherer G (1992). A familial mutation in the testis-determining gene *SRY* shared by both sexes. *Hum Genet* 90:350–352.

Kan A K S, Abdalla H I, Oskarsson T. (1997). Case report: two successful pregnancies in a 46,XY patient. *Hum Reprod* 12:1434–1435.

Kwok C, Tyler-Smith C, Mendonca B B, Hughes I, Berkovitz G D, Goodfellow P N, Hawkins J R (1996). Mutation analysis of the 2 kb 5' to *SRY* in XY females and XY intersex subjects. *J Med Genet* 33:465–468.

Lida T, Nakahori Y, Komaki R, Mori E, Hayashi N. Tsutsumi O, Taketani Y, Nakagome Y (1994). A novel nonsense mutation in the HMG box of the *SRY* gene in a patient with XY sex reversal. *Hum Mol Genet* 3:1437–1438.

McElreavey K, Vilain E, Abbas N, Costa J-M, Souleyreau N, Kucheria K, Boucekkine C, Thibaud E, Brauner R, Flamant F, Fellous M (1992a). XY sex reversal associated with a deletion 5' to the *SRY* "HMG box" in the testis-determining region. *Proc Natl Acad Sci USA* 89:11016–11020.

McElreavey K D, Vilain E, Boucekkine C, Vidaud M, Jaubert F, Richaud F, Fellous M (1992b). Short communication: XY sex reversal associated with a nonsense mutation in *SRY*. *Genomics* 13:838–840.

McElreavey K D, Vilain E, Barbaux S, Fuqua J S, Fechner P Y. Souleyreau N, Doco-Fenzy M, Gabriel R, Quereux C, Fellous M, Berkovitz G D (1996). Loss of sequences 3' to the testis-determining gene, *SRY*, including the Y pseudoautosomal boundary associated with partial testicular determination. *Proc Natl Acad Sci USA* 93:8590–8594.

Müller J, Schwartz M, Skakkebaek N (1992). Analysis of the sex-determining region of the Y chromosome (*SRY*) in sex reversed patients: point-mutation in *SRY* causing sex-reversion in a 46,XY female. *J Clin Endocrinol Metab* 75:331–333.

Poulat F, Girard F, Chevron M-P, Gozé C, Rebillard X, Calas B, Lamb N, Berta P (1995). Nuclear localization of the testis determining gene product *SRY*. *J Cell Biol* 128:737–748.

Poulat F, Soullier S, Gozé C, Heitz F, Calas B, Berta P (1994). Description and functional implications of a novel mutation in the sex-determining gene *SRY*. *Hum Mutat* 3:200–204.

Sauer M V, Lobo R A, Paulson P J (1989). Successful twin pregnancy after embryo donation to a patient with XY gonadal dysgenesis. *Am J Obstet Gynecol* 161:380–381.

Schmitt-Ney M, Thiele H, Kaltwaber P, Bardoni B, Cisternino M, Scherer G (1995). Two novel missense mutations reducing DNA binding identified in XY females and their mosaic fathers. *Am J Hum Genet*: 56:862–869.

Swyer G I M (1955). Male pseudohermaphroditism: a hitherto undescribed form. *Br Med J* 2: 709–712.

Tajima T, Nakae J, Shinohara N, Fujieda K (1994). A novel mutation localized in the 3' non-HMG box region of the *SRY* gene in 46,XY gonadal dysgenesis. *Hum Mol Genet*: 3:1187–1189.

Tsuchiya K, Reijo R, Page D C, Disteche C M (1995). Gonadoblastoma: molecular definition of the susceptibility region on the Y chromosome. *Am J Hum Genet* 57:1400–1407.

Veitia R, Ion A, Barbaux S, Jobling M A, Souleyreau N, Ennis K, Ostrer H, Tosi M, Meo T, Chibani J, Fellous M, McElreavey K (1997). Mutations and sequence variants in the testis-determining region of the Y chromosome in individuals with a 46,XY female phenotype. *Hum Genet* 99:648–652.

Vilain E, McElreavey K, Jaubert F, Raymond J-P, Richaud F, Fellous M (1992). Familial case with sequence variant in the testis-determining region associated with two sex phenotypes. *Am J Hum Genet* 50:1008–1011.

Vilain E, Jaubert F, Fellous M, McElreavey K (1993). Pathology of 46,XY pure gonadal dysgenesis: absence of testis differentiation associated with mutations in the testis-determining factor. *Differentiation* 52:151–159.

Zeng Y, Ren Z, Zhang M, Huang Y, Zeng F, Huang S (1993). A new de novo mutation (A113T) in HMG box of the *SRY* gene leads to XY gonadal dysgenesis. *J Med Genet* 30: 655–657.

SRY⁺, *ZFY*⁻ INDIVIDUALS

In the initial report proposing *ZFY* as a candidate gene for the testis-determining factor (*TDF*), one 46,XX male's Y complement did not include this gene (Page et al., 1987). The phenotype of that patient was not provided. Verga and Erickson (1989) soon reported another 46,XX male who was *ZFY*-negative. The finding of more such males was important in rejecting *ZFY* as *TDF* and the cloning of *SRY* as the definitive testis-determining factor gene (see Chapter 2). Although rare, these patients indicate a possible role of *ZFY* in several aspects of sex differentiation.

Clinical and Imaging Presentation.   As previously described by Palmer and colleagues (1989), the phenotypes in four 46,XX*SRY*⁺*ZFY*⁻ males ranged from a "normal male" (with cryptorchidism) to one patient with a uterus. The patient with the uterus had "posterior" hypospadias (the degree of severity was not indicated; was it perineoscrotal?); another two males had "anterior" hypospadias (distal), one of whom also had a vaginal pouch. In addition, the patient with the uterus also had bilateral ovotestis. Nonetheless, even this patient (who would otherwise fit the phenotype of 46,XX true hermaphroditism) had Y-positive sequences from near the pseudoautosomal boundary, as did the other three patients. These Y sequences were eventually shown to include *SRY*. Another patient with normal male external genitalia and no cryptorchidism was, nonetheless, short and infertile (López et al., 1995). Thus, a minimal phenotype may be infertility (expected with the loss of Y fertility genes, see Chapter 5), although the short stature in this last case raises the question of other possible birth defects.

Laboratory Studies.   For one subject, testosterone levels were low (López et al., 1995). This individual had azoospermia, hyperplasia of tubules, and absence of germ cells. In the four males described by Palmer and colleagues (1989), the testicular biopsies revealed Leydig cells and Sertoli cells, but no spermatogonia.

Genotyping.   These patients are characterized as *SRY*-positive, *ZFY*-negative although full *SRY* sequencing has not yet been performed. It is nonetheless probable that the various departures from a normal male phenotype are caused by the absence of ZFY (see Chapter 2 for positive data on role of ZFY in sexual differentiation).

Management. Surgical repair of hypospadias and cryptorchidism should be performed. Counseling is indicated for the cause of infertility.

Discussion. As discussed in Chapter 2, ZFY is widely expressed, although its expression pattern overlaps that of the very similar gene product, ZFX. The expression of ZFY in the epididymis may help to account for its development in the absence of testosterone (Chapter 13) or the androgen receptor (Chapter 2). The extreme lack of evolutionary variation in the gene (Burrows and Ryder, 1997) also argues for a functional role for ZFY. One such role may be as a gene involved in height attainment (Chapter 6) and another may be in the differentiation of secondary sexual structures. The SRY^+, ZFY^- patients already described support a role for ZFY in sex-specific development. The discovery of more patients will better help to delineate this role.

REFERENCES

Burrows W, Ryder O A (1997). Y-chromosome variation in great apes. *Nature* 385:125–126.

López M, Torres L, Mendéz J P, Cervantes A, Perez-Palacios G, Erickson R P, Alfaro G, Kofman-Alfaro S (1995). Clinical traits and molecular findings in 46,XX males. *Clin Genet* 48:29–34.

Page D C, Mosher R, Simpson E M, Fisher E M C, Mardon G, Pollack J, McGillivray B, de la Chapelle A, Brown L G (1987) The sex-determining region of the human Y chromosome encodes a finger protein. *Cell* 51:1091–1104.

Palmer M S, Sinclair A H, Berta P, Ellis N A, Goodfellow P N, Abbas N E, Fellous M (1989). Genetic evidence that ZFY is not the testis-determining factor. *Nature* 342:937–939.

Verga V, Erickson R P (1989). An extended long-range restriction map of the human sex-determining region on Yp, including ZFY, finds marked homology on Xp and no detectable Y sequences in an XX male. *Am J Hum Genet* 44:756–765.

AZOOSPERMIA AND YQ ALTERATIONS

Infertility is an anguishing problem that affects up to 17% of couples. Male infertility is frequently the result of a lack of spermatozoa, azoospermia or severe oligospermia, which frequently has a genetic cause. The first report that associated Yq deletions with azoospermia was by Tiepolo and Zuffardi in 1976. Because of the findings of microscopic deletions of Yq in six men with azoospermia, they proposed that an *Azoospermia Factor* mapping to this region was required for spermatogenesis (Tiepolo and Zuffardi, 1976). Recent work has identified candidate genes in this region (see below). Although affected persons do not show gonadal maldevelopment, in the sense of showing alterations of somatic or secondary sexual structures, their gonads are very maldeveloped in the sense of not successfully making the mature product of the gonad.

Clinical and Imaging Presentation. Men with Yq alterations are found through infertility clinics when a standard semen analysis discloses azoospermia or severe oligospermia. The testes may sometimes be small but also can be of normal size.

Laboratory Features.   High-resolution karyotype analyses frequently disclose Yq deletions, although the deletions are sometimes submicroscopic. Results of hormonal studies are usually normal, although FSH is sometimes elevated (Pryor et al., 1997).

Genotyping.   The original findings of Tiepolo and Zuffardi (1976) were confirmed by further molecular analyses in a series of deletion or translocation Yq patients (Koenig et al., 1985; Vergnaud et al., 1986; Affara et al., 1986). As more probes were defined on the Y, and more patients were collected, the region became more finely delimited (Disteche et al., 1986; Gal et al., 1987; Andersson et al., 1988). Bardoni and colleagues. (1991) studied 23 persons bearing structural abnormalities in the long arm of the Y chromosome and mapped *AZF* to a specific interval within Yq11.23.

Further work has defined three subregions: AZF*a* (subinterval 5C), *AZFb* (distal 5 and proximal 6 subintervals) and *AZFc* (subinterval 6D to heterochromatin) (Vogt et al., 1996). The first candidate gene was cloned from the *AZFb* region. Ma and colleagues (1992) used 30 DNA probes in a series of 21 patients: they found two non-overlapping deletions in azoospermic men. They then cloned a gene from the DNA corresponding to the more distal of the two deletions (Ma et al., 1993) and suggested it as a candidate for *AZF*. The gene belongs to a family that includes a minimum of three members; it was named *YRRM* (*Y* RNA *r*ecognition *m*otif) when the DNA sequence revealed a motif shared by proteins that bind to RNA. The gene family has been renamed the *RBM* (RNA-*b*inding *m*otif) family and *RBM-1* has been extensively characterized (Najmabadi et al., 1996). The argument that this was a good candidate gene for *AZF* depended on its mapping to a region that had been deleted in three patients with azoospermia or severe oligospermia, its testis-specificity and conserved sequence, and finding that all or part of one of these genes was contained within microdeletions of two oligospermic patients in whom molecular defects had not previously been found (Ma et al., 1993). An antibody directed to the RBM-unique repeats has been used on testicular sections taken from normal subjects and men with a variety of microdeletions to show that the members of this multigene family located in *AZFb* are expressed (Elliott et al., 1997). The conservation and amplification of the repeats on the marsupial Y also argues for a primal role in mammalian spermatogenesis (Delbridge et al., 1997). Studies by other groups (Kobayashi et al., 1994) found *RBM-1* to be involved only in three of 10 men with microdeletions and azoospermia or severe oligospermia, and the investigators argued that a second locus must be required for spermatogenesis. One group (Nakahori et al., 1994) also found that *RBM-2* is commonly absent in fertile Japanese males.

A second candidate gene for *AZF* was found (Reijo et al., 1995) in the *AZFc* region. The researchers studied a collection of 12 overlapping deletions in azoospermic or oligospermic males that did not include *RBM* genes. From this region, they cloned a gene, *DAZ* (*D*eleted in *AZ*oospermia), that is transcribed in the adult testis and also appears to encode an RNA-binding protein (Reijo et al., 1995). The gene has an interesting pattern of expression: it apparently is expressed in spermatocytes and yet is limited to testis—most genes with spermatocytic expression previously identified have not been limited to the testis (Reijo et al., 1996). The highly homologous mouse gene with similar expression patterns (although including ovary) is autosomal rather than Y-linked (Cooke et al., 1996) and there is a human homologue, *DAZLA* (Seboun et al., 1997). It appears that the Y copy has been recruited from the autosome and modified and amplified (Saxena et al., 1997). The *DAZ* homologous, Y-chromosomal gene *SPGY* also has an autosomal copy, which is only expressed in the testis (Shan et al., 1996; Yen et al., 1996). This gene shows homology to the *Drosophila* gene *boule* which is also a spermatogenic gene, a second example (the chromosome 9/C. *elegans DMT1* being the other) of marked evolutionary conservation of male sexual differentiation genes. To date, no point mutations in *DAZ* or *RBM* have been identified as a cause of azoospermia or oligospermia. This group of Y-chromosomal genes encoding RNA-binding proteins that may have a role in spermatogenesis has recently been reviewed (Cooke and Elliott, 1997).

A candidate spermatogenesis gene has been identified in the *AZFa* interval. The homologue of the *Drosophila* developmental gene *fat facets (faf)* is located on the sex chromosomes (Jones et al., 1996). There is an X-linked copy (*DFFX*) mapping to Xp11.4, which escapes X-inactivation, and related sequences (*DFFRY*) have been mapped to Yq11.2. The murine homologue of this gene (*Dffry*) is expressed exclusively in the testes and maps to the *Sxr*[b] deletion interval that is associated with an early block of spermatogenesis (Brown et al., 1998). Analysis of tissue from three azoospermic male patients has shown that *DFFRY* is deleted from their Y chromosomes (Brown et al., 1998). The *faf* gene, and its homologues, are members of a family of deubiquitinating genes whose products remove ubiquitin from protein-ubiquitin conjugates. The possible importance of the *AZFa* regions is indicated by the deletion of *DAZ* or *YRRM* in only 6 of 11 patients with Y deletions and azoospermia or severe oligoospermia (Foresta et al., 1997). Thus, the three regions on Yq whose deletions are associated with infertility appear to contain spermatogenesis genes of diverse functions: RNA-binding proteins and an enzyme involved in the control of protein degradation. Amplification, diversification and rearrangement of these Y gene families has been frequent during the evolution of primates (Gläser et al., 1998).

Management.   The common clinical problem present is infertility due to azoospermia or severe oligospermia, although Y deletions can be associated with normospermia—idiopathic infertility (Pryor et al., 1997). If there is oligospermia, single sperm can be used for egg injection. This procedure has a high level of success and is currently popular with *in vitro* fertilization programs (Schlegel and Girardi, 1997). However, one will be perpetuating the genetic defect when that sperm carries the deleted Y chromosome and genetic counselling should precede such procedures (In't Veld et al., 1997). Spermatids can be recovered from testicular biopsies in azoospermic men and fused with eggs for successful fertilization, as has been demonstrated in mice (Brinster and Zimmermann, 1994) and in men with Klinefelter Syndrome (Palermo et al., 1998).

Discussion.   An interesting feature of the deletions in *DAZ* has been the great phenotypic variability. The patients' testicular biopsies have shown morphology

ranging from complete absence of germ cells to evidence of much greater comple-
tion of spermatogenesis—for example, spermatogenic arrest with occasional production of condensed spermatids (Reijo et al., 1995). The cause of this clinical variation is unknown but may be the result of variation in the size of deletions, in
modifying genes, or in variable numbers of copies of *YRRM* or *DAZ*. A recent,
thorough study of 200 infertile men found 7% with deletions but only 10 of the 14
deletions were etiologically related to the infertility, because four were also found
in fertile fathers (Pryor et al., 1997). However, the enlargement of a deletion, with
consequent oligospermia, during transmission from father to son has been found
(Stuppia et al., 1996). In the study of Pryor and colleagues (1997), more deletions
were found for *YRRM* than for *DAZ*, and there was a poor correlation of deletion
location with specific signs.

REFERENCES

Affara N A, Florentin L, Morrison N, Kwok K, Mitchell M, Cook A, Jamieson D, Glasgow
   L, Meredith L, Boyd E, Ferguson-Smith M A (1986). Regional assignment of Y-linked
   DNA probes by deletion mapping and their homology with X-chromosome and autoso-
   mal sequences. *Nucleic Acids Res* 14:5353–5373.
Andersson M, Page D C, Pettay D, Subrt I, Turleau C, de Grouchy J, de la Chapelle A (1988).
   Y-autosome translocations and mosaicism in the aetiology of 45, X maleness: assignment
   of fertility factor to distal Yq11. *Hum Genet* 79:2–7.
Bardoni B, Zuffardi O, Guioli S, Ballabio A, Simi P, Cavalli P, Grimoldi M G, Fraccaro M,
   Camerino G (1991). A deletion map of the human Yq11 region: implications for the ev-
   olution of the Y chromosome and tentative mapping of a locus involved in spermatogenesis. *Genomics* 11:443–451.
Brinster R L, Zimmermann J W (1994). Spermatogenesis following male germ cell transplantation. *Proc Natl Acad Sci USA* 91:11298–11302.
Brown G M, Furlong R A, Sargent C A, Erickson, R P, Longepied G, Mitchell M, Jones M H,
   Hargreave T B, Cooke H J, Affara N A (1998). Deletion of the *DFFRY* gene in patients
   with the *AZFa* phenotype and of the murine homologue (*Dffry*) in XO *Sxr*^b mice correlated
   with an early failure of spermatogenesis and infertility. *Hum Mol Genet.* 7:97–107.
Cooke H J, Elliott D J (1997). RNA-binding proteins and human male infertility. *Trends Genet*
   13:87–89.
Cooke H J, Lee M, Kerr S, Ruggiu M (1996). A murine homologue of the human *DAZ* gene
   is autosomal and expressed only in male and female gonads. *Hum Mol Genet* 5:513–516.
Delbridge M L, Harry J L, Toder R, O'Neill R J W, Ma K, Chandley A C, Graves J A M (1997).
   A human candidate spermatogenesis gene, *RBM1*, is conserved and amplified on the
   marsupial Y chromosome. *Nat Genet* 15:131–136.
Disteche C M, Brown L, Saal H, Friedman C, Thuline H C, Hoar D I, Pagon R A, Page D C
   (1986). Molecular detection of a translocation (Y;15) in a 45, X male. *Hum Genet* 74:372–
   377.
Elliott D J, Millar M R, Oghene K, Ross A, Kiesewetter F, Pryor J, McIntyre M, Hargreave
   T B, Saunders P T K, Vogt P H, Chandley A C, Cooke H (1987). Expression of RBM in the
   nuclei of human germ cells is dependent on a critical region of the Y chromosome long
   arm. *Proc Natl Acad Sci USA* 94:3848–3853.
Foresta C, Ferlin A, Garolla A, Rossato M, Barbaux S, De Bortoli A (1997). Y-chromosome
   deletions in idiopathic severe testiculopathies. *J Clin Endocrinol Metab* 82:1075–1080.
Gal A, Weber B, Neri G, Serra A, Muller U, Schempp W, Page D C (1987). A 45, X male with
   Y-specific DNA translocated onto chromosome 15. *Am J Hum Genet* 40:477–488.
Gläser B, Grützner F, Willmann U, Stanyon R, Arnold N, Taylor K, Rietschel W, Zeitler S,
   Toder R, Schempp W (1998). Simian Y chromosomes: species-specific rearrangements of
   DAZ, *RBM*, and *TSPY* versus contiguity of PAR and *SRY*. *Mamm Genome* 9:226–231.

In't Veld P A, Halley D J J, van Hemel J O, Niermeijer M F, Dohle G, Weber RFA (1997). Genetic counselling before intracytoplasmic sperm injection. *Lancet* 350:490–493.

Jones M H, Furlong R A, Burkin H, Chalmers I J, Brown G M, Khwaja O, Affara N A (1996). The *Drosophila* developmental gene fat facets has a human homologue in Xp11.4 which escapes X-inactivation and has related sequences on Yq11.2 *Hum Mol Genet* 5:1693–1702.

Kobayashi K, Mizuno K, Hida A, Komaki R, Tomita K, Matsushita I, Namiki M, Iwamoto T, Tamura S, Minowada S, Nakahori Y, Nakagome Y (1994). PCR analysis of the Y chromosome long arm in azoospermic patients: evidence for a second locus required for spermatogenesis. *Hum Mol Genet* 3:1965–1967.

Koenig M, Moisan J P, Heilig R, Mandel J L (1985). Homologies between X and Y chromosomes detected by DNA probes: localization and evolution. *Nucleic Acids Res* 13:5485–5501.

Ma K, Inglis J D, Sharkey A, Bickmore W A, Hill R E, Prosser E J, Speed R M, Thomson E J, Jobling M, Taylor K, Wolfe J, Cooke H J, Hargreave T B, Chandley A C (1993). A Y-chromosome gene family with RNA-binding protein homology: candidates for the azoospermia factor *AZF* controlling human spermatogenesis. *Cell* 75:1287–1295.

Ma K, Sharkey A, Kirsch S, Vogt P, Keil R, Hargreave T B, McBeath S, Chandley A C (1992). Towards the molecular localisation of the *AZF* locus: mapping of microdeletions in azoospermic men within 14 subintervals of interval 6 of the human Y chromosome. *Hum Mol Genet* 1:29–33.

Najmabadi H, Chai N, Kapali A, Subbarao M N, Bhasin D, Woodhouse E, Yen P, Bhasin S (1996). Genomic structure of a Y-specific ribonucleic acid binding motif-containing gene: a putative candidate for a subset of male infertility. *J Clin Endocrinol Metab* 81:2159–2164.

Nakahori Y, Kobayashi K, Komaki R, Matsushita I, Nakagome Y (1994). A locus of the candidate gene family for azoospermia factor (*YRRM2*) is polymorphic with a null allele in Japanese males. *Hum Mol Genet* 3: 1709.

Palermo G D, Schlegel P N, Sills E S, Veeck L L, Zaninovic N, Menendez S, Rosenwaks Z (1998). Births after intracytoplasmic injection of sperm obtained by testicular extraction from men with nonmosaic Klinefelter's syndrome. *N Engl J Med* 338:588–590.

Pryor J L, Kent-First M, Muallem A, Van Bergen A H, Nolton W E, Meisner L, Roberts K P (1997). Microdeletions in the Y chromosome of infertile men. *N Engl J Med* 336:534–539.

Reijo R, Lee T-Y, Alagappan R, Brown L G, Rosenberg M, Rozen S, Jaffe T, Straus D, Hovatta O, de la Chapelle A, Silber S, Page D C (1995). Diverse spermatogenic defects in humans caused by Y chromosome deletions encompassing a novel RNA-binding protein gene. *Nat Genet* 10:383–393.

Reijo R, Seligman J, Dinulos M D, Jaffe T, Brown L G, Disteche C M, Page D C (1996). Mouse autosomal homolog of *DAZ*, a candidate male sterility gene in humans, is expressed in male germ cells before and after puberty. *Genomics* 35:346–352.

Saxena R, Brown L G, Hawkins T, Alagappan R K, Skaletsky H, Reeve M P, Reijo R, Rozen S, Dinulos M B, Disteche C M, Page D C (1996). The *DAZ* gene cluster on the human Y chromosome arose from an autosomal gene that was transposed, repeatedly amplified and pruned. *Nat Genet* 14:292–299.

Schlegel P N, Girardi S K (1997). *In vitro* fertilization for male factor infertility. *J Clin Endocrinol Metab* 82:701–716.

Seboun E, Barbaux S, Bourgeron T, Nishi S, Algonik A, Egashira M, Nikkawa N, Bishop C, Fellous M, McElreavey K, Kasahara M (1997). Gene sequence, localization, and evolutionary conservation of *DAZLA*, a candidate male sterility gene. *Genomics* 41:227–235.

Shan Z, Hirschmann P, Seebacher T, Edelmann A, Jauch A, Morrell J, Urbitsch P, Vogt P H (1996). A *SPGY* copy homologous to the mouse gene *Dazzla* and the Drosophila gene *boule* is autosomal and expressed only in the human male gonad. *Hum Mol Genet* 5:2005–2011.

Stuppia L, Calabrese G, Franchi P G, Mingarelli R, Gatta V, Palka G, Dallapiccola B (1996). Widening of a Y-chromosome interval-6 deletion transmitted from a father to his infertile son accounts for an oligozoospermic critical region distal to the *RBM*1 and *DAZ* genes. *Am J Hum Genet* 59:1393–1395.

Tiepolo L, Zuffardi O (1976). Localization of factors controlling spermatogenesis in the non-fluorescent portion of the human Y-chromosome long arm. *Hum Genet* 34:119–124.

Vergnaud G, Page D C, Simmler M C, Brown L, Rouyer F, Noel B, Botstein D, de la Chapelle A, Weissenbach J (1986). A deletion map of the human Y chromosome based on DNA hybridization. *Am J Hum Genet* 38:109–124.

Vogt P H, Edelmann A, Kirsch S, Henegariu O. Hirschmann P, Kiesewetter F, Kohn F M, Schill W B, Farah S, Ramos C, Hartmann M, Hartschuh W, Meschede D, Behre H M, Castel A, Nieschlag E, Weidner W, Grone H J, Jung A, Engel W, Haidl G (1996). Human Y chromosome azoospermia factors (*AZF*) mapped to different subregions in Yq11. *Hum Mol Genet* 5:933–343.

Yen P H, Chai N N, Salido E C (1996). The human autosomal gene, *DAZLA*: testis specificity and a candidate for male infertility. *Hum Mol Genet* 5:2013–2017.

6

X Chromosome Aberrations

In this chapter we consider gonadal maldevelopment caused by X-chromosome aberrations. As in Chapter 5, "gonadal maldevelopment" is defined broadly so that it includes defective spermatogenesis due to an extra X chromosome in XXY males and gonadal dysgenesis due to accelerated oocyte attrition in XO females. These two conditions, and XX/XY mosaics, are discussed under the heading, "Genomic Mutations"—an abnormal number of whole X chromosomes. This is followed by a section on gonadal maldevelopment due to abnormality in parts of an X chromosome, under the heading "Chromosomal Mutations." Next we discuss the consequences of X chromosomes that bear a *SRY*-containing portion of the Y chromosome. Finally, we treat a prototypic example of gonadal maldevelopment due to mutation of a single X-linked gene.

Genomic Mutations

Turner Syndrome

The syndrome associated with a 45,X karyotype is generally named after Henry Hubert Turner, based on his 1938 description of seven quite uniform cases (Turner, 1938), although Ullrich gave a clear description of a case marked by congenital lymphedema nine years earlier (Ullrich, 1930). The Turner syndrome phenotype is now a well-recognized identity of female gonadal failure and maldevelopment, with variations known to be caused by several different chromosomal constitutions [e.g., 46X,r(X)] (Van Dyke et al., 1992); our focus will be on the gonadal abnormalities. Although in Turner syndrome the ovaries are frequently considered "dysgenetic," their condition is really the result of fetal/neonatal degeneration, as emphasized by Opitz and Pallister (1979). And even though 98% of conceptuses with the 45,X karyotype die *in utero*, it remains one of the more common causes of female gonadal failure and maldevelopment.

Clinical and Imaging Presentations.   Short stature, absent secondary sex characteristics, and primary amenorrhea are the most constant features, but facial dysmorphism consisting of micrognathia, webbed neck, low posterior hairline, and posteriorly rotated ears is frequently found, as reviewed in Grumbach and Conte (1992). Congenital heart defects and great vessel disease are present in about 55% of patients; left-sided defects (e.g., coarctation of the aorta) are the most common abnormalities. Renal structural anomalies are found in 60%, but these do not usually have clinical consequences. Lymphedema, especially of the posterior neck, hands, and feet, is common at birth but decreases during childhood. The *in utero* lymphedema may be involved in the pathogenesis of skeletal, cardiac, and renal defects (Ogata and Matsuo, 1995). The lymphedema may recur when estrogen therapy is begun and lymphangiectasia can occur in a variety of locations. Autoimmune disorders, such as Hashimoto's lymphocytic thyroiditis, ulcerative colitis, Crohn's disease, and diabetes mellitus, have an increased frequency. Imaging studies reveal the cardiovascular and renal abnormalities when they are present. Notably, pelvic ultrasound does not always disclose a "streak" gonad—findings in one third of cases range from small ovaries, sometimes containing minute cysts, to ovaries indistinguishable from those normal for patient age (Massarano et al., 1989). Although primary amenorrhea due to ovarian dysgenesis is considered a hallmark, patients with marked somatic features of Turner syndrome caused by structural X-chromosomal changes (see below) may be fertile (Fryns et al., 1982; Fitzgerald et al., 1984; Fryns et al., 1988; Blumenthal and Allanson, 1997).

Particular cognitive problems, especially visuospatial (Rovet and Netley, 1980), cause patients to achieve lower performance IQ scores than verbal IQ scores (Bender et al., 1993). Performance may improve with age (Waber, 1979; Swillen and Fryns, 1996) and be related to increased levels of sex steroids, the absence of which also affects spatial ability in men (Hier and Crowley, 1982).

Laboratory Studies.   Ovarian endocrine function is deficient and serum gonadotropin levels are usually markedly elevated. Low serum T_4 and elevated TSH will be found if autoimmune hypothyroidism develops. Karyotype is 45,X or one of its variants (see below).

Genotyping.   About 65% of patients are 45,X; 20% have structural abnormalities of X; and at least 20% are mosaic (see below), including 45,X/46,XY (usually about 5% of the total; reviewed in Grumbach and Conte, 1992). If Xp is absent, short stature is prominent, and ovarian dysgenesis is seen in only about two thirds of the patients. The variation may occur among individuals within a family who have the same deletion (Zinn et al., 1997). If Xq is lost, a smaller percentage of patients are short but nearly 100% have ovarian dysgenesis, unisomy for Xq13-q26 being particularly critical (Cunniff et al., 1991; see Chromosomal Mutations, below), although a recent study of 14 partial Xq monosomies found no correlation between the size of the deletion and gonadal dysfunction (Maraschio et al., 1996). X isochromosome Xq (XiXq) patients are also profoundly sterile, which supports the notion that the degree of X-chromosomal nonpairing may strongly influence oocyte failure (Ogata and Matsuo, 1995). Patients with 46,X r(X) are usually mentally retarded (Van Dyke et al., 1991); this seems to reflect partial functional disomy due to impaired inactivation of this second X (Migeon et al., 1994).

X-chromosomal polymorphisms have been used to study the parental origin of the single X chromosome (Hassold et al., 1985). Although one report suggested a strong tendency for it to be maternal (Loughlin et al., 1991), other studies have found parental ratios consistent with the expected proportion for equal parental meiotic or mitotic nondisjunction products, taking into account the inviability of 45,Y (Cockwell et al., 1991; Mathur et al., 1991). Parental age does not affect parental origin of the X chromosome (Loughlin et al., 1991; Mathur et al., 1991), and no clinical differences can be related to parental origin of the single X (Mathur et al., 1991). Differences in imprinting of X^p and X^m are known to affect triplo-X, triploid fetuses and could differentially affect Turner fetuses, depending on the parental source of the X (Epstein, 1990); however, the parental X origin ratio is identical in aborted and liveborn 45,X individuals (Jacobs et al., 1992). The parental source of the X does affect cognitive function, however; patients with a maternal X have significant deficiencies in social abilities and verbal IQ (Skuse et al., 1997). Mother/daughter pairs of "classic" Turner syndrome with mosaicism (Ayuso et al., 1984; Verschraegen-Spae et al., 1992) or partial Turner syndrome, with alterations not eliminating fertility (Fitzgerald et al., 1984; Massa et al., 1992; Aller et al., 1995), can occur. Another mechanism that can lead to familial Turner syndrome is an X-autosome translocation. In the balanced carrier, there is a strong selection pressure among the cells of the early embryo for the intact X to be inactivated such that inactivation has not spread into the autosomal components. However, in an offspring with an unbalanced karyotype, selective inactivation of the abnormal X with spreading into otherwise trisomic autosomal material may be selected and lead to functional monosomy X. In one family, three generations were affected by Turner syndrome because of an X;1 translocation (Leichtman et al., 1978).

Mosaicism with 46,XY or 46,XX lines is much discussed in Turner syndrome—the former because of the risk of gonadoblastoma (see Chapter 6 for a discussion of this risk), the latter because of its implications for fertility and for survival of the

XO fetus. In regard to the former, mosaic Turner patients who are fertile are not surprising (Ayuso et al., 1984; Fitzgerald et al., 1984); fertility only after hormonal replacement is perhaps more surprising (Blumenthal and Allanson, 1997). In regard to the latter, Held and colleagues (1992) have argued that only fetuses with a 46,XX line present during early development, possibly with a requirement for the extra X in extra-embryonic tissues, survive. Modern techniques (FISH and PCR) disclose much higher rates of 45X/46XX or 45X/46+ altered X mosaicism—up to 90% (Fernandez et al., 1996). However, the second cell line(s) is frequently present only at levels of 1% or 2%. Thus, the essential role for a second X in fetal survival is still moot.

Management.   Management is multifaceted and several health supervision guidelines have been published (Saenger, 1996; Rosenfeld et al., 1994). These include thyroid function screening and sensitivity to symptoms of diabetes mellitus because of the increased incidence of autoimmune disorders. Psychological and educational screening are recommended because of the unique cognitive problems. Cosmetic surgery (e.g., to correct marked neck webbing) may decrease a negative self-image.

Renal and/or cardiovascular abnormalities require special attention. The former should be evaluated by ultrasonography and urological repair of appropriate lesions performed. Coarctation of the aorta occurs in less than 20% of patients and should be surgically corrected (Saenger, 1996). Bicuspid aortic valve occurs in 30% and warrants prophylactic antibiotics for subacute bacterial endocarditis (Rosenfeld et al., 1994). Idiopathic hypertension is common and should be screened.

The role of gonadal steroids in stimulating growth and sexual development is clear, but arguments exist about which hormones are best, the time for starting replacement, and the role of recombinant human growth hormone (rHGH). Early treatment with ethynyl estradiol has been proposed (Ross et al., 1986), whereas oxandrolone (Rosenbloom and Frias, 1973), with or without rHGH, is commonly used. Although the combination is better than either alone (Rosenfeld et al., 1988), the slight increment in height obtained by the addition of expensive rHGH may not be warranted. More recent data suggest better results with rHGH when estrogen replacement is delayed (Rosenfeld et al., 1994). Turner patients can conceive with ovum donation with as high a degree of success as patients with other causes of ovarian failure (Press et al., 1995).

Discussion.   A major question in the pathogenesis of Turner syndrome is the identity of the genes that are needed in two copies. A primary candidate anti-Turner gene is a gene (or genes) located in the pseudoautosomal region that is involved in statural growth. Patients with deletions of the pseudoautosomal region often have short stature (Ballabio et al., 1989; Henke et al., 1991; Ogata et al., 1992; Joseph et al., 1996). One patient with short stature had a pseudoautosomal deletion that encompassed only 700 kb (Ogata et al., 1995). Candidate genes for the pseudoautosomal growth factor anti-Turner gene included two growth factor receptor genes: the granulocyte-macrophage colony-stimulating factor receptor, CSF2R (Gough et al., 1990), and an interleukin-3 receptor, IL3RA (Milatovich et al., 1993); a mitochondrial nucleotide translocase that is important for general energy metabolism

(Slim et al., 1993); and two widely expressed proteins of unknown function, MIC2 (Goodfellow et al., 1986) and XE7 (Ellison et al., 1992). Recent evidence suggests that a novel homeobox gene, *SHOX*, which is sometimes deleted in short women without Turner syndrome, is this gene (Rao et al., 1997). A second growth factor is non-pseudoautosomal and is homologous to a Yq growth factor gene (see Chromosomal Mutations, below).

A candidate anti-Turner gene is RPS4 (Fisher et al., 1990; Zinn et al., 1994). This structural gene for a ribosomal protein maps close to *SRY* and *ZFY*—near the pseudoautosomal border. In some 46,XY females, this gene is deleted and they have had congenital lymphedema (Blagowidow et al., 1989; Levilliers et al., 1989). The functional equivalence of RPS4X and RPS4Y has been demonstrated (Watanabe et al., 1993). Major arguments against this gene as an anti-Turner gene have been the mapping of the X homologue to proximal Xq (given that persons with 46,X,i(Xq) show most features of the Turner phenotype), the lack of Turner features in a 46,XY female with a deletion of RPS4Y (Muller et al., 1992), and the finding of two active copies of RPS4X in cell lines from Turner patients with structurally abnormal Xs (Just et al., 1992).

Ogata and colleagues (1993) have argued that the Turner stigmata in 46,XY females with Xp deletions are caused by the deletion of ZFX rather than RPS4Y. The *ZFY*/*ZFX* pair are candidate anti-Turner genes based on their expression pattern and map location. Initial studies of *ZFY* expression detected expression by Northern analyses in all Y-chromosome positive cell lines studied (T-cell leukemia, neuroblastoma, fibroblast, and lymphoblastoid lines; Schneider-Gadicke et al., 1989). Palmer and colleagues (1990) used RT-PCR to demonstrate expression of *ZFY* in fetal brain and adult liver as well as testis. Lau and Chan (1989) found the apparently same minor transcript in fetal testis. *ZFX* (human) was expressed in all the tissues in which they had found *ZFY* to be expressed, and also in adult testes, by Schneider-Gadicke and colleagues (1989). Palmer and colleagues (1990) found *ZFY* to be expressed in all adult or fetal tissues studied, and Lau and Chan (1989) found *ZFX* to be expressed in the ovary. *ZFX* was well expressed from the inactivated X (Schneider-Gadicke et al., 1989; Palmer et al., 1990). Thus, two copies of this highly homologous pair are expressed in most tissues, and single dosage might be expected to affect many functions. Ogata and colleagues (1993) point out that "there has been no report documenting a patient with characteristic Turner stigmata in the presence of two copies of *ZFX, ZFY*." The knockout of *Zfx* showed growth deficiency, decreased viability, and lower numbers of germ cells, both in homozygous deficient females and in hemizygous males (Luoh et al., 1997). These data strongly support the notion that ZFX is an anti-Turner gene.

Ogata and Matsuo (1995) have extensively reviewed the literature on X chromosome aberrations and argue that a primary lymphogenic gene, which may be crucial for much of the pathology in Turner syndrome, is located in the middle of Xp and distally on Yp, a location also suggested by Fechner and colleagues (1992). However, multiple genes that are active on the inactive X and on the Y are involved in preventing the Turner phenotype. We have recently described a male infant with Turner-like neonatal lymphedema and a balanced Y:16 translocation with the Y breakpoint distal in the Yq euchromatin (Erickson et al., 1995). This case suggests the possibility that a gene involved in fetal, but not adult lymphatic function, maps to this Yq region.

REFERENCES

Aller V, Gargallo M, Abrisqueta J A (1995). Familial transmission of a duplication-deficiency X chromosome associated with partial Turner syndrome. *Clin Genet* 48:317–320.

Ayuso M C, Bello M J, Benitez J, Sanchez-Cascos A, Mendoza G (1984). Two fertile Turner women in a family. *Clin Genet* 26:591–596.

Ballabio A, Bardoni B, Carrozzo R, Andria G, Bick D, Campbell L, Hamel B, Ferguson-Smith M A, Gimelli G, Fraccaro M, Maraschio P, Zuffardi O, Guioli S, Camerino G (1989). Contiguous gene syndromes due to deletions in the distal short arm of the human X chromosome. *Proc Natl Acad Sci USA* 86:10001–10005.

Bender B G, Linden M G, Robinson A (1993). Neuropsychological impairment in 42 adolescents with sex chromosome abnormalities. *Am J Med Genet* 48:169–173.

Blagowidow N, Page D C, Huff D, Mennuti M T (1989). Ullrich-Turner syndrome in an XY female fetus with deletion of the sex-determining portion of the Y chromosome. *Am J Med Genet* 34:159–162.

Blumenthal A L, Allanson J E (1997). Turner syndrome in a mother and daughter: r(X) and fertility. *Clin Genet* 52:189–191.

Cockwell A, MacKenzie M, Youings S, Jacobs P (1991). A cytogenetic and molecular study of a series of 45,X fetuses and their parents. *J Med Genet* 28:151–155.

Cunniff C, Jones K L, Benirschke K (1991). Ovarian dysgenesis in individuals with chromosome abnormalities. *Hum Genet* 86:552–556.

Ellison J W, Ramos C, Yen P H, Shapiro L J (1992). Structure and expression of the human pseudoautosomal gene XE7. *Hum Mol Genet* 1:691–696.

Epstein C J (1990). Mechanisms leading to the phenotype of Turner syndrome. In: Rosenfeld R G, Grumbach M M (eds). *Turner Syndrome*. Marcel Dekker, NY, pp. 13–28.

Erickson R P, Hudgins L, Stone J F, Schmidt S, Wilke C, Glover T W (1995). A "balanced" Y;16 translocation associated with Turner-like neonatal lymphedema suggests the location of a potential anti-Turner gene on the Y chromosome. *Cytogenet Cell Genet* 71:163–167.

Fechner P Y, Smith K D, Jabs E W, Migeon C J, Berkovitz G D (1992). Partial gonadal dysgenesis in a patient with a marker Y chromosome. *Am J Med Genet* 42:807–812.

Fernández R, Méndez J, Pásaro E (1996). Turner syndrome: a study of chromosomal mosaicism. *Hum Genet* 98:29–35.

Fisher E M, Beer-Romero P, Brown L G, Ridley A, McNeil J A, Lawrence J B, Willard H F, Bieber F R, Page D C (1990). Homologous ribosomal protein genes on the human X and Y chromosomes: escape from X inactivation and possible implications for Turner syndrome. *Cell* 63:1205–1218.

Fitzgerald P H, Donald R A, McCormick P (1984). Reduced fertility in women with X chromosome abnormality. *Clin Genet* 25:301–309.

Fryns J P, Kleczkowska A, Petit P, VanDenBerghe H. (1982). Fertility in patients with X chromosome deletions. *Clin Genet* 22:76–79.

Fryns J P, Kleczkowska A, Debucquoy P, VanDenBerghe H (1988). Fertility and X chromosome rearrangements: isodicentric X chromosome formation in the mother and Xp deletion in her daughter. *Clin Genet* 34:321–324.

Goodfellow P J, Darling S, Thomas N S, Goodfellow P N (1986). A pseudoautosomal gene in man. *Science* 234:740–743.

Gough N M, Gearing D P, Nicola N A, Baker E, Pritchard M, Callen D F, Sutherland G R (1990). Localization of the human GM-CSF receptor gene to the X-Y pseudoautosomal region. *Nature* 345:734–736.

Grumbach M M, Conte F A (1992) Disorders of sexual differentiation. In: Wilson J D, Foster

D W (eds.). *Williams Textbook of Endocrinology*, 8th ed., W. B. Saunders, Philadelphia, PA, pp. 853–952.

Hassold T, Kumlin E, Takaesu N, Leppert M (1985). Determination of the parental origin of sex-chromosome monosomy using restriction fragment length polymorphisms. *Am J Hum Genet* 37:965–972.

Held K R, Kerber S, Kaminsky E, Singh S, Goetz P, Seemanova E, Goedde H W (1992). Mosaicism in 45,X Turner syndrome: does survival in early pregnancy depend on the presence of two sex chromosomes? *Hum Genet* 88:288–294.

Henke A, Wapenaar M, van Ommen G-J, Maraschko P, Camerino G, Rappold G. (1991). Deletions within the pseudoautosomal region help map three new markers and indicate a possible role of this region in linear growth. *Am J Hum Genet* 49:811–819.

Hier D B, Crowley W F Jr. (1982). Spatial ability in androgen-deficient men. *N Engl J Med* 306:1202–1205.

Jacobs P A, Betts P R, Cockwell A E, Crolla J A, MacKenzie M J, Robinson D O, Youings S A (1992). A cytogenetic and molecular reappraisal of a series of patients with Turner syndrome. *Ann Hum Genet* 54:209–223.

Joseph M, Cantú E S, Pai G S, Willi S M, Papenhausen P R, Weiss L (1996). Xp pseudoautosomal gene haploinsufficiency and linear growth deficiency in three girls with chromosome Xp22q11 translocation. *J Med Genet* 33:906–911.

Just W, Geerkens C, Held K R, Vogel W (1992). Expression of RPS4X in fibroblasts from patients with structural aberrations of the X chromosome. *Hum Genet* 89:240–242.

Lau Y-FC, Chan K (1989). The putative testis-determining factor and related genes are expressed as discrete-sized transcripts in adult gonadal and somatic tissues. *Am J Hum Genet* 45:942–952.

Levilliers J, Quack B, Weissenbach J, Petit C (1989). Exchange of terminal portions of X-and Y-chromosomal short arms in human XY females. *Proc Natl Acad Sci USA* 86:2296–2300.

Leichtman D A, Schmickel R D, Gelehrter T D, Judd W J, Woodbury M C, Meilinger K L (1978). Familial Turner syndrome. *Ann Int Med* 89:473–476.

Loughlin S A R, Redha A, McIver J, Boyd E, Carothers A, Connor J M (1991). Analysis of the origin of Turner's syndrome using polymorphic DNA probes. *J Med Genet* 28:156–158.

Luoh S-W, Bain P A, Polakiewicz R D, Goodheart M L, Gardner H, Jaenisch R, Page D C (1997). *Zfx* mutation results in small animal size and reduced germ cell number in male and female mice. *Development* 124:2275–2284.

Maraschio P, Tupler R, Barbierato L, Dainotti E, Larizza D, Bernardi F, Hoeller A, Garau A, Tiepolo L (1996). An analysis of Xq deletions. *Hum Genet* 97:375–381.

Massa G, Vanderschueren-Lodeweyckx M, Fryns J-P (1992). Deletion of the short arm of the X chromosome: a hereditary form of Turner syndrome. *Eur J Pediatr* 151:893–894.

Massarano A A, Adams J A, Preece M A, Brook C G D (1989). Ovarian ultrasound appearances in Turner syndrome. *J Pediatr* 114:568–573.

Mathur A, Stekol L, Schatz D, MacLaren N K, Scott M L, Lippe B (1991). The parental origin of the single X chromosome in Turner syndrome: lack of correlation with parental age or clinical phenotype. *Am J Hum Genet* 48:682–686.

Migeon B R, Luo S, Jani M, Jeppesen P (1994). The severe phenotype of females with tiny ring X chromosomes is associated with inability of these chromosomes to undergo X inactivation. *Am J Hum Genet* 55:497–504.

Milatovich A, Kitamura T, Miyajima A, Francke U (1993). Gene for the alpha-subunit of the human interleukin-3 receptor (IL3RA) localized to the X-Y pseudoautosomal region. *Am J Hum Genet* 53:1146–1153.

Muller U, Kirkels V G H J, Scheres J M J (1992). Absence of Turner stigmata in a 46, XYp-female. *Hum Genet* 90:239–242.

Ogata T, Matsuo N (1995). Turner syndrome and female sex chromosome aberrations: deduction of the principal factors involved in the development of clinical features. *Hum Genet* 95:607–629.

Ogata T, Petit C, Rappold G, Matsuo N, Matsumoto T, Goodfellow P (1992). Chromosomal localization of a pseudoautosomal growth gene(s). *J Med Genet* 29:624–628.

Ogata T, Tyler-Smith C, Purvis-Smith S, Turner G (1993). Chromosomal localization of a gene(s) for Turner stigmata on Yp. *J Med Genet* 30:918–922.

Ogata T, Yoshizawa A, Muroya K, Matsuo N, Fukushima Y, Rappold G, Yokoya S (1995). Short stature in a girl with partial monosomy of the pseudoautosomal region distal of DXYS15: further evidence for the assignment of the critical region for a pseudoautosomal growth gene(s). *J Med Genet* 32:831–834.

Opitz J M, Pallister P D (1979). Brief historical note: The concept of "gonadal dysgenesis." *Am J Med Genet* 4:333–343.

Palmer M S, Berta P, Sinclair A H, Pym B, Goodfellow P N (1990). Comparison of human ZFY and ZFX transcripts. *Proc Natl Acad Sci USA* 87:1681–1685.

Press F, Shapiro H M, Cowell C A, Oliver G D (1995). Outcome of ovum donation in Turner's syndrome patients. *Fertil Steril* 64:995–998.

Rao E, Weiss B, Fukami M, Rump A, Niesler B, Mertz A, Muroya K, Binder G, Kirsch S, Winkelmann M, Nordsiek G, Heinrich U, Breuning M H, Ranke M B, Rosenthal A, Ogata T, Rappold G A (1997). Pseudoautosomal deletions encompassing a novel homeobox gene cause growth failure in idiopathic short stature and Turner syndrome. *Nat Genet* 16: 54–63.

Rosenbloom A L, Frias J L (1973). Oxandrolone for growth promotion in Turner syndrome. *Am J Dis Child* 125:385–387.

Rosenfeld R G, Hintz R L, Johanson M J, Sherman B, Brasel J, Burstein S, Chenausek S, Compton P, Frane J, Gotlin R W, Kuntze J, Lippe B M, Mahoney P C, Moore W V, New M I, Saenger P, Sybert V (1988). Three-year results of a randomized prospective trial of methionyl human growth hormone and oxandrolone in Turner syndrome. *J Pediatr* 113:393–400.

Rosenfeld R G, Tesch L G, Rodriguez-Rigau L J, McCauley E, Albertsson-Wikland K, Asch R, Cara J, Conte F, Hall J G, Lippe B, Nagel T C, Neely E K, Page D C, Ranke M, Saenger P, Watkins J M, Wilson D M (1994). Recommendations for diagnosis, treatment, and management of individuals with Turner syndrome. *Endocrinologist* 4:351–358.

Ross J L, Long L M, Skerda M, Cassorla F, Kurtz D, Loriaux D L, Cutler G B (1986). Effect of low doses of estradiol on 6-month growth rates and predicted height in patients with Turner syndrome. *J Pediatr* 109:950–953.

Rovet J, Netley C (1980). The mental rotation task performance of Turner syndrome subjects. *Behav Genet* 10:437–439.

Saenger P (1996). Turner's syndrome. *N Engl J Med* 335:1749–1754.

Schneider-Gadicke A, Beer-Fomero P, Brown L G, Nussbaum R, Page D C (1989). ZFX has a gene structure similar to ZFY, the putative sex determinant and escapes X inactivation. *Cell* 57:1247–1258.

Skuse D H, James R S, Bishop D V, Coppin B, Dalton P, Aamodt-Leeper G, Bacarese-Hamilton M, Creswell C, McGurk R, Jacobs P A (1997). Evidence from Turner's syndrome of an imprinted X-linked locus affecting cognitive function. *Nature* 387:705–708.

Slim R, Levilliers J, Ludecke H-J, Claussen U, Nguyen V C, Gough N M, Horsthemke B, Petit C (1993). A human pseudoautosomal gene encodes the ANT3 ADP/ATP translocase and escapes inactivation. *Genomics* 16:26–33.

Swillen A, Fryns J-P (1996). Neurodevelopmental changes with age in Ullrich-Turner syndrome. Letter to the Editor. *Am J Med Genet* 61:198.

Turner H H (1938). A syndrome of infantilism, congenital webbed neck, and cubitus valgus. *Endocrinology* 23:566–574.

Ullrich O Uber typische Kombinationsbilder multipler Abartungen (1930). *Z Kinder* 49:271–276.

Van Dyke D L, Wiktor A, Palmer C G, Miller D A, Witt M, Babu V R, Worsham M J (1992). Ullrich-Turner syndrome with a small ring X chromosome and presence of mental retardation. *Am J Med Genet* 43:996–1005.

Van Dyke D L, Wiktor A, Roberson J R, Weiss L. (1991). Mental retardation in Turner syndrome. *J Pediatr* 118:415–417.

Verschraegen-Spae M-R, Depypere M, Speleman F, Dhondt M, DePaepe A. (1992). Familial Turner syndrome. *Clin Genet* 41:218–220.

Waber D P (1979). Neuropsychological aspects of Turner's syndrome. *Dev Med Child Neurol* 21:58–70.

Watanabe M, Zinn A R, Page D C, Nishimoto T (1993). Functional equivalence of human X- and Y-encoded isoforms of ribosomal protein S4, consistent with a role in Turner syndrome. *Nat Genet* 4:268–271.

Zinn A R, Alagappan R K, Brown L G, Wool I, Page D C (1994). Structure and function of ribosomal protein S4 genes on the human and mouse sex chromosomes. *Mol Cell Biol* 14: 2485–2492.

Zinn A R, Ouyang B, Ross J L, Varma S, Bourgeois M, Tonk V (1997). Del (X) (p 21.2) in a mother and two daughters with variable ovarian function. *Clin Genet* 52:235–239.

KLINEFELTER SYNDROME

Klinefelter, Reifenstein, and Albright initially described the syndrome now known by Klinefelter's name in 1942. It was not until 1959 that Jacobs and Strong (1959) discovered that these patients are 47,XXY. This condition is now a well-recognized entity, surrounded with some controversy about the effects of the extra X on mental and behavioral function. Our focus will be on the gonadal aspects. Although the testes in Klinefelter syndrome are usually lacking in spermatogenesis because of the failure of inactivation of the second X chromosome (see below), the hormonal function of the testis varies from near normal to severely deficient. The cause of this variability is unknown.

Clinical and Imaging Presentation.   The presence of Klinefelter syndrome is detected in most patients at adolescence because of the lack of sexual maturation. Others with this syndrome are identified through infertility clinics. The syndrome may be suspected in prepubertal boys with the triad of relatively long legs, small external genitalia, and behavioral disorders. The phenotype of Klinefelter syndrome is not markedly different from that of normal males, although—relevant to the effect of the Y chromosome on height discussed in Chapter 6—Klinefelter males have heights well above average, with proportionally long legs and decreased arm span to height ratio (reviewed in Mandoki et al., 1991). Gynecomastia occurs fairly frequently and may be possibly related to a reported increase in incidence of male breast cancer (Evans and Crichlow, 1987). There is an increased incidence of other tumors, especially extragonadal germ cell tumors, including ones in the central nervous system (Schimke et al., 1983). An increased incidence of birth defects has not been noted in this condition. Sexual precocity, sometimes associated with thoracic teratocarcinoma and sometimes idiopathic (von Muhlenbahl and Heinrich, 1994), has an increased frequency (Chaussain et al., 1980). The incidence is about 1 in 1000 births, an incidence similar to that of 47,XXX, a karyotype which is not associated with problems of sexual development but is accompanied by similar psychological problems (Linden et al., 1988).

The question of behavioral abnormalities and mild developmental delay in Klinefelter syndrome has engendered an extensive controversy. Early studies (Netley, 1986, 1987; Salbenblatt et al., 1987) emphasized deficiencies in verbal, but not performance, IQ. More precise psychometric testing seems to implicate a distinct deficiency in the rate of accessing verbal information from memory (i.e., a deficiency in verbal fluency) (Bender et al., 1989). Despite these deficiencies, however, it was found that adults with Klinefelter syndrome appeared to do as well as a control group in terms of socioeconomic status and degree of education (Porter et al., 1988). Amniocentesis permits the diagnosis of many patients *in utero*, a mode of ascertainment that is unbiased by altered school performance. Such patients have tended to compare very favorably with matched-sib controls (Robinson et al., 1992). Nevertheless, decreased verbal fluency and reading ability of patients with Klinefelter syndrome has been confirmed in several studies (Bender et al., 1993; Rovet et al., 1995). The remaining question concerns the severity of these deficits. Definite mental retardation occurs with sex chromosome tetrasomy and pentasomy (Linden et al., 1995).

Laboratory Studies.   Luteinizing hormone (LH) values are within the normal range before the onset of puberty but are usually elevated by midway through the second decade (Robinson et al., 1992). Puberty commences with a rise in serum testosterone that frequently plateaus below normal levels. Hypergonadotropism is usually necessary to maintain near normal levels of testosterone. This is confirmed by the elevated plasma LH response to GnRH simulation after puberty (De Behar et al., 1975; Salbenblatt et al., 1985). Even if testosterone levels are normal, a measurement of testicular testosterone reserve following human chorionic gonadotropin (hCG) stimulation can help in the decision of when, or if, to start testosterone replacement therapy (Topper et al., 1982). Estradiol levels are usually elevated, as are the estrogen to androgen ratios (Garbrilove et al., 1980); these account for the increased incidence of gynecomastia mentioned above.

Genotyping.   Most patients are pure 47,XXY. Mosaicism is sometimes found, and partly explains rare fertile cases: in one study that looked at peripheral blood (Foss and Lewis, 1971), only one of four fertile males with Klinefelter syndrome was found to be a 47,XXY/46,XY mosaic. Of course, this does not discount the possibility that the testes contained 46,XY lines. A variant with 47,XY,i(Xq) that does not cause increased height has been reported by several groups (Donland et al., 1987; Fryns et al., 1990; Arps et al., 1996). A 47,XY,i(Xq) patient who was actually isodicentric for Xq (i.e., including a centromeric proximal portion of Xp) with a normal height suggests that double dosage of Xp is responsible for the increased height in Klinefelter syndrome (Zelante et al., 1991). Parent-of-origin studies have shown that the ratio of maternal to paternal additional Xs is about equal (MacDonald et al., 1994). In the latter study, paternal age did not affect the frequency of Klinefelter syndrome, but maternal age did. One case of familial Klinefelter syndrome due to recurrent paternal nondisjunction has been described (Woods et al., 1997).

Management.   As already discussed under laboratory studies, the major treatment is testosterone replacement when it is needed. There has been some evidence that testosterone replacement improves behavior (Nielsen et al., 1988). As emphasized by Graham and coworkers (1988), a knowledge of the reading and related language problems that have an increased incidence in Klinefelter syndrome males may lead to specific educational interventions that can help maximize their potential. Testicular sperm extraction and intracytoplasmic sperm injection into an ovum *in vitro* has led to healthy births (Palermo et al., 1998). However, these sperm may have an extra sex chromosome that is detectable by preimplantation testing.

Discussion. The mechanism by which an extra X inhibits germ cell development in the testis seems clear-cut: persistence of one active X chromosome. The inactivation of one X chromosome in the somatic cells of mammalian females is well known and is a much-studied phenomenon, but the inactivation of the single X chromosome during mammalian male gamete formation (Lifschytz, 1972) is less well known and the implications of this X-inactivation for the biochemical genetics of spermatogenesis have not generally been explored. A study of spermatozoal glucose-6-phosphate dehydrogenase (G6PD) in mice found it to be identical by several criteria to the erythrocytic, X-linked form rather than the autosomal, hexose-6-phosphate dehydrogenase (Erickson, 1975). A study of the specific activities of G6PD in mouse testes during the first wave of spermatogenesis and in spermatogenic cells suggested that it might well be synthesized premeiotically and be stable enough to persist into sperm (Erickson, 1976). This is now known to be incorrect in mice, because they, but not most other mammals, use an autosomal, retroposon-captured G6PD during spermatogenesis (Hendriksen et al., 1997). Nonetheless, both studies concluded that X-linked G6PD did not continue to be synthesized; and based on this one enzyme, X-inactivation during spermatogenesis might involve the same loci that are inactivated in female somatic cells. It has now been shown that *Xist*, the gene transcribed from the inactive X, is expressed during spermatogenesis, starting in spermatogonia—that is, before the visible manifestations of X-inactivation (Richler et al., 1992; Salido et al., 1992; McCarrey and Dilworth, 1992).

It was originally believed that X-chromosome inactivation was complete. This delayed acceptance of the finding that X-linked steroid sulfatase remains active on the inactive chromosome in humans (Shapiro et al., 1979). Steroid sulfatase is on Xp near the terminal, pseudoautosomal region. A more general acceptance of lack of inactivation of the Xp terminus developed with the finding of expressed genes including *MIC2* (Goodfellow et al., 1984) and the GM-CSF receptor (Gough et al., 1990) in the pseudoautosomal region. More recently, the discovery that another region of non-X-inactivation was separated from Xp by a region of X-inactivation demonstrated that X-inactivation is patchy (Brown and Willard, 1990). *ZFX* provides another patch of non-X-inactivation in humans (but not in mice). In addition, the *Xist* gene, which is only expressed on the inactive X, has now been found to be located near the X-inactivation center, still another region noncontiguous with the other regions of active genes on the inactive X (Brown et al., 1991). In fact, duplications of portions of the X chromosome that are not inactivated suggest that extra dosage of genes that are normally noninactivated is sometimes tolerated in males (Schmidt et al., 1991), but duplications of proximal Xq are usually associated with multiple congenital anomalies and mental retardation (Apacik et al., 1996).

It remains to be seen if "patchy" X-inactivation is also present during spermatogenesis. The expression of *Xist* during spermatogenesis suggests that the mechanism of inactivation may be the same in female somatic and male germ cells. However, X:Y pairing during spermatogenesis (see Chromosomal Mutations, below), does not have a corollary in female somatic cells. Mice show *Zfx* inactivation (Ashworth et al., 1991; Adler et al., 1991). They also have an almost identical, autosomal homologue, *Zfa*, recruited by retrotransposon-like activity, which is only expressed during spermatogenesis. This scenario also suggests that the pattern of X-inactivation in males during spermatogenesis might be similar to that of females in somatic cells.

REFERENCES

Adler D A, Bessler S L, Chapman V M, Page D C, Disteche C M (1991). Inactivation of the Zfx gene on the mouse X chromosome. *Proc Natl Acad Sci USA* 88:4592–4595.

Apacik C, Cohen M, Jakobeit M, Schmucker B, Schuffenhauer S, Thurn und Taxis E, Genzel-Boroviczeny O, Stengel-Rutkowski S (1996). Two brothers with multiple congenital anomalies and mental retardation due to disomy (X) (q12 →q13.3) inherited from the mother. *Clin Genet* 50:63–73.

Arps S, Koske-Westphal T, Meinecke P, Meschede D, Nieschlag E, Harprecht W, Steuber E, Back E, Wolff G, Kerber S, Held K R (1996). Isochromosome Xq in Klinefelter syndrome: report of 7 new cases. *Am J Med Genet* 64:580–582.

Ashworth A, Rastan S, Lovell-Badge R, Kay G (1991). X-chromosome inactivation may explain the difference in viability of XO humans and mice. *Nature* 351:406–408.

Bender B G, Linden M G, Robinson A (1989). Verbal and spatial processing efficiency in 32 children with sex chromosome abnormalities. *Pediatr Res* 25:577–579.

Bender B G, Linden M G, Robinson A (1993). Neuropsychological impairment in 42 adolescents with sex chromosome abnormalities. *Am J Med Genet* 48:169–173.

Brown C J, Willard H F (1990). Localization of a gene that escapes inactivation to the X chromosome proximal short arm: implications for X inactivation. *Am J Hum Genet* 46:273–279.

Brown C J, Ballabio A, Rupert J L, Lafreniere R G, Grompe M, Tonlorenzi R, Willard H F (1991). A gene from the region of the human X inactivation centre is expressed exclusively from the inactive X chromosome. *Nature* 349:38–44.

Chaussain J-L, Lemerle J, Roger M, Canlorbe P, Job J-C (1980). Klinefelter syndrome, tumor, and sexual precocity. *J Pediatr* 97:607–609.

DeBehar B R, Mendilaharzu H, Rivarola M A, Bergada C (1975). Gonadotropin secretion in prepubertal and pubertal primary hypogonadism: response to LHRH. *J Clin Endocrinol Metab* 41:1070–1075.

Donland M A, Dolan C R, Metcalf M J, Bradley C M, Salk D (1987). Trisomy Xq in a male: the isochromosome X Klinefelter syndrome. *Am J Med Genet* 27:189–194.

Erickson R P (1975). Mouse spermatozoal glucose-6-phosphate dehydrogenase is the X-linked form. *Biochem Biophys Res Commun* 63:1000–1004.

Erickson R P (1976). Glucose-6-phosphate dehydrogenase activity changes during spermatogenesis: possible relevance to X-chromosome inactivation. *Dev Biol* 53:134–137.

Evans D B, Crichlow R W (1987). Carcinoma of the male breast and Klinefelter's syndrome: is there an association? *CA-A Cancer J Clin* 37:246–250.

Foss G L, Lewis F J W (1971). A study of four cases with Klinefelter's syndrome, showing motile spermatozoa in their ejaculates. *J Reprod Fertil* 25:401–408.

Fryns J P, Kleczkowska A, Steeno O (1990). Isochromosome Xq in Klinefelter syndrome. *Am J Med Genet* 36:365.

Garbrilove J L, Freiberg E K, Nicolis G L (1980). Testicular function in Klinefelter's syndrome. *J Urol* 124:825–826.

Goodfellow P, Pym B, Mohandas T, Shapiro L J (1984). The cell surface antigen locus, M1C2X, escapes X-inactivation. *Am J Hum Genet* 36:777–782.

Gough N M, Gearing D P, Nicola N A, Baker E, Pritchard M, Callen D F, Sutherland G R

(1990). Localization of the human GM-CSF receptor gene to the X-Y pseudoautosomal region. *Nature* 345:734–736.

Graham J M Jr, Bashir A S, Stark R E, Silbert A, Walzer S (1988). Oral and written language abilities of XXY boys: implications for anticipatory guidance. *Pediatrics* 81:795–806.

Hendriksen P J M, Hoogerbrugge J W, Baarends W M, de Boer P, Vreeburg J T M, Vos E A, van der Lende T, Grooteyoed J A (1997). Testis-specific expression of a functional retroposon encoding glucose-6-phosphate dehydrogenase in the mouse. *Genomics* 41:350–359

Jacobs P A, Strong J A (1959). A case of human intersexuality having a possible XXY sex-determining mechanism. *Nature* 183:302–303.

Klinefelter H F Jr, Reifenstein E C Jr, Albright F (1942). Syndrome characterized by gynecomastia, aspermatogenesis without A-leydigism, and increased excretion of follicle-stimulating hormone. *J Clin Endocrinol* 2:615–627.

Lifschytz E (1972). X-chromosome inactivation: an essential feature of normal spermiogenesis in male heterogametic organisms. In: Beaty R A, Gluecksohn-Waelsch S (eds). *Proceedings of the International Symposium of the Genetics of the Spermatozoon*. Copenhagen: Bogtrykkeriet Forum, pp 223–232.

Linden M G, Bender B G, Harmon R J, Mrazek D A, Robinson A (1988). 47,XXX: What is the prognosis? *Pediatrics* 82:619–630.

Linden M G, Bender B G, Robinson A (1995). Sex chromosome tetrasomy and pentasomy. *Pediatrics* 96:672–682.

MacDonald M, Hassold T, Harvey J, Wang L H, Morton N E, Jacobs P (1994). The origin of 47,XXY and 47,XXX aneuploidy: heterogeneous mechanisms and role of aberrant recombination. *Hum Mol Genet* 3:1365–1371.

Mandoki M W, Summer G, Hoffman R P, Riconda D L (1991). Review of Klinefelter's syndrome in children and adolescents. *J Am Acad Child Adolesc Psychiatry* 30:167–172.

McCarrey J R, Dilworth D D (1992). Expression of *Xist* in mouse germ cells correlates with X-chromosome inactivation. *Nat Genet* 2:200–203.

Netley C T (1986). Summary overview of behavioral development in individuals with neonatally identified X and Y aneuploidy. *Birth Defects: Orig Art Ser* 22:293–306.

Netley C (1987). Predicting intellectual functioning in 47,XXY boys from characteristics of sibs. *Clin Genet* 32:24–27.

Nielsen J, Pelsen B, Sorensen K (1988). Follow-up of 30 Klinefelter males treated with testosterone. *Clin Genet* 33:262–269.

Palermo G D, Schlegel P N, Sills E S, Veeck L L, Zaninovic N, Menendez S, Rosenwaks Z (1998). Births after intracytoplasmic injection of sperm obtained by testicular extraction from men with nonmosaic Klinefelter's syndrome. *N Engl J Med* 338:588–590.

Porter M E, Gardner H A, DeFeudis P, Endler N S (1988). Verbal deficits in Klinefelter (XXY) adults living in the community. *Clin Genet* 33:246–253.

Richler C, Soreq H, Wahrman J (1992). X Inactivation in mammalian testis is correlated with inactive X-specific transcription. *Nat Genet* 2:192–195.

Robinson A, Bender B G, Linden M G (1992). Prognosis of prenatally diagnosed children with sex chromosome aneuploidy. *Am J Med Genet* 44:365–368.

Rovet J, Netley C, Bailey J, Keenan M, Stewart D (1995). Intelligence and achievement in children with extra X aneuploidy: a longitudinal perspective. *Am J Med Genet* 60:356–363.

Salbenblatt J A, Bender B G, Puck M H, Robinson A, Faiman C, Winter J S D (1985). Pituitary-gonadal function in Klinefelter syndrome before and during puberty. *Pediatr Res* 19:82–86.

Salbenblatt J A, Meyers D C, Bender B G, Linden M G, Robinson A (1987). Gross and fine motor development in 47,XXY and 47,XYY males. *Pediatrics* 80:240–244.

Salido E C, Yen P H, Mohandas T K, Shapiro L J (1992). Expression of the X-inactivation-associated-gene *Xist* during spermatogenesis. *Nat Genet* 2:196–199.

Schimke R N, Madigan C M, Silver B J, Fabian C J, Stephens R L (1983). Choriocarcinoma, thyrotoxicosis, and the Klinefelter syndrome. *Cancer Genet Cytogenet* 9:1–8.

Schmidt M, DuSart D, Kalitsis P, Leversha M, Dale S, Sheffield L, Toniolo D (1991). Duplications of the X chromosome can be active in two copies. *Hum Genet* 86:519–521.

Shapiro L J, Mohandas T, Weiss T, Romeo G (1979) Non-inactivation of an X-chromosome locus in man. *Science* 204:1224–1226.

Topper E, Dickerman Z, Prager-Lewin R, Kaufman H, Maimon Z, Laron Z (1982).Puberty in 24 patients with Klinefelter syndrome. *Eur J Pediatr* 139:8–12.

von Muhlendahl K, Heinrich U (1994). Sexual precocity in Klinefelter syndrome: report on two new cases with idiopathic central precocious puberty. *Eur J Pediatr* 153:322–324.

Woods C G, Noble J, Falconer A R (1997). A study of brothers with Klinefelter syndrome. *J Med Genet* 34:702.

Zelante L, Calvano S, Dallapiccola B (1991). Isodicentric Xq in Klinefelter syndrome. *Am J Med Genet* 41:267–268.

XX/XY MOSAIC TRUE HERMAPHRODITISM AND X/XY MOSAICISM

Although a rare cause of sexual ambiguity, true hermaphroditism due to 46,XX/46,XY mosaicism has been multiply described (Fitzgerald et al., 1970; Park et al., 1970; Kakati et al., 1971; Benirschke et al., 1972; Shanfield et al., 1973; de La Chapelle et al., 1974). 45,X/46,XY mosaicism (mixed gonadal dysgenesis) is found in patients whose phenotype is that of Turner syndrome and who have ambiguous genitalia (Bisat et al., 1993; Knudtzon and Aarskog, 1987); it is discovered even more frequently through amniocentesis and other prenatal studies (Hsu 1989; Wheeler et al., 1988). Perhaps the major importance of these entities is the implications of a 46,XY line in a gonad for the risk of gonadoblastoma (Simpson and Photopoulos, 1976).

Clinical and Imaging Presentation.　Most patients have ambiguous external genitalia, which leads to postnatal ascertainment. On the other hand, if the condition is diagnosed prenatally, most of the patients will be phenotypically normal males (Wheeler et al., 1988; Hsu, 1989). In one study of 75 prenatal diagnoses of 45,X/46,XY mosaicism, 95% of the fetuses had normal male genitalia, although 27% had abnormal gonadal histology (Chang et al., 1990). Alternating gonadal hermaphroditism, usually with the testicular portion on the right side, is much more common than bilateral ovotestis (van Niekerk, 1974). Ultrasound studies will frequently identify a uterus and a fallopian tube on the side of the ovary or ovotestis. Other birth defects, such as renal hypoplasia and renal agenesis (Wax et al., 1994), and other tumors, such as testicular juvenile granulosa cell tumor (Tanaka et al., 1994), may be associated with 45,X/46,XY mosaicism. Any phenotypic female who shows spontaneous virilization almost certainly has a Y chromosome–containing cell line (and a tumor).

Laboratory Studies.　Karyotypes will, of course, show the mosaicism that has led to this classification. The routine blood karyotype may not reflect the degree of mosaicism in the most relevant tissues and may not correlate well with the phenotype. The karyotype of gonadal cell lines may be more helpful. The Y chromosome need not be intact. For instance, isodicentric Y chromosomes may be involved in the second cell line and result in similar phenotypes (Stuppia et al., 1996).

Genotyping.　Not relevant.

Management. Perhaps the most important aspect of this entity is the need to diagnose cell lines containing a Y chromosome in gonads because of the risk of gonadoblastoma. Although it has been long appreciated that gonadal tumors are more likely to occur in dysgenetic gonads (reviewed in Scully, 1970), with post-1957 developments in cytogenetics, it was realized that gonadoblastoma or dysgerminoma is a risk when a Y chromosome is present (Ionescu and Maximilian, 1977). Although most of the tumors do not occur until patients reach puberty (Manuel et al., 1976), they have occurred in much younger patients (e g , aged 5 years) (Khodr, et al., 1979). Thus, prophylactic removal of the dysgenetic gonad is usual. In one case, a successful pregnancy occurred before dysgerminoma arising from a gonadoblastoma necessitated hysterectomy, bilateral salpingectomy, and unilateral gonadectomy (Talerman et al., 1990).

Discussion. The association with the Yq arm in patients with translocations has tentatively mapped the portion of the Y responsible for gonadoblastoma to Yq (De Arce et al., 1992). Tyrkus and colleagues (1984) studied two cases of atypical gonadal dysgenesis and also postulated that the regulatory locus causing malignancy was on the long arm of the Y. David Page (1987) argued that this gene is located either near the centromere or on the long arm of the Y chromosome on the basis of two reported cases of females with dysgenic gonads, deleted Y chromosome, and gonadoblastoma (Disteche et al., 1986; Magenis et al., 1984; Magenis et al., 1987). Another recent report (Petrovic et al., 1992) also localizes the Y malignancy-determining region as paracentromeric. Thus, all available evidence suggests that the Y "malignancy gene" is in proximal Yq.

REFERENCES

Benirschke K, Naftolin F, Gittes R, Khudr G, Yen S S C, Allen F H Jr (1972). True hermaphroditism and chimerism: a case report. *Am J Obstet Gynecol* 113:449–458.

Bisat T, May K, Litwer S, Broecker B (1993). Y chromosome mosaicism in the gonads, but not in the blood, of a girl with the Turner phenotype and virilized external genitalia. *Clin Genet* 44:142–145.

Chang J H, Clark R D, Bachman H (1990). The phenotype of 45,X/46,XY mosaicism: an analysis of 92 prenatally diagnosed cases. *Am J Hum Genet* 46:156–167.

De Arce M A, Costigan C, Gosden J R, Lawler M, Humphries P (1992). Further evidence consistent with Yq as an indicator of risk of gonadal blastoma in Y-bearing mosaic Turner syndrome. *Clin Genet* 41:28–32.

de la Chapelle A, Schroder J, Rantanen P, Thomasson B, Niemi M, Tiilikainen A, Sanger R, Robson E B (1974). Early fusion of two human embryos? *Ann Hum Genet* 38:63–75.

Disteche C M, Casanova M, Saal H, Friedman C, Sybert V, Graham J, Thuline H, Page D C, Fellous M (1986). Small deletions of the short arm of the Y chromosome in 46,XX females. *Proc Natl Acad Sci USA* 83:7841–7844.

Fitzgerald P H, Brehaut L A, Shannon F T, Angus H B (1970). Evidence of XX/XY sex chromosome mosaicism in a child with true hermaphroditism. *J Med Genet* 7:383–388.

Hsu Y L E (1989). Prenatal diagnosis of 45,X/46,XY mosaicism—a review and update. *Prenat Diagn* 9:31–48.

Ionescu B, Maximilian C (1977). Three sisters with gonadoblastoma. *J Med Genet* 14:194–199.

Kakati S, Sharma T, Udupa K N, Chaudhuri S P R (1971). A true hermaphrodite with XX/XY mosaicism. *Indian J Med Res* 59:104–106.

Khodr G S, Cadena G D, Ong T C, Siler-Khodr T (1979). Y-autosome translocation, gonadal dysgenesis, and gonadoblastoma. *Am J Dis Child* 133:277–282.

Knudtzon J, Aarskog D (1987). 45,X/46,XY mosaicism. *Eur J Pediatr* 146:266–271.

Magenis R E, Casanova M, Fellow M, Olson S, Sheey R (1987). Further cytologic evidence for Xp-Yp translocation in XX males using *in situ* hybridization with Y-derived probe. *Hum Genet* 75:228–233.

Magenis R E, Tochen M L, Holohan K P, Carey T, Allen L, Brown M G, (1984). Turner syndrome resulting from partial deletion of Y chromosome short arm; localization of male determinants. *J Pediatr* 105:916–919.

Manuel M, Katayama K P, Jones H W Jr (1976). The age of occurrence of gonadal tumors in intersex patients with Y chromosome. *Am J Obstet Gynecol* 124:293–300.

Page D C (1987). Hypothesis: A Y chromosomal gene causes gonadoblastoma in dysgenetic gonads. *Development* 101 (suppl):151–155.

Park I J, Jones H W Jr, Bias W B (1970). True hermaphroditism with 46,XX/46,XY chromosome complement: report of a case. *Obstet Gynecol* 36:377–387.

Petrovic V, Nasioulas S, Chow C W, Voullaire L, Schmidt M, Dahl H (1992). Minute Y chromosome derived marker in a child with gonadoblastoma: cytogenetic and DNA studies. *J Med Genet* 29:542–546.

Scully R E (1970). Gonadoblastoma. A review of 74 cases. *Cancer* 6:1340–1356.

Shanfield I, Young R B, Hume D M (1973). True hermaphroditism with XX/XY mosaicism: report of a case. *J Pediatr* 83:471–473.

Simpson J L, Photopoulos G (1976). The relationship of neoplasia to the disorders of abnormal sexual differentiation. *Birth Defects* 12:15–50.

Stuppia L, Calabrese G, Franchi P G, Mingarelli R, Morizio E, Sabatino G, Palka G (1996). Molecular studies in three patients with isodicentric Y chromosome. *Hum Genet* 98:691–695.

Talerman A, Verp M S, Senekjian E, Gilewski, T, Volgelzang N (1990). True hermaphrodite with bilateral ovotestes, bilateral gonadoblastomas and dysgerminomas, 46,XX/46,XY karyotype, and a successful pregnancy. *Cancer* 66:2668–2672.

Tanaka Y, Sasaki Y, Tachibana K, Suwa S, Terashima K, Nakatani Y (1994). Testicular juvenile granulosa cell tumor in an infant with X/XY mosaicism clinically diagnosed as true hermaphroditism. *Am J Surg Pathol* 18:316–322.

Tyrkus M, McCorquodale M, Postellon D, Franco-Saenz R (1984). Atypical gonadal dysgenesis: the role of Yq in determining phenotype and malignancy risk. *Clin Genet* 25:259–266.

van Niekerk W A (1974). *True Hermaphroditism*. Harper, New York.

Wax J R, Prabhakar G, Giraldez R A, Hutchins G M, Stetten G, Blakemore K J (1994). Unilateral renal hypoplasia and contralateral renal agenesis: a new association with 45,X/46,XY mosaicism. *Am J Perinatol* 11:184–186.

Wheeler M, Peakman D, Robinson A, Henry G (1988). 45,X/46,XY mosaicism: contrast of prenatal and postnatal diagnosis. *Am J Med Genet* 29:565–571.

Chromosomal Mutations

XP21 DUPLICATIONS IN 46,XY FEMALES

A number of causes for the occurrence of 46,XY females are described in this book. Among them are *SRY*-positive individuals with duplications of Xp21 who illuminate the complexity of the testis-determination pathway. Bernstein and colleagues (1980) first described the occurrence of Xp duplications in some 46,XY females and hypothesized that a gene suppressing the Y-linked testis-determining factor might be involved. Because ZFX is included in many of the duplications, it was considered a candidate for the gene involved (Scherer et al., 1989). However, with the realization that ZFX escapes inactivation (normal females already have two expressed doses of the gene), this hypothesis was discarded. As more sex-reversed patients with Xp21 duplications were gathered and the region was more closely delimited, DAX1 (see also Chapter 3) became a candidate gene: its role in development (as discussed in Chapter 2) provides a workable hypothesis for a mechanism whereby Xp21 duplications suppress testes formation.

Clinical and Imaging Presentation.   As with many other causes of 46,XY females, the external genitalia look normal and the 46,XY karyotype is discovered only when a chromosome study is performed for some other reason, usually the presence of other congenital abnormalities. These abnormalities include neurological defects (hypotonia and mental retardation) cardiac abnormalities, oral-facial clefting, and other facial malformations (Bernstein et al., 1980; Scherer et al., 1989; Rao et al., 1994). Two patients described by Arn and colleagues (1994) had fewer malformations; mildly ambiguous genitalia in the first offspring of a woman carrying the duplication led to the diagnosis in this 46,XY female and a less ambiguous second daughter. Their carrier mother was apparently normal. Features suggestive of Turner syndrome were seen in one patient with 46,X,dup(X) (p11.4-p22.1) (Wyandt et al., 1991).

Ultrasonography or other imaging studies usually show normal müllerian derivatives. In some patients the intactness of müllerian derivatives has been confirmed at necropsy. The patients of Arn and colleagues (1994) were atypical: the müllerian derivatives were absent, although the gonads were dysgenetic.

Laboratory Features.   A variety of laboratory abnormalities related to the various congenital malformations have been described. Endocrine workups have been relatively sparse and have shown prepubertal levels of testosterone that do not increase with gonadotropin stimulation. To date, only visible Xp21 duplications have been described; differential genome hybridization in 46,XY females would probably disclose more cases of this entity.

Genotyping.   A series of patients, carefully characterized by Ogata and Matsuo (1994), had a small critical region with Xp21.2-p21.3. This was further refined to a 160-kb region by Bardoni and colleagues (1994). This region was shown to contain DAX1, a gene whose mutations cause adrenal hypoplasia congenita (Muscatelli et al., 1994; Zanaria et al., 1994); the treated survivors also have hypothalamic and pituitary defects (Habiby et al., 1996) but the hypothalmic-pituitary-gonadal axis is normal in infancy (Takahashi et al., 1997). Other genes are also found in this critical region (see Chapter 2). Nevertheless, the discovery that the mouse homologue of DAX1, Dax1, shows a pattern of expression in testes compatible with a requirement for DAX1 inactivation during testicular development (Swain et al., 1996) suggests that DAX1 is the gene responsible for the dosage-sensitive sex reversal (DSS) mapping to this region. This hypothesis is strengthened by the results of mice overexpressing Dax1 as the result of transgenesis (Swain et al., 1998). One transgenic line expressed five-fold normal levels of DAX1 at the proper developmental stage and location because the *Dax*1 promoter was used. This overexpression did not cause sex reversal (compared to frequent sex reversal in humans with assumed two-fold increases in expression) but did result in delayed testes development. When the transgene was expressed with a "weakened" *Sry* from a Y^POS (Eicher et al., 1982), about 20% of the mice showed sex reversal and another 20% were hermaphroditic (Swain et al., 1998). These results suggested that *DAX1* is the gene responsible for Xp21 duplication sex reversal, but the finding that the mouse knockout of *Dax1* has no gonadal abnormalities raises questions as to its overall importance (Yu et al., 1998).

One might predict that promoter mutations up-regulating expression of *DAX1* will eventually be found. The finding that apparently comparable duplications do not always lead to sex reversal (Arn et al., 1994; Baumstark et al., 1996) suggests that position effects or modifying genes influence the phenotype. Monosomy in this region (46,X,delX) is compatible with fertility (Fitzgerald et al., 1984). Hypogenitalism in a boy with an Xp duplication 2 mbp distal to DSS is unlikely to be caused by a position effect acting on *DAX1* (Telvi et al., 1996).

Management. When the genitalia of newborns are mildly or moderately ambiguous, surgical correction and sex assignment as a female are usually indicated. Because the portion of the Y chromosome with the potential to stimulate gonadoblastoma formation is present (when a gonad is at the 37°C internal temperature), streak gonads should be removed as in other cases of Y chromosome–containing, intra-abdominal gonadal tissue. Management includes treatment of the congenital malformations that usually lead to the diagnosis of the condition. Finally, hormonal replacement to obtain optimal growth and secondary sexual characteristics is indicated.

Discussion. Among 46,XY females, Xp21 duplications are one among many causes of this female karyotype. As with many of the other causes, Xp21 duplication is likely to be an unexpected finding when a karyotype is done for some other reason, usually to elucidate the etiology of multiple congenital malformations. Occasionally, it is discovered accidentally. One would expect a number of 46,XY females to be discovered from karyotypes performed for primary amenorrhea. However, at least in our experience, most cases have been discovered from karyotypes performed by pediatric geneticists, not endocrinologists.

The importance of this cause of sex reversal is the information it provides about the complexity of multiple pathways involved in gonadal differentiation. The evidence that the mouse homologue *Dax1* is expressed and then extinguished in the early developing testis while expression continues to increase in the developing ovary (Swain et al., 1996) suggests that continued expression in the testes is harmful for testicular development. Furthermore, the gonads would be dysgenic because XY germ cells have low potential for forming the oocytes essential for normal ovary development. Much remains to be learned about the etiology of this disorder. Why have some cases not had müllerian derivatives? Would promoter mutations sometimes result in overexpression of *DAX1* without a duplication, hence, result in sex reversal? The *DAX1* promoter contains an SF-1 binding element (Guo et al., 1996), so could alterations in SF-1 result in overexpression of *DAX1*? Finally, what is the interaction between *DAX1* and *SRY* (or genes controlled by *SRY*) that leads to arrest of testicular development?

REFERENCES

Arn P, Chen H, Tuck-Muller C M, Mankinen C, Wachtel G, Li S, Shen C C, Wachtel S S (1994). *SRX*, a sex reversing locus in Xp21.2-p22.11. *Hum Genet* 93:389–393.

Bardoni B, Zanaria E, Guioli S, Floridia G, Worley K C, Tonini G, Ferrante E, Chiumello G, McCabe E R B, Fraccaro M, Zuffardi O, Camerino G (1994). A dosage sensitive locus at chromosome Xp21 is involved in male to female sex reversal. *Nat Genet* 7:497–501.

Baumstark A, Barbi G, Djalali M, Geerkens C, Mitulla B, Mattfeldt T, de Almeida J C C, Vargas F R, Llerena J C Jr Vogel W, Just W (1996). Xp-duplications with and without sex reversal. *Hum Genet* 97:79–86.

Bernstein R, Jenkins T, Dawson B, Wagner J, Dewald G, Koo G C, Wachtel S S (1980). Female phenotype and multiple abnormalities in sibs with a Y chromosome and partial X chromosome duplication: H-Y antigen and Xg blood group findings. *J Med Genet* 17:291–300.

Eicher E M, Washburn L L, Whitney B, Morrow K E (1982). *Mus poschiavinus* Y chromosome in the C57BL/6J murine genome causes sex reversal. *Science* 217:535–537.

Fitzgerald P H, Donald R A, McCormick P (1984). Reduced fertility in women with X chromosome abnormality. *Clin Genet* 25:301–304.

Guo W, Burris T P, Zhang Y-H, Huang B-L, Mason J, Copeland K C, Kupfer S R, Pagon R A, McCabe E R B (1996). Genomic sequence of the *DAX1* gene: an orphan nuclear receptor responsible for X-linked adrenal hypoplasia congenita and hypogonadotropic hypogonadism. *J Clin Endocrinol Metab* 81:2481–2486.

Habiby R L, Boepple P, Nachtigall L, Sluss P M, Crowley, W F Jr, Jameson J L (1996). Adrenal hypoplasia congenita with hypogonadotropic hypogonadism evidence that *DAX-1* mutations lead to combined hypothalamic and pituitary defects in gonadotropin production. *J Clin Invest* 98:1055–1062.

Muscatelli F, Strom T M, Walker A P, Zanaria E, Récan D, Meindl A, Bardoni B, Guioli S, Zehetner G, Rabl W, Schwarz H P, Kaplan J-C, Camerino G, Meitinger T, Monaco A P (1994). Mutations in the *DAX-1* gene give rise to both X-linked adrenal hypoplasia congenita and hypogonadotropic hypogonadism. *Nature* 372:672–676.

Ogata T, Matsuo N (1994). Testis-determining gene(s) on the X chromosome short arm: chromosomal localisation and possible role in testis determination. *J Med Genet* 31:349–350.

Rao P N, Klinepeter K, Stewart W, Hayworth R, Grubs R, Pettenati M J (1994). Molecular cytogenetic analysis of a duplication Xp in a male: further delineation of a possible sex influencing region on the X chromosome. *Hum Genet* 94:149–153.

Scherer G, Schempp W, Baccichetti C, Lenzini E, Bricarelli F D, Carbone L D L, Wolf U (1989). Duplication of an Xp segment that includes the ZFX locus causes sex inversion in man. *Hum Genet* 81:291–294.

Swain A, Zanaria E, Hacker A, Lovell-Badge R, Camerino G (1996). Mouse *DAX1* expression is consistent with a role in sex determination as well as in adrenal and hypothalamus function. *Nat Genet* 12:404–409.

Swain A, Narvaez V, Burgoyne P, Camerino G, Lovell-Badge R (1998). *Dax1* antagonizes *Sry* action in mammalian sex determination. *Nature* 391:761–767.

Takahashi T, Shoji Y, Shoji Y, Haraguchi N, Takahashi I, Takada G (1997). Active hypothalamic-pituitary-gonadal axis in an infant with X-linked adrenal hypoplasia congenita. *J Pediatr* 130:485–488.

Telvi L, Ion A, Carel J-C, Desguerre I, Piraud M, Boutin A M, Feingold J, Ponsot G, Fellous M, McElreavey K. (1996). A duplication of distal Xp associated with hypogonadotrophic hypogonadism, hypoplastic external genitalia, mental retardation, and multiple congenital abnormalities. *J Med Genet* 33:767–771.

Wyandt H E. Bugeau-Michaud L, Skare J C, Milunsky A. (1991). Partial duplication of Xp: a case report and review of previously reported cases. *Am J Med Genet* 40:280–283.

Yu R N, Ito M, Saunders T L, Camper S A, Jameson J L (1998). Role of *Ahch* in gonadal development and gametogenesis. *Nat Genet* 20:353–357.

Zanaria E, Muscatelli F, Bardoni B, Strom T M, Guioli S, Guo W, Lalli E, Moser C, Walker A P, McCabe E R. (1994). An unusual member of the nuclear hormone receptor superfamily responsible for X-linked adrenal hypoplasia congenita. *Nature* 372:635–641.

OVARIAN FAILURE WITH CHROMOSOMAL MUTATIONS OF XQ

It has long been known that deletions of the short arm of X are associated with features of Turner syndrome. Deletions of Xq are frequently associated with infertility (see Chapter 6; Goldman et al., 1982). As discussed in Chapter 2, it has been hypothesized that there is a critical region at Xq13-q27 that must be intact in both X chromosomes for normal ovarian development to occur (Sarto et al., 1973; Summitt et al., 1978). Distal Xq deletions seem to have milder degrees of infertility (Kaiser et al., 1984). This cause of ovarian failure is the subject of this section.

Clinical and Imaging Presentation.   Many of these patients present with primary amenorrhea, but oligomenorrhea and early menopause (secondary amenorrhea) also occur (Kaiser et al., 1984; Krauss et al., 1987). Those in the latter group may transmit their condition to their daughters (Krauss et al., 1987; Bates and Howard, 1990; Veneman et al., 1991). Mild, Turner-like features are sometimes described, such as cubitus valgus (Dar et al., 1988), but this may represent an ascertainment bias—patients with menstrual irregularities who have some features of Turner syndrome are probably more likely to be karyotyped.

Laboratory Features.   A wide variety of deletions has been reported; Kaiser and colleagues (1984) reviewed 24 cases from the literature with different deletions of Xq. Paracentric inversions have also been reported (Dar et al., 1988). Plasma gonadotropin levels are usually high and estradiol low or normal. In patients with low estradiol, the response to hCG may sometimes be normal—see, for example, Kaiser and colleagues (1984).

Genotype.   The great variety of deletion and translocation or inversion (Madariaga and Rivera, 1997) breakpoints suggests that there is not a single gene involved in ovarian development. In fact, one study of the location of eleven X-autosome breakpoints associated with secondary amenorrhea concluded that at least eight genes in Xq21 are involved (Sala et al., 1997). These include genes located at Xq 13.3–q21.1 (Powell et al., 1994), Xq21.3–q27 (Krauss et al., 1987), and Xq 26.1–q27 (Thorapel et al., 1993). The early menopause found in fragile X carriers suggests that *FRX-1* might be one of the genes involved in ovarian function (Cronister et al., 1991; Partington et al., 1996; Vianna-Morgante et al., 1996).

Management.   Because the amenorrhea, oligomenorrhea, and/or early menopause is the result of a primary ovarian failure, there is no treatment. These women, like other women with ovarian failure, could carry pregnancies from donated eggs.

Discussion.   As discussed in Chapter 2, the variability of both the effects and the locations of deletions suggest that there are multiple X genes involved in female fertility. It seems probable that absence or decreased expression of a single gene may be compatible with years of ovarian function followed by early menopause. A loss of more than one gene may be associated with oligomenorrhea or amenorrhea (Fitzgerald et al., 1984). There are also autosomal genes that can cause 46,XX, hypogonadotropic-hypogonadism (Aittomäki, 1994), one of which maps to 3q22–q23 and may be associated with eyelid malformations (Amati et al., 1996); thus it is clear that, as with testes determination, both X-linked and autosomal genes are required for normal ovarian development.

REFERENCES

Aittomäki K (1994). The genetics of XX gonadal dysgenesis. *Am J Hum Genet* 54:844–851.

Amati P, Gasparini P, Zlotogora J, Zelante L, Chomel J C, Kitzis A, Kaplan J, Bonneau D (1996). A gene for premature ovarian failure associated with eyelid malformation maps to chromosome 3q22-q23. *Am J Hum Genet* 58:1089–1092. Letter to the Editor.

Bates A, Howard P J (1990). Distal long arm deletions of the X chromosome and ovarian failure. *J Med Genet* 27:722–723.

Cronister A, Schreiner R, Wittenburger M, Amiri K, Harris K, Hagerman R J (1991). Heterozygous fragile X female: historical, physical, cognitive, and cytogenetic figures. *Am J Med Genet* 38:269–274.

Dar H, Tal J, Bar-el I I, Halpern I, Sharf M (1988). Paracentric inversion of Xq and ovarian dysfunction. *Am J Med Genet* 29:167–170.

Fitzgerald P H, Donald R A, McCormick P (1984). Reduced fertility in women with X chromosome abnormality. *Clin Genet* 25:301–309.

Goldman B, Polani P E, Daker M G, Angell R R (1982) Clinical and cytogenetic aspects of X-chromosome deletions. *Clin Genet* 21:36–52.

Kaiser P, Harprecht W, Steuernagel P, Daume E (1984). Long arm deletions of the X chromosome and their symptoms: a new case (bp q24) and a short review of the literature. *Clin Genet* 16:433–439.

Krauss C M, Turksoy R N, Atkins L, McLaughlin C, Brown L G, Page D C (1987). Familial premature ovarian failure due to an interstitial deletion of the long arm of the X chromosome. *N Eng J Med* 317:125–131.

Madariaga M L, Rivera H (1997). Familial inv(X) (p22q22): ovarian dysgenesis in two sisters with del Xq and fertility in one male carrier. *Clin Genet* 52:180–183.

Partington M W, Moore Dy, Turner G M (1996). Confirmation of early menopause in fragile X carriers. *Am J Med Genet* 64:370–372.

Powell, C M, Taggart R T, Drumheller T C, Wangsa D, Qian C, Nelson L M, White B J (1994). Molecular and cytogenetic studies of an X: autosome translocation in a patient with premature ovarian failure and review of the literature. *Am J Med Genet* 52:19–26.

Sala C, Arrigo G, Torri G, Martinazzi F, Riva P, Larizza L, Philipe C, Jonveaux P, Sloan F, Labella T, Toniolo D (1997). Eleven X chromosome breakpoints associated with premature ovarian failure (POF) map to a 15-Mb YAC contig spanning Xq21. *Genomics* 40:123–131.

Sarto G E, Therman E, Patau K (1973). X inactivation in man: a woman with t(Xq−; 12q+). *Am J Hum Genet* 25:262–270.

Summitt R L, Tipton R E, Wilroy Jr. R S, Martens P R, Phelan J P (1978). X-autosome translocations: a review. *Birth Defects* 14:219–247.

Tharapel A T, Anderson K P, Simpson J L, Martens P R, Wilroy Jr R S, Llerene Jr J C, Schwartz C E (1993). Deletion (X)(q26.−>q28) in a proband and her mother: molecular characterization and phenotypic-karyotypic deductions. *Am J Hum Genet* 52:463–471.

Veneman T F, Beverstock G C, Exalto N, Mollevanger P (1991). Premature menopause because of an inherited deletion in the long arm of the X chromosome. *Fertil Steril* 55:631–633.

Vianna-Morgante A M, Costa S S, Pares A S, Verreschi I T N (1996). FRAXA premutation associated with premature ovarian failure. *Am J Med Genet* 64:373–375.

46,XX MALES WITH *SRY*

Therkelsen (1964) and Ferguson-Smith (1966) proposed that 46,XX males were the result of an X-Y interchange such that a small piece of the Y chromosome that contained the testes-determining factor was translocated to the X. This hypothesis explained other data on anomalous inheritance of Xg[a], an X-linked blood group found by de la Chapelle and colleagues (1964). With improvements in karyotypic techniques, there were reports of 46,XX males with altered length or altered banding patterns of one X's short arm (Evans et al., 1979; Magenis et al., 1982). The ability to clone segments of the Y chromosome confirmed the presence of Y-derived single-copy DNA in 46,XX males (Guellaen et al., 1984; Müller et al., 1985; Page et al., 1985; Affara et al., 1986). The two levels of observations were joined by *in situ* hybridization showing that the Y-derived sequences were indeed in the extra material on Xp (Andersson et al., 1986; Magenis et al., 1987). A full historical perspective is provided by de la Chapelle (1986). A subgroup of 46,XX males who present in infancy with congenital malformations are clinically and molecularly distinct (no *SRY*; Fechner et al., 1993) and may best be considered with 46,XX true hermaphroditism (see Chapter 7).

Clinical and Imaging Presentation.   46,XX males tend to be identified at one of two stages in the life cycle. As do some patients with Klinefelter syndrome (Chapter 6), they may produce inadequate testosterone and show incomplete virilization at puberty. Thus, about one third have gynecomastia, and facial hair may be scant (Wachtel and Bard, 1981). External genitalia are usually normal, although one of the first cases was notable for a small penis and scrotum (de la Chapelle et al., 1964); undermasculinization, in the form of hypospadias, has been reported in other cases (de la Chapelle, 1972; Kasdan et al., 1973; López, et al., 1995). The second period of ascertainment is among azoospermic males seen at infertility clinics. In our experience, the ratio of men found in infertility clinics to teenagers identified by incomplete virilization is also about 2 to 1 (Stalvey et al., 1989; Verga and Erickson, 1989; López et al., 1995). Familial 46,XX males are usually true hermaphrodites and will be discussed under 46,XX true hermaphroditism in Chapter 7.

46,XX males are shorter than XY males, indicating that the Y chromosome codes for a "growth factor." The identity of the growth factor is not known, but it is not related to the ordinary androgen/estrogen differences between the two sexes. Chromosomally male individuals who lack androgen receptors are, on the average, taller than normal females and average for males (Ferguson-Smith, 1991). Likewise, a

TABLE 6–1. Heights of XX and XY Individuals with Various Conditions*

	Height in CM	
	XY Individuals	*XX Individuals*
Normal	174.7 ± 6.7	162.2 ± 6.0
Testicular feminization (androgen insensitivity)	172.2 ± 6.5	—
Pure gonadal dysgenesis	172 ± 7	164.3 ± 7.7
XX males	—	166.4 ± 7.4

*Taken from Ogata and Matsuo, 1993.

male who lacked estrogen receptors continued growing well into adulthood (Korach, 1994) (and to a height of seven feet) indicating that in humans, as in mice
(Lubahn et al., 1993), estrogens are needed to stop growth. However, lower female
heights are not solely due to elevated estrogens: in the absence of estrogen, XY
patients with pure gonadal dysgenesis (PGD) are taller than XX patients with PGD
(Ogata and Matsuo, 1992), just as XY males are taller than XX males (see Table 6–
1; Ogata and Matsuo, 1993). The mechanism by which XXY Klinefelter patients
become taller than normal XY men has not been shown, but it cannot be a simple
consequence of disturbed andogen:estrogen balance, because increased stature often
becomes apparent before puberty and because their body proportions differ from
the classical ones associated with simple eunuchoidism.

These differences are due to a Y-specific gene that has been tentatively mapped
to different Y chromosome intervals by different groups, each comparing heights
of patients with various Yq deletions: 4B-5A (Barbaux et al., 1995; Salo et al., 1995a;
Rousseaux-Prévost et al., 1996) or 5C-5D (Ogata et al., 1995). This gene has been
named growth control Y (GCY). Thus, there may be two Yq loci for GCY but patients
with similar deletions can have quite variable features (Salo et al., 1995b). It has
been hypothesized that the gene is primarily involved in prepubertal growth and
possibly fetal growth (Ogata and Matsuo, 1997).

Laboratory Studies.   By definition, cytogenetic studies should reveal a 46,XX karyotype (after an extensive chromosomal analysis to exclude mosaicism and autosomal structural abnormalities); high-resolution karyotype (Evans et al., 1979) or
flow karyotype analysis (Carter et al., 1990) may disclose a size difference in the
two Xs. Gonadotropin values range from prepubertal concentrations to hypergonadotropic levels, depending on the probands' developmental stage. As in Klinefelter
syndrome (see above), persistently elevated serum gonadotropin levels are usually
found in postpubertal subjects; prepubertal subjects have age-appropriate gonadotropin levels. In the postpubertal subjects, basal serum testosterone is below or at
normal values whereas prepubertal subjects have age-appropriate basal testosterone
concentrations (La Franchi et al., 1980). Estradiol concentrations have been within
normal ranges. In adults, semen analysis reveals azoospermia, and gonadal biopsies
show Leydig cell hyperplasia, seminiferous tubule hypoplasia, and absence of germ
cells. 47,XXX males also occur (Scherer et al., 1989).

Genotyping.   By definition, molecular studies for *SRY* are positive in these individuals. *ZFY* is not always present (see Chapter 5). The molecular basis for the
abnormal X-Y interchange has been extensively studied (Fig. 6–1). The normal pairing of the human X and Y chromosomes during meiosis is initiated within the
pseudoautosomal (homologous) region (Pearson and Bobrow, 1970; Rappold, 1993).
This pairing was observed to extend beyond the homologous region in some cases
(Chandley et al., 1984), predisposing to an unequal X-Y interchange. Sex vesicle
"entrapment" during the first meiotic prophase may promote association of the Yp
fragment with the X pseudoautosomal region (Stalvey et al., 1989). Many studies
of the breakpoints involved have been reported. These studies reveal the importance of X:Y homology outside the pseudoautosomal region, both in unique sequence and shared tandem repeats. Molecular analyses of the breakpoints in the
DNA of one patient indicated homologous recombination between *Alu* sequences

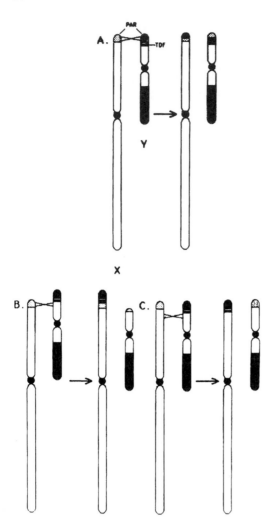

FIGURE 6–1. Hypothetical representation of the interaction between Xp and Yp in the pseudoautosomal region (PAR) during meiosis (A) resulting in normal inheritance of the testis-determining factor (TDF) on the Y; (B) resulting in a nonhomologous interchange moving TDF to the X; or (C) resulting in an illegitimate crossing over moving TDF to the X. (From Stalvey et al., *Am J Med Genet* 32:564–572, 1989; by permission.)

that were surrounded by otherwise non-homologous regions (Rouyer et al., 1987). Müller and colleagues (1989) identified two blocks of 20 kb, tandemly repeated Y-chromosome-specific DNA sequences between which chromosomal breaks occurred in the translocations found in five of six 46,XX males positive for the repeat sequences and in the deletions of Yp in two of three 46,XY females. Petit and colleagues (1990) also identified a repeated DNA element, which was not only shared by the X and Y in the pseudoautosomal region but was also found centromeric to the pseudoautosomal region on the X-specific part of Xp22.3, as a potential site of interchange. In further studies, this group has provided extensive molecular analyses of breakpoints in XX males, concluding that the presence of the repeated elements is not essential—rather, the high homology of X and Y loci at the breakpoints is causative (Weil et al., 1994; Wang et al., 1995). Although a L1 (long-interspersed repeat) element was involved in one patient and an *Alu* repeat, left monomer, in another, the 98.7% sequence homology in one case at and near the breakpoint, and a 96% sequence homology in another, emphasized the importance of overall homology rather than these repeat elements (Weil et al., 1994). A newly described protein kinase gene with Xp22.3 and Yp copies sharing the same orientation is also a frequent site for exchanges (Schiebel et al., 1997). The presence of Yq sequences in a 46,XX male was surprising but could be explained by an unequal interchange between an X and an inverted Y chromosome presumed present in the patient's father (Donlon and Müller, 1991).

Management. Testosterone replacement is appropriate for patients with hypergonadotropic hypogonadism. Artificial insemination by donor may be offered to the partners of the azoospermic males.

Discussion. If pairing is not accurate during some meioses, misaligned, not perfectly homologous regions on the X and Y chromosomes may be entrapped by the formation of the synaptonemal complex or the sex vesicle, the term for the condensed X:Y seen during spermatogenesis. The pseudoautosomal region has a frequency of crossing over during male meiosis that is 10 to 20-fold greater than the rest of the genome (Rouyer et al., 1986). As presented above, juxtaposition of like sequences within otherwise nonhomologous regions may provide enough homology to create an "effective" pairing in a "hot spot" region and allow crossing over to occur (Weil et al., 1994; Wang et al., 1995).

Fryns and colleagues (1985) reviewed the literature on Y:autosome translocations from the early 1970s; they found approximately 40 cases and divided them into two general types. The first class included translocations with familial transmission, most of which were detected accidentally because there were few phenotypic effects. Of these, the most common type involved chromosome 15 (10 of 17 families) and chromosome 22 (3 of 17 families). The other group of translocations were *de novo* Y:autosome translocations that had more serious phenotypic effects: all patients were sterile. The physical isolation provided by the sex vesicle might be expected to largely prevent translocation of broken fragments of Yp to autosomes and, instead, enhance the possibility of their attachment to Xp. If one compares the Y:autosome translocation frequency with the frequency of XX males, the putative role of the sex vesicle in enhancing X:Y exchanges seems clear. As mentioned earlier, the frequency of XX males is approximately one in 20,000 phenotypic males. Therefore, assuming a birth rate of approximately 10 million/year for the years and countries covered in the review by Fryns and colleagues (1985), and with a sex ratio of about 50%, in any one year approximately five million males would be born, of which 250 might be expected to be XX males. Thus, for any one year, six times more XX males should be present than the total number of Y:autosome translocations reported in the over-10-year study period (Fryns et al., 1985). Of course, reporting of patients is not complete and additional Y:autosome translocations with no phenotypic effect probably go undetected. Nonetheless, there does seem to be at least an order of magnitude difference between Y:autosome and X:Y translocations. This argues for a role of the sex vesicle in maintaining X:Y proximity during the later stages of meiosis. Such proximity could lead to preferential translocation of Yp to Xp during meiosis and thus increase the incidence of XX males compared with other Y:X or Y:autosome translocations. The incidence of 46, XY females (i.e., the reciprocal crossover product) appears to be lower than the incidence of these 46, XX males (Levilliers et al., 1989). If this is not merely an ascertainment bias, if could reflect the loss of a lymphogenesis gene (see Chapter 6) leading to prenatal lethality as seen in Turner syndrome (Ogata and Matsuo, 1995).

REFERENCES

Affara N A, Ferguson-Smith M A, Tolmie J, Kwok K, Mitchell M, Jamieson D, Cooke A, Florentin L (1986). Variable transfer of Y-specific sequences in XX males. *Nucleic Acids Res* 14:5375–5387.

Andersson M, Page D C, de la Chapelle A (1986) Chromosome Y-specific DNA is transferred to the short arm of X chromosome in human XX males. *Science* 233:786–788.

Barbaux S, Vilain E, Raoul O, Gilgenkrantz S, Jeandidier E, Chadenas D, Souleyreau N, Fellous M, McElreavey K (1995). Proximal deletions of the long arm of the Y chromosome suggest a critical region associated with a specific subset of characteristic Turner stigmata. *Hum Mol Genet* 4:1565–1568.

Carter N P, Ferguson-Smith M E, Affara N A, Briggs H, Ferguson-Smith M A (1990). Study of X chromosome abnormality in XX males using bivariate flow karyotype analysis and flow sorted dot blots. *Cytometry* 11:202–207.

Chandley A C, Goetz P, Hargreave T B, Joseph A M, Speed R M (1984). On the nature and extent of XY pairing at meiotic prophase in man. *Cytogenet Cell Genet* 38:241–247.

de la Chapelle A, Hortling H, Niemi M, Wennstrom J (1964). XX Sex chromosomes in a human male: first case. *Acta Med Scand (Suppl)* 412:25–28. 1964.

de la Chapelle A. (1972) Analytic review: nature and origin of males with XX sex chromosomes. *Am J Hum Genet* 24:71–105.

de la Chapelle A (1986) Genetic and molecular studies on 46, XX and 45, X males. *Cold Spring Harbor Symp Quant Biol* 51:249–255.

Donlon T A, Müller U (1991). Deletion mapping of DNA segments from the Y chromosome long arm and their analysis in an XX male. *Genomics* 10:51–56.

Evans H J, Buckton K E, Spowart G, Carothers A D (1979). Heteromorphic X chromosomes in 46, XX males: evidence for the involvement of X-Y interchange. *Hum Genet* 49:11–31.

Fechner P Y, Marcantonio S M, Jaswaney V, Stetten G, Goodfellow P N, Migeon C J, Smith K D, Berkowitz G D (1993). The role of the sex-determining region Y gene in the etiology of 46,XX maleness. *J Clin Endocrinol Metab* 76:690–695.

Ferguson-Smith M A (1966). X-Y chromosomal interchange in the aetiology of true hermaphroditism and of XX Klinefelter's syndrome. *Lancet* 2:475–476.

Ferguson-Smith M A (1991). Genotype-phenotype correlations in individuals with disorders of sex determination and development including Turner's syndrome. *Semin Dev Biol* 2: 265–276.

Fryns J P, Kleczkowska A, van den Berghe H (1985). Clinical manifestations of Y/autosome translocations in man. In: Sandberg AA (ed.). The Y Chromosome, Part B: *Clinical Aspects of Y Chromosome Abnormalities*. New York: Alan R. Liss, pp 213–243.

Guellaen G, Casanova M, Bishop C, Geldworth D, Andre G, Fellous M, Weissenbach J (1984). Human XX males with Y single-copy DNA fragments. *Nature* 307:172–173.

Kasdan R, Nankin H R, Troen P, Wald N, Pan S, Yanaihara T (1973). Paternal transmission of maleness in XX human beings. *N Engl J Med* 288:539–545.

Korach K S (1994). Insights from the study of animals lacking functional estrogen receptor. *Science* 193:1134–1135.

LaFranchi S, Magenis E R, Prescott G H (1980). Variation in pituitary-gonadal function in two adolescent boys with 46XX male syndrome. *J Pediatr* 97:960–962.

Levilliers J, Quack B, Weissenbach J, Petit C (1989). Exchange of terminal portions of X and Y chromosomal short arms in human XY females. *Proc Natl Acad Sci USA* 86:2296–2300.

López M, Torres L, Méndez J P, Cervantes A, Pérez-Palacios G, Erickson R P, Alfaro G, Kofman-Alfaro S (1995). Clinical traits and molecular findings in 46, XX males. *Clin Genet* 48:29–34.

Lubahn D B, Moyer J S, Golding T S, Couse J F, Korach K S, Smithies O (1993). Alteration of reproductive function but not prenatal sexual development after insertional disruption of the mouse estrogen receptor gene. *Proc Natl Acad Sci USA* 90:11162–11166.

Magenis R E, Webb M J, McKean R S, Tomar D, Allen L J, Kammer H, VanDyke D L, Lovrien E (1982). Translocation (X:Y) (p 22.33; p 11.2) in XX males: etiology of male phenotype. *Hum Genet* 62:271–276.

Magenis R E, Casanova M, Fellous M, Olson S, Sheehy R (1987). Further cytologic evidence for Xp-Yp translocation in XX males using in situ hybridization with Y-derived probe. *Hum Genet* 75:228–233.

Müller U, Lalande M, Donlon T, Latt S A (1985). Moderately repeated DNA sequences specific for the short arm of the human Y chromosome are present in XX males and reduced in copy number in an XY female. *Nucleic Acids Res* 14:1325–1340.

Müller U, Lalande M, Donlon T A, Heartlein M W (1989). Breakage of the human Y-chromosome short arm between two blocks of tandemly repeated DNA sequences. *Genomics* 5:153–156.

Ogata T, Matsuo N (1992). Comparison of adult height between patients with XX and XY gonadal dysgenesis: support for a Y specific growth gene(s). *J Med Genet* 29:539–541.

Ogata T, Matsuo N (1993). Sex chromosome aberrations and stature: deduction of the principal factors involved in the determination of adult height. *Hum Genet* 91:551–562.

Ogata T, Matsuo N (1995). Turner syndrome and female sex chromosome aberrations: deduction of the principal factors involved in the development of clinical features. *Hum Genet* 95:607–629.

Ogata T, Matsuo N (1997). The Y specific growth gene(s): how does it promote stature? *J Med Genet* 34:323–325.

Ogata T, Tomita K, Hida A, Matsuo N, Nakahori Y, Nakagome Y (1995). Chromosomal localisation of a Y specific growth gene(s). *J Med Genet* 32:572–575.

Page D C, de la Chapelle A, Weissenbach J (1985). Chromosome Y-specific DNA in related human XX males. *Nature* 315:224–226.

Pearson P L, Bobrow M (1970). Definitive evidence for the short arm of the Y chromosome associating with the X chromosome during meiosis in the human male. *Nature* 226:959–961.

Petit C, Levilliers J, Rouyer F, Simmler M C, Herouin E, Weissenbach J (1990). Isolation of sequences from Xp22.3 and deletion mapping using sex chromosome rearrangements from human X-Y interchange sex reversals. *Genomics* 6:651–658.

Rappold G A (1993). The pseudoautosomal regions of the human sex chromosomes. *Hum Genet* 92:315–324.

Rousseaux-Prévost R, Rigot J-M, Delobel B, Lesur P, Collier F, Croquette M-F, Gauthier A, Mazeman E, Rousseaux J (1996). Molecular mapping of a Yq deletion in a patient with normal stature. *Hum Genet* 98:505–507.

Rouyer F, Simmler M C, Johnson C, Vergnaud G, Cooke H, Weissenbach J (1986). A gradient of sex linkage in pseudoautosomal region of the human sex chromosomes. *Nature* 319:291–295.

Rouyer R, Simmler M C, Page D C, Weissenbach J (1987). A sex chromosome rearrangement in a human XX male caused by *Alu-Alu* recombination. *Cell* 51:417–425.

Salo P, Kääriäinen H, Page D C, de la Chapelle A (1995). Deletion mapping of stature determinants on the long arm of the Y chromosome. *Hum Genet* 95:283–286.

Salo P, Ignatius J, Simola K O J, Tahvanainen E, Kääriäinen H (1995b). Clinical features of nine males with molecularly defined deletions of the Y chromosome long arm. *J Med Genet* 32:711–715.

Scherer G, Schempp W, Fraccaro M, Bausch E, Bigozzi V, Maruschio P, Montali E, Simon G, Wolf U (1989). Analysis of two 47,XXX males reveals X-Y interchange and maternal or paternal nondisjunction. *Hum Genet* 81:247–251.

Schiebel K, Winkelmann M, Mertz A, Xu X, Page D C, Weil D, Petit C, Rappold G A (1997). Abnormal XY interchange between a novel isolated protein kinase gene, *PRKY*, and its homologue, *PRKX*, accounts for one third of all (Y+)XX males and (Y-)XY females. *Hum Mol Genet* 6:1985–1989.

Stalvey J R D, Durbin E J, Erickson R P (1989). Sex vesicle "entrapment": translocation or nonhomologous recombination of misaligned Yp and Xp as alternative mechanisms for abnormal inheritance of the sex-determining region. *Am J Med Genet* 32:564–572.

Therkelsen A J (1964). Sterile man with chromosomal constitution, 46, XX. *Cytogenetics* 3:207–218.

Verga V, Erickson R P (1989). An extended long range restriction map of the human sex-determining region on Yp, including *ZFY*, finds marked homology on Xp and no detectable Y sequences in a XX male. *Am J Hum Genet* 44:756–765.

Wachtel S S, Bard J (1981). The XX testis. *Pediatr Adoles Endocrinol* 8:116–132.

Wang I, Weil D, Levilliers J, Affara N A, de la Chapelle A, Petit C (1995). Prevalence and molecular analysis of two hot spots for ectopic recombination leading to XX maleness. *Genomics* 28:52–58.

Weil D, Wang I, Dietrich A, Poustka A, Weissenbach J, Petit C (1994). Highly homologous loci on the X and Y chromosomes are hot spots for ectopic recombinations leading to XX maleness. *Nat Genet* 7:414–419.

X-linked Single-Gene Disorders:
Male Pseudohermaphroditism in the X-linked
α-Thalassemia/Mental Retardation Syndrome

The association of α-thalassemia and mental retardation is a rare event. Sometimes this is due to deletions of the tip of chromosome 16p where the α-globin cluster is located. In contrast, an X-linked form, which sometimes includes 46,XY females, has been mapped to Xq12-q21.31 (Gibbons et al., 1992). This entity, ATR-X, has been associated with point mutations in *XH2* (or *ATRX*), a gene showing homology to the SNF2 superfamily (named after the yeast SW12/SNF2 protein, a DNA-dependent ATPase with putative DNA helicase domains) that includes transcriptional regulators (Gibbons et al., 1995b). This entity has been reviewed recently (Gibbons et al., 1995a). Another X-linked single gene disorder at Xq28 is suggested by the finding of two patients with extended deletions at the myotubular myopathy locus who also had micropenis and severe hypospadias, but the histology of the gonads was not described (Hu et al., 1996). Nonetheless, these sex-reversed patients indicate the possibility of additional gene(s) located in this chromosomal region.

Clinical and Imaging Presentation.   The most striking feature of these patients is the severe mental retardation, which presents in the neonatal period (Weatherall et al., 1981). Hypotonia and feeding difficulties are common. Walking is greatly delayed and toilet training is seldom achieved. The characteristic facial appearance includes a flat nasal bridge, a short up-turned nose, and a "carp-shaped" mouth (Wilkie et al., 1990, 1991). Partial ocular albinism without alpha-thalassemia was

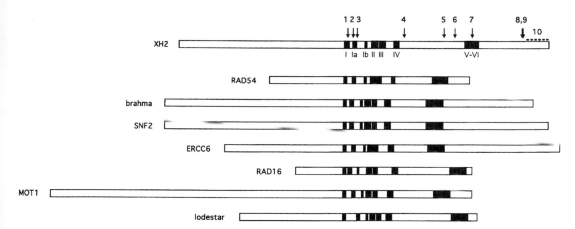

FIGURE 6–2. *XH2* (or *ATRX*) is a member of a putative DNA helicase family. The black bars (I–VI) show the helicase domains common to this group. The position of some *XH2* mutations (1–10) that have been characterized in ATR-X patients are shown: 1–7 are missense mutations; 8 and 9 are in-frame premature stop codons; 10 is a deletion. (From Gibbons et al., *Hum Mol Genet* 4:1705–1709, 1995a; by permission.)

recently reported in one pedigree (see below; Ion et al., 1996). The severity of the sexual ambiguity ranges from undescended testes and hypogenitalism to hypospadias and even to female external genitalia despite a 46,XY karyotype (McPherson et al., 1995; Reardon et al., 1995). The male pseudohermaphrodites have dysgenetic testes, but no female internal organs.

Laboratory Features. The hematological abnormalities include the form of α-thalassemia termed hemoglobin H (B^4) disease, with smaller amounts of hypochromia and lower levels of hemoglobin H than found in other forms of this condition (McPherson et al., 1995). The hematological abnormalities may include no more than a small percentage of red blood cells with hemoglobin H inclusions that are detected by incubating the red blood cells with 1% brilliant cresyl blue (McPherson et al., 1995): in one family, there was no evidence of hematological abnormalities (Ion et al., 1996). Mild hematological abnormalities may be found in female carriers of ATR-X. A skewed X-inactivation pattern with the mutant X inactivated has been seen in cells from a variety of tissues in the carriers (Gibbons et al., 1992). These findings suggest that a hematological workup should be considered in mentally retarded boys with ambiguous genitalia.

Genotyping. The locations of 25 mutations have been defined (Gibbons et al., 1995a; Picketts et al., 1996; Gibbons et al., 1997) (Fig. 6–2). One familial splice site junction mutation was always associated with mental retardation and the characteristic facial dysmorphism but α-thalassemia was not present in a mutant individual with 30% normal transcripts (Villard et al., 1996a). The mutations causing sexual ambiguity are predominantly located in the C-terminal portion of the molecule, close to, or in the helicase domains common to, the SNH2 family. Originally, premature stop codons and deletions were found only at the extreme C-terminus of the molecule, but extension of the sequence in the N-terminus identified a zinc finger domain that was also highly mutated (Gibbons et al., 1997). These N-terminal mutations are associated with less sexual ambiguity (R. J. Gibbons, personal communication). A separate syndrome, the Juberg-Marsidi syndrome, has also been found to be caused by mutations in *XH2* (or *ATRX*; Villard et al., 1996b). This is a syndrome of severe mental retardation, growth failure, sensorineural deafness, microgenitalism (severe hypogenitalism), and early death. This mutation was located in the helicase V domain of the gene (see Fig. 6–2).

Management.   This is a disorder of severe mental retardation for which there is no special management. The hematological abnormalities have not generally required transfusions or other special treatment.

Discussion.   The *steel* and *W* (white spotting) mutations in mice affect both germ cell and hematological stem cell movements, and it might be tempting to think of ATR-X as having a similar spectrum of abnormalities, but germ cells are not necessary for normal testicular differentiation (see Chapter 2). It seems more likely that *XH2* is a transcriptional factor that is necessary for some aspects of neuronal/glial development in the brain, for regulation of α-globin loci, and for regulation of some aspects of male sexual development, including testis differentiation. It is of great interest that the mutations found to date have mostly been nonsense mutations with frameshifts and deletions limited to the extreme C-terminus. The mutation found in Juberg-Marsidi syndrome is in a domain that is highly conserved among helicases. The more severe phenotype of Juberg-Marsidi syndrome suggests that other (e.g., early truncating) mutations would not be compatible with life. Studies of the role in development of *XH2* are no doubt in progress.

REFERENCES

Gibbons R J, Suthers G K, Wilkie A O, Buckle V J, Higgs D R (1992). X-linked alpha-thalassemia/mental retardation (ATR-X) syndrome: localization to Xq12-q21.31 by X inactivation and linkage analysis. *Am J Hum Genet* 51:1136–1149.

Gibbons R J, Picketts D J, Higgs D R (1995a). Syndromal mental retardation due to mutations in a regulator of gene expression. *Hum Mol Genet* 4:1705–1709.

Gibbons R J, Picketts D J, Villard L, Higgs D R. (1995b). Mutations in a putative global transcriptional regulator cause X-linked mental retardation with alpha-thalassemia (ATR-X syndrome). *Cell* 80:837–845.

Gibbons R J, Bachoo S, Picketts D J, Aftimos S, Asenbauer B, Bergoffen J A, Berry S A, Dahl N, Fryer A, Keppler K, Kurosawa K, Levin M L, Masuno M, Neri G, Pierpont M E, Slaney S F, Higgs D R (1997). Mutations in transcriptional regulator *ATRX* establish the functional significance of a PHD-like domain. *Nat Genet* 17:146–148.

Hu, L-J, Laporte J, Kress W, Kioschis P, Siebenhaar R, Poustka A, Fardeau M, Metzenberg A, Janssen E A, Thomas N, Mandel J L, Dahl N (1996). Deletions in Xq28 in two boys with myotubular myopathy and abnormal genital development define a new contiguous gene syndrome in a 430 kb region. *Hum Mol Genet* 5:139–143.

Ion A, Telvi L, Chaussain J L, Galacteros F, Valayer J, Fellous M, McElreavey K (1996). A novel mutation in the putative DNA helicase *XH2* is responsible for male-to-female sex reversal associated with an atypical form of the ATR-X syndrome. *Am J Hum Genet* 58:1185–1191.

McPherson E W, Clemens M M, Gibbons R J, Higgs D R (1995). X-linked alpha-thalassemia/mental retardation (ATR-X) syndrome: a new kindred with severe genital anomalies and mild hematologic expression. *Am J Med Genet* 55:302–306.

Picketts D J, Higgs D R, Bachoos Blake D J, Quarrell O W J, Gibbons R J (1996). *ATRX* encodes a novel member of the SNF2 family of proteins: mutations point to a common mechanism underlying the ATR-X syndrome. *Hum Mol Genet* 5:1899–1907.

Reardon W, Gibbons R J, Winter R M, Baraitser M. (1995). Male pseudohermaphroditism in sibs with the alpha-thalassemia/mental retardation (ATR-X) syndrome. *Am J Med Genet* 55:285–287.

Villard L, Toutain A, Lossi A-M, Gecz J, Houdayer T, Moraine C, Fontés M (1996a). Splicing mutations in the ATR-X gene can lead to a dysmorphic mental retardation phenotype without alpha-thalassemia. *Am J Hum Genet* 58.499 505.

Villard L, Gecz J, Mattéi J F, Fontés M, Saugier-Veber P, Munnich A, Lyonnet S (1996b). *XNP* mutation in a large family with Juberg-Marsidi syndrome. *Nat Genet* 12:359–360.

Weatherall D J, Higgs D R, Bunch C, Old J M, Hunt D M, Pressley L, Clegg J B, Bethlenfalvay N C, Sjolin S, Koler R D, Magenis E, Francis J L, Bebbington D (1981). Hemoglobin H disease and mental retardation: a new syndrome or a remarkable coincidence? *N Engl J Med* 305:607–612.

Wilkie A O, Zeitlin H C, Lindenbaum R H, Buckle V J, Fischel-Ghodsian N, Chui D H, Gardner-Medwin D, MacGillivray M H, Weatherall D J, Higgs D R (1990). Clinical features and molecular analysis of the alpha-thalassemia mental retardation syndromes. II. Cases without detectable abnormality of the alpha-globin complex. *Am J Hum Genet* 46: 1127–1140.

Wilkie A O, Gibbons R J, Higgs D R, Pembrey M E (1991). X-linked alpha-thalassemia/mental retardation: spectrum of clinical features in three related males. *J Med Genet* 28:738–741.

7

Autosomal Disorders

Genomic/Chromosomal Disorders

CHROMOSOME 9 ALTERATIONS

Several cases of 46,XY sexual reversal associated with deletions of the distal region of chromosome 9p have been reported. As discussed in Chapter 2, the possible localization of an autosomal copy of ZFY in this region of 9p suggests one candidate gene that might be involved; a very conserved gene involved in male sex differentiation in *Caenorhabditis elegans* and *Drosophila* suggests another. Although the number of cases is small, one can expect that rapid progress will be made in delimiting a gene, or genes, on 9p involved in testis differentiation.

Clinical and Imaging Presentations. These XY patients have presented with normal female external genitalia and a variety of birth defects. The associated birth defects may be due to other chromosomal alterations, for several of the cases have been associated with unbalanced autosomal translocations. Thus, Fryns and colleagues (1986) presented the case of a 26-year-old severely mentally retarded woman with striking facial dysmorphism and hand changes; partial trisomy 3p was also present. Crocker and colleagues (1988) reported a child with a quite different array of facial dysmorphism (cloudy cornea and cleft palate) who developed heart failure and hydrocephalus, but, in this case, there was partial trisomy for half of the long arm of chromosome 7. Short stature, micrognathia, low-set ears, and ambiguous genitalia were associated with a ring chromosome 9 (Melaxotou and Kalpini-Mavrou, 1977), which suggests a distal location of the gene(s). A patient with a pure 9p deletion had no facial dysmorphism but was noted to have microcephaly and widely spaced nipples (Bennett et al., 1993). Imaging studies have shown normal müllerian derivatives when only 9p was deleted (Bennett et al., 1993), and a vestigial uterus with a 3 mm diameter cervix was found at postmortem examination in the $9p^-$, $7q^+$ patient (Crocker et al., 1988). In contrast, trisomy 9p is associated with few genital abnormalities; the latter are seen quite frequently in tetrasomy 9p (Leichtman et al., 1996).

Laboratory Studies.   Karyotypic investigations have shown that the deletion can be at p23.05 (Bennett et al., 1993; Ogata et al., 1997) although other cases (Veitia et al., 1997; McDonald et al., 1997) have been as distal as p24.1. Endocrine studies have shown normal adrenal steroids (Crocker et al., 1988) and normal pituitary function (Bennett et al., 1993), but abnormal gonadal steroids (Bennett et al., 1993). The histology of gonads has ranged from streak gonads ("a few epididymal tubules, islands of interstitial cells, and wolffian duct remnants") in the pure $9p^-$ situation (Bennett et al., 1993) through testicles with seminiferous tubules lined by Sertoli cells only in the $9p^-$, $7q^+$ patient (Crocker et al., 1988) to gonads with both ovary-like and testicular-like portions in a patient who also had trisomy for the distal part of 13q (Jotterand and Juillard, 1976).

Genotyping.   No specific chromosomal locus has been identified; as mentioned, however, an autosomal copy of ZFY maps to the distal portion of the short arm of chromosome 9 from p22 to pter (Affara et al., 1989). Recently, the male sexual regulatory gene, *mab-3*, was cloned from C. *elegans* and found to be homologous to the important sex cascade pathway gene, *doublesex*, in *Drosophila* (Raymond et al., 1998). A human homologue, expressed only in testis, was found to map to distal 9p (Raymond et al., 1998). Thus, this gene is an important candidate gene for this form of sex reversal. Surveys for 9p deletions in patients with ambiguous genitalia have commenced (Fuqua et al., 1996). Indeed, Ferguson-Smith and colleagues (1998) have just reported that seven of 11 patients with XY gonadal dysgenesis not attributable to known causes had complete or mosaic deletion of the *DMT1* orthologue. This finding needs confirmation (D. Zarkower, University of Minnesota, personal communication).

Management.   A large part of the clinical management of the patients that have survived with trisomy for other chromosomes, as well as the 9p deletion, has focused on their various birth defects. The patient with pure 9p deletion did not require special treatment other than surgical removal of the gonads because of the high risk of gonadal malignancy. There was no evidence of gonadoblastoma detected in the gonads in this patient at 2 years and 8 months of age (Bennett et al., 1993). One would envision steroid replacement for both height and secondary sexual characteristics as this patient becomes older.

Discussion. In sections of the previous chapter, X-chromosome aberrations and X-linked genes that are involved in testis differentiation were discussed. The chromosome 9p gene is merely one of several autosomal regions implicated in testis differentiation. Subsequent chapters will discuss chromosomes 10 and 22, as well as a variety of autosomal single-gene disorders. Thus, the small number of cases with chromosome 9p deletions and 46,XY sexual reversal are part of a larger story, implicating a large number of genes in the testis differentiation pathway.

REFERENCES

Affara N A, Chambers D, O'Brien J, Habeebu S S M, Kalaitsidaki M, Bishop C E, Ferguson-Smith M A (1989). Evidence for distinguishable transcripts of the putative testis-determining gene (ZFY) and mapping of homologous cDNA sequences to chromosomes X, Y and 9. *Nucleic Acids Res* 17:2987–2999.

Bennett C P, Docherty Z, Robb S A, Ramani P, Hawkins J R, Grant D (1993). Deletion 9p and sex reversal. *J Med Genet* 30:518–520.

Crocker M, Coghill S B, Cortinho R (1988). An unbalanced autosomal translocation (7;9) associated with feminization. *Clin Genet* 34:70–73.

Fryns J P, Kleczkowska A, Casaer P, van den Berghe H (1986). Double autosomal chromosomal aberration (3p trisomy/9p monosomy) and sex reversal. *Ann Genet* 29:49–52.

Fuqua J S, Sher E S, Perlman E J, Urban M D, Ghahremani M, Pelletier J, Migeon C J, Brown T R, Berkovitz G D (1996). Abnormal gonadal differentiation in two subjects with ambiguous genitalia, Müllerian structures, and normally developed testes: evidence for a defect in gonadal ridge development. *Hum Genet* 97:506–511.

Ferguson-Smith M A, Sanoudou D, Lee C (1998). Microdeletion of DMT1 at 9p24.3 is the commonest cause of 46,XY females. *Am J Hum Genet* 63 (Suppl): A162, Abstract 919.

Jotterand M, Juillard E (1976). A new case of trisomy for the distal part of 13q due to maternal translocaton, (t9;13) (p21;q21). *Hum Genet* 33:213–222.

Leichtman L G, Zackowski J L, Storto P D, Newlin A (1996). Non-mosaic tetrasomy 9p in a liveborn infant with multiple congenital anomalies: case report and comparison with trisomy 9p. *Am J Med Genet* 63:433–437.

McDonald, M T, Flejter W, Sheldon S, Putzi M J, Gorski J L. XY sex reversal and gonadal dysgenesis due to 9p24 monosomy. *Am J Med Genet* 73:321–326.

Metaxotou C, Kalpini-Mavrou A (1977). Ring Chromosome 9. 46,XY,r(9) in a male with ambiguous external genitalia. *Hum Genet* 37:351–354.

Ogata T, Muroya K, Matsuo N, Hata J, Fukushima Y, Suzuki Y (1997). Impaired male sex development in an infant with molecularly defined partial 9p monosomy: implication for a testis forming gene(s) on 9p. *J Med Genet* 34:331–334.

Raymond C S, Shamu C E, Shen M M, Seifert K J, Hirsch B, Hodgkin J, Zarkower D (1998). Evidence for evolutionary conservation of sex-determining genes. *Nature* 391:691–695.

Veitia R, Nunes M, Brauner R, Doco-Fenzy M, Joanny-Flinois O, Jaubert F, Lortal-Jacob S, Fellous M, McElreavey K (1997). Deletions of distal 9p associated with 46,XY male to female sex reversal: definition of the breakpoints at 9p23-3-p24.1. *Genomics* 41:271–279.

CHROMOSOME 10 ALTERATIONS

Monosomy 10qter creates a recognizable clinical phenotype in which 46,XY individuals display sexual ambiguity or even sex reversal. The molecular defect is not known but it presumably resides in a gene whose product is needed during development of secondary sexual structures and external genitalia, for testicular hormones and histology have appeared normal when examined. It is not known if testicular differentiation is delayed in these cases.

Clinical and Imaging Presentation.   As reviewed by Wulfsberg and colleagues (1989), even when results are corrected for the frequent prematurity, about one third of the affected infants were growth retarded at birth; at older ages most were growth retarded, and all were developmentally retarded. The craniofacial features are fairly distinctive: microcephaly, a broad-based nose with a beak-like tip, somewhat large and frequently malformed ears, down-slanting of palpebral fissures, hypertelorism, and micrognathia. A short neck can also be found. Other external manifestations include fifth-finger clinodactyly in about one half of cases and limited elbow extension and/or toe syndactyly in about one fifth of cases. Congenital heart defects are frequent and urogenital anomalies, such as posterior urethra, were found in females as well as males. At the time of the review by Wulfsberg and colleagues (1989), six out of six males had undescended testes and two of the six males had ambiguous genitalia. More severe cases of ambiguous genitalia in XY individuals have since been reported (Wilkie et al., 1993). In the first case, an ultrasound exam showed an apparently normal cervix with a very small uterus. The second patient had a perineoscrotal hypospadias, which has also been described by Fryns and colleagues (1989).

Laboratory Features.   Karyotypes have shown deletions of chromosome 10 with their proximal location ranging from q25.3 to q26.2. Many of the patients have other chromosomal anomalies as well, resulting from unbalanced gametes produced by balanced carrier parents. Hormonal studies have corresponded to the degree of sex reversal. For instance, the patient in case 1 of Wilkie and colleagues (1993), who displayed sex reversal, had low basal gonadotropin levels and low testosterone that did not respond to human chorionic gonadotropin stimulation, implying a major defect in the hypothalamic-pituitary-gonadal axis. In contrast, the patient in case 2 of the same investigators, who had ambiguous genitalia, had normal plasma testosterone and gonadotropin levels. Testicular histology performed on tissue from this patient showed a normal distribution of germ, Sertoli, and Leydig cells (Wilkie et al., 1993). The big difference in endocrine parameters between cases 1 and 2 implies causal heterogeneity.

Genotyping.   The molecular defect is not yet known. Studies on X-and Y-linked genes have been normal in several cases studied: in case 1 of Wilkie and colleagues there was normal-length *SRY* product; the androgen receptor showed normal binding and thermolability in case 2. Several candidate genes related to sexual differentiation are located on chromosome 10q but seem to be proximal to the deletion site. Thus, P450c17, which is involved in testosterone synthesis (see Chapter 3), maps to band 10q24-25 (Sparkes et al., 1991). The mouse gene homologous to *PAX2*, *Pax-2*, is expressed in the developing mesonephros and in the mesonephric duct in a transient pattern (Phelps and Dressler, 1993; Dressler et al., 1990). Elegant antisense experiments have shown that *Pax-2* is required for epithelial mesenchymal conversion in the developing kidney (Rothenpieier and Dressler, 1993). It is conceivable that alterations in expression of *PAX2* in the developing mesonephros could influence the development of the adjacent gonads. Although initial evidence localized *PAX2* to 10q22.1-24.3 (Eccles et al., 1992), more recent analyses have suggested a 10q24-25 localization (Sanyanusin et al., 1995a). Heterozygosity, caused by a deletion that includes *Pax-2* in the mouse, results in retinal abnormalities but not genital abnormalities (Keller et al., 1994) and human mutations, including a translocation breakpoint, in *PAX2* show optic nerve colobomas, renal anomalies, and vesicoureteral reflux (Sanyanusin et al., 1995a, 1995b; Narahara et al., 1997). Thus, hemizygosity for *PAX2* mutations or deletions is unlikely to explain the urogenital abnormalities seen with 10q deletions.

Management.   The more severely ambiguous patients can be raised as girls with appropriate surgical treatment. If gonads are intra-abdominal, they should be removed because of the risk of gonadoblastoma. These patients are severely retarded and many do not survive the neonatal period. Thus, aggressive treatment may not be warranted.

Discussion.   Correct dosage for one or more genes located on distal 10q is important for sexual development. The finding of clitoromegaly in a XX, female patient with triploidy for this chromosomal region also suggests that there is a dosage-sensitive gene related to sex differentiation located here (Halpern et al., 1996). The presence of a uterus in a patient with only a 10qter deletion (and no other chromosomal abnormalities; Wilkie et al., 1993) indicates that the product of this gene(s) must act early in development such that in its absence, the developing testes do not produce sufficient müllerian-inhibiting substance (MIS) to cause regression of paramesonephric structures. As already discussed, the candidate genes we know of seem proximal to the usual deletions. It can be expected that continued mapping of genes involved in sex differentiation in the mouse, which can then be mapped to the human genome by homology mapping, will eventually disclose other candidate genes that are deleted.

REFERENCES

Dressler G R, Deutsch U, Chowdhury K, Nornes H O, Gruss P. (1990). *Pax-2*, a new murine paired-box-containing gene and its expression in the developing excretory system. *Development* 109:787–795.

Eccles M R, Wallis L J, Fidler A E, Spurr N K, Goodfellow P J, Reeve A E (1992). Expression of the *PAX2* gene in human fetal kidney and Wilms' tumor. *Cell Growth Differ* 3:279–289.

Fryns J P, Kleczkowska A, Fivez H, Van Den Berghe H (1989). Severe midline fusion defects in a newborn with 10q26 → qter deletion. *Ann Genet* 32:124–125.

Halpern G J, Shohat M, Merlob P (1996). Partial trisomy 10q: further delineation of the clinical manifestations involving the segment 10q23 → 10q24. *Annal Genet* 39:181–183.

Keller S A, Jones J M, Boyle A, Barrow L L, Killen P D, Green D G, Kapousta N V, Hitchcock P F, Swank R T, Meisler M H (1994). Kidney and retinal defects (*Krd*), a transgene-induced mutation with a deletion of mouse chromosome 19 that includes the *Pax2* locus. *Genomics* 23:309–320.

Narahara K, Baker E, Ito S, Yokoyama Y, Yu S, Hewitt D, Sutherland G R, Eccles M R, Richards R I (1997). Localisation of a 10q breakpoint within the PAX2 gene in a patient with a de novo t(10;13) translocation and optic nerve coloboma-renal disease. *J Med Genet* 34:213–216.

Phelps D E, Dressler G R (1993). Aberrant expression of *Pax2* in Danforth's short tail (Sd) mice. *Dev Biol* 157:251–258.

Rothenpieier U W, Dressler G R (1993). *Pax-2* is required for mesenchyme-to-epithelium conversion during kidney development. *Development* 119:711–720.

Sanyanusin P, Schimmenti, L A, McNoe L A, Ward T A, Pierpont M E M, Sullivan M J, Dobyns W B, Eccles M R (1995a). Mutation of the *PAX2* gene in a family with optic nerve colobomas, renal anomalies and vesicoureteral reflux. *Nat Genet* 9:358–363.

Sanyanusin P, McNoe L A, Sullivan M J, Weaver R G, Eccles M R (1995b). Mutation of *PAX2* in two siblings with renal-coloboma syndrome. *Hum Mol Genet* 4:2183–2184.

Sparkes R S, Klisak I, Miller W L (1991). Regional mapping of genes encoding human steroidogenic enzymes: P450scc to 15q23→q-24, adrenodoxin to 11q22; adrenodoxin reductase to 17q24→q25; and P450c17 to 10q24-25. *DNA Cell Biol* 10:359–365.

Wilkie A O M, Campbell F M, Daubeney P, Grant D B, Daniels R J, Mullarkey M, Affara N A, Fitchett M, Huson S M (1993). Complete and partial XY sex reversal associated with terminal deletion of 10q: report of 2 cases and literature review. *Am J Med Genet* 46:597–600.

Wulfsberg E A, Weaver R P, Cunniff C M, Jones M C, Jones K L (1989). Chromosome 10qter deletion syndrome: a review and report of three new cases. *Am J Med Genet* 32:364–367.

46,XX TRUE HERMAPHRODITISM AND SEX REVERSAL IN THE ABSENCE OF *SRY*; TRISOMY 22 IS SOMETIMES INVOLVED

46,XX true hermaphroditism is not rare and occurs in both sporadic and familial forms (Fraccaro et al., 1979). The latter occur with higher frequency in particular ethnic subgroups (especially South African blacks; Ramsay et al., 1988) suggesting that genetic determination is important. In many cases, 46,XX males (with testes, not ovotestes) have also occurred in the familial forms (Berger et al., 1970; Kasdan et al., 1973; Skordis et al., 1987; Ostrer et al., 1989; Kuhnle et al., 1993; Ramos et al., 1996; Zentano et al., 1997), indicating that ovotestes can be considered an intermediate, if more common, degree of sexual differentiation in these cases. Searches for Y-chromosomal sequences in these individuals have frequently been performed, always with negative results (Waibel et al., 1987; Raine et al., 1989; Pereira et al., 1991; Fechner et al., 1993; Spurdle et al., 1995; Turner et al., 1995; Zentano et al., 1997). The other common cause of true hermaphroditism, 46,XX/46,XY mosaicism, is discussed in Chapter 6.

Clinical and Imaging Presentation. These patients usually present at the time of birth because of ambiguous genitalia; the 46,XX true males in the same families are frequently found when more severely affected family members are studied. Rarely, the patients have other congenital anomalies (Fechner et al., 1993). In one review of 38 cases (from 152 ascertained in a 10-year-period; Ramsay et al., 1988), an enlarged clitoris or small phallus was found in all 38; 33 of 35 had hypospadias, and 14 of 24 had a separate vaginal opening with a formed vagina. Not unexpectedly, because of the known asymmetry of testicular development, testicular tissue was identified on the right side much more frequently than on the left: 32 cases versus 15 cases (Ramsay et al., 1988). Laparoscopy and/or imaging studies frequently show the presence of uterine and fallopian tube differentiation. Sometimes nothing more than rudimentary round ligaments are identified (Skordis et al., 1987). Psychological problems of confused gender identity may be present (reviewed in Krob et al., 1994). Ovarian fertility may occur but successful fatherhood is unlikely.

Laboratory Features.   Karyotypes are routinely 46,XX, as the definition requires. Basal plasma testosterone levels are usually high for females in the first 6 months; later, hCG-stimulated testosterone values indicate the presence of testicular tissue (Hadjiathanasiou et al., 1994)

Genotyping.   *SRY* and other Y chromosomal sequences are not found (Spurdle et al., 1995) even in the 46,XX males (Vilain et al., 1994). This fits the finding that *SRY* is not necessary for male sexual differentiation in all species of mammals, as exemplified by species of voles that don't need *SRY* to make males (Just et al., 1995; see Chapter 2); a similar condition is found in pigs (Pailhoux et al., 1994) and all females of four species of moles (Sánchez et al., 1996). No specific mutations in any gene have yet been identified for this condition, but trisomy 22 has sometimes been associated with it (see below). One case associated with multiple birth defects occurred with a distal Xp deletion (Tar et al., 1995).

Management.   Surgical management will reflect the need for hypospadias repair and removal of gonads if they cannot be reduced to the scrotum. Gonadal removal, phallic reduction, and rearing as a female are common; masculinizing genitoplasty may be indicated in individuals with significant testosterone production (Hadjiathanasiou et al., 1994).

Discussion.   The familial occurrence of 46,XX true hermaphroditism (frequently these families also have 46,XX males) and a high frequency in certain ethnic subgroups suggests genetic causation. One chromosomal region that might be involved is chromosome 22.

Abnormalities of genital and gonadal formation with chromosome 22 aneuploidy have been reported. Kim and colleagues (1977) noted a phenotypically male infant with duplications of chromosomes 22 (pter → q11) and 13 (pter → q11) who manifested somatic features of both these aneuploidies but, in addition, had normal genital organs of both sexes. At autopsy, testes, a penis, as well as a hypoplastic uterus and vagina were seen. Cantu and colleagues (1981) reported a female with duplication 22 (q12 →ter) who had ovarian dysgenesis; this may reflect the negative effects of partial testicular differentiation. Nicholl and colleagues (1994) reported a patient with 47,XX,+ chromosome 22 who manifested clear evidence of intersex. They reported a cytogenetically female infant with multiple somatic abnormalities, including intrauterine growth retardation, microcephaly, low-set ears, cleft palate, and congenital heart disease. The child was phenotypically male and had cryptorchidism and a small penis. Internal examination revealed a rudimentary vagina and uterus with histologically male gonads. No ovarian tissue was noted. Y-specific probes for the centromere and GMGY10 did not reveal Y material.

We have recently seen another patient with partial trisomy 22 and 46,XX true hermaphroditism. In our case, *SRY* was not found in DNA prepared from blood, from cell culture lines started with tissue from both the right and left gonads, and from DNA of the testicular portion of the right gonad (Aleck et al., 1999).

The presence of true hermaphroditism with trisomy for all or part of chromosome 22, in the absence of *SRY*, *ZFY* or other evidence for Y-chromosomal genes, suggests that there are genes on chromosome 22 that are involved in sexual determination. It is unclear whether the true hermaphroditism seen in these patients represents a gene dosage effect in which three copies of a normal gene product alters the sexual expression of an XX individual, or whether the duplication had resulted in a novel gene such as a fusion gene that alters sexual determination. We suspect that gene dosage is the more likely explanation.

REFERENCES

Aleck K, Stone J, Argueso L, Erickson R P (1999) True hermaphroditism without SRY associated with partial duplication of chromosome 22. *Am. J. Med. Genet.*, under revision.

Berger R, Abonyi D, Nadot A, Vialatte J, Lejeune J (1970). Hermaphdrodisme vrai et "garcon XX' dans une fratrie. *Rev Eur Etud Clin Biol* 15:330.

Cantu J M, Hernandez A, Vaca G, Plascencia L, Martinez-Basalo C, Ibarra B, Rivera H (1981). Trisomy 22q12 leads to qter: "aneusomie de recombinaison" of a pericentric inverstion. *Ann Genet (Paris)* 24:37–40.

Fechner P Y, Marcantonio S M, Jaswancy V, Stetten G, Goodfellow P N, Migeon C J, Smith K D, Berkovitz G D (1993). The role of the sex-determining region Y gene in the etiology of 46,XX maleness. *J Clin Endocrinol Metab* 76:690–695.

Fraccaro M, Tiepolo L, Zuffardi O. Chiumello G, Di Natale B, Gargantini L, Wolf U (1979). Familial XX true hermaphroditism and the H-Y antigen. *Hum Genet* 48:45–52.

Hadjiathanasiou C G, Brauner R, Lortat-Jacob S, Nivot S, Jaubert F, Fellous M, Nihoul-Fekete C, Rappaport R (1994). True hermaphroditism: genetic variants and clinical management. *J Pediatr* 125:738–744.

Just W, Rau W, Vogel W, Akhverdian M, Fredga K, Graves J A M, Lyapunova E (1995). Absence of Sry in species of the vole Ellobius. *Nat Genet* 11:117–118.

Kasdan R, Nankin H R, Troen P, Wald N, Pan S, Yanaihara T (1973). Paternal transmission of maleness in XX human beings. *N Engl J Med* 288:539–545.

Kim H J, Hsu L Y F, Goldsmith L C, Strauss L, Hirschhorn K (1977). Familial translocation with partial trisomy of 13 and 22: evidence that specific regions of chromosomes 13 and 22 are responsible for the phenotype of each trisomy. *J Med Genet* 14:114–119.

Krob G, Braun A, Kuhnle U (1994). True hermaphroditism: geographical distribution, clinical findings, chromosomes and gonadal histology. *Eur J Pediatr* 153:2–10.

Kuhnle U, Schwarz H P, Lohrs U, Stengel-Ruthkowski S, Cleve H, Braun A (1993). Familial true hermaphroditism: paternal and maternal transmission of true hermaphroditism (46,XX) and XX maleness in the absence of Y-chromosomal sequences. *Hum Genet* 92:571–576.

Nicholl R M, Grimsley L, Butler L, Palmer R W, Fees H C, Savage M O, Costeloe K (1994). Trisomy 22 and intersex. *Arch Dis Child* 71:F57–F58.

Ostrer H, Wright G, Clayton M, Skordis N, MacGillivray M H (1989). Familial XX chromosomal maleness does not arise from a Y chromosomal translocation. *J Pediatr* 114:977–982.

Pailhoux E, Popescu P C, Parma P, Boscher J, Legault C, Molten J L, Fellous M, Cotinot C (1994). Genetic analysis of 38,XX males with genital ambiguities and true hermaphrodites in pigs. *Anim Genet* 25:299–305.

Pereira E T, de Almeida J C C, Gunha A C Y R G, Patton M, Taylor R, Jeffery S (1991). Use of probes for ZFY, SRY and the Y pseudoautosomal boundary in XX males, XX true hermaphrodites, and an XY female. *J Med Genet* 28:591–595.

Raine J, Robertson M E, Malcolm S, Hoey H, Grant D B (1989). Absence of Y specific DNA sequences in two siblings with 46,XX hermaphroditism. *Arch Dis Child* 64:1185–1187.

Ramos E S, Moreira-Filho C A, Vicente Y A M V A, Llorach-Velludo M A S, Tucci S Jr, Duarte M H O, Araujo A G, Martelli L (1996). SRY-negative true hermaphrodites and an XX male in two generations of the same family. *Hum Genet* 97:596–598.

Ramsay M, Bernstein R, Zwane E, Page D C, Jenkins T (1988). XX true hermaphroditism in South African Blacks: an enigma of primary sexual differentiation. *Am J Hum Genet* 43:4–13.

Sánchez A, Bullejos M, Burgos M, Hera C, Stamatopoulos C, Díaz de la Guardia R, Jiménez R. (1996) Females of four mole species of genus *Talpa* (insectivora, mammalia) are true hermaphrodites with ovotestes. *Mol Reprod Dev* 44:289–294.

Skordis N A, Stetka D G, MacGillivray M H, Greenfield S P (1987). Familial 46,XX males coexisting with familial 46,XX true hermaphrodites in same pedigree. *J Pediatr* 110:244–248.

Spurdle A B, Shankman S, Ramsay M (1995). XX true hermaphroditism in South African Blacks: exclusion of *SRY* sequences and uniparental disomy of the X chromosome. *Am J Med Genet* 55:53–56.

Tar A, Solyom J, Gyorvari B, Ion A, Telvi L, Barbaux S, Souleyreau N, Vilain E, Fellous M, McElreavey K (1995). Testicular development in an *SRY*-negative 46,XX individual harboring a distal Xp deletion. *Hum Genet* 96:464–468.

Turner B, Fechner P Y, Fuqua J S, Marcantonio S M, Perlman E J, Vondermark J S, Berkovitz G D (1995). Combined Leydig cell and Sertoli cell dysfunction in 46,XX males lacking the sex-determining region Y gene. *Am J Med Genet* 57:440–443.

Vilain E, LeFiblec B, Morichon-Delvallez N, Brauner R, Dommergues M, Dumez Y, Jaubert F, Boucekkine C, McElreavey K, Vekemans M, Fellous M (1994). *SRY*-negative XX fetus with complete male phenotype. *Lancet* 343:240–241.

Waibel F, Scherer G, Fraccaro M, Hustinx T W J, Weissenbach J, Wieland J, Mayerova A, Back E, Wolf U (1987). Absence of Y-specific DNA sequences in human 46,XX true hermaphrodities and in 45,X mixed gonadal dysgenesis. *Hum Genet* 76:332–336.

Zenteno J C, López M, Vera C, Méndez J P, Kofman-Alfaro S (1997). Two *SRY*-negative XX male brothers without genital ambiguity. *Hum Genet* 100:606–610.

Autosomal Single-Gene Disorders

DENYS-DRASH AND FRASIER SYNDROMES AND *WT1*

The triad of nephropathy, genital abnormalities, and Wilms tumor was first described in a child with 46,XY/XX mosaicism by Denys and colleagues (1967). Further cases were published in English by Drash and colleagues (1970), hence Denys-Drash syndrome. The association of Wilms' tumor, aniridia, genitourinary abnormalities, and mental retardation (the so-called *WAGR* syndrome), associated with deletions on 11p13, also pointed toward the potential association of Wilms tumor with genitourinary abnormalities (Gessler et al., 1989). When chromosomal changes on 11p associated with Wilms tumor led to the isolation of a Wilms tumor ogene (*WT1*; Call et al., 1990; Gessler et al., 1990; Haber et al., 1990), it was not long before mutations in *WT1* were found in Denys-Drash syndrome (Pelletier et al., 1991a). Mutations in *WT1* were also found in the Frasier syndrome, which shares two of the Denys-Drash syndrome's major features, nephropathy and male pseudohermaphroditism (Barbaux et al., 1997). The alterations of *WT1* associated with abnormal genital development will be the focus of this section.

Clinical and Imaging Presentation.   The initial presentation of Denys-Drash syndrome usually includes nephropathy or Wilms tumor. Of affected persons, only about 13% present as phenotypic males; the vast majority appear female or have ambiguous genitalia. Of the "females," about one half actually have a 46,XY karyotype (Müeller, 1994). Because *WT1* is an autosomal locus, the mutation should occur equally in either sex, and the slight deficiency of patients with Denys-Drash syndrome and 46,XX karyotypes probably reflects an under-ascertainment bias. If nephropathy is used as the key element of the diagnosis, nine of 12 patients showed genital abnormalities as well (Jadresic et al., 1990). Gonads are frequently dysgenic and true hermaphroditism may occur (Edidin, 1985; Eddy and Mauer, 1985). Both müllerian and wolffian derivatives may be present, and sometimes wolffian structures may be found in persons with female external genitalia (Müeller, 1994). Imaging studies of the urinary system reveal abnormalities in about half the patients: blunted caliceal systems (absent or small renal pelves, and sometimes even vesicoureteral reflux). Gonadoblastoma has also occurred (Fisher et al., 1983; Pelletier et al., 1991b).

Frasier syndrome consists of chronic renal failure due to glomerulopathy and male pseudohermaphroditism (Frasier et al., 1964; Moorthy et al., 1987). It has also been reported in 46,XX females (Bailey et al., 1992)—other 46,XX cases may have been dismissed as amenorrhea secondary to renal failure.

Laboratory Studies.   The nephropathy of Denys-Drash consists of proteinuria, frequently resulting in nephrotic syndrome, associated with hypertension and rapid development of end-stage renal failure (Jadresic et al., 1990). Hematuria is not usual. Renal histopathology usually discloses hypertrophy of the podocyte layer of the glomerulus and mesangial sclerosis in a diffuse manner, although focal lesions are sometimes found instead (Jadresic et al., 1990). The histological features of Wilms tumor are usually favorable for cure (Jadresic et al., 1990). Gonadotropin levels have been high and testosterone low in those cases in which it has been studied. A partial androgen receptor deficiency in cultured genital skin fibroblasts has been reported in one case (Turleau et al., 1987), but this observation has not yet been confirmed. The renal findings are quite similar to those in Frasier syndrome (Moorthy et al., 1987).

Genotyping.   Very shortly after *WT1* was cloned, two types of evidence were provided for its potential role in Denys-Drash syndrome. Expression studies by *in situ* RNA hybridization to sections of human embryos demonstrated that the *WT1* gene was expressed in the developing kidney and in the genital ridge, fetal gonad, and surrounding mesothelium (Pritchard-Jones et al., 1990). Studies of developing mice showed that the levels of *WT1* mRNA in the gonads were greater than those detected in the embryonic kidney (Pelletier et al., 1991c). Second, although deletions of *WT1* in the WAGR syndrome result in mild aberrations of sexual differentiation, point mutations have been found in the Denys-Drash syndrome (Pelletier et al., 1991a; Pelletier et al., 1991b; Baird et al., 1992; Bruening et al., 1992; Ogawa et al., 1993).

It seemed likely that Denys-Drash syndrome is caused by dominant-negative mutations in the *WT1* gene: mutations in this protein may prevent it from binding in its normal DNA site but permit it to interact with other transcriptional activators or the product of its normal allele so as to perturb testicular differentiation (Hastie, 1992). Wilms tumor is thought to occur when alterations leading to homozygosity or hemizygosity for the mutant locus occurs—normal *WT1* can suppress growth of Wilms tumor cells (Haber et al., 1993). The *WT1* gene product belongs to the class of zinc finger, DNA-binding proteins and nine of the 10 initial mutations were in zinc finger III, and one in zinc finger II (Pelletier et al., 1991b). Recent tabulations (Coppes et al., 1993; Müeller, 1994) show that half of 34 mutations have occurred in the codon for amino acid 394 in exon 9. Of the remaining mutations, all are in the zinc fingers, have altered splice sites, or have created a stop codon that would severely alter the C-terminal portion of the protein (Müeller, 1994). Those mutations not reviewed by Coppes and colleagues (1993) and Müeller (1994) also fit this pattern—for example, Baird and Cowell (1993). Binding to four candidate DNA targets by glutathione-S-transferase *WT1* fusion proteins containing *WT1* Denys-Drash mutations from the three major categories was abrogated (Little et al., 1993, 1995). Two alternative splice sites in the *WT1* transcript lead to four messages, of which two code for proteins co-localizing with nuclear splicing factors (Larsson et al., 1995); thus the Denys-Drash mutations could be acting by creating dominant-negative proteins competing with the normal *WT1* gene product in forming complexes typical of transcription factors, or by altering the dosage of the multiple isoforms. The dominant-negative model fits the lack of nephropathy and milder genital defects found in *WAGR* (deletion) patients or genital anomalies in mice heterozygous for a stem cell knockout of *WT1* (Kriedberg et al., 1993). In addition, *WT1* mutations were not found in control 46,XY patients with various forms of genital abnormalities but without nephropathy (Clarkson et al., 1993). The mutations found in Frasier syndrome are in the donor splice site in intron 9 of WT1 and result in the loss of isoforms with lys-thr-ser (+KTS) between zinc fingers 3 and 4 (Barbaux et al., 1997). Such mutations had also been reported in Denys-Drash syndrome, but they occurred in patients without Wilms tumor. These data also suggest that the -KTS isoform is the tumor-suppressing form of *WT1*.

Management.   The management of patients with Denys-Drash syndrome requires more attention to the potential malignancies and nephropathy than to the sexual ambiguity. Frequent ultrasound scans to search for Wilms tumor are essential. When the nephropathy is far advanced, nephrectomy acts as a step toward hemodialysis or renal transplantation and is also indicated in order to remove the possible source of the Wilms tumor. The progressive nature of the nephropathy means that hemodialysis or renal transplantation will usually be needed. However, if this has not occurred and Wilms tumor is found, successful treatment of the Wilms tumor is the usual outcome because the Wilms tumor has low-grade histopathology. Given that gonadoblastoma has also occurred, as in other cases of Y-containing abdominal gonads, gonadectomy should also be considered, and it is easily performed at the time of nephrectomy. Finally, surgical correction of ambiguous genitalia will be usual. For the management of Frasier syndrome, one needs to focus on the renal failure and hormone replacement.

Discussion.   Although rare disorders, the Denys-Drash and Frasier syndromes provide an excellent example of the advances in molecular genetics at work. Unlike the *ret* oncogene—where dominant mutations are associated with endocrine tumors and recessive mutations are associated with Hirschsprung disease (for review, see Erickson and Lewis 1995)—dominant mutations of the *WT1* gene are associated with urogenital abnormalities and nephropathy, whereas recessive mutations are associated only with Wilms tumor and/or genitourinary abnormalities. Many questions, of course, remain to be answered. The great heterogeneity in the genital abnormalities in Denys-Drash syndrome has so far not been clarified by the range of mutations—the most common mutation, of the codon for amino acid 394 in exon 9, has been associated with a variety of urogenital abnormalities (Müeller, 1994). Thus, as in many of the other disorders discussed in this book, modifying genes, perhaps some of them once described in other chapters, may be involved in the varying presentations of Denys-Drash syndrome.

REFERENCES

Bailey W A, Zwingman T A, Reznik V M, Griswold W R, Mendoza S A, Jones K L, Freidenberg G R (1992). End-stage renal disease and primary hypogonadism associated with a 46,XX karyotype. *Am J Dis Child* 146:1218–1223.

Baird P N, Cowell J K, (1993). A novel zinc finger mutation in a patient with Denys-Drash syndrome. *Hum Mol Genet* 2:2193–2194.

Baird P N, Santos A, Groves N, Jadresic L, Cowell J K (1992). Constitutional mutations in the *WT1* gene in patients with Denys-Drash syndrome. *Hum Mol Genet* 1:301–305.

Barbaux S, Niaudet P, Gubler M-C, Grünfeld J-P, Jaubert F, Kuttenn F, Fékéte C N, Souleyreau-Therville N, Thibaud E, Fellous M, McElreavey K (1997). Donor splice-site mutations in *WT1* are responsible for Frasier syndrome. *Nat Genet* 17:467–470.

Bruening W, Bardeesy N, Silverman B L, Cohn R A, Machin G A, Aronson A J, Housman D, Pelletier J (1992). Germline intronic and exonic mutation in the Wilms' tumor gene (*WT1*) affecting urogenital development. *Nat Genet* 1:144–149.

Call K M, Glaser T, Ito C Y, Buckler A J, Pelletier J, Harber D A, Rose E A, Kral A, Yeger H, Lewis W H, Jones C, Housman D E (1990). Isolation and characterization of a zinc finger polypeptide gene at the human chromosome 11 Wilms' tumor locus. *Cell* 60:509–520.

Clarkson P A, Davies H R, Williams D M, Chaudhary R, Hughes I A, Patterson M N (1993). Mutational screening of the Wilms' tumour gene, *WT1*, in males with genital abnormalities. *J Med Genet* 30:767–772.

Coppes M J, Huff V, Pelletier J (1993). Denys-Drash syndrome: relating a clinical disorder to genetic alterations in the tumor suppressor gene *WT1*. *J Pediatr* 123:673–678.

Denys P, Malvaux P, Van den Berghe H, Tangue W, Proesmans W (1967). Association d'un syndrome anatomo-pathologique de pseudohermaphrodisme masculin, d'une tumeur de Wilms, d'une nephropathie parenchymateuse et d'un mosaicism XX/XY. *Arch Fr Pediatr* 24:729–739.

Drash A, Sherman F, Hartmann W H, Blizzard R M (1970). A syndrome of pseudohermaphroditism, Wilms' tumor, hypertension, and degenerative renal disease. *J Pediatr* 76:585–593.

Eddy A, Mauer S M (1985). Reply. *J Pediatr* 107:988.

Edidin D V (1985) Pseudohermaphroditism, glomerulopathy, and Wilms' tumor (Drash syndrome). *J Pediatr* 107:988.

Erickson R P, Lewis S E (1995). The new human genetics. *Environ Mol Mutagen* 25 (suppl 26): 7–12.

Fisher J E, Andres G A, Cooney D R, MacDonald M A (1983). A syndrome of pure gonadal dysgenesis: gonadoblastoma, Wilms' tumour and nephron disease. *Lab Invest* 48:4P–5P.

Frasier S, Bashore R A, Mosier H D (1964). Gonadoblastoma associated with pure gonadal dysgenesis in monozygotic twins. *J Pediatr* 64:740–745.

Gessler M, Poustka A, Cavenee W, Neve R I, Orkin S H, Bruns G A P (1990). Homozygous deletion in Wilms' tumours of a zinc-finger gene identified by chromosome jumping. *Nature* 343:774–778.

Gessler M, Thomas G H, Couillin P, Junien C, McGillivray B C, Hayden M, Jaschek G, Bruns

G A P (1989) A deletion map of the WAGR region on chromosome 11. *Am J Hum Genet* 44:486–495.

Haber D, Buckler A, Glaser T, Call K M, Pelletier J, Sohn R L, Douglass E C, Housman D E (1990). An internal deletion within an 11p13 zinc finger gene contributes to the development of Wilms' tumour. *Cell* 61:1257–1269.

Haber D A, Park S, Maheswaran S, Englert C, Re G G, Hazen-Martin D J, Sens D A, Garvin A J (1993). WT1-mediated growth suppression of Wilms' tumor cells expressing a WT1 splicing variant. *Science* 262:2057–2060.

Hastie N D (1992) Dominant-negative mutations in the Wilms' tumour (*WT1*) gene cause Denys-Drash syndrome—proof that a tumour-suppressor gene plays a crucial role in normal genitourinary development. *Hum Mol Genet* 1:293–295.

Jadresic L, Leake J, Gordon I, Dillon M J, Grant D B, Pritchard J, Risdon R A, Barratt T M. (1990). Clinicopathologic review of twelve children with nephropathy, Wilms' tumor, and genital abnormalities (Drash syndrome). *J Pediatr* 117:717–725.

Kreidberg J A, Sariola H, Loring J M, Maeda M, Pelletier J, Housman D, Jaenisch R (1993). WT1 is required for early kidney development. *Cell* 74:679–691.

Larsson S H, Charlieu J-P, Miyagawa K, Engelkamp D, Rassoulzadegan M, Ross A, Cuzin F, van Heyningen V, Hastie N D (1995). Subnuclear localization of WT1 in splicing or transcription factor domains is regulated by alternative splicing. *Cell* 81:391–401.

Little M, Holmes G, Bickmore W, Van Heyningen V, Hastie N, Wainwright B (1995). DNA binding capacity of the WT1 protein is abolished by Denys-Drash syndrome WT1 point mutations. *Hum Mol Genet* 4:351–358.

Little M H, Williamson K A, Mannens M, Kelsey A, Gosden C, Hastie N D, van Heyningen V (1993). Evidence that WT1 mutations in Denys-Drash syndrome patients may act in a dominant-negative fashion. *Hum Mol Genet* 2:259–264.

Moorthy A V, Chesney R W, Lubinsky M (1987). Chronic renal failure and XY gonadal dysgenesis: "Frasier" syndrome—a commentary on reported cases. *Am J Med Genet* 3:297–302.

Müeller R F (1994). Syndrome of the month: the Denys-Drash syndrome. *J Med Genet* 31:471–477.

Ogawa O, Eccles M R, Yun K, Mueller R F, Holdaway M D D, Reeve A E (1993). Novel insertional mutation at the third zinc finger coding region of the WT1 gene in Denys-Drash syndrome. *Hum Mol Genet* 2:203–204.

Pelletier J, Bruening W, Kashtan C E, Mauer S M, Manivel J C, Striegel J E, Houghton D C, Junien C, Habib R, Fouser L, Fine R N, Silverman B L, Haber D A, Housman D (1991a). Germline mutations in the Wilms' tumor suppressor gene are associated with abnormal urogenital development in Denys-Drash syndrome. *Cell* 67:437–447.

Pelletier J, Bruening W, Li F P, Haber D A, Glaser T, Housman D E (1991b). WT1 mutations contribute to abnormal genital system development and hereditary Wilms' tumour. *Nature* 353:431–434.

Pelletier J, Schalling M, Buckler A J, Rogers A, Haber D A, Housman D (1991c). Expression of the Wilms' tumor gene WT1 in the murine urogenital system. *Genes Dev* 5:1345–1356.

Pritchard-Jones K, Fleming S, Davidson D, Bickmore W, Porteous D, Gosden C, Bard J, Buckler A, Pelletier J, Housman D, van Heyningen V, Hastie N (1990). The candidate Wilms' tumour gene is involved in genitourinary development. *Nature* 346:194–196.

Turleau C, Niaudet P, Sultan C, Rault G, Mahfoud A, Nichoul-Fekete C, Iris L, deGrouchy J (1987). Partial androgen receptor deficiency and mixed gonadal dysgenesis in Drash syndrome. *Hum Genet* 75:81–83.

CAMPTOMELIC DYSPLASIA AND *SOX9*

Camptomelic dysplasia has gone from naming (from Greek *kamptos* meaning "bent") to cloning in three and a half decades. Many unanswered questions remain. Although it seems clear that the "standard" form of camptomelic dysplasia is due

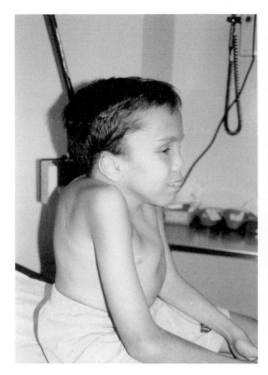 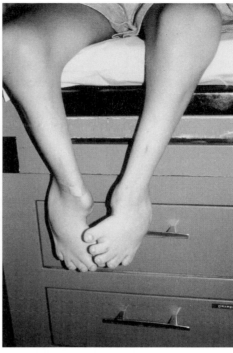

FIGURE 7–1. (A) Lateral view of 14-year-old boy with camptomelic dysplasia showing characteristic facies and abnormal chest/shoulder configuration including pectus carinatum. (B) View of lower extremities of same patient showing distal tibial displacement and mild camptodactyly of the tibia.

to haplo-insufficiency of *SOX9*, some patients have not been found to have mutations in the coding sequence. Although some of these patients may reflect the effects of promoter mutations or position effects (to be discussed below), some may reflect mutations in other genes—there may be locus as well as allelic heterogeneity. Such heterogeneity may be reflected in clinical variation, such as the possibility of normal IQ form, and possibly in mode of inheritance (there may be an autosomal recessive form). However, the major focus of this chapter is the relationship of the *SOX9* mutations to the 46,XY sex reversal that frequently occurs in this disorder.

Clinical and Imaging Presentation. Patients with camptomelic dysplasia present at birth with bowed legs, abnormal facies, and other birth defects (Fig. 7–1). One of the two original descriptions (Lee et al., 1972) said it well with this subtitle: "short life-span dwarfism with respiratory distress, hypotonia, peculiar facies, and multiple skeletal and cartilaginous deformities." The original reports (Maroteaux et al., 1971; Lee et al., 1972) were followed by confirmatory cases (Schmickel et al., 1973) and reports of familial involvement (Thurmon et al., 1973). The occurrence of sex reversal was reported (Hovmoller et al., 1977; Hoefnagel et al., 1978); definitive clinical delineation started with the articles of Hall and Spranger, (1980a) and Houston and colleagues (1983) but has continued (Mansour et al., 1995). On the basis of these reports, one can generate the following generalized clinical description. The infant with camptomelic dysplasia typically presents at birth with bowed tibia and respiratory distress. The respiratory distress is of a much greater degree than expected from the frequently small thorax and is associated with evidence of diffuse laryngotracheobronchomalacia (Grad et al., 1978). Radiological studies will reveal hypoplastic scapulae, vertically narrow iliac wings, and hypoplastic pedicles of many of the thoracic vertebrae. There may be only 11 pairs of ribs. Clinical examination will find macrocephaly and micrognathia frequently and cleft palate in about two thirds of the cases. Sex reversal occurs frequently, with about two thirds of 46,XY patients appearing female. There is a a high frequency of flat nasal bridge and low-set ears. The external manifestations of the skeletal abnormalities include talipes equinovarus and congenital dislocation of the hip. The bowed tibia are not an essential part of the diagnosis. As presented by Houston and colleagues (1983), in one of the early descriptions of cases now known to fit the condition, Middleton (1934) argued that the tibial bowing is the secondary result of a primary shortness of the calf muscles that first cause the talipes equinovarus and then, with continued stress, cause tibial bending. The frequent dimpling over the anterior angulation of the tibial bowing is due to the lack of fat beneath the skin.

Camptomelic dysplasia is not the only cause of congenital bowing of long bones. Hall and Spranger (1980b) reviewed about 20 entities that can have congenital bowing of long bones and placed 13 cases that did not fit any of those entities into three groups.

Most of the patients die in the neonatal period because of respiratory insufficiency, so many come to postmortem exam and, if diagnosis has not occurred prior to death, findings at postmortem can help establish the diagnosis. Absent or hypoplastic olfactory bulbs, heart defects in about 20%, and hydronephrosis in about 40% are useful additional findings (Hall and Spranger, 1980a). Hypoplastic trachea or cartilaginous rings that suggest tracheomalacia are frequently found. Some patients spontaneously survive the neonatal respiratory difficulties; Houston and colleagues (1983) provided follow-up on one of the initial cases reported by Maroteaux and colleagues (1971), finding the patient to be moderately retarded with an IQ of about 45 at 17 years of age. Children can be supported through these neonatal respiratory difficulties and, although at least one patient has been reported to have died early on discharge, at 11 months (Ninomiya et al., 1995), others have had longer term survival and also seem to be only moderately retarded (Benjamin Wilfond, personal communication, 1995).

XY sex reversal in syndromal association with spastic paraplegia and other features of nonreproductive maldevelopment has recently been reported (Spastic Paraplegia and Sex Reversal in Chapter 15).

Laboratory Features.   Most patients have died in the newborn period and laboratory investigations have been limited to diagnosing/monitoring the respiratory disease. To our knowledge, the few surviving older patients have not undergone endocrine investigations. The gonads may have an ovarian appearance with primary follicles (Mansour et al., 1995). In a case report arguing for autosomal dominant inheritance (Lynch et al. 1993), a minimally affected female was fertile and had a child with classic features of the disease.

Genotyping. Camptomelic dysplasia was classically considered to be an autosomal recessive disorder because of the occasional occurrence of families with affected sibs. The recent discovery of mutations in *SOX9* leading to haplo-insufficiency for this gene as the cause of camptomelic dysplasia with frequent sex reversal argues that some of the disorders in these families may have been caused by gonadal mosaicism and this has been documented in one family (Cameron et al., 1996). However, the presence of consanguinity in at least two families also suggests that there may be a separate autosomal recessive form.

In the early 1990s, a series of patients with cytogenetic abnormalities helped to identify the 17q24.3-q25.1 region as the likely localization of a candidate gene for camptomelic dysplasia (Maraia et al., 1991; Young et al., 1992; Tommerup et al., 1993). Soon it was discovered that mouse *Sox9*, a gene whose expression is consistent with a primary role of skeletal formation, maps to mouse chromosome 11, in a region homologous to the q24.3-q25.1 region of chromosome 17 (Wright et al., 1995). This made *SOX9* an excellent candidate for the defective gene in camptomelic dysplasia. *SOX9* mutational analysis detected heterozygous mutations in many, but not all, patients with camptomelic dysplasia (Foster et al., 1994; Wagner et al., 1994). Most of the mutations lead to truncation of the transactivating domain (Foster et al., 1994; Kwok et al., 1995; Sudbeck et al., 1996), although two nonsense mutations in the HMG box (which is a putative DNA-binding domain) have also been described (Kwok et al., 1995). Mutations distinguishing patients with and without sex reversal have not yet been found (Meyer et al., 1997)—an identical frameshift mutation has been associated in one case with 46,XY sex reversal and in another case without it (Kwok et al., 1995). Thus, modifier genes, perhaps affecting rates of gonadal growth as discussed in Chapter 2, may play a major role in determining the presence or absence of sex reversal. Mutations in *SOX9* have not been found in 46,XY sex reversal without the skeletal manifestations of camptomelic dysplasia (Kwok et al., 1996).

As well as showing expression patterns appropriate for a role in testis differentiation (da Silva et al., 1996), the pattern of expression of *Sox9* suggests a role for it in many of the structures that are abnormal in camptomelic dysplasia (Wright et al., 1995). Besides a major role in the developing skeleton, *Sox9* is expressed in otocysts, nasal cartilage (perhaps related to the abnormal structure of the nose), ventricular cells of the brain and spinal cord and ectoderm cells overlying the spinal cord (perhaps related to the mental retardation in survivors), and in "tubular structures in the heart" (perhaps related to the high incidence of congenital heart disease). *Sox9* is coexpressed with (Ng et al., 1997), and directly regulates the type II collagen gene that is expressed in chondrocytes (Bell et al., 1997), and a role in testis formation seems likely even in birds (Kent et al., 1996). Marshall Graves (1997) has suggested that *Sox9* may be regulated by *Sry* through suppression of *Sox3*, the sex gene most homologous to *Sry* (Collignon et al., 1996).

An intriguing aspect of the relationship of *SOX9* to camptomelic dysplasia is the likelihood that position effects, reviewed in Milot and colleagues (1996), can be involved. The breakpoint in the translocation study by Foster and colleagues (1994) is located 88 kb from *SOX9*. The roughly one third of patients in whom mutations in *SOX9* have not been found (Foster et al., 1994) might be examples of further mutations localized outside the coding region of the gene. Thus, it is quite possible that *SOX9* lies in a region of chromatin with a high propensity for causing position effects. Alternatively, a second, nearby gene may be involved (Ninomiya et al., 1996).

Management. As previously discussed, ventilatory support will lead to survival of patients with camptomelic dysplasia who are likely not to be ventilation-dependent by 1 year of age. However, it is expected that they will be moderately retarded. Although one can envision mutations in *SOX9* that might affect the skeleton without affecting the central nervous system, there is no evidence of such a differential developmental role as yet. Although one child died not long after being taken off ventilatory support, others have survived to mid-childhood and are capable of semi-independent living. Standard orthopedic support for their limb deformities is appropriate.

Discussion. Although camptomelic dysplasia has been classified as an autosomal recessive disorder as recently as 1992 (McKusick, 1992), autosomal dominant (Lynch et al., 1993), and even X-linked (Schimke, 1979) patterns of inheritance have been considered. With the discovery that camptomelic dysplasia is usually associated with heterozygous mutations in *SOX9*, it seems likely that gonadal mosaicism is frequently the cause of multiple affected sibs. However, consanguinity has been reported in some families with multiple cases, so allelic or locus heterogeneity associated with autosomal recessive inheritance may still be a possibility.

REFERENCES

Bell D M, Leung K K H, Wheatley S C, Ng L J, Zhou S, Ling K W, Sham M H, Koopman P, Tam P P L, Cheah K S E (1997). *SOX9* directly regulates the type-II collagen gene. *Nat Genet* 16:174–178.

Cameron F J, Hageman R M, Cooke-Yarborough C, Kwok C, Goodwin L L, Sillence D O, Sinclair A H (1996). A novel germ line mutation in *SOX9* causes familial campomelic dysplasia and sex reversal. *Hum Mol Genet* 5:1625–1630.

Collignon J, Sockanathan S, Hacker A, Cohen-Tannoudji M, Norris D, Rastan S, Stevanovic M, Goodfellow P N, Lovell-Badge R (1996). A comparison of the properties of *Sox-3* with *Sry* and two related genes, *Sox-1* and *Sox-2*. *Development* 122:509–520.

da Silva S M, Hacker A, Harley V, Goodfellow P, Swain A, Lovell-Badge R (1996). *SOX9* expression during gonadal development implies a conserved role for the gene in testis differentiation in mammals and birds. *Nat Genet* 14:62–68.

Foster J W, Dominguez-Steglich M A, Guioll S, Kwok C, Weller P A, Stevanovic M, Weissenbach J, Mansour S, Young I D, Goodfellow P N, Brook J D, Schafer A J (1994). Campomelic dysplasia and autosomal sex reversal caused by mutations in an *SRY*-related gene. *Nature* 372:525–530.

Grad R, Sammut P H, Britton J R, Goodrich P, Hoyme H E, Dambro N N (1987). Bronchoscopic evaluation of airway obstruction in campomelic dysplasia. *Pediatr Pulmonol* 3:364–367.

Hall B D, Spranger J (1980a). Congenital bowing of the long bones: a review and phenotype analysis of 13 undiagnosed cases. *Eur J Pediatr* 133:131–138.

Hall B D, Spranger J W (1980b). Campomelic dysplasia: further elucidation of a distinct entity. *Am J Dis Child* 134:285–289.

Houston C S, Opitz J M, Spranger J W, Macpherson R I, Reed M H, Gilbert E F, Hermann J, Schinzel A (1983). The campomelic syndrome: review, report of 17 cases, and follow-up on the currently 17-year-old boy first reported by Maroteaux et al. in 1971. *Am J Med Genet* 15:3–28.

Hoefnagel D, Wurster-Hill D H, Dupree W B, Beinirschke K, Fuld G L (1978). Camptomelic dwarfism associated with XY-gonadal dysgenesis and chromosome anomalies. *Clin Genet* 13:489–499.

Hovmoller M L, Osuna A, Eklof O, Fredga K, Hjerpe A, Lindsten J, Ritzen M, Stanescu V, Svenningsen N (1977). Camptomelic dwarfism: a genetically determined mesenchymal disorder combined with sex reversal. *Hereditas* 86:51–62.

Kent J, Wheatley S C, Andrews J E, Sinclair A H, Koopman P (1996). A male-specific role for *SOX9* in vertebrate sex determination. *Development* 122:2813–2822.

Kwok C, Weller P A, Guioli S, Foster J W, Mansour S, Zuffardi O, Punnett H H, Dominguez-Steglich M A, Brook J D, Young I D, Goodfellow P N, Schafer A J (1995). Mutations in *SOX9*, the gene responsible for campomelic dysplasia and autosomal sex reversal. *Am J Hum Genet* 57:1028–1036.

Kwok C, Goodfellow P N, Hawkins J R. (1996). Evidence to exclude *SOX9* as a candidate gene for XY sex reversal without skeletal malformation. *J Med Genet* 33:800–801.

Lee F A, Isaacs H, Strauss J (1972). The "Campomelic" syndrome: short life-span dwarfism with respiratory distress, hypotonia, peculiar facies, and multiple skeletal and cartilaginous deformities. *Am J Dis Child* 124:485–496.

Lynch S A, Gaunt M L, Minford A M B (1993). Campomelic dysplasia: evidence of autosomal dominant inheritance. *J Med Genet* 30:683–686.

Mansour S, Hall C M, Pembrey M E, Young I D. (1995). A clinical and genetic study of campomelic dysplasia. *J Med Genet* 32:415–420.

Maraia R, Saal H M, Wangsa D. (1991). A chromosome 17q de novo paracentric inversion in a patient with campomelic dysplasia; case report and etiologic hypothesis. *Clin Genet* 39:401–408.

Maroteaux T, Spranger J, Opitz J M, Kuchera J, Lowry R B, Schimke R N, Kagan S M (1971). The campomelique syndrome. *Presse Med* 79:1157.

Marshall Graves J A (1997). Two uses for old SOX. *Nat Genet* 16:114–115.

McKusick V A. Camptomelic dwarfism MIM No 211970. In: *Mendelian Inheritance in Man.* Johns Hopkins University Press, Baltimore, MD. 1992.

Meyer J, Sudbeck P, Held M, Wagner T, Schmitz M L, Bricarelli F D, Eggermount E, Friedrich U, Haas O A, Kobelt A, Leroy J G, Maldergem L V, Michel E, Mitulla B, Pfeiffer R A, Schnizel A, Schmidt H, Scherer G (1997). Mutational analysis of the *SOX9* gene in campomelic dysplasia and autosomal sex reversal: lack of genotype/phenotype correlations. *Hum Mol Genet* 6:91–98.

Middleton D S (1934). Studies in prenatal lesions of striated muscle as a cause of congenital deformity. I. Congenital tibial kyphosis; II. Congenital high shoulder; III. Myodystrophia foetalis deformans. *Edinburgh Med J* 41:401–442.

Milot E, Fraser P, Grosveld F (1996). Position effects and genetic disease. *Trends Genet* 12:123–126.

Ng L-J, Wheatley S, Muscat G E O, Conway-Campbell J, Bowles J, Wright E, Bell D M, Tam P P L, Cheah K S E, Koopman P (1997). SOX9 binds DNA, activates transcription, and coexpresses with Type II collagen during chondrogenesis in the mouse. *Dev Biol* 183:108–121.

Ninomiya S, Narahara K, Tsuji K, Yokoyama Y, Ito S, Seino Y (1995). Acampomelic campomelic syndrome and sex reversal associated with de novo t(12;17) translocation. *Am J Med Genet* 56:31–34.

Ninomiya S, Isomura M, Narahara K, Seino Y, Nakamura Y (1996). Isolation of a testis-specific cDNA on chromosome 17q from a region adjacent to the breakpoint of t(12;17) observed in a patient with acampomelic campomelic dysplasia and sex reversal. *Hum Mol Genet* 5:69–72.

Schimke R N (1979). Letter to the Editor: XY sex-reversed campomelia: possibly an X-linked disorder? *Clin Genet* 16:62–63.

Schmickel R D, Heidelberger K P, Poznanski A K (1973). The campomelique syndrome. *J Pediatr* 82:299–302.

Sudbeck P, Schmitz M L, Baeuerle P A, Scherer G (1996). Sex reversal by loss of the C-terminal transactivation domain of human *SOX9*. *Nat Genet* 13:230–232.

Thurmon T F, DeFraites E B, Anderson E E (1973). Familial camptomelic dwarfism. *J Pediatr* 83:841–843.

Tommerup N, Schempp W, Meinecke P, Pederson S, Bolund L, Brandt C, Goodpasture C, et al. (1993). Assignment of an autosomal sex reversal locus (SRA1) and campomelic dysplasia (CMPD1) to 17q24.3-q25.1. *Nat Genet* 4:170–174.

Wagner T, Wirth J, Meyer J, Zabel B, Held M, Zimmer J, Pasantes J, Icarelli F D, Keutel J, Hustert E (1994). Autosomal sex reversal and campomelic dysplasia are caused by mutations in and around the *SRY*-related gene *SOX9*. *Cell* 79:1111–1120.

Wright E, Hargrave M R, Christiansen J, Cooper L, Kun J, Evans T, Gangadharan U, Greenfield A, Koopman P (1995). The *Sry*-related gene *Sox9* is expressed during chondrogenesis in mouse embryos. *Nat Genet* 9:15–20.

Young I D, Zuccollo J M, Maltby E L, Broderick N J (1992). Campomelic dysplasia associated with a de novo 21;17q reciprocal translocation. *J Med Genet* 29:251–252.

OVARIAN DYSGENESIS (WITH DEAFNESS; PERRAULT SYNDROME)

Phenotype females with a 46,XX karyotype, streak gonads, hypoplastic internal genitalia, and no stigmata of the Turner syndrome are classified as having a special form of gonadal dysgenesis (see also Chapter 5 for discussion of XY gonadal dysgenesis). The condition is often familial in consanguineous families such that autosomal recessive inheritance seems assured (Elliott et al., 1959; Vesaly et al., 1980; Aleem, 1981; Meyers et al., 1996). A normal-appearing azoospermic male sib of affected sisters was described on one occasion (Granat et al., 1983). In another family, one female sib had ovarian dysgenesis whereas another had delayed-to-infrequent menses, perhaps indicative of a broader spectrum of ovarian dysfunction or the presence of modifying factors (Boczkowski, 1970).

Several families have also been reported in which affected individuals had other features, especially sensorineural deafness (the Perrault syndrome) (Perrault et al., 1951; Bosze et al., 1983). In some families, apparently sexually normal male sibs were deaf (Pallister and Opitz, 1979). Others have described additional neurologic features—ataxia, neuropathy, mild mental retardation, dyspraxia (Nishi et al., 1988; Linssen et al., 1994). In another sib pair, the typical ovarian lesion was accompanied by microcephaly, short stature, and arachnodactyly and no deafness (Maximilian et al., 1970). Autosomal recessive inheritance also seems likely for these more complex forms of XX, gonadal dysgenesis.

REFERENCES

Aleem F A (1981). Familial 46,XX gonadal dysgenesis. *Fertil Steril* 35:317–320.

Boczkowski K (1970). Pure gonadal dysgenesis and ovarian dysplasia in sisters. *Am J Obstet Gynecol* 106:626–628.

Bosze P, Skripezcky K, Gaal M, el al. (1983). Perrault's syndrome in two sisters. *Am J Med Genet* 16:237–241.

Elliott G A, Sandler A, Rabinowitz D (1959). Gonadal dysgenesis in three sisters. *J Clin Endocrinol* 19:995–1003.

Granat M, Amar A, Mor-Yosef S, et al. (1983). Familial gonadal germinative failure: endocrine and human leukocyte antigen studies. *Fertil Steril* 40:215–219.

Linssen W H, Van den Bent M J, Brunner H G, et al. (1994). Deafness, sensory neuropathy, and ovarian dysgenesis: a new syndrome or a broader spectrum of Perrault syndrome. *Am J Med Genet* 51:81–82.

Maximilian C, Ionescu B, Bucur S (1970). Deux soeurs avec dysgénésie gonadique majeure, hypotrophic staturale, microcéphalie, arachnodactylie et caryotype 46,XX. *J Génét Hum* 18:365 378.

Meyers C M, Boughman J A, Rivas M, et al. (1996). Gonadal (ovarian) dysgenesis in 46,XX individuals; frequency of the autosomal recessive form. *Am J Med Genet* 63:518–524.

Nishi Y, Hamamoto K, Kajiyama M, et al. (1988). The Perrault syndrome: clinical report and review. *Am J Med Genet* 31:623–628.

Pallister P D, Opitz J M (1979). The Perrault syndrome: autosomal recessive ovarian dysgenesis with facultative, non-sex-limited sensorineural deafness. *Am J Med Genet* 4:239–246.

Perrault M, Klotz B, Housset E (1951). Deux cas de syndrome de Turner avec surdi-mutite dans une meme fratrie. *Bull Mem Soc Med Hop Paris* 16:79–84.

Vesely D L, Bower R H, Kohler P O et al. (1980). Familial ovarian dysgenesis in 46,XX females. *Am J Med Sci* 280:157–166.

8

Absence of the Gonads

"Absent gonads" may reflect failure of gonad formation or failure of gonad retention. The gonads that are absent may have been meant to become, or once were, either ovaries (Overzier and Linden, 1956; Medina et al., 1982) or testes (Cunningham, 1960). This chapter deals primarily with conditions in which the gonads were formed and then disappeared. Two examples in males are testicular regression syndromes and congenital anomalies presumably due to testicular torsion. 46,XX females with no gonads have also been described (Levinson et al., 1976; Kennerknecht et al., 1993; Medina et al., 1982; Mendonca et al., 1994; Kennerknecht et al., 1997). Gonads may also be absent in Turner syndrome (Chapter 6) and other forms of gonadal dysgenesis. Our focus will be on testicular regression syndromes. This group of conditions is characterized by embryonic or fetal formation of testicular tissue and later gonadal regression in 46,XY individuals with ambiguous genitalia. Individuals with female external genitalia, and those with partially masculinized genitalia are sometimes found in the same family and are considered to show different manifestations of the same autosomal recessive disorder that can also cause absent gonads in 46,XX individuals.

Clinical and Imaging Presentations.   The initial case reports were of individuals with ambiguous genitalia without other major birth defects (Sarto and Opitz, 1973; Kofman-Alfaro et al., 1976; Rosenberg et al., 1984). These patients were all 46,XY, and various surgical interventions, commonly attempting to correct cryptorchidism, did not find gonads. As familial cases were found (Jusso and Briard, 1980) in which one affected individual was a phenotypic male with micropenis and a 46,XY sibling was a phenotypic female without significant sexual ambiguity, it was realized that expressivity could vary significantly. An early loss of the gonads will lead to phenotypic females with normal müllerian ducts, whereas testicular insufficiency during the second half of the pregnancy will lead to micropenis without structural abnormalities of the genital tract. Recently, 46,XY individuals with female external genitalia, absent gonads, and a variety of other birth defects have been found. Thus, two "sisters" with 46,XY karyotype, mental retardation, short stature, severely retarded bone age, and a characteristic facies, but discordant visceral malformations (agenesis of the kidney with malrotated colon in one sister, but not in the second) were described as a new autosomal recessive syndrome (Kennerknecht et al., 1995). Agonadism has also been described in a 46,XY patient with the CHARGE association (Coloboma, Heart defects, Atresia choanae, Retardation, Genital anomalies, and Ear abnormalities/deafness).

Another association seems to be with severe motor and physical retardation in the absence of multiple birth defects (Maciel-Guerra et al., 1991; Sybert et al., 1995). Currently, ultrasonography is used to delineate the absence of gonads; surgical exploration is confirmatory.

Laboratory Features.   Because of the mode of ascertainment described above, karyotypes are usually 46,XY; however, familial cases of agonadism in which one sib is 46,XY and the other 46,XX have been reported (Kennerknecht et al., 1993; Mendonca et al., 1994), and one case of agonadism in a singleton 46,XX individual has been described (Levinson et al., 1976). As expected, gonadotropin levels are high and sex steroids undetectable. The measurement of serum müllerian inhibiting substance is a better indicator of absent testes than is the measurement of serum testosterone (Lee et al., 1997). *SRY* was expectedly normal in four cases of bilateral congenital anorchia (Lobaccaro et al., 1993) and five cases of testicular regression syndrome (Marcantonio et al., 1994).

Genotyping.   Monozygotic twins are usually discordant for testicular regression syndrome (only two out of nine pairs in one review were concordant; Ruvalcaba et al., 1981). This argues against a common genetic causation. On the other hand, a consanguinity rate of approximately 5% (Rosenberg et al., 1984) and the multiple familial cases argue that an autosomal recessive gene can also cause this condition. Indeed, there are likely to be mutations in several genes that cause gonadal regression, some with multiple congenital anomalies (as described above), and some causing isolated testicular regression. To our knowledge, no gene has yet been identified. Testicular torsion causing infarction of the testes may also be familial (Cunningham, 1960; Castella et al., 1975).

Management.   In those patients with female or near-female external genitalia, rearing as a female, perhaps with surgical support, and with appropriate hormonal replacement, will be appropriate. In those patients with ambiguous genitalia, surgical construction toward the male phenotype may be appropriate. For them, androgen replacement will be necessary. In either situation, genetic counseling for sterility should be available.

Discussion.   A variety of genetic disorders seem to cause testicular regression syndrome, with and without associated birth defects; many cases, however (as evidenced in the discordance among monozygotic twins), are thought not to have a genetic etiology. In this regard, the possibility of testicular torsion or strangulation due to lack of stabilizing ligamentous attachments of the testes (related to its need to descend through the inguinal canal to the scrotum) are likely explanations. Damaged embryonic structures are frequently absorbed leaving little residual "scar" tissue. Atrophy *in utero* would be the likely consequence of testicular demise due to torsion or strangulation.

REFERENCES

Castella E E, Sod R, Anzorena O, Texido J. (1975). Neonatal testicular torsion in two brothers. *J Med Genet* 12:112–113.

Cunningham R F. (1960). Familial occurrence of testicular torsion. *JAMA* 174:1330.

Josso N, Briard, M-L (1980). Embryonic testicular regression syndrome: variable phenotypic expression in siblings. *J Pediatr* 97:200–204.

Kennerknecht I, Sorgo W, Oberhoffer R, Teller M T, Mattfeldt T, Negri G, Vogel W (1993). Familial occurrence of agonadism and multiple internal malformations in phenotypically normal girls with 46,XY and 46,XX karyotypes, respectively: a new autosomal recessive syndrome. *Am J Med Genet* 47:1166–1170.

Kennerknecht I, von Saurma P, Brenner R, Just W, Barbi G, Sorgo W, Heinze E, Wolf A S, Schneider V, Gunther K-P, Teller W M, Vogel W (1995). Agonadism in two sisters with XY gonosomal constitution, mental retardation, short stature, severely retarded bone age, and multiple extragenital malformations: a new autosomal recessive syndrome. *Am J Med Genet* 59:62–67.

Kennerknecht I, Mattfeldt T, Paulus W, Nitsch C, Negri G, Barbi G, Just W, Schwemmle S, Vogel W (1997). XX-agonadism in a fetus with multiple dysraphic lesions: a new syndrome. *Am J Med Genet* 70:413–414.

Kofman-Alfaro S, Saavedra D, Ochoa S, Scaglia H, Perez-Palacios G (1976). Pseudohermaphroditism due to XY gonadal absence syndrome. *J Med Genet* 13:242–246.

Kushnick T, Wiley J E, Palmer S M (1992). Agonadism in a 46,XY patient with CHARGE association. *Am J Med Genet* 42:96–99.

Lee M M, Konahoe P K, Silverman B L, Hasegawa T, Hasegawa Y, Gustafson M L, Chang Y, MacLaughlin D T (1997). Measurements of serum Müllerian inhibiting substance in the evaluation of children with nonpalpable gonads. *N Engl J Med* 336:1480–1486.

Levinson G, Zarate A, Guzman-Toledano R, Canales E S, Jimenez M (1976). An XX female with sexual infantilism, absent gonads, and lack of Müllerian ducts. *J Med Genet* 13:68–69.

Lobaccaro J-M, Medlej R, Berta P, Belon C, Galifer R B, Guthmann J P, Chevalier C, Czernichow P, Dumas R, Sultan C (1993). PCR analysis and sequencing of the *SRY* sex determining gene in four patients with bilateral congenital anorchia. *Clin Endocrinol* 38:197–201.

Maciel-Guerra A T, Farah S B, Garmes H M, Pinto Jr W, da Silva J M B, Baptista M T, Marques-de-Faria A P, Guerra Jr G, de Mello M P (1991). Brief clinical report. True agonadism: report of a case analyzed with Y-specific DNA probes. *Am J Med Genet* 41:444–445.

Marcantonio S M, Fechner P Y, Migeon C J, Perlman E J, Berkovitz G D (1994). Embryonic testicular regression sequence: a part of the clinical spectrum of 46,XY gonadal dysgenesis. *Am J Med Genet* 49:1–5.

Medina M, Kofman-Alfaro S, Pérez-Palacios G (1982). 46,XX gonadal absence: a variant of the XX pure gonadal dysgenesis? *Acta Endocrinol* 90:585–587.

Mendonca B B, Barbosa A S, Arnhold I J P, McElreavey K, Fellous M, Moreira-Filho C A (1994). Gonadal agenesis in XX and XY sisters: evidence for the involvement of an autosomal gene. *Am J Med Genet* 52:39–43.

Overzier C, Linden H (1956). Echter Agonadismus (Anorchismus) bei Geschwistern. *Gynaecologia* 142:215–233.

Rosenberg C, Mustacchi Z, Braz A, Arnhold I J P, Chu T H, Carnevale J, Frota-Pessoa O (1984). Testicular regression in a patient with virilized female phenotype. *Am J Med Genet* 19:183–188.

Ruvalcaba R H A, Gogue H P, Kelley V C (1981). Discordance of congenital bilateral anochia in uniovular twins: 17 years of observations on growth and development. *Pediatrics* 67:276–280.

Sarto G E, Opitz J M. (1973). The XY gonadal agenesis syndrome. *J Med Genet* 10:288–293.

Sybert V P, Pagon R A, Ramsdell L, Marymee K (1995). Re: True agonadism: report of a case analyzed with Y-specific DNA probes. *Am J Med Genet* 55:113. Letter to the Editor.

IV

SEXUAL MALDEVELOPMENT

9

Genetic Disorders of the Anti-Müllerian Hormone (AMH) and Its Receptor

AMH, also known as müllerian inhibitory substance (MIS) or factor (MIF) is secreted by Sertoli cells from the eighth fetal week (Josso et al., 1993; Lee and Donahoe, 1993). It causes regression of the müllerian ducts (MD) in males. Failure of the MD to regress permits their development into the uterus and fallopian tubes. Persistence of MD derivatives among subjects with a male sexual phenotype occurs in three main clinical settings: a "pure" form in which the synthesis or action of AMH is defective; a complicated form, often unilateral, in which the primary problem is one or another type or degree of testicular dysgenesis; and, inauthentically, before proper diagnosis of female pseudohermaphroditism. Persistent müllerian duct derivatives have also been reported in syndromal association with nonreproductive anomalies (Urioste Syndrome in chapter 15).

About 50% of subjects with the pure form have deficient or defective AMH production, usually due to a point mutation in the AMH gene; the other half have normal AMH genes and AMH production, implying target organ insensitivity to AMH (Josso et al., 1996).

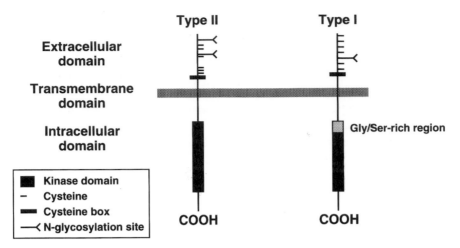

FIGURE 9–1. The generic structural features of type II and type I receptors for members of the TGF-β family of growth-inhibitory proteins such as anti-müllerian hormone (AMH). (Reproduced from Josso et al., *Frontiers in Endocrinology* 20:55–60, 1996, with permission.)

The AMH gene is located on 19p. Its expression is regulated by the nuclear receptor SF-1 (Shen et al., 1994). Its product, 560 amino acids, is organized into a dimeric, 145-kilodalton glycoprotein, and is a member of the transforming growth factor–β (TGF-β) superfamily (Josso et al., 1993; Lee and Donahoe, 1993). Like TGF-β itself, AMH is processed proteolytically to yield a bioactive C-terminal fragment (Pepinsky et al., 1988) that shares amino acid homology with that of TGF-β, and a N-terminal fragment that is not itself necessary for bioactivity. Interestingly, however, their N-terminal and C-terminal cleavage products can reassociate noncovalently, and this reunion potentiates bioactivity of AMH (Wilson et al., 1993).

The AMH receptor (AMHR) gene is located on 12q. Its product, 573 amino acids, is a serine/threonine protein kinase with a single transmembrane domain encoded by exon 4 (Imbeaud et al., 1995). Exons 1–3 yield the signal sequence and the extracellular domain; exons 5–11, the intracellular domain (Fig. 9–1). Its promoter lacks a CAAT box and a functional TATA box. There is a single Sp 1 site at -47, and a canonical SRY response element at -525. The AMHR belongs to the family of so-called type II receptors for TGF-β-related proteins. Signals initiated by ligand–type II receptor interaction must be transduced to downstream targets by phosphorylated type I receptors (Massagué, 1992).

Clinical and Laboratory Features.   In the pure form of the persistent müllerian duct syndrome (PMDS), otherwise normally virilized men are usually identified during surgery for unilateral inguinal hernia (herniorrhaphy) or cryptorchidism (orchidopexy). Usually, one testis is in the scrotum while the other, the uterus, and the ipsilateral fallopian tube are in the inguinal hernia (*hernia uteri inguinalis*). Occasionally, the contralateral testis and fallopian tube are in the same inguinal sac (transverse testicular ectopia). Uncommonly, the cryptorchidism is bilaterally intra-abdominal and the uterus is entirely pelvic. Occasionally, the uterus is considered hypoplastic. Rarely, the presenting complaint is male infertility. Nevertheless, aplasia of the epididymis and upper vas deferens are common, and the lower part of the vas deferens is often stuck to the uterine wall or embedded in it. Disturbed anatomic relations resulting from persistent müllerian duct structures prevents the gubernaculum from fixing the testis to the base of the scrotum (Hutson and Baker, 1994). The resulting increase in scrotal mobility may lead to torsion and consequent testicular atrophy.

The serum level of AMH (by ELISA), or the anti-müllerian activity of a testicular biopsy (by bioassay) is either unmeasurable or very low, indicating the likelihood of an AMH gene mutation, or normal to slightly elevated, indicating the likelihood of an AMHR mutation. However, testicular regression secondary to testicular torsion may yield spuriously low levels of AMH in some patients with AMHR mutations.

Genotyping and Ethnic Considerations of AMH Gene Mutations. The AMH gene contains five exons. The first three encode the N-terminal fragment and are relatively mutation-rich, although they are relatively CpG-poor. The other two exons encode the C-terminal fragment whose bioactivity is potentiated by association with the N-terminal fragment.

In the largest single series (Imbeaud et al. 1994), point mutations in the AMH gene were discovered in 13 of 15 patients with AMH deficiency. Nine of the 13 were novel. Ten mutations were in exons 1–3 (659 bp), even though exons 4 and 5 contain 1023 bp. Most affected males were homozygous; only three were compound heterozygotes, yet consanguinity was recognized in only one family. These data were obtained from a total of 19 families accumulated over a 4-year period by a laboratory in France, and the patients were predominantly of Mediterranean ethnicity. In a recent update, four of eight new patients had mutations in exon 1, and four were in the 3' half of exon 5 (Imbeaud et al., 1996). Thus, the PMD syndrome is not as rare as once thought, particularly among some ethnic groups.

Genotyping and Ethnic Consideration of AMHR Gene Mutation. The first AMHR mutation discovered was a $G^{+1} \rightarrow A$ transition at the donor-splice site of intron 2 (Imbeaud et al., 1995). This caused either skipping of exon 2 or in-frame intronic inclusion due to use of a cryptic downstream donor-splice site, and impaired a ligand-binding portion of the AMHR. The most common mutation, accounting for 50% of cases with AMHR mutation, is a 27-bp deletion in exon 10. The 27-bp deletion removes a portion of the AMHR just N-terminal of the region in the type II TGF-β receptor that is essential for normal kinase activity (Wieser et al., 1993). AMHR mutations are found predominantly in subjects from the northern parts of France and Europe, and less than half are homozygous. Because the 27-bp deletion occurs on the background of a single haplotype, the frequency of this mutation is likely to represent a founder effect.

Discussion and Speculation on AMH and AMHR Gene Mutations. There are several interesting characteristics of AMH gene mutation as a whole. First, the low rate of consanguinity, the high rate of compound heterozygosity, and the recognition of several benign polymorphisms suggest that the locus has a relatively high mutation rate. This is reinforced by the relatively high prevalence of the AMH-deficient syndrome, and by the low frequency of AMH gene mutation at CpG sites. Usually these are mutational hot spots. In the AMH gene, pathogenic missense mutations are more common in the CpG-poor exons 1–3 than in the CpG-rich exons 4 and 5. Imbeaud and colleagues (1994) have suggested that the high CG content of exons 4 and 5 may reflect a relatively low propensity to methylation and therefore a relatively low susceptibility to mutation of its CpG sites. However, the reason for low methylation remains to be explained. The apparently paradoxical mutational behavior of the AMH gene is magnified by the fact that exons 1–3 encode the N-terminal portion of AMH, the portion that is bio-inactive after proteolytic processing. Thus, the mutations in exon 1–3 probably act by destabilizing the AMH protein before it is proteolytically processed at its target sites of action.

The failure to find an AMH gene mutation in a subject with immuno-undetectable AMH in his serum might represent decreased mRNA synthesis or stability due to mutation in a regulatory region of the AMH gene.

All AMH and AMHR mutations described to date have behaved in an autosomal recessive fashion. However, by inference from other TGFβR-family members, mutations that truncate the AMHR just downstream of the transmembrane domain could produce dominant-negative phenotypes.

Although AMH has depressive effects on granulosa cells, decreasing their aromatase and luteinizing hormone receptor activity (Lee and Donahoe, 1993), it is not necessary for normal ovarian function in humans: AMH-deficient females can reproduce normally.

It may be difficult to identify mutations responsible for PMD syndrome in two situations: when the mutation affects proteolytic processing of AMH and when the mutation affects a downstream step of the signaling pathway that is initiated by AMH-AMHR interaction.

Interestingly, excessive AMH has adverse developmental effects on transgenic mice of both sexes: females are masculinized; males are feminized (Behringer et al., 1990). Whether either or both mechanisms are pathogenic in human fetuses is an open question.

REFERENCES

Behringer R R, Cate R L, Froelick G J, Palmiter R D, Brinster R L (1990). Abnormal sexual development in transgenic mice chronically expressing mullerian inhibiting substance. *Nature* 345:167–170.

Hutson J M, Baker M L (1994). A hypothesis to explain abnormal gonadal descent in persistent Müllerian duct syndrome. *Pediatr Surg Int* 9:542–543.

Imbeaud S, Belville C, Messika-Zeitoun L, Rey R, di Clemente N, Josso N, Picard J Y (1996). A 27 base-pair deletion of the anti-Müllerian type II receptor gene is the most common cause of the persistent Müllerian duct syndrome. *Hum Mol Genet* 5:1269–1277.

Imbeaud S, Carré-Eusebe D, Rey R, Belville C, Josso N, Picard J Y (1994). Molecular genetics of the persistent Müllerian duct syndrome: a study of 19 families. *Hum Mol Genet* 3:125–131.

Imbeaud S, Faure E, Lamarre I, Mattei M G, di Clemente N, Tizard R, Carre-Eusebe D, Belville C, Tragethon L, Tonkin C, et al. (1995). Insensitivity to anti-Müllerian hormone due to a mutation in the human anti-Müllerian hormone receptor. *Nat Genet* 11:382–388.

Josso N, Cate R L, Picard J Y, Vigier B, di Clemente N, Wilson C, Imbeaud S, Pepinsky R B, Guerrier D, Boussin L, et al. (1993). Anti-müllerian hormone: the Jost factor. *Recent Prog Horm Res* 48:1–59.

Josso N, Picard J-Y, di Clemente N, Imbeaud S, Faure E, Belville C. (1996). Anti-Müllerian hormone and its receptor in sex differentiation. In:*Sex Differentiation: Clinical and Biological Aspects*, Hughes I A (ed), Cambridge, Frontiers in Endocrinology 20:55–60.

Lee M, Donahoe P K (1993). Müllerian inhibiting substance: a gonadal hormone with multiple functions. *Endocr. Rev.* 14:152–164.

Massagué J (1992). Receptors for the TGF-β family. *Cell* 69:1067–1070.

Pepinsky R B, Sinclair L K, Chow E P, Mattaliano R J, Manganara T F, Donahoe P K, Cate R L (1988). Proteolytic processing of müllerian inhibiting substance produces a transforming growth factor-β-like fragment. *J Biol Chem* 263:18961–18964.

Shen W-H, Moore C C D, Ikeda Y, Parker K L, Ingraham H A (1994). Nuclear receptor steroidogenic factor 1 regulates the Müllerian inhibiting substance gene: a link to the sex determination cascade. *Cell* 77:651–661.

Wieser R, Attisano L, Wrana J L, Massagué J (1993). Signaling activity of transforming growth factor-β type II receptors lacking specific domains in the cytoplasmic region. *Mol Cell Biol* 13:7239–7247.

Wilson C A, di Clemente N, Ehrenfels E, Pepinsky R B, Josso N, Vigier B, Cate R L (1993). Müllerian Inhibiting substance requires its N-terminal domain for maintenance of biological activity, a novel finding within the transforming growth factor-β superfamily. *Mol Endocrinol* 7:247–257.

10

Genetic Disorders Expressed by Gonadotropin Insufficiency

MOLECULAR BIOLOGY OF THE GONADOTROPINS, THE GONADOTROPIN-RELEASING HORMONE, AND ITS RECEPTOR

The two pituitary gonadotropins, follicle-stimulating hormone (FSH) and luteinizing hormone (LH), as well as chorionic gonadotropin (CG) belong to the glycoprotein hormone family. A closely related member is thyroid-stimulating hormone (TSH). All four are heterodimers that share a common α subunit bound noncovalently to a hormone-distinct β subunit (Fig. 10–1). The regulation of both LH-and FSH-subunit expression is under the complex control of gonadal steroids, gonadal peptides (inhibins and activins), and the hypothalamic gonadotropin-releasing hormone (GnRH) (Albanese et al., 1996). Certain regions of both subunits participate in receptor recognition, but the β subunits are primarily responsible for interaction with specific (cognate) receptors that belong to the family of receptors whose effects are transduced by coupling to G proteins (Fig. 11–2). LH and CG are so similar that they bind to the same receptor. The function of each subunit depends on internal disulfide bonds that form between specific cysteine residues. Their stability

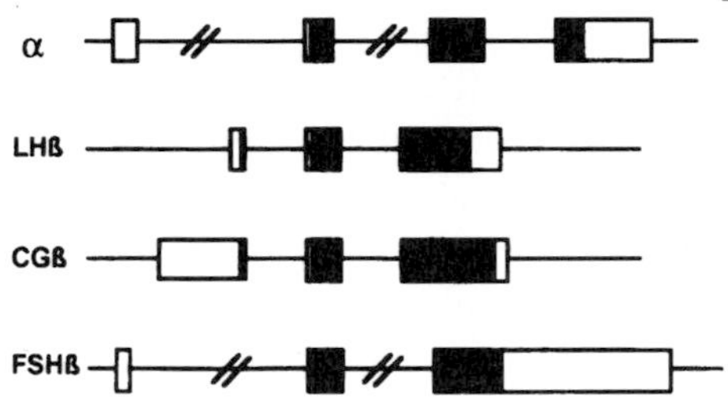

	Gene Length (Kb)	mRNA (bp)	Chromosome Location	Gene Copy#
α	9.4	800	6p21.1-23	1
LHβ	1.1	700	19q13.3	1
CGβ	1.5	1000	19q13.3	6
FSHβ	4.2	1800	11p13	1

FIGURE 10–1. The genomic organization of the glycoprotein hormone family α monomer, and of its three hormone-distinct β monomer partners. (Reproduced from Jameson J L, *Mol Cell Endocrinol* 125:143–149, 1996, with permission.)

and signal transduction ability, but not their receptor-binding activity, are also influenced by glycosylation at certain asparagine residues of both subunits.

The human (h) FSHβ gene is at 11p13 (Fig. 10–1). It has three exons: the first, 5' untranslated, of 33 or 63 nucleotides; the second encodes an 18-amino-acid propeptide plus active residues 1–35; the third encodes the remaining 76 amino acids of the full peptide. Alternative 5' splicing and 3' polyA-site usage yield four different mRNAs with very different stabilities (Gharib et al., 1990).

The hLHβ gene is on chromosome 19q13 adjacent to a cluster of homologous CGβ genes and pseudogenes (Fig. 10–1). It also has three exons. The first is untranslated; the second encodes a signal propetide plus active residues 1–41; the third encodes the remaining 80 amino acids of the full peptide (Gharib et al., 1990).

The hGnRH (gonadotropin-releasing hormone) gene is at 8p (Yang-Feng et al., 1986). It contains four exons. The first exon encodes a 5' untranslated region; the second exon encodes the signal peptide, the GnRH decapeptide, and the beginning of the GnRH-associated peptide (GAP). Exons 3 and 4 encode the remainder of the GAP peptide and the 3'-untranslated region (Radovick et al., 1990). GnRH is secreted into the hypothalamic-pituitary portal circulation in a pulsatile fashion by neurons of the anterior hypothalamus. In turn, GnRH stimulates synthesis and secretion of the pituitary gonadotropins.

Homozygous or compound heterozygous mutations of the FSHβ gene cause amenorrhea and hypogonadism in women, and oligo/azoospermia in otherwise eugonadal men with normal testosterone levels (Fig. 10–2).

Homozygous or compound heterozygous mutations of the LHβ gene are known to cause pubertal failure in males and probably would do so in females because LH contributes to ovarian estrogen biosynthesis.

Homozygous or compound heterozygous mutations of the GnRH gene would be expected to cause combined LH and FSH deficiency, resulting in male and female pubertal failure. No human examples have been published, but the hypogonadal mouse is homozygous for a deleted GnRH gene (Mason et al., 1986).

The human GnRH-receptor (GnRHR) gene is on 4q and has three exons. It yields a mature mRNA of 5 kb that encodes a protein of 328 amino acids (Kaker et al.,

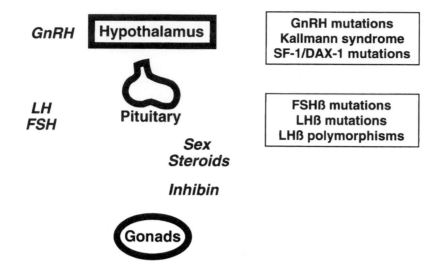

FIGURE 10–2. Some mutations (boxed) affecting the endocrine hypothalamus and the pituitary gonadrotropins that are discussed in this chapter. (Reproduced from Jameson J L *Mol Cell Endocrinol* 125:143–149, 1996, with permission.)

1992). The GnRHR is a member of the superfamily of G protein–coupled receptors (GPCR; Arora et al., 1995). Typically (Fig. 11–1), it has seven helical transmembrane (TM) domains, three intracellular (i) and three extracellular (e) loops, an N-terminal extracellular tail, and Leu at the conserved hydrophobic position, 147, in the middle of i2. Atypically, it lacks an intracellular tail. In addition, its i1 loop is highly basic, its i2 loop has Ser in place of Tyr in the GPCR signature sequence [Asp(D), Arg(R), Tyr(Y)] at the TM three-i2 loop junction), and it has Asn87 and Asp318 in TM two and three, respectively, instead of the more frequent reciprocal arrangement among members of the GPCR superfamily. After GnRHR binds agonist, it initiates a G protein–mediated signaling sequence (Fig. 11–2) that involves phospholipase C activation, hydrolysis of phosphoinositide to diacylglycerol and inositol triphosphate, calcium mobilization, and protein kinase C activation. The receptor is then internalized and down-regulated by endocytotic processing. Down-regulation of GnRHR after exposure of the pituitary gland to long-acting GnRH agonists is a prominent feature of its cell biology. It causes gonadotropin secretion to decrease markedly, and this effect is the basis for using such agonists to treat prostate cancer, precocious puberty, and other conditions.

REFERENCES

Arora K K, Sakai A, Catt K J. (1995). Effects of second intracellular loop mutations on signal transduction and internalization of the gonadotropin-releasing hormone receptor. *J Biol Chem* 270:22820–22826.

Albanese C, Colin I M, Crowley W F, Ito M, Pestell R G, Weiss J, Jameson J L (1996). The gonadotropin genes: evolution of distinct mechanisms for hormonal control. *Recent Prog Horm Res* 51:23–61.

Gharib S D, Weirman M E, Shupnik M A, Chin W W. (1992). Molecular biology of the pituitary gonadotropins. *Endocrinol Rev* 11:177–199.

Kakar S S, Musgrove L C, Devor D C, Sellers J C, Neill J D (1992). Cloning, sequencing, and expression of human gonadotropin releasing hormone (GnRH) receptor. *Biochem Biophys Res Commun* 189:289–295.

Mason A J, Hayflick J S, Zweller T, Young W S, Phillips H A, Nikolics K, Seeburg P H (1986). A deletion truncating the gonadotropin-releasing hormone gene is responsible for hypogonadism in the HPG mouse. *Science* 235:1366–1371.

Radovick S, Wondisford F E, Nakayama Y, Yamada M, Cutler Jr G B, Weintraub B D (1990) Isolation and characterization of the human gonadotropin-releasing hormone gene in the hypothalamus and placenta. *Mol Endocrinol* 4:476–480.

Yang-Feng T L, Seeburg P H, Franke U (1986). Human luteinizing hormone-releasing hormone gene is located on the short arm of chromosome 8 (region 8p 11.2>p21). *Somat Cell Mol Genet* 12:95–100.

HYPOTHALAMIC HYPOGONADISM DUE TO DEFECTIVE MIGRATION OF GnRH NEURONS FROM THE OLFACTORY PLACODE TO THE HYPOTHALAMUS: KALLMANN SYNDROME

Clinical and Imaging Features.   Kallmann syndrome (KS) is a combination of hypogonadism and anosmia inherited as a X-linked trait. Autosomal variants (dominant or recessive) may be more common (White et al., 1983; Santen and Paulsen 1973; Georgopoulos et al. 1997); in fact, various *de novo* autosomal rearrangements have been described in three patients (Schinzel et al., 1995). The hypogonadism is due to GnRH deficiency, and the anosmia (or hyposmia) to aplasia (hypoplasia) of the olfactory bulbs and tract. GnRH deficiency results from failure of GnRH neurons to migrate from the olfactory placode in the nose through the forebrain, and finally to the hypothalamus. Abnormal development of the olfactory bulbs presumably reflects abnormal axonal extension of olfactory neurons and failure to form synapses with cells within the olfactory bulbs.

At birth, affected males may have cryptorchidism and small but normally formed external genitalia. If not, penile growth may be subnormal during childhood, or at puberty. A variety of other defects occur in patients with X-linked Kallmann syndrome: the most notable are renal agenesis, often unilateral (Hardelin et al., 1992), and bimanual synkinesis (involuntary movement of the distal upper limbs that mirrors voluntary contraction of identical muscles on the opposite side; Conrad et al., 1978). Others include pes cavus, cleft lip and palate, and visual-spatial perception disorder (Bick et al., 1992). Variable expressivity is prominent in X-linked KS: in some families, olfaction and pubertal development are concordantly mild or severe (Parenti et al., 1995); in other families discordance for synkinesis or olfactory sulcus anomaly has been noted. In some individuals, complete anosmia is associated with mild hypogonadism (Wortsman and Hughes, 1996). In some families, GnRH deficiency and anosmia occur in different individuals. Hence, it may be impossible to distinguish between KS and the normosmic form of idiopathic hypogonadotropic hypogonadism (Dean et al., 1990; Pawlowitzki et al., 1987) even with sophisticated immunofluorescence technology (Quinton et al., 1997).

Magnetic resonance imaging (MRI) has been used to demonstrate absence or hypoplasia of the olfactory bulbs and sulci; it is especially useful for diagnosing KS in young children whose olfactory status is difficult to assess. However, MRI is not fully sensitive for detecting olfactory abnormalities, and it is insensitive for detecting the morphologic anomalies presumably associated with bimanual synkinesis (Quinton et al., 1996).

The KS locus (*KAL 1*) is at Xp 22.3. Some patients have KS together with other diseases (ichthyosis due to steroid sulfatase deficiency; chrondrodysplasia punctata) whose loci are nearby: these patients have a "contiguous gene syndrome" due to a chromosome deletion that eliminates several adjacent genes on Xp (Bick et al., 1992).

Laboratory Features.   Serum levels of LH, FSH, and testosterone are low basally, but respond to the administration of pulsatile GnRH.

Genotyping and Mutant Gene Expression.   The *KAL* gene has 14 exons that encode a protein of 680 amino acids. It contains several fibronectin type III repeats that allude to the property of cellular adhesion (Franco et al., 1991; Legouis et al., 1991). Such a property would be essential for axonal pathfinding. It is also predicted to have anti-protease activity. There is a highly homologous pseudogene on the Y chromosome. The promoter of the *KAL* gene (Cohen-Salmon et al., 1995) is GC-rich, has a CAAT box but not a TATA box, and contains two binding sites for each of the SP1 and AP2 transcription factors. There may be two transcription start sites. A 5' flanking fragment extending to −435 has weak, but tissue-specific, transcriptional activity. A fragment extending further upstream loses this activity, implying the existence of an upstream negative regulatory element.

Deletion of one degree or another is a frequent mode of mutation of *KAL*: It may affect adjacent loci, the entire *KAL* gene alone, a single exon, or a single base leading to frameshift and premature translation termination. Single-base changes leading to missense substitutions are relatively common. A recurrent mutation, Glu 514 Lys in exon 11, has been discovered in a Mexican population (Maya-Nuñez et al., 1998) The absence of other coding sequence mutations or mutations in splice junctions in pedigrees with clear X-linked inheritance suggests mutations in regulatory portions of the gene. In one patient, an X/Y translocation produced a mutant fusion product containing portions of *KAL* and its Y-linked homologue (Guioli et al., 1992).

Management.   Patients with KS are successfully treated by pulsatile administration of GnRH. This requires a portable mini-infusion pump. Treatment should begin before the expected onset of puberty. Treatment delay is associated with delayed restoration of spermatogenesis and fertility (Nachtigall et al., 1997). The same treatment, or administration of gonadotropins, has successfully restored fertility in KS females (Sungurtekin et al., 1995).

Discussion.   It is clear that functionally mature (Rawson et al., 1995) GnRH neurons normally find their way from temporary residence in the olfactory epithelium to their final destination in the hypothalamus by moving along avenues created by growing axons of the olfactory neurons. It is also clear that these axons depend on the product of the *KAL* gene in order that they themselves can find their way through the olfactory tract to the olfactory bulbs. These two facts solve the "mysterious association of disordered olfaction and gonadal incompetence" (Caviness, 1992) that defines KS. The neuropathologic basis for bimanual synkinesis remains to be discovered, but the renal agenesis that occurs in about 40% of KS patients is clearly related to the normal appearance of the *KAL* mRNA in mesonephros and metanephros as early as 45 days post-fertilization (Duke et al., 1995), when it is not yet present in the brain. Remarkably, however, the frequent unilaterality of the renal agenesis implies that the *KAL* product participates in one or more subtle morphogenetic thresholds that determine normal kidney development. At 11 weeks of gestation, the *KAL* transcription product is found in the olfactory bulb. This observation fits with the projection that GnRH neuron migration would be completed by the thirteenth to the fifteenth week of gestation.

REFERENCES

Bick D, Franco B, Sherins R J, Heye B, Pike L, Crawford J, Maddalena A, Incerti B, Pragliola A, Meitnger T, Ballabio A (1992). Brief report: intragenic deletion of the Kalig-1 gene in Kallmann's syndrome. *N Engl J Med* 326:1752–1755.

Caviness VS (1992). Kallmann's syndrome-beyond "migration." *N Engl J Med* 326:1775–1775.

Cohen-Salmon M, Tronche F, del Castillo I, Petit C (1995). Characterization of the promoter of the human KAL gene, responsible for the X-chromosome-linked Kallmann syndrome. *Gene* 164:235–242.

Conrad B, Kriebel J, Hetzel W D (1978). Hereditary bimanual synkinesis combined with hypogonadotropic hypogonadism and anosmia in four brothers. *J Neurol* 218:263–274.

Dean J C S, Johnston A W, Klopper A I (1990). Isolated hypogonadotrophic hypogonadism: a family with autosomal dominant inheritance. *Clin Endocrinol* 32:341–347.

Duke V M, Winyard P J, Thorogood P, Soothill P, Bouloux P M, Woolf A S (1995). KAL, a gene mutated in Kallmann's syndrome, is expressed in the first trimester of human development. *Mol Cell Endocrinol* 110:73–79.

Franco B, Guioli S, Pragliola A, Hardelin J P, Levilliers J, del Castillo I, Cohen-Salmon M, Legouis R, Blanchard S, Compain S, Bouloux P, Kirk J, Moraine C, Chaussain J L, Weissenbach J, Petit C (1991). A gene detected in Kallmann's syndrome shares homology with neural cell adhesion and axonal path-finding molecules. *Nature* 353:529–536.

Hardelin J P, Levilliers J, del Castillo I, Cohen-Salmon M, Legouis R, Blanchard S, Compain S, Bouloux P, Kirk J, Moraine C, Chaussain J L, Weissenbach J, Petit C (1992). X chromosome-linked Kallmann syndrome: stop mutations validate the candidate gene. *Proc Natl Acad Sci* 89:8190–8194.

Georgopoulos N, Pralong F P, Seidman C E, Seidman J G, Crowley W F, Vallejo M (1997). Genetic heterogeneity evidenced by low incidence of Kal-1 mutations in sporadic cases of gonadotropin releasing hormone (GnRH) deficiency: evidence for the existence of autosomal genes involved in GnRH expression. *J Clin Endocrinol Metab* 82:213–217.

Guioli S, Incerti B, Zanaria E, Bardone B, Franco B, Taylor K, Ballabio A, Camerino G (1992). Kallmann syndrome due to a translocation in an X/Y fusion gene. *Nat Genet* 1:337–340.

Legouis R, Hardelin J P, Levilliers J, Hardelin J P, Levilliers J, del Castillo I, Cohen-Salmon M, Legouis R, Blanchard S, Compain S, Bouloux P, Kirk J, Moraine C, Chaussain J L, Weissenbach J, Petit C (1991). The candidate gene for the X-linked Kallmann syndrome encodes a protein related to adhesion molecules. *Cell* 67:423–435.

Maya-Nuñez G, Zenteno J C, Ulloa-Aguirre A, Kofman-Alfaro S, Mendez J P (1998). A recurrent missense mutation in the KAL gene in patients with X-linked Kallmann's syndrome. *J Clin Endocrinol Metab* 83:1650–1653.

Nachtigall L B, Boepple P A, Pralong F P, Crowley W F (1997). Adult-onset idiopathic hypogonadotropic hypogonadism—a treatable form of male infertility. *N Engl J Med* 336: 410–415.

Parenti G, Rizzolo M G, Ghezzi M, Di Maio S, Sperandeo M P, Incerti B, Franco B, Ballabio A, Andria G (1995). Variable penetrance of hypogonadism in a sibship with Kallmann syndrome due to a deletion of the KAL gene. *Am J Med Genet* 57:476–478.

Pawlowitzki I H, Diekstall P, Schadel A, Miny P (1987). Estimating frequency of Kallmann syndrome among hypogonadic and among anosmic patients. *Am J Med Genet* 26:473–479.

Quinton R, Duke V M, de Zoysa P A, Platts A D, Valentine A, Kendal B, Pickman S, Kirk J M W, Besser G M, Jacobs H S, Bouloux P M G (1996). The neuroradiology of Kallmann's syndrome: a genotypic and phenotypic analysis. *J Clin Endocrinol Metab* 81:3010–3017.

Quinton R, Hasan W, Grant W, Thrasivoulou C, Quiney R E, Besser G M, Bouloux P-M G (1997). Gonadotropin-releasing hormone immunoreactivity in the nasal epithelia of adults with Kallman's syndrome and isolated hypogonadotropic hypogonadism and in the early midtrimester human fetus. *J Clin Endocrinol Metab* 82:309–314.

Rawson N E, Brank J G, Cowart B J, Lowry L D, Pribitkin E A, Rao V M, Restrepo D (1995). Functionally mature olfactory neurons from two anosmic patients with Kallmann syndrome. *Brain Res* 681:58–64.

Santen R J, Paulsen C A (1973). Hypogonadotropic eunuchoidism. I. Clinical study of the mode of inheritance. *J Clin Endocrinol Metab* 36:47–54.

Schinzel A, Lorda-Sanchez I, Binkert F, Carter N P, Bebb C E, Ferguson-Smith M A, Eiholzer U, Zachmann M, Robinson W P (1995). Kallmann syndrome in a boy with a t(1;10) translocation detected by reverse chromosome painting. *J Med Genet* 32:957–961.

Sungurtekin U, Fraser I S, Shearman R P (1995). Pregnancy in women with Kallmann's syndrome. *Fertil Steril* 63:494–499.

White B J, Rogol A D, Brown K S, Lieblich J M, Rosen S W (1983). The syndrome of anosmia with hypogonadotropic hypogonadism: a genetic study of 18 new families and review. *Am J Med Genet* 15:417–435.

Wortsman J, Hughes L F (1996). Case report: olfactory function in a fertile eunuch with Kallmann syndrome. *Am J Med Sci* 311:135–138.

HYPOGONADOTROPIC HYPOGONADISM (HHG): A PUBERTAL EXPRESSION OF *DAX1* MUTATION CAUSING X-LINKED ADRENAL HYPOPLASIA CONGENITA (AHC)

Clinical and Laboratory Features. AHC causes early infantile adrenal insufficiency and is associated with hypogonadism at puberty. The hypothalamic-pituitary-gonadal axis is normal in infancy (Takahashi et al., 1997). The serum levels of glucocorticoids, mineralocorticoids, and androgens are low, and resistant to ACTH stimulation. The adrenal glands are dysplastic, and the permanent zone of the adrenal cortex is absent. Lethality is prevented by proper replacement therapy. Some patients with AHC have a contiguous gene syndrome that includes glycerol kinase deficiency and Duchenne muscular dystrophy. Pubertal hypogonadotropic hypogonadism was once thought to be a distinct component of the contiguous syndrome. Now, it is known to be an independent consequence of mutant *DAX1* expression, and the evidence for its combined hypothalamic and pituitary origin has become substantive (Habiby et al., 1996). As expected, all the postpubertal patients have low serum levels of LH, FSH, and testosterone. However, their responses to a stimulatory challenge of GnRH are varied. This implies that in particular patients, the pituitary and the hypothalamus may both contribute to the HHG, but to different extents. The variable clinical presentation of *DAX1* mutations has recently been emphasized by Reutens and colleagues (1999).

Genotyping and Mutant Gene Expression. The *DAX1* gene contains only two exons that span 5 kb of the X chromosome. It encodes a 470-amino-acid protein that strongly resembles the nuclear hormone receptor superfamily. Its C-terminal portion has homology to the ligand-binding domain of the superfamily. Its N-terminal portion contains 3.5 repeats of a 67-amino acid domain that has DNA-binding activity. In other words, the putative protein has the structural attributes of a transcriptional regulatory factor whose ligand(s) (if any) and target gene(s) remain to be identified.

In the study of Muscatelli and colleagues (1994) of 26 unrelated patients with AHC, 14 had *DAX1* deletions and 12 had point mutations in the gene's coding region. Interestingly, of the 12 point mutations, five were nonsense and five were frameshift in type. They clustered around the middle of the coding region, about equally in the ligand-binding–like and DNA-binding–like portions. Likewise, of five unrelated Japanese patients in the report of Nakae and colleagues (1996), three had nonsense mutations and two mutations were of the frameshift variety. Furthermore, only two of eight additional Japanese families with AHC had missense mutations (Yanase et al., 1986; Nakae et al., 1997)—Lys382Asn and Trp291Cys. Clearly, missense mutation is relatively underrepresented among all mutations of the DAX-1 gene. Importantly, of the patients studied by Muscatelli and colleagues, all those with point mutations who were at least 14 years old (eight patients, six families) also had HHG, thus excluding the contiguous syndrome hypothesis for the conjunction of AHC with HHG. It is noteworthy, also, that pubertal HHG occurred in a maternal uncle with Ala300Val whose affected nephew was documented to have a normal hypothalamic-pituitary-testis axis in infancy (Takahashi et al., 1997).

Management.   Aside from replacement therapy to compensate for deficiency of glucocorticoids and mineralocorticoids, these patients will need pulsatile GnRH (as for those with Kallmann syndrome) or both gonadotropins (Finkel et al., 1985).

Discussion.   Developmental studies of *Dax1* in the mouse (Swain et al., 1996), and in the human (Burris et al., 1996), have revealed that the gene is expressed not only early in the development of the adrenal, the pituitary, and the hypothalamus, but also in the gonads. It had previously been shown that *DAX1* is one of the expressed genes in the critical region of the so-called dosage-sensitive sex reversal (DSS) locus at Xp21. Indeed, there is growing circumstantial evidence that *DAX1* may be the *DSS* locus. This evidence is discussed in Chapter 2.

REFERENCES

Burris T P, Guo W, McCabe E R (1996). The gene responsible for adrenal hypoplasia congenita, DAX-1, encodes a nuclear hormone receptor that defines a new class within the superfamily. *Recent Prog Horm Res* 51:241–259.

Finkel D M, Phillips J L, Snyder P J (1985). Stimulation of spermatogenesis by gonadotropins in men with hypogonadotropic hypogonadism. *N Engl J Med* 313:651–655.

Habiby R L, Boepple P, Nachtigall L, Sluss P M, Crowley Jr W F, Jameson J L (1996). Adrenal hypoplasia congenital with hypogonadotropic hypogonadism: evidence that DAX-1 mutations lead to combined hypothalamic and pituitary defects in gonadotropin production. *J Clin Invest* 98:1055–1062.

Muscatelli F, Strom T M, Walker A, Zanaria E, Recans D, Meindl A, Bardoni B, Guioli S, Zehetner G, Rabl W, et al. (1994). Mutations in the DAX-1 gene give rise to both X-linked adrenal hypoplasia congenital hypogonadotropic hypogonadism. *Nature* 372:672–676.

Nakae J, Abe S, Tajima T, Shinohara N, Murashita M, Igarashi Y, Kusuda S, Suzuki J, Fujieda K (1997). Three novel mutations and a *de novo* deletion mutation of the DAX-1 gene in patients with X-linked adrenal hypoplasia congenita. *J Clin Endocrinol Metab* 82:3835–3841.

Nakae J, Tajima T, Kusuda S, Kohda N, Okabe T, Shinohara N, Kato M, Murashita M, Mukai T, Imanaka K, Fujieda K (1996). Truncation at the C-terminus of the DAX-1 protein impairs its biological actions in patients with X-linked adrenal hypoplasia congenita. *J Clin Endocrinol Metab* 81:3680–3685.

Reutens A T, Achermann J C, Ito M, Ito M, Gu W-X, Habiby R L, Donohoue P A, Pang S, Hindmarsh P C, Jameson J L (1999). Clinical and functional effects of mutations in the *DAX-1* gene in patients with adrenal hypoplasia congenita. *J Clin Endocrinol Metab* 84: 504–511.

Swain A, Zanaria E, Kacker A, Lovell-Badge R, Camerino G (1996). Mouse Dax1 expression is consistent with a role in sex determination as well as in adrenal and hypothalamus function. *Nat Genet* 12:404–409.

Takahashi T, Shoji Y, Shoji Y, Haraguchi N, Takahashi I, Takada G (1997). Active hypothalamic-pituitary-gonadal axis in an infant with X-linked adrenal hypoplasia congenita. *J Pediatr* 130:485–488.

Yanase T, Takayanagi R, Oba K, Nishi Y, Ohe K, Nawata H (1996). New mutations of DAX-1 genes in two Japanese patients with X-linked congenital adrenal hypoplasia and hypogonadotropic hypogonadism. *J Clin Endocrinol Metab* 81:530–535.

PARTIAL HYPOGONADOTROPIC HYPOGONADISM DUE TO MUTATION OF THE GNRH RECEPTOR

Clinical and Imaging Features (based primarily on a single pair of affected male and female young adult siblings; de Roux et al., 1997). Puberty in the male was delayed to age 16 and was subnormal: at 22 years, his facial and pubic hair were scant, penis length was only 6 cm, and testes were each 8 mL in volume. Libido was low. Gynecomastia was not present; neither was anosmia nor any other facultative sign of Kallmann syndrome. The patient's arm span (186 cm) exceeded his height by 6 cm. His sister experienced thelarche at 14 years, despite primary amenorrhea. At 37 years, her secondary sexual characteristics were normal. Pelvic ultrasonography exposed a normal uterus and two small ovaries without a single dominant follicle. Both parents, and another sister of intermediate age, were sexually normal. In contrast to the female described above, none of three affected sisters (17, 21, and 30 years of age) in the family described by Layman and colleagues (1998) experienced thelarche.

Laboratory Findings. The brother's serum testosterone level was only 2.8 nM (lower normal: 9), but his LH and FSH concentrations were normal, both basally and in response to GnRH challenge. Frequent LH sampling revealed normal pulse frequency but decreased pulse amplitude. Semen fructose and citrate (markers of androgenicity) were markedly reduced in concentration, despite low semen volume. Sperm density was normal, but motility and morphology were subnormal. Six weeks after the sister discontinued maintenance therapy with a combined oral contraceptive, her plasma estradiol level was normal (for the early follicular phase), and so were her LH and FSH concentrations. In the sibship reported by Layman and colleagues, the affected brother's serum testosterone level was also only about 2 nM; his basal LH level was very low, but it did respond normally, nearly three-fold, to GnRH stimulation. All three of his sisters had low serum LH and FSH levels that responded adequately, or briskly (three-to-five-fold for LH), to GnRH challenge.

Frequency. Judging from the recency of the first reported family with partial hypogonadotropic hypogonadism due to GnRH receptor mutation, it would appear that such families are very uncommon. However, the true frequency of such mutation may be concealed, somewhat, by even milder expression than in the first

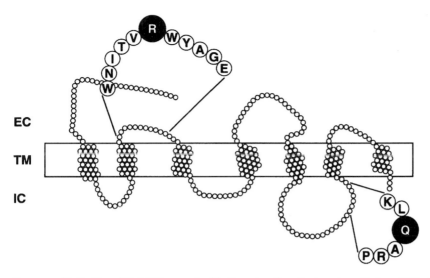

EC

TM

IC

FIGURE 10–3. The Gln106Arg substitution in the first extracellular (EC) loop, and the Arg262Gln mutation in the third intracellular (IC) loop of the GnRH receptor in one family with hypogonadotropic hypogonadism. TM is a transmembrane domain composed of seven helices. (Reproduced from de Roux et al., *N Engl J Med* 337:1597–1601, 1997, with permission.)

family, and by the fact that the conventional dose of GnRH used in the challenge test (100 μg IV) may be sufficient to overcome partial defects in binding or in subsequent steps of G protein–coupled signal transduction, as exemplified in families reported by de Roux and colleagues and Layman and colleagues. Furthermore, most patients with idiopathic hypogonadotropic hypogonadism (IHH) eventually respond to sufficient exogenous GnRH, a situation suggesting resistance to GnRH at one level or another. In fact, Layman and colleagues (1998) recently screened the *GNRHR* of 46 unrelated patients with normosmic IHH (32 males, 14 females, all older than 17 years) in order to find one female who had two affected sisters and one affected brother, all with the same pair of mutations on genomic sequencing.

Genotyping and Gene Expression. Both affected siblings described by de Roux and colleagues are compound heterozygotes for point mutations in the *GnRHR*: an A-G transition at nt 317 giving a Gln106Arg substitution in the 1e loop; a G-A transition at nt 785 causing an Arg262Gln substitution in the i3 loop (Fig. 10–3). Their mother carried the 106 mutation; their father and sister, the 262 mutation. Both mutated amino acids are absolutely conserved in the GnRH receptors of various species. COS cells transfected with the normal or the 262 mutant receptor had normal specific GnRH binding; those with the 106 mutant had only about 12.5% of normal binding. Cells transfected with either mutant receptor had 50% of normal maximal inositol phosphate accumulation, and they required 50-fold more GnRH to achieve a half-maximal response. These behaviors in the laboratory mirror the partial defectiveness of the patients' mutations *in vivo*.

The four affected siblings of Layman and colleagues are also compound heterozygotes for two missense mutations that alter conserved amino acids. One, in exon 3, is Arg262Gln, the same mutation found previously by de Roux and colleagues; the other, Tyr284Cys, is in TM helix 6. When Layman and colleagues transfected

COS cells with the Arg262Gln mutant, they also found normal binding affinity and near-normal binding capacity of the GnRH receptor. However, the transfected cells produced about 60% of normal maximal inositol phosphate (IP), and required about 10-fold more agonist to do so. In contrast, cells transfected with the Tyr284Cys mutant not only had impaired binding affinity and capacity, but also required approximately 20-fold more agonist to reach about 25% of maximal IP production.

Management.   Effective strategies for the treatment of GnRH receptor deficiency remain to be defined. Conceivably, pulsatile administration of GnRH might overcome a partial receptor deficiency. In those with complete deficiency, LH, FSH, or their substitutes will be necessary. In the foregoing context, it is remarkable that one sister in the family of Layman and colleagues did ovulate in response to exogenous gonadotropins, whereas the second did not, even after receiving adequate doses of pulsatile GnRH for 46 days.

Discussion.   The Gln106Arg mutation described above mimics the action of a nearby artificial mutation (Asn102Ala) in reducing ligand binding (Davidson et al., 1996). Likewise, the natural mutant Arg262Gln described here recalls the fact that artificial mutation of Ala 261 causes impaired G-protein coupling and internalization (Myburgh et al., 1997). Furthermore, the i3 loop is known to be important for signal transmission in a variety of GPCR. On the other hand, it is still not known whether the 102–106 amino acid portion of the e1 loop participates in ligand binding directly or conformationally. Artificial mutations in the i2 loop have clarified the roles of certain amino acids in the GPCR signature motif and of the hydrophobic site at position 147 in agonist binding, internalization and signaling. For instance, Ser140Tyr, which restores the usual signature sequence, Asp, Arg, Tyr, had increased ligand affinity and internalization, but not increased signaling. In contrast, Leu147Ala or Asp had unchanged binding affinity but less internalization and less signal transduction (Arora et al., 1995). Likewise, replacement of Tyr by a nonaromatic residue in the conserved sequence Asn318, Pro319, X, X, Tyr322 did not lower agonist binding, but it eliminated G-protein coupling and inositol phosphate production, and it reduced internalization by 50%. Appropriately, Tyr322Phe behaved entirely normally (Arora et al., 1996). Interestingly, restoration of Asp87 and Asn318, the usual combination in the GPCR superfamily, in place of Asn87 and Asp318, as found in the GnRHR, had no effect on ligand binding but abolished the receptor down-regulation response in cultured GH_3 cells. Moreover, inositol triphosphate production was impaired, but that of cAMP was not. This dissociative effect on the two G protein–coupled signaling systems should help to elucidate the factors that determine which signaling system is used by a given G protein–coupled receptor under different conditions (Awara et al., 1996).

REFERENCES

Arora K K, Sakai A, Catt K J (1995). Effects of second intracellular loop mutations on signal transduction and internalization of the gonadotropin-releasing hormone receptor. *J Biol Chem* 270:22820–22826.
Arora K K, Cheng Z, Catt K J (1996). Dependence of agonist activation on an aromatic moiety in the DPLIY motif of the gonadotropin-releasing hormone receptor. *Mol Endocrinol* 10: 979–986.

Awara W M (1996). Effects of Asn318 and Asp87Asn318 mutations on signal transduction by the gonadotropin-releasing hormone and receptor regulation. *Endocrinology* 137:655–662.

Davidson J S, McArdle C A, Davies P, Elario R, Flanagan C A, Millar R P (1996). Asn102 of the gonadotropin-releasing hormone receptor is a critical determinant of potency for agonists containing C-terminal glycinamide. *J Biol Chem* 271:15510–15514.

de Roux N, Young J, Misrahi M, Genet R, Chanson P, Schaison G, Milgrom E (1997). A family with hypogonadotropic hypogonadism and mutations in the gonadotropin-releasing hormone receptor. *N Engl J Med* 337:1597–1601.

Layman L C, Cohen D P, Jin M, Xie J, Li Z, Reindollar R H, Bolbolan S, Bick D P, Sherins R R, Duck L W, Musgrove L C, Sellers J C, Neill J D (1998). Mutations in gonadotropin-releasing hormone receptor gene cause hypogonadotropic hypogonadism. *Nat Genet* 18: 14–15.

Myburgh D B, Pawson A J, Davidson J S, Millar R P, Hapgood J P (1997). Ala261 of intracellular loop 3 of the GnRH receptor is involved in G-protein coupling and internalization. In: Program of the 79th Annual Meeting of the Endocrine Society, Minneapolis, June, 1997 Abstract No. P 1–132, p 167.

PRIMARY AMENORRHEA AND OLIGO/AZOOSPERMIA DUE TO FSH DEFICIENCY THAT CAUSES GRANULOSA CELL DYSFUNCTION IN WOMEN AND SERTOLI CELL DYSFUNCTION IN MEN: FSH β GENE MUTATION

Clinical and Imaging Considerations.   Females present with incoordinate puberty: axillary and pubic hair appear because androgenesis is intact, but menarche does not occur, and breast development is poor because estrogenesis is impaired. The body proportions are eunuchoid. Males identified biochemically, before the advent of DNA diagnosis, presented with infertility, small testes, or both, but secondary sexual development could be otherwise normal (Maroulis et al., 1977; Al-Ansari et al., 1984). The single male whose diagnosis was recently affirmed by DNA analysis (Phillip et al., 1998) had a puberty that, at 18 years, was impaired unevenly: he reported normal potency and ejaculation, penile length was unremarkable, and pubic hair reached Tanner stage 4, but axillary hair was scant, facial hair was absent, skeletal musculature was deficient, bone age was 16 years, and his testes were soft and very small. Yet he did not have any gynecomastia. Computed tomography or magnetic resonance imaging is used to rule out a pituitary tumor.

The mother of the patient of Matthews and colleagues (1993) was infertile for 6 years and had frequent menstrual irregularity, punctuated by periods of amenorrhea. In contrast, the mothers of the patients described by Layman and colleagues (1997), and Phillip and colleagues (1998) had no reproductive or menstrual problems, even though all three mothers carried the same mutation heterozygously.

Laboratory Features.   Normal (Matthews et al., 1993) or supranormal (Layman et al., 1997) levels of LH, but low or undetectable levels of FSH, both basally and after GnRH stimulation, are typical of the two women with genetically proven FSH deficiency (Matthews et al., 1993; Layman et al., 1997). Provocatively, the male with genetically proven FSH deficiency (Phillip et al., 1998) also had elevated levels of LH, before and after stimulation. Nevertheless, his total and free testosterone levels were low. One possible reason for this set of discordant laboratory values is discussed below.

Serum from the patient of Matthews and colleagues failed to stimulate aromatase activity in cultured Sertoli cells, indicating absence of FSH bioactivity, as well as absent FSH immunoreactivity. Also, the patient lacked anti-FSH autoantibodies, thereby excluding a pauciglandular form of autoimmune disease. The mother of the patient of Matthews and colleagues had low basal levels of FSH and LH, and GnRH elicited a subnormal response of FSH but not of LH. Her residual FSH level had a normal ratio of bioactivity to immunoreactivity and was considered to reflect haploinsufficiency, but her abnormal LH levels were not explained. Semen analysis reveals variably low sperm concentration and reduced motility, or azoospermia, as in the patient of Phillip and colleagues (1998). Testicular biopsy exposes spermatogenetic arrest, in some cases at the level of spermatids (Maroulis et al., 1977). In the female patient described by Rabin and colleagues (1972), primordial follicles were abundant, graafian follicles were infrequent, and mature follicles were apparently absent.

Genotyping and Mutant Gene Expression. The proband described by Matthews and colleagues (1993) was homozygous for a two-nucleotide deletion in codon 61 of exon 3 that frameshifts to a premature termination codon. Her mother and brother were heterozygous. Her father, deceased, and mother were not knowingly consanguineous, but came from the same isolated community. The mutation predicts an altered amino acid sequence for residues 61–86, and truncation thereafter. The C-terminal portion of the hFSHβ subunit (residues 93–99 in particular) is known to be involved in FSHR binding (Lindau-Shepard et al., 1994). Therefore, the mutation would be predicted to interdict normal binding to the FSHR. Furthermore, the C-terminus of FSHβ is involved in α-β subunit association, and subunit association is a prerequisite for normal secretion of these heterodimeric hormones.

The proband investigated by Layman and colleagues (1997) was a compound heterozygote: she shared one mutation, Val61→X, with the proband of Matthews and colleagues (1993); the second, Cys51Gly, would prevent the formation of internal disulfide bonds that are conformationally essential. Chinese hamster ovary (CHO) cells stably transfected with single vectors carrying wild-type α-subunit sequence and either mutant type of β-subunit sequence yielded no FSH by immunoradiometric assay.

Management. FSH replacement in the female patient of Matthews and colleagues evoked inhibin and estrogen responses, follicular maturation, ovulation and a postovulatory progesterone response. Eventually, she had a successful pregnancy. Indeed, pregnancy was achieved by supraphysiologic doses of FSH even in the patient of Rabinowitz and colleagues (1979), who developed anti-FSH antibodies after her initial exposure to therapeutic FSH. FSH treatment, or treatment with GnRH, has also been successful for men with isolated FSH deficiency (Al-Ansari et al., 1984).

Discussion. Male mice homozygous for *FSHβ* "knockouts" are oligospermic but fertile; their female counterparts are hypoestrogenic and infertile (Kumar et al., 1997); Kumar et al., 1998. These phenotypes mimic those in humans without FSH, or without the effect of FSH because of FSH receptor deficiency (Chapter 11). Ovarian estrogenesis depends on the biosynthetic synergy of theca and granulosa cells. Theca cells make androgen primarily under the influence of LH, enhanced by FSH. These androgens are transferred to granulosa cells. FSH acts on granulosa cells to promote follicle development and aromatase activity; the latter catalyzes the conversation of androgen to estrogen.

The low serum testosterone in the male patient of Phillip and colleagues (1998) is very likely to reflect deficient FSH-dependent Sertoli cell–Leydig cell interaction (Carreau, 1996, Rivarola et al., 1995). The patient's low serum level of inhibin B affirms Sertoli cell hypofunction, and his elevated levels of LH reflect a compensatory response to testosterone deficiency.

Despite the small number of biochemically and genetically proven cases, the apparently appreciable phenotypic variability of males with FSH deficiency recalls the same situation in men with FSH receptor deficiency (Tapanainen et al., 1997).

Five of six mutant alleles in three patients with FSHβ deficiency have been identical GT deletions in codon 61 of exon 3. If this does not reflect ancestral relatedness among the affecteds, it will demand an explanation at the level of DNA synthesis.

Male or female infertility due to isolated FSH deficiency appears to be unusual: in the study of Avril-Ducarne and colleagues (1990), only two of 57 men with oligospermia had this finding. Provocatively, however, up to 30% of infertile men have low ratios of FSH bioactivity to immunoactivity. Some of these men may have a genetic basis for this abnormal ratio. The possibility of subfertility due to heterozygosity for a FSHβ mutation needs to be evaluated systematically.

REFERENCES

Al-Ansari A A K, Khalil T H, Kalani Y, Mortimer C H (1984). Isolated follicle-stimulating hormone deficiency in men: successful long-term gonadotrophin therapy. *Fertil Steril* 42: 618–626.

Avril-Ducarne D, et al. (1990) Apport de l'enquete hormonale au choix therapeutique d'une sterilite masculine. *J Gynecol Obstet Biol Reprod* 19:881–888.

Carreau S (1996), Paracrine control of human Leydig cell and Sertoli cell functions. *Folia Histochem Cytobiol* 34:111–119.

Kumar T R, Low M J, Matzuk M M (1998). Genetic rescue of follicle-stimulating hormone β-deficient mice. *Endocrinology* 139:3289–3295.

Kumar T R, Wang Y, Lu N, Matzuk M M (1997). Follicle stimulating hormone is required for ovarian follicle maturation but not male fertility. *Nat Genet* 15:201–204.

Layman L C, Lee E J, Peak D B, Namnoum A B, Vu K V, van Lingen B L, Gray M R, McDonough P G, Reindollar R H, Jameson J L (1997). Delayed puberty and hypogonadism caused by mutation in the follicle-stimulating hormone β-subunit gene. *N Engl J Med* 337: 607–611.

Lindau-Shepard B, Roth K E, Dias J A (1994). Identification of amino acids in the C-terminal region of human follicle-stimulating hormone (FSH) β-subunit involved in binding to human FSH receptor. *Endocrinology* 135:1235–1240.

Maroulis G B, Parlow A F, Marshall J R (1977). Isolated follicle stimulating hormone deficiency in man. *Fertil Steril* 28:818–822.

Matthews C H, Borgato S, Beck-Peccoz P, Adams M, Tone Y, Gambino G, Casagrande S, Tedeschini G, Benedetti A, Chatterjee V K (1993). Primary amenorrhoea and infertility due to a mutation in the β-subunit of follicle-stimulating hormone. *Nat Genet* 5:83–86.

Phillip M, Arbelle J E, Segev Y, Parvari R (1988). Male hypogonadism due to a mutation in the gene for the β-subunit of follicle-stimulating hormone. *N Engl J Med* 338:1729–1732.

Rabin D, Spitz I, Bercovici B, Bell J, Laufer A, Benveniste R, Polishuk W (1972). Isolated deficiency of follicle-stimulating hormone: clinical and laboratory features. *N Engl J Med* 287:1313–1317.

Rabinowitz D, Benveniste R, Lindner J, Lorber D, Daniell J (1979). Isolated FSH deficiency revisited. *N Engl J Med* 300:126–128.

Rivarola M A, Belgorosky A, Berensztein E, de Davila M T (1995). Human prepubertal testicular cells in culture: steroidogenic capacity, paracrine and hormone control. *J Steroid Biochem Mol Biol* 53:119–125.

Tapanainen J S, Aittomaki K, Min J, Vaskivuo T, Huhtaniemi I T (1997). Men homozygous for an inactivating mutation of the follicle-stimulating hormone (FSH) receptor gene present variable suppression of spermatogenesis and fertility. *Nat Genet* 15:205–206.

LHβ GENE MUTATION THAT DISABLES LH BINDING TO THE LH RECEPTOR AND CAUSES TOTAL PUBERTAL FAILURE IN HOMOZYGOUS MALES BUT APPARENTLY ISOLATED INFERTILITY IN HETEROZYGOUS MALES

Clinical Considerations.   In the first such family described (Weiss et al., 1992), the proband was the offspring of a consanguineous marriage; he presented with delayed puberty. After 2 years of testosterone therapy had ended for the patient, puberty did not resume spontaneously. Although he virilized well in response to chronic CG treatment, including a boost in spermatogenesis, he never became fertile. Three maternal uncles were infertile despite otherwise normal secondary sexual development: they also had consanguineous parents (Weiss et al., 1992). The mother and sister of the proband, both heterozygotes, were fertile. The proband was previously reported to have hypogonadism due to an immunologically active, but biologically inactive LH (Beitins et al., 1981).

Laboratory Features.   The proband had twice-normal serum LH level by immunoassay, but undetectable levels by radioreceptor assay. His testosterone level was low but his FSH level was normal. Testicular biopsy disclosed arrested spermatogenesis and no Leydig cells. His infertile uncles had low or low-normal serum testosterone levels and normal or high-normal immuno-assayable LH levels. The ratio of LH measured by radioimmunoassay and by radioreceptor assay in the serum of the proband's mother indicated that she had about equal parts of normal and mutant LH in her blood. Curiously, the proband's sister and one of his maternal uncles had undetectable levels of LH in their sera by the radioreceptor assay.

Genotyping and Mutant Gene Expression.   In the family described by Weiss and colleagues. (1992), the fully affected male was homozygous for Gln54Arg in the β subunit. When an expression vector encoding the mutant LHβ gene was cotransfected into CHO cells that also contained a LHα gene, mutant dimeric hormone in the culture medium was undetectable by radioreceptor assay but was easily detectable by radioimmunoassay. Thus, the biological inactivity of the mutant LH was attributable to its loss of receptor-binding ability.

Management.   The patient reported by Weiss and colleagues (1992) responded well, but suboptimally, to chronic CG replacement. He virilized normally and his sperm count rose to 11 million per milliliter, with 50 % motility. However, he never became fertile despite repeated courses of CG supplemented with testosterone. As discussed below, there is good reason to believe that early replacement of LH or CG is necessary to prevent infertility.

Discussion.   The first lesson of the experiment of nature created by homozygosity for Gln54Arg in the LHβ gene is that primary male sexual differentiation can be normal without the action of LH. Indeed, there is independent evidence that the fetal testes initiate secretion of testosterone spontaneously; that is, even without the stimulus of CG. The absence of Leydig cells in the patient's testis biopsy is consistent with Leydig cell hypoplasia (or aplasia) in patients with LH receptor mutations. The failure of chronic CG therapy to restore the patient's fertility may mean that prenatal/prepubertal exposure to CG/LH may be necessary to imprint or prime Leydig cells in a manner that allows them to achieve their full testosterone biosynthetic capacity postpubertally. From this point of view, it is important to recall that a high intratesticular concentration of testosterone is necessary for normal spermatogenesis. Indeed, the patient's three heterozygous maternal uncles may well have been infertile because of their low serum levels of testosterone. Yet the patient's father, presumably heterozygous, was fertile, as were his heterozygous mother and sister.

"Fertile eunuch syndrome" is an outmoded term for adult males who appear to have isolated LH deficiency. Their serum testosterone levels are low, their habitus is hypogonadal (eunuchoid), and, inexplicably, they usually have gynecomastia. Spermatogenesis may be impaired variably. Serum FSH levels are normal basally, but do not respond to clomiphene stimulation. Hence, FSH reserve is low. The "syndrome" may be one form of partial hypogonadotropic hypogonadism (see previous section), but there is little evidence that it is genetic (Faiman et al., 1968).

REFERENCES

Beitins I Z, Axelrod L, Ostrea T, Little R, Badger T M (1981). Hypogonadism in a male with an immunologically active, biologically inactive luteinizing hormone: characterization of the abnormal hormone. *J Clin Endocrinol Metab* 52:1143–1149.

Faiman C, Hoffmann D L, Ryan R J, Albert A (1968). The "fertile eunuch" syndrome: demonstration of isolated luteinizing hormone deficiency by radioimmunoassay technique. *Mayo Clin Proc* 43:661–667.

Weiss J, Axelrod L, Whitcomb R W, Harris P E, Crowley W F, Jameson J L (1992). Hypogonadism caused by a single amino acid substitution in the β subunit of luteinizing hormone. *N Engl J Med* 326:179–183.

LHβ GENE MUTATION POSSIBLY ASSOCIATED WITH MENSTRUAL DISORDER AND INFERTILITY IN JAPAN

Clinical Considerations.   Three Japanese women with various degrees of ovarian dysfunction and infertility were targeted for LHβ gene analysis because their serum levels of LH were widely disparate when measured by radioimmunoassays using different monoclonal antibodies (Furui et al., 1994). One of the women had polycystic ovaries. Two more such Japanese women were identified among 51 patients examined to estimate the frequency of the association between immunologically anomalous LH and menstrual disorder (Suganuma et al., 1995). None of the 50 control subjects had the association. This suggested that immunologically anomalous LH could be pathogenic among Japanese women. In contrast, Pettersson and colleagues (1990; 1992) had previously found the same anomalous LH immunotrait in 3.5% of healthy individuals of both sexes in Finland, indicating that the trait is a benign polymorphism in that country.

Laboratory Features.   The Japanese and Finnish groups have performed a number of comparable studies to characterize this immunovariant of LH. For instance, Furui and colleagues (1994) found a lesser degree of the immunoaberrant LH in some first-degree relatives, and in both parents of their first three patients with the severe phenotype, suggesting that they are heterozygous. In like manner, Haavisto and colleagues (1995) found that 24% of healthy Finnish males and females had the presumably heterozygous phenotype. They also showed no difference between the variant and normal LH in pulsatility, or in response to GnRH stimulation. However, they did find that the mutant LH had a faster clearance rate from the rat circulation, and higher biopotency, than the normal (Haavisto et al., 1995). Notably, in contrast, the Japanese group found increased LH responses to GnRH in some proven homozygotes (Suganuma et al., 1995).

Rajkhowa and colleagues (1995) assessed the prevalence of the LHβ variant in a United Kingdom population of healthy women (controls) and those with polycystic ovary syndrome (PCOS). They found the variant in 15% of all controls, in 12% of obese controls, and in 26% of PCOS subjects that were obese, but in only 5% if non-obese. Control subjects, but not PCOS subjects, with the variant had higher serum estradiol, testosterone, and sex hormone–binding globulin. This may reflect higher biopotency of the variant. But if so, the increment did not affect the clinical or laboratory phenotype in PCOS subjects, and its relevance to non-PCOS individuals is not apparent.

Genotyping and Mutant Gene Expression.   First, the Finnish (Pettersson et al., 1994), then the Japanese group found the same set of point mutations in the subjects with the LH immunovariant: Trp8Arg and Ile 15Thr in codons 8 and 15, respectively, of the LHβ gene. These two substitutions yield the amino acids that normally occupy the homologous positions in the CGβ chain. The introduction of Thr15 renders Asn13 a potential site for N-glycosylation. In fact, in CGβ, the site is glycosylated. Interestingly, Suganuma and colleagues (1996) constructed LHβ expression vectors containing one or both mutations, cotransfected them into CHO cells with normal LHα genes, and compared the mutant forms of LH, with normal LH produced likewise, after extraction from CHO culture medium. They found that Trp8Arg is primarily responsible for the immunologically anomalous behavior of the mutant LH, that Ile 15Thr does engender additional Asn-linked glycosylation, and that neither mutation, or both, affects the ability of the mutant LH to bind to the LHR on the MA-10 mouse Leydig tumor cell line, or to induce ovulation in rats. However, the Try8Arg mutation alone, or with Ile15Thr, rendered the mutant LH more biopotent than normal as measured by maximum progesterone secretion from MA-10 cells. Furthermore, all three forms of mutant LH had a faster clearance rate from the rat circulation—an observation made previously by Haavisto and colleagues (1995) using samples of mutant LH derived from patient serum.

Management.   In the absence of evidence for a distinct pathogenetic contribution of the LH immunovariant to any disease process, women with a possibly related disorder should be treated for the disorder as if their LH is not variant.

Discussion.   The shortened circulatory half-life, and the augmented steroidogenetic biopotency of the variant LH are both explainable by its additional carbohydrate chain. At this writing there is little to incriminate immunovariant LH as a decisive determinant of any menstrual or ovulatory disorder in the human. At most, perhaps in Japan, it may be one factor in the multifactorial causation of one or another menstrual/ovulatory disorder. On the other hand, conceivably the LH variant could, somehow, protect against disorders associated with abnormal LH, or FSH secretion or action.

REFERENCES

Furui K, Suganuma N, Tsukahara S-I, Asada Y, Kikkawa F, Tanaka M, Ozawa T, Tomoda Y (1994). Identification of two point mutations in the gene coding luteinizing hormone (LH) β-subunit, associated with immunologically anomalous LH variants. *J Clin Endocrinol Metab* 78:107–113.

Haavisto A-M, Pettersson K, Bergendahl M, Virkamaki A, Huhtaniemi I. (1995). Occurrence and biological properties of a common genetic variant of luteinizing hormone. *J Clin Endocrinol Metab* 80:1257–1263.

Pettersson K, Ding Y, Huhtaniemi I (1992). An immunologically anomalous luteinizing hormone variant in a healthy woman. *J Clin Endocrinol Metab* 74:164–171.

Pettersson K, Soderholm J (1990). Individual differences in LH immunoreactivity revealed by monoclonal antibodies. *Clin Chem* 37:333–340.

Pettersson K, Makela M M, Dahlen P, Lamminen T, Huoponen K, Huhtaniemi I (1994). gene polymorphism found in the LH beta gene of an immunologically anomalous variant of human luteinizing hormone. *Eur J Endocrinol* 130 (Suppl 2): 65.

Rajkhowa M, Talbot J A, Jones P W, Pettersson K, Haavisto A M, Huhtaniem I, Clayton R N. (1995). Prevalence of an immunological LH β-subunit variant in a UK population of healthy women and women with polycystic ovary syndrome. *Clin Endocrinol* 43:297–303.

Suganuma N, Furui K, Furuhashi M (1995). Screening of the mutations in luteinizing hormone β-subunit in patients with menstrual disorders. *Fertil Steril* 63:989–995.

Suganuma N, Furui K, Kikkawa F, Tomoda Y, Furuhashi M (1996). Effects of the mutations (Trp^8→Arg and Ile^{15}→Thr) in human luteinizing hormone (LH) β-subunit on LH bioactivity *in vitro* and *in vivo*. *Endocrinology* 137:831–838.

11

Genetic Disorders of Gonadotropin Action

MOLECULAR AND CELLULAR BIOLOGY OF THE GONADOTROPIN RECEPTORS

The chorionic gonadotropin/luteinizing hormone receptor (henceforth, LHR), and the follicle-stimulating hormone receptor (FSHR) belong to the subfamily of G protein–coupled receptors for glycoprotein hormones. They share a very long ($\sim$ 350 amino acids) N-terminal extracellular domain devoted primarily to high-affinity ligand binding, seven membrane-spanning α-helices with six intervening loops (three each, internal and external), and a relatively short C-terminal intracellular domain (Fig. 11–1). The genes for both receptors map to a small region, p21, on chromosome 2 (Gyapay et al., 1994). The first 10 exons of the *LHR*, and the first 9 exons of the *FSHR* encode most of their respective extracellular domains. The last exon of each gene yields a small segment of the extracellular domain and the entire remaining portion of each receptor. For either receptor to work normally, it must do three things: integrate into the membrane of a cell that is the target of a hormone; bind the cognate hormone with sufficient affinity to initiate the signal; and couple

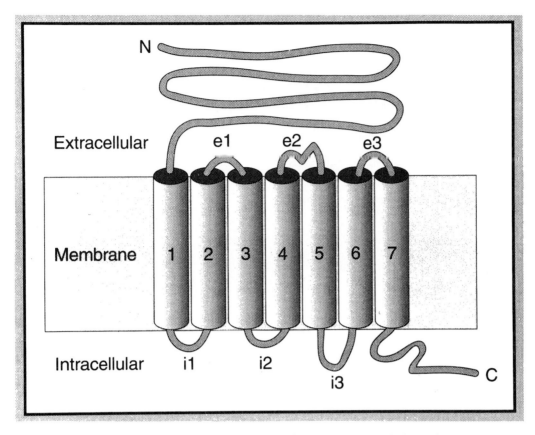

FIGURE 11–1. The common structural attributes of a G protein–coupled membrane receptor. There are extracellular and intracellular tails, and a transmembranous barrel composed of seven hydrophobic α-helices that are connected by three extracellular (e) and three intracellular (i) loops. N, is the amino terminus of receptor protein and C, its carboxy terminus (Reproduced from Shenker A, *Growth Genet Horm* 12:33, 1996, with permission.)

with the G protein, adenylyl cyclase system to transduce the signal generated by hormone-receptor binding (Fig. 11–2). In addition to high-affinity hormone binding by the N-terminal halves of the LHR and FSHR, the LHR has a low-affinity hormone-binding site in its membrane-associated C-terminal half. In truncation experiments, occupancy of the latter site is sufficient to activate the LHR. To explore differences between LHR and FSHR in the number and location of hormone-binding sites, and in their mechanisms of activation, amino acid substitution experiments have recently been done on five amino acids (Asp 405–Lys 409) of the FSHR, at the junction between helix 2 and exoloop 1, that are weakly conserved among the LHR, FSHR, and TSHR (Ji and Ji, 1995). His 407 is involved in high-affinity ligand binding, whereas Asp 405, Thr 408, and Lys 409 are necessary for FSHR activation and, thereby, for G-protein coupling to the adenylyl cyclase system.

Normal CG or LH binding to the LHR stimulates Leydig or theca cell androgenesis acutely by increasing transport of cholesterol from the outer to the inner mitochondrial membrane (a process dependent on the StAR protein; see Chapter

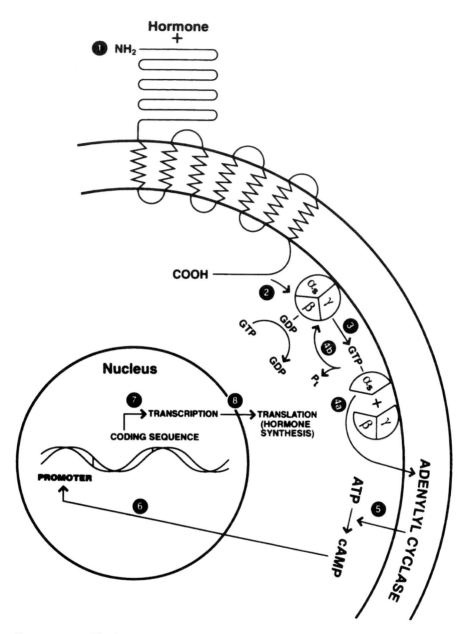

Figure 11–2. The basic mechanism of gonadotropin-initiated, G protein–mediated, sex hormone synthesis in Leydig or granulosa cells. LH or FSH induces (or favors) the activated state of the receptor. This state somehow stimulates the inactive membrane-bound, heterotrimeric G protein to become active by displacing its GDP (guanosine diphosphate) with GTP (guanosine triphosphate). The GTP-bound Gαs subunit dissociates from the trimer, stimulates cAMP formation, and ultimately sex steroid synthesis. The cycle is autoregulated by the intrinsic GTPase activity of the GTP-Gαs complex. (Reproduced from DiMeglio L A, Pescovitz O H, *J Pediatr* 131: S8–12, 1997, with permission.)

13), and chronically by increasing transcriptional expression of androgenic enzymes. The acute and chronic stimuli are both mediated by cAMP. Some LHR mutations prevent Leydig cell or theca lutein cell proliferation, nullify or impair ligand-dependent androgenesis, and interfere with normal male sexual differentiation before birth and at puberty. They also obstruct theca lutein cell proliferation and, therefore, female reproductive maturation at puberty. Other LHR mutations provoke ligand-independent (autonomous) receptor activity: these cause precocious puberty in males by constitutive Leydig cell hyperplasia and hypersecretion of testosterone.

In pubertal females, normal FSH binding to the FSHR stimulates estrogen synthesis in granulosa cells, rescues follicles from atresia, and initiates normal ovulatory cycles. In pubertal males, FSH contributes to initiation of spermatogenesis, probably by promoting Sertoli cell proliferation. It also helps to maintain spermatogenesis in adult males. FSHR mutation arrests ovarian folliculogenesis in pubertal females, and impairs spermatogenesis variably in pubertal males.

REFERENCES

Gyapay G, Morissette J, Vignal A, Dib C, Fizames C, Millasseau P, Marc S, Bernardi G, Lathrop M A, Weissenbach J (1994). The 1993–1994 Genethon human genetic linkage map. *Nat Genet* 7:246–339.

Ji I, Ji T H (1995). Differential roles of exoloop 1 of the human follicle-stimulating hormone receptor in hormone binding and receptor activation. *J Biol Chem* 270:15970–15973.

Genetic Disorders of the Chorionic Gonadotropin (CG)/Luteinizing Hormone (LH) Receptor

IMPAIRED MASCULINIZATION OF MALES AND OVARIAN DYSFUNCTION IN FEMALES DUE TO CG/LH RECEPTOR MUTATIONS THAT CAUSE TESTICULAR AND OVARIAN RESISTANCE TO CG/LH

Clinical and Imaging Presentations. At birth, severely affected XY subjects have female external genitalia (possibly with slight posterior labial fusion); those mildly affected may simply have micropenis without hypospadias (Toledo, 1992; Latronico et al., 1996); those moderately affected will have some degree of external genital ambiguity (Schwartz et al., 1981). At puberty, XY subjects with a female phenotype develop eunuchoid body proportions and appreciable pubic hair, but they do not have breast development or menses. Their gonads are scrotal (if mildly affected), and inguinal or intraabdominal (if moderately or severely affected). Two XX patients have been documented. One (Latronico et al., 1996) had primary amenorrhea, but otherwise near-normal pubertal development, except for cystic ovaries and a small uterus on ultrasonography. The second (Toledo et al., 1996) also had primary amenorrhea with an otherwise normal puberty. Ultrasonography exposed a large cyst in the right ovary and a small uterus; densitometry revealed reduced bone mass. Other putatively affected XX adult subjects have also had primary amenorrhea despite otherwise normal female pubertal development (Kremer et al., 1995; Saldanha et al., 1987). XY females have normal müllerian duct regression; hence they may not have satisfactory vaginal intercourse without vaginal elongation-dilation. All affected subjects have a heterosexual orientation.

Laboratory Features. All affected individuals respond normally to ACTH stimulation. XY subjects have low basal blood testosterone (and testosterone precursor) levels that do not rise after hCG stimulation. In early infancy and at puberty, their basal LH and, inconstantly, their FSH levels are high (hypergonadotropic hypogonadism), but neither of these values rises unduly after a standard gonadotropin-releasing hormone (GnRH) stimulus. Conventional testicular histology usually reveals interstitial fibroblasts with only a few immature Leydig cells, and basal laminar thickening of seminiferous tubules that contain only Sertoli cells. However, immunocytochemistry may expose reactivity to LHR or P450c17 antibodies and, thus, Leydig cell ancestry in an appreciable portion of them (Misrahi et al., 1997). The adult XX subject described by Latronico and colleagues (1996) had elevated LH, but normal FSH and estradiol in the blood. Her serum progesterone concentrations were low inconsistently, but those of testosterone, androstenedione, and 17-hydroxyprogesterone were normal. The second adult XX subject (Toledo et al., 1996) had elevated plasma LH and FSH levels that reacted normally to a GnRH stimulus. Estradiol and progesterone levels were low-or mid-normal, respectively, did not respond to hCG challenge, and did not fluctuate as in normal ovulatory cycles. Ovarian histology revealed all stages of follicle development (up to preovulatory) including large antral follicles with a layer of luteinized theca cells; corpora lutea or albicans were absent.

Genotyping and Mutant Gene Expression. In one family with three severely affected XY siblings, a homozygous nonsense mutation was found at a triplet that normally encodes Arg554 in the third intracellular loop of the LH receptor (Latronico et al., 1996). In a second family, a boy with a normally formed but small penis was homozygous for Ser616Tyr in the seventh transmembrane helix of the LH receptor (Fig. 11–3; Latronico et al., 1996). The parents of neither family were aware of consanguinity, but each set came from small isolated villages in different parts of the world. In a third family with parental consanguinity (Kremer et al., 1995), two XY siblings with female phenotypes had Ala593Pro in the sixth transmembrane α-helix of the LH receptor (Fig. 11–4). In a fourth family, a nonsense mutation in the paternal allele occurred at position 545 in the fifth transmembrane helix (Laue et al., 1995); later, the maternal allele was found to contain a 33-bp in-frame insertion in exon 1 (Wu et al., 1997). More recently, Stavrou and colleagues (1998) reported homozygosity for a Glu354Lys mutation in the extracellular domain close to the first transmembrane helix, and they alluded to two other inactivating mutations (one of them Cys131Arg) that are embedded more deeply in the extracellular domain. Expression studies in embryonic kidney cells showed that Ser616Tyr seriously impairs LH binding to the LH receptor and, expectedly, the production of cAMP. Comparable *in vitro* studies on the mutant LH receptor bearing Ala593Pro disclosed a markedly reduced B_{max} but a normal K_d for hCG binding, with essentially no cAMP response even to 1 μg/mL of hCG. The lack of cAMP response

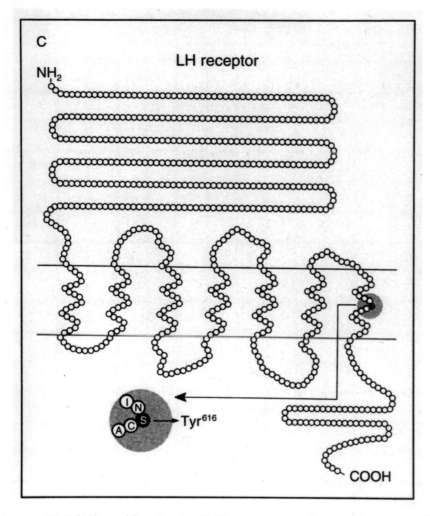

FIGURE 11–3. A loss-of-function Ser616Tyr mutation in the seventh transmembrane α-helix of the LH receptor. (Reproduced from Latronico AC, et al., *N Engl J Med* 334:507–512, 1996, with permission.)

occurred despite an adequate level of binding, indicating defective receptor-activation or coupling with G protein. The low B_{max} is attributable to faulty folding of the mutant receptor, and its consequent impaired translocation to the cell membrane. LHR-Cys545X had 10-fold less than normal affinity for hCG (Laue et al., 1995), and its expression was reduced at the cell surface. Expectedly, Cys131Arg in the extracellular domain impaired hCG binding markedly, and the patient was born with sufficient external genital ambiguity that she was reared as a female (Misrahi et al., 1997).

Management. After gonadectomy, adult female XY subjects with severely deficient or defective LH receptor activity are treated with estrogen to promote breast development. Affected XY subjects with micropenis benefit from androgen therapy both in infancy and at the time of puberty. Following affirmation of biparental heterozygosity, genetic counseling would proffer a 25% recurrence risk. In the fu-

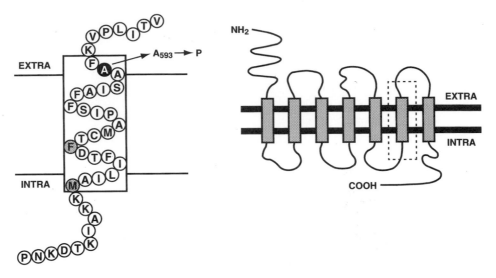

FIGURE 11–4. A loss-of-function Ala593Pro mutation at the junction of the sixth transmembrane α-helix and the third intracellular loop of the LH receptor. In contrast, missense mutations at Asp578 and Met 571 yield a gain of function that results in male-limited precocious puberty (see also Fig 11–6). (Reproduced from Kremer H, et al., *Nat Genet* 9:160–164, 1995, with permission.)

ture, preimplantation diagnosis and prophylaxis by fetal androgen replacement may be feasible.

Discussion.   Early studies on impaired masculinization associated with Leydig cell hypoplasia (Schwartz et al., 1981; David et al., 1984; Martinez-Mora et al., 1991) revealed impaired testicular CG/LH binding, but could not distinguish which was "cause" and which "effect." Molecular-genetic analysis has proven causality and has permitted the initiation of efforts to define the structure-function properties that allow a LH receptor to function as a G protein–coupled signal transducer. Different degrees and, perhaps, the different timing of LH receptor insufficiency will yield different degrees of impaired masculinization in affected subjects. Alternatively, different mutations of the LH receptor may have differential consequences for the binding or action of hCG or LH. Conceivably, therefore, hCG-dependent *morphogenesis* of the penis may be normal, only to be followed by impaired *growth* of the penis under the influence of defective LH activity (Toledo 1992; Latronico et al., 1996). Remarkably, in XX subjects even a severe LH receptor defect does not interfere with pubic hair or breast development—presumably, in part, because of adrenal androgenesis, and basal ovarian or peripheral aromatization of androgen precursors to estradiol, respectively. Interestingly, however, one LH receptor defect did interfere with follicular maturation, ovulation, luteinization, and progesterone biosynthesis (Latronico et al., 1996), whereas a different one only blocked ovulation (Toledo et al., 1996). Furthermore, the XX patient described by Toledo and colleagues (1996) had not only a small uterus but an immature vagina and reduced bone mass, a triad indicating chronic hypoestrogenism. Nonetheless, both XX patients with a LHR defect had sufficient circulating estradiol to suppress the development of very high LH and FSH levels, like those observed in XX patients who have very low estradiol and inhibin levels because of FSHR defects (Aittomaki et al., 1996). Data from rats and rabbits imply that the initiation of androgenesis by human Leydig cells may be hCG-independent, even if Leydig cell division may not be (Huhtaniemi, 1994; George et al., 1978). This implication is supported by the fact that some XY subjects with severe LH receptor defects have epididymes and vasa deferentia (Berthezene et al., 1976; Brown et al., 1978; Schwartz et al., 1981; Kremer et al., 1995; Misrahi et al., 1997). A different school of thought holds that development of these wolffian derivatives is not fully testosterone-independent.

REFERENCES

Aittomäki K, Herva R, Stenman U H, Juntunen K, Ylöstalo P, Hovatta O, de la Chapelle A (1996). Clinical features of primary ovarian failure caused by a point mutation in the follicle-stimulating hormone receptor gene. *J Clin Endocrinol Metab* 81:3722–3726.

Berthezene F, Forest M G, Grimaud J A, Claustrat B, Mornex R (1976). Leydig-cell agenesis: a cause of male pseudohermaphroditism. *N Engl J Med* 295:969–972.

Brown D M, Markland C, Dehner L P (1976) Leydig cell hypoplasia: a cause of male pseudohermaphroditism. *J Clin Endocrinol Metab* 46:1–7.

David R, Yoon D J, Landin L, Lew L, Sklar C, Schinella R, Golimbu M (1984). A syndrome of gonadotropin resistance possibly due to a luteinizing hormone receptor defect. *J Clin Endocrinol Metab* 59:156–160.

George F W, Catt K J, Neaves W B, Wilson J D (1978). Studies on the regulation of testosterone synthesis in the fetal rabbit testis. *Endocrinology* 102:665–673.

Huhtaniemi I (1994). Fetal testis—a very special endocrine organ. *Eur J Endocrinol* 130:25–31.

Kremer H, Kraaij R, Toledo S P A, Post M, Fridman J B, Hayashida C Y, van Reen M, Milgrom E, Ropers H H, Mariman E, Themmen A P N, Brunner H C (1995). Male pseudohermaphroditism due to a homozygous missense mutation of the luteinizing hormone receptor gene. *Nat Genet* 9:160–164.

Latronico A C, Anasti J, Arnhold I J P, Rapaport R, Mendonca B B, Bloise W, Castro M, Tsigos C, Chrousos G P (1996). Brief report: testicular and ovarian resistance to luteinizing hormone caused by inactivating mutations of the luteinizing hormone-receptor gene. *N Engl J Med* 334:507–512.

Laue L, Wu S M, Kudo M, Hsueh A J W, Cutler Jr G B, Griffin J E, Wilson J D, Brain C, Berry A C, Grant D B, Chan W Y (1995). A nonsense mutation of the human luteinizing hormone receptor gene in Leydig cell hypoplasia. *Hum Mol Genet* 4:1429–1433.

Martinez-Mora J, Saz J M, Toran N, Isnard R, Perez-Iribarne M M, Egozcue J, Audi L (1991). Male pseudohermaphroditism due to Leydig cell agenesis and absence of testicular L H receptors. *Clin Endocrinol* 34:485–491.

Misrahi M, Meduri G, Pissard S, Bouvattier C, Beau I, Loosfelt H, Jolivet A, Rappaport E, Milgrom E, Bougneres P (1997). Comparison of immunocytochemical and molecular features with the phenotype in a case of incomplete male pseudohermaphroditism associated with a mutation of the luteinizing hormone receptor. *J Clin Endocrinol Metab* 82:2159–2165.

Saldanha P H, Arnhold I J P, Mendonca B B, Bloise W, Toledo S P A (1987). A clinicogenetic investigation of Leydig cell hypoplasia. *Am J Med Genet* 26:337–344.

Schwartz M, Imperato-McGinley J, Peterson R E, Cooper G, Morris P L, MacGillivray M, Hensle T (1981). Male pseudohermaphroditism secondary to an abnormality in Leydig cell differentiation. *J Clin Endocrinol Metab* 53:123–127.

Stavrou S S, Zhu Y-S, Cai L-Q, Katz M D, Herrera C, Defillo-Ricart M, Imperato-McGinley J (1998). A novel mutation of the human luteinizing hormone receptor in 46XY and 46XX sisters. *J Clin Endocrinol Metab* 83:2091–98.

Toledo S P A (1982). Leydig cell hypoplasia leading to two different phenotypes: male pseu-
    dohermaphroditism and primary hypogonadism not associated with this. *Clin Endocrinol*
    36:521–522.
Toledo S P A, Brunner H G, Kraaij R, Post M, Dahia P L M, Hayashida C Y, Kremer H, Them-
    men A P N (1996). An inactivating mutation of the luteinizing hormone receptor causes
    amenorrhea in a 46,XX female. *J Clin Endocrinol Metab* 81:3850–3854.
Wu S M, Hallermeier K, Laue L, Griffin J E, Wilson J D, Grant D B, Brain C, Berry E C, Culter
    G B Jr, Chan W Y (1997). Insertional mutation in exon 1 inactivates the LH/hCG receptor
    in a patient with Leydig cell hypoplasia. *Program, 79th Annual Meeting, Endocrine Society*,
    553 (Abstract).

PSEUDOPRECOCIOUS PUBERTY IN MALES: CONSTITUTIVE LEYDIG CELL HYPERACTIVITY DUE TO LH RECEPTOR MUTATIONS THAT PROVOKE LIGAND-INDEPENDENT RECEPTOR ACTIVITY (FAMILIAL TESTOTOXICOSIS)

Clinical and Imaging Presentations. Typically, there is a vertical family history of precocious puberty, limited to males, that is transmitted by males or females. Onset of phallic and testicular enlargement, and the appearance of pubic hair, usually occurs between 3 and 4 years of age, but external genitomegaly has been noted at birth. Axillary hair is delayed in relation to pubic hair. Acne may be present, and so may aggressive behavior, spontaneous erection, and masturbatory activity. Because of premature epiphyseal fusion, untreated affected adults are shorter than their normal male relatives. The condition is labeled pseudoprecocious puberty because it does not involve premature activation of the hypothalamic-pituitary axis, and it is gonadotropin-independent; true (central) precocious puberty is dependent on gonadotropins that are secreted as the result of premature activation of the axis.

Laboratory Features. Affected boys, less than 4 years of age, have pubertal concentrations of testosterone in the blood despite low, nonpulsatile basal gonadotropin levels, a prepubertal gonadotropin response to a GnRH stimulus, and a failure of long-acting GnRH analogue-agonist to suppress testosterone secretion. Interestingly, at puberty GnRH release does stimulate LH production and testosterone secretion, indicating that the Leydig cell constitutivity imposed by the LHR mutation is usually submaximal (Laue et al., 1993; Egli et al., 1985; Rosenthal et al., 1996). This fact has management implications, as discussed below. Testicular histology ranges from normal adult to excessive Leydig cell maturation for a given degree of spermatogenesis.

Genotyping and Mutant Gene Expression. Kremer and colleagues (1993) and Shenker and colleagues (1993) each predicted that familial male peripheral precocious puberty (FMPPP) might be caused by LH receptor mutations that conferred activity on the LH receptor in the absence of LH binding (Fig. 11–5). They fulfilled their predictions initially by finding heterozygous missense mutations in the portion of the LH gene that encodes amino acids in or near the sixth transmembrane helix— a segment of the LH receptor that is involved in the binding of G protein (Fig. 11–6). Kremer and colleagues (1993) found Met575lle and Asp582Gly in two European families. In nine American families, seven from the southeastern United States,

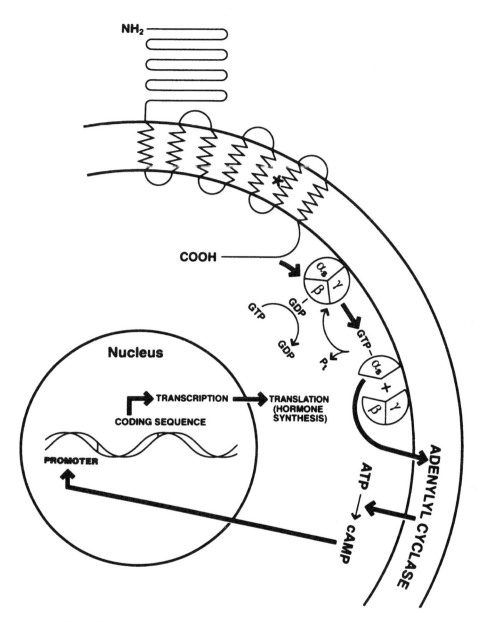

FIGURE 11–5. The mechanism of gonadotropin-independent testosterone synthesis in a Leydig cell due to constitutive activation of the LH receptor by a mutation (*) such as Asp578Gly. The thick solid arrows connote hyperactivity of the signal transduction pathway culminating in excessive hormone synthesis. (Reproduced from DiMeglio L A, Pescovitz O H, *J Pediatr* 131:S8–12, 1997, with permission).

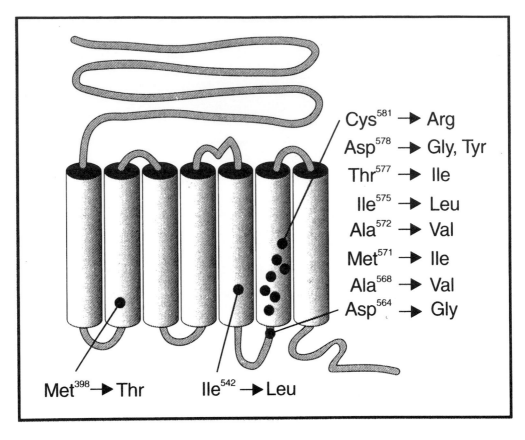

FIGURE 11–6. The concentration of LH receptor–activating mutations in or near the sixth transmembrane α-helix. (Reproduced from Shenker A, *Growth Genet Horm* 12:33–48, 1996, with permission.)

Shenker and colleagues (1993) found Asp578Gly (corresponding to Asp582Gly as numbered by Kremer et al.). In two of six additional families (five European), Kosugi and colleagues (1995) found Met571Ile (corresponding to Met575Ile) in one (European) family, and Thr577Ile in the other. In two sporadic cases, Japanese patients have Ala572Val, further incriminating transmembrane helix 6 (Yano et al., 1995). On the other hand, Met398Thr in the second transmembrane helix (Kraaij et al., 1995; Evans et al., 1996), and Leu457Arg in the third helix (Latronico et al., 1998) also cause FMPPP, so other parts of the LHR can probably interact with coupled G proteins. Kremer and colleagues (1993) used linkage analysis and inference from amino acid changes to support the pathogenic significance of the mutations they discovered. Shenker and colleagues (1993) and Kosugi and colleagues (1995) constructed mutant expression vectors and demonstrated agonist-independent cAMP production in transfected host cells. Indeed, the mutations they studied did not affect the affinity of the LHR for agonist, or the degree of agonist responsiveness (Yano et al., 1995); in contrast, Met398Thr did decrease maximal agonist-induced cAMP production (Kraaij et al., 1995). Müller and colleagues (1998) recently reported Asp578Tyr as the cause of unusually severe testotoxicosis. Appropriately, they found that cells transfected with Asp578Tyr LHR had nearly twice as much basal cAMP production as those expressing the more common Asp578Gly mutation. In fact, this represented 65% of the maximal agonist-induced level. Furthermore, Asp578Tyr also doubled basal activation of the phosphoinositide pathway. Asp578 is conserved in all glycoprotein hormone receptors, and it has been predicted to play a key role in maintaining an inactive conformation of the hLHR (Kosugi et al., 1996). This prediction is substantiated by the comparative genotype–phenotype observations on patients with Asp578Tyr.

Management. The earliest efforts at therapy of FMPPP used a progestin, medroxyprogesterone acetate, or an anti-androgen, cyproterone acetate. More recently, excessive androgen synthesis by the diseased Leydig cells, and the consequences thereof, have been controlled by treatment with ketoconazole, an inhibitor of several steps in the pathway of androgen biosynthesis. However, this drug carries the risk of serious hepatotoxic side effects and, at the doses used, its efficacy is overridden by the pubertal increase of gonadotropin secretion (Holland et al., 1987). Another effective therapeutic regimen (Laue et al., 1989) has consisted of spironolactone (an androgen antagonist that competes for the androgen receptor) in combination with testolactone (an aromatase inhibitor). The latter was incorporated on the rationale that estrogens contribute to the normal pubertal growth spurt in boys. The superimposition of a pubertal GnRH stimulus on the mutant LHR-induced Leydig cell constitutivity requires the addition of a long-acting GnRH agonist to the basic combined-treatment regimen. The latter desensitizes pituitary gonadotropes to GnRH stimulation by down-regulating their GnRH receptors (Laue et al., 1993).

Discussion. Mutations in exon 11 of the LHR gene that cause amino acid substitution at or near its fifth and sixth transmembrane helices are, by far, the most common causes of gonadotropin-independent male sexual precocity that is not due to an androgen-secreting tumor. In fact, one such mutation, Asp578Gly, accounted for the disorder in 24 of 28 affected families.

The reason why heterozygous females are asymptomatic is presumably manifold. First, Leydig cell androgenesis is strictly LHR-dependent, whereas ovarian steroidogenesis is codependent on LHR and FSHR; this explanation coincides with the fact that tumorigenic hCG causes precocious puberty only in males. Second, 17,20-lyase activity is apparently more rate-limiting for androgen biosynthesis in theca than in Leydig cells. Third, intraovarian down-regulatory mechanisms seem to buffer the effects of LHR constitutivity.

The Asp578Gly mutation and several of the others increase basal cAMP production without affecting other properties of LH/CG binding by the LHR, and without affecting basal or agonist-induced inositol phosphate production. Evidently, in these cases, the mutant LHR effects Gαs coupling to activate adenylyl cyclase, but not Gαq coupling to activate phospholipase C.

Paradoxically, LHRs carrying the Ile542Leu and Cys581Arg mutations are ligand-unresponsive, despite their ligand independence (Laue et al., 1995), whereas the Ala572Val mutation creates constitutivity and altered responsiveness as measured by both inositol phosphate and cAMP (Yano et al., 1995). Themmen and Brunner (1996) have optimized the transient transfection assay system by using mouse tumor Leydig cells as hosts in order to demonstrate LHR constitutivity by increased pregnenolone production.

A "gain-of-function" mechanism is often the explanation for heterozygous (dominant) expression of an autosomal gene. The gain may be in the amount or in the effect of a usual function (whether positive or negative), or in the acquisition of a novel noxious function. FMPPP is a perfect example of an increase in a usual positive function to the point that it is harmful. Presumably, the mutant amino acid substitutions change receptor conformation in a way that is normally agonist-dependent. Not surprisingly, other human genetic diseases have been shown to result from constitutivity of G protein–coupled receptors, respectively: retinitis pigmentosa, rhodopsin (Robinson et al., 1992); thyroid hyperplasia, TSHR (Duprez et al., 1994); and hypocalcemia, calcium-sensing receptor (Pollak et al., 1994).

REFERENCES

Duprez L, Parma J, Van Sande J, Allgeier A, Leclere J, Schwartz C, Delisle M J, Decoulx M, Oriazzi J, Dumont J, Vassart G (1994). Germline mutations in the thyrotropin receptor gene cause non-autoimmune autosomal dominant hyperthyroidism. *Nat Genet* 7:396–401.

Evans B A J, Bowen D J, Smith P J, Clayton P E, Gregory J W (1996) a new point mutation in the luteinising hormone receptor gene in familial and sporadic male limited precocious puberty: genotype does not always correlate with phenotype. *J Med Genet* 33:143–147.

Egli C A, Rosenthal S M, Grumbach M M, Montalvo J M, Gondos B (1985). Pituitary gonadotropin-independentmale-limited autosomal dominant sexual precocity in 4 generations: "familial testotoxicosis." *J Pediatr* 106:33–40.

Holland F J, Kirsch S E, Selby R (1987). Gonadotropin-independent precocious puberty ("testotoxicosis"): influence of maturational status on response to ketoconazole. *J Clin Endocrinol Metab* 64:328–333.

Kosugi S, Van Dop C, Geffner M E, Rabl W, Carel J C, Chaussain J L, Mori T, Merendino J J, Shenker A (1995). Characterization of heterogeneous mutations causing constitutive activation of the luteinizing hormone receptor in familial male precocious puberty. *Hum Mol Genet* 4:183–188.

Kosugi S, Mori T, Shenker A (1996). The role of Asp[578] in maintaining the inactive conformation of the human lutropin/choriogonadotropin receptor. *J Biol Chem* 271:31813–31813.

Kraaij R, Post M, Kremer H, Milgrom E, Epping W, Brunner H G, Grootegoed J A, Themmen A P N (1995). A missense mutation in the second transmembrane segment of the luteinizing hormone receptor causes familial male-limited precocious puberty. *J Clin Endocrinol Metab* 80:3168–3172.

Kremer H, Mariman E, Otten B J, Moll G W, Stoelinga G B A, Wit J, Jansen M, Drop S L, Fass B, Ropers H H, Brunner H G (1993). Cosegregation of missense mutations of the luteinizing hormone receptor gene with familial male-limited precocious puberty. *Hum Mol Genet* 2:1779–1783.

Latronico A C, Abell A N, Arnhold I J P, Liu X, Lins S S, Brito V N, Billerbeck A E, Segaloff D L, Mendonca B B (1998). A unique constitutively activating mutation in third transmembrane helix of luteinizing hormone receptor causes sporadic male gonadotropin-independent precocious puberty. *J Clin Endocrinol Metab* 83:2435–2440.

Laue L, Kenigsberg D, Pescovitz O H, Hench K D, Barnes K M, Loriaux D L, Cutler Jr G B (1989). Treatment of familial male precocious puberty with spironolactone and testolactone. *N Engl J Med* 320:496–502.

Laue L, Jones J, Barnes K M, Cutler G B Jr (1993). Treatment of familial male precocious puberty with spironolactone, testolactone, and deslorelin. *J Clin Endocrinol Metab* 76:151–155.

Laue L, Chan W Y, Hsueh A J W, Kudo M, Hsu S Y, Wu S M, Blomberg L A, Cutler G B Jr (1995). Genetic heterogeneity of constitutively activating mutations of the human luteinizing hormone receptor in familial male-limited precocious puberty. *Proc Natl Acad Sci USA* 92:1906–1910.

Müller J, Gondos B, Kosugi S, Mori T, Shenker A (1998). Severe testotoxicosis phenotype associated with Asp[578] → Tyr mutation of the lutrophin/choriogonadotrophin receptor gene. *J Med Genet* 35:340–341.

Pollak M R, Brown E M, Estep H L, McLaine P N, Kofor O, Park J, Hebert S C, Seidman C E, Seidman J G (1994). Autosomal dominant hypocalcaemia caused by a calcium-sensing receptor gene mutation. *Nat Genet* 8:303–307.

Robinson P R, Cohen G B, Zhukovsky E A, Oprian D D (1992). Constitutively active mutants of rhodopsin. *Neuron* 9:719–725.

Rosenthal I M, Refetoff S, Rich B, Barnes R B, Sunthornthepvarakul T, Parma J, Rosenfield R L (1996). Response to challenge with gonadotropin-releasing hormone agonist in a mother and her two sons with a constitutively activating mutatuion of the luteinizing hormone receptor—a clinical research center study. *J Clin Endocrinol Metab* 81:3802–3806.

Shenker A, Laue L, Kosugi S, Merendino J J, Minegishi T, Cutler G B Jr (1993). A constitutively activating mutation of the luteinizing hormone receptor in familial male precocious puberty. *Nature* 365:652–654.

Themmen A P N, Brunner H G (1996). Luteinizing hormone receptor mutations and sex differentiation. *Eur J Endo* 134:533–540.

Yano K, Saji M, Hidaka A, Moriya N, Okuno A, Kohn L D, Cutler G B Jr (1995). A new constitutively activating point mutation in the luteinizing hormone/choriogonadotropin receptor gene in cases of male-limited precocious puberty. *J Clin Endocrinol Metab* 80: 1162–168.

Genetic Disorders of the Post-LH Receptor Cascade

UNDERACTIVITY OF Gsα LEADING TO MULTIHORMONE, INCLUDING GONADOTROPIN, RESISTANCE IN PSEUDOHYPOPARATHYROIDISM 1A; ALBRIGHT'S HEREDITARY OSTEODYSTROPHY

Pseudohypoparathyroidism (PHP) is clinical and biochemical hypoparathyroidism in the face of elevated circulating parathormone and failure to mount a calcemic or phosphaturic response to exogenous parathormone (PTH). In type 1, there is impaired renal adenylate cyclase responsiveness to PTH; in type 2, there is a normal renal cAMP response to PTH without an appropriate phosphaturic response. Patients with type 1a have a set of physical features that constitute Albright's hereditary osteodystrophy (AHO), and decreased Gsα activity in multiple cell types. They are, therefore, prone to resist multiple hormones (Levine et al., 1983) whose receptors must couple with Gsα in order to augment cAMP, and thereby a given target cell action. First-degree relatives of patients with PHP1a may have AHO without overt hormone resistance (pseudoPHP). In type 1b, the defect is limited to the PTH receptor, and Gsα activity is normal (Silve et al., 1986). The remainder of this section is concerned with resistance to gonadotropins that may occur as part of the clinical and biochemical syndrome known as PHP, type 1a/ pseudoPHP.

Clinical and Imaging Presentation.   The clinical expressions of hypocalcemia and hyperphosphatemia include paraesthesias, convulsions, tetany, Q-T interval prolongation, enamel hypoplasia, delayed tooth eruption, cataract, and basal ganglia calcification. In addition, affected individuals have short stature, obesity, round facies, brachydactyly (particularly of the fourth and fifth metacarpals), mild to moderate mental retardation, and subcutaneous ossification. Occasionally, hypothyroidism is the presenting sign because of resistance to TSH (Weisman et al., 1985; Levine et al., 1985). Furthermore, 10 of 13 women studied by Levine and colleagues (1983) had sexual immaturity, amenorrhea, or oligomenorrhea presumably due to gonadotropin resistance. Single case reports of sexual immaturity in an affected male (Shapiro et al., 1980) and two females (Wolfsdorf et al., 1978; Shima et al., 1988) have also appeared. In a larger, recent study, Namnoum and colleagues (1998) noted that 14 of 17 adult female patients were oligomenorrheic or amenorrheic and hypoestrogenic.

Laboratory Features.   There is hypocalcemia, hyperphosphatemia, normal renal function, and increased circulating immunoreactive PTH. Most patients with PHP 1a have about a 50% decrease of Gsα activity in cell membranes of many cell types. The activity is measured by the extent to which an extract of a patient's cell membranes is able to restore inducibility of adenyl cyclase to membranes prepared from a mutant line of murine lymphoma cells that is Gsα-depleted. Those female patients with severe gonadotropin resistance (Wolfsdorf et al., 1978) have high basal levels of LH and FSH, and an accentuated increment in these hormones after a GnRH stimulus. However, most female patients have normal or only slightly increased serum gonadotropin levels, and they respond normally to GnRH challenge (Namnoum et al., 1998). This indicates partial gonadotropin resistance in theca and granulosa cells of the adult ovary.

Genotyping and Gene Expression.   There is a single Gsα gene on the distal long arm of human chromosome 20 (Gejman et al., 1991). It spans approximately 20 Kb, contains 13 exons, and encodes a protein of 396 amino acids (Patten et al., 1990). Four types of Gsα mRNA can be derived by alternative splicing (Kozasa et al., 1988). There are multiple transcriptional initiation sites. The promoter has four GC-rich boxes, but neither a CAAT nor a TATA sequence. A variety of different point mutations has been discovered in the Gsα gene of patients with PHP 1a (Weinstein et al., 1992; Miric et al., 1993; Schwindinger and Levine, 1994; Shapira et al., 1996). Many of these mutations yield reduced levels of Gsα mRNA. The R385H mutation is noteworthy because it occurs near the C-terminus of Gsα, an area involved in coupling to the receptor (Conklin et al., 1996).

Management.   It is necessary to treat hypocalcemia with vitamin D, occasionally supplemented with oral calcium. The use of acetazolamide to decrease phosphatemia may be helpful. Patients with multiple forms of endocrine resistance may need additional therapy for hypothyroidism, or for hypogonadism.

Discussion.   It is not understood why haploinsufficiency of Gsα protein causes parathormone resistance frequently but resistance to other G-coupled hormones much less commonly. Nor is it clear why an autosomal dominant disease appears to affect females twice as often as males. One contributing factor may be the menstrual-ovulatory expressions that occur in many affected females. Paradoxically, Fitch (1982) pointed out that the great majority of families with AHO in the literature demonstrate transmission by females. She also listed numerous case reports illustrating impaired male reproductive function. More recently, several groups (Davies and Hughes, 1993; Wilson et al., 1994) have discovered that maternally transmitted cases are more likely to have full phenotypic expression (PHP type 1a) than paternally transmitted cases (pseudoPHP). This form of transmission distortion (parent-of-origin effect) has also been observed among members of a three-generation family (Nakamoto et al., 1998). It implies that genomic imprinting determines expressivity of the disorder, and this is fortified by the fact that the h*GNAS1* gene is found at 20q13.11, a location syntenic with a mouse chromosome region that is also imprinted (Cattanach and Kirk, 1985). Indeed, only the paternal mouse *Gnas* gene is expressed in renal glomeruli (Williamson et al., 1996).

REFERENCES

Cattanach B M, Kirk M (1985). Differential activity of maternally and paternally derived chromosome regions in mice. *Nature* 315:496–498.

Conklin B R, Herzmark P, Ishida S, Voyno-Yasenetskaya T A, Sun Y, Farfel Z, Bourne H R (1996). Carboxyl-terminal mutations of $G_{q\alpha}$ and $G_{s\alpha}$ that alter the fidelity of receptor activation. *Mol Pharmacol* 50:885–890.

Davies S J, Hughes H E (1993). Imprinting in Albright's hereditary osteodystrophy. *J Med Genet* 30:101–103.

Fitch N. Albright's hereditary osteodystrophy: a review. *Am J Med Genet* 11:11–29.

Gejman P V, Weinstein L S, Martinez M, Spiegel A M, Cao Q, Hsieh W T, Hoehe M R, Gershon E S (1991). Genetic mapping of the Gs-α subunit gene (GNASI) to the distal long arm of chromosome 20 using a polymorphism detected by denaturing gradient gel electrophoresis. *Genomics* 9:782–783.

Kozasa T, Itoh H, Tsukamoto T, Kaziro Y (1988). Isolation and characterization of the human Gsα gene. *Proc Natl Acad Sci USA* 85:2081–2085.

Levine M A, Downs R W, Moses A M, Breslau N A, Marx S J, Lasker R D, Rizzoli R E, Aurbach G D, Spiegel A M (1983). Resistance to multiple hormones in patients with pseudohypoparathyroidism: association with deficient activity of guanine nucleotide regulatory protein. *Am J Med* 74:545–556.

Levine M A, Jap T S, Hung W (1985). Infantile hypothyroidism in two sibs: An unusual presentation of pseudohypoparathyroidism type Ia. *J Pediatr* 107:919–922.

Miric A, Bechio J D, Levine M A (1993). Heterogeneous mutations in the gene encoding the stimulatory G protein of adenylyl cyclase in Albright hereditary osteodystrophy. *J Clin Endocrinol Metab* 76:1560–1568.

Nakamoto J M, Sandstrom A T, Brickman A S, Christenson R A, Van Dop C (1998). Pseudohypoparathyroidism type Ia from maternal but not paternal transmission of a $G_s\alpha$ gene mutation. *Am J Med Genet* 77:261–267.

Namnoum A B, Merriam G R, Moses A M, Levine M A (1998). Reproductive dysfunction in women with Albright's hereditary osteodystrophy. *J Clin Endocrinol Metab* 83:824–829.

Patten J L, Johns D R, Vale D, Eil C, Gruppuso P A, Steele G, Smallwood P M, Levine M A (1990). Mutation in the gene encoding the stimulatory G protein of adenylate cyclase in Albright's hereditary osteodystrophy. *N Engl J Med* 322:1412–1419.

Shapira H, Mouallem M, Shapiro M S, Weisman Y, Farfel Z (1996). Pseudo-hypoparathyroidism type Ia: two new heterozygous frameshift mutations in exons 5 and 10 of the Gsα gene. *Hum. Genet* 97:73–75.

Schwindinger W F, Levine M A (1994). Albright hereditary osteodystrophy. *Endocrinologist* 4: 17–27.

Silve C, Santora A, Breslau N, Moses A, Spiegel A (1986). Selective resistance to parathyroid hormone in cultured skin fibroblasts from patients with pseudohypoparathyroidism Type Ib. *J Clin Endocrinol Metab* 62:640–644.

Shapiro M S, Bernheim J, Gutman A, Arber I, Spitz I M (1980). Multiple abnormalities of anterior pituitary hormone secretion in association with pseudo-hypoparathyroidism. *J Clin Endocrinol Metab* 51:483–487.

Shima M, Nose O, Shimizu K, Seino Y, Yabuuchi H, Saito T (1988). Multiple associated endocrine abnormalities in a patient with pseudohypoparathyroidism type 1a. *Eur J Pediatr* 147:536–538.

Weinstein L S, Gejman P V, de Mazancourt P, American N, Spiegel A M (1992). A heterozygous 4-bp deletion mutation in the Gsα gene (GNAS1) in a patient with Albright hereditary osteodystrophy. *Genomics* 13:1319–1321.

Weisman Y, Golander A, Spirer Z, Farfel Z (1985). Pseudohypoparathyroidism type 1a presenting as congenital hypothyroidism. *J. Pediatr.* 107:413–415.

Williamson C M, Schofield J, Dutton E R, Seymour A, Beechey C V, Edwards Y H, Peters J (1996). Glomerular-specific imprinting of the mouse Gsα gene: how does this relate to hormone resistance in Albright hereditary osteodystrophy? *Genomics* 36:280–287.

Wilson L C, Oude Luttikhuis M E, Clayton P T, Fraser W D, Trembath R C (1994). Parental origin of Gs alpha gene mutations in Albright's hereditary osteodystrophy. *J Med Genet* 31:835–839.

Wolfsdorf J I, Rosenfield R L, Fang V S, Kobayashi R, Razdan A K, Kim M H (1978). Partial gonadotrophin-resistance in pseudohypoparathyroidism. *Acta Endocrinol* 88:321–328.

UNDERACTIVITY OF Gsα LEADING TO PHP 1A COMBINED WITH CONSTITUTIVELY ACTIVE LEYDIG CELL Gsα LEADING TO MALE PRECOCIOUS PUBERTY

The apparently paradoxical coexistence of these two disorders was found in two unrelated boys with the same single missense mutation of Gsα (Iiri et al., 1994).

Clinical and Imaging Features.   In combination, these features are those observed in male subjects with PHP 1a alone, or testotoxicosis alone (this chapter).

Genotyping and Gene Expression.   The Gsα missense mutation in both boys was Ala366 Ser. This is a temperature-sensitive mutation. *In vitro*, at 33°, the mutant Gsα releases GDP constitutively, in the absence of LH-activated receptor, resulting in autonomous testosterone production (Fig. 11–7). This situation mimics the one in the testes *in situ*. At 37°, the mutant Gsα protein is labile physically and functionally, hence the loss of parathormone action that is responsible for PHP 1a.

REFERENCE
Iiri T, Herzmark P, Nakamoto J, Van Dop C, Bourne H R (1994). Rapid GDP release from Gs alpha in patients with gain and loss of endocrine function. *Nature* 371:164–168.

SOMATIC Gsα-ACTIVATING MUTATIONS IN McCUNE-ALBRIGHT SYNDROME

McCune-Albright syndrome (MAS) is a sporadic disorder that comprises various foci of endocrine hyperfunction, a form of bone disease, and increased skin pigmentation.

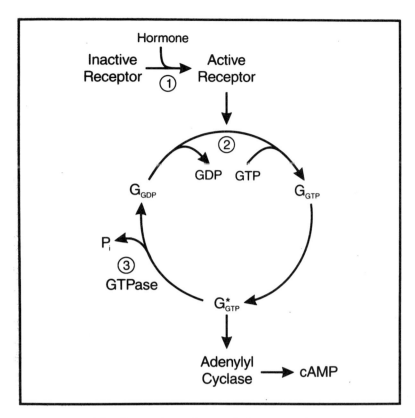

FIGURE 11–7. The G protein cycle coupled to an active receptor (top) and to an adenylyl cyclase: cAMP effector (bottom). The cycle can be driven by (1) hormone binding or constitutive activation of the receptor, (2) constitutive GDP:GTP exchange in the absence of activated receptor or (3) decreased GTPase activity. (Reproduced from Shenker A, *Growth Genet Horm* 12:34, 1996, with permission.)

Clinical and Imaging Features.   The main endocrine hyperfunction is that of the gonads, leading to precocious puberty due to increased synthesis of sex steroids by Leydig or granulosa cells; the bone lesion is polyostotic fibrous dysplasia; and the skin pigmentation takes the form of irregular café-au-lait spots. The skin and bone involvement are usually asymmetrical and may be ipsilateral. They may precede precocious puberty. Affected females have sexual precocity more often than affected males (Giovanelli et al., 1978) and vaginal bleeding often precedes premature thelarche or pubarche. Other glands that may function autonomously are the thyroid, the adrenal cortex, and the anterior pituitary, particularly its growth hormone–and prolactin-secreting cells (D'Armiento et al., 1983). Occasional manifestations of MAS include thymic hyperplasia, liver disease, and gastrointestinal polyps.

Genotyping and Gene Expression.   Somatic missense substitution of Arg201 by His or Cys has been identified in multiple tissues from multiple patients (Weinstein et al., 1991). These mutations are constitutively activating because they inhibit the GTPase activity of the Gsα subunit (Fig. 11–8). The reader will recall that activation of adenylyl cyclase is terminated by the GTPase activity that is intrinsic to Gsα. The heterogenous phenotype of MAS is most likely the result of different densities of

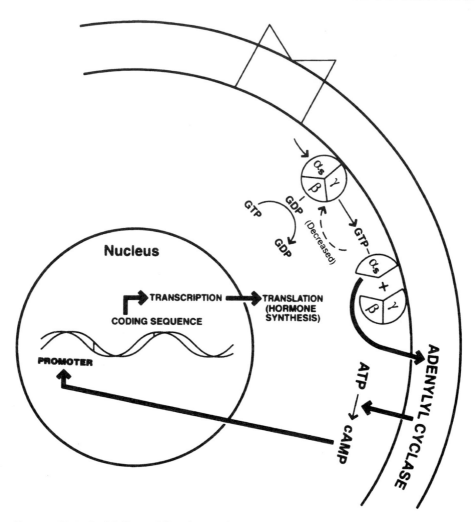

FIGURE 11–8. In McCune-Albright syndrome, Arg201His or Cys in Ga$_s$ reduces GTPase activity. This hyperactivates adenylylyl cylase, increases cAMP, and elevates sex steroid production. (Reproduced from DiMeglio L A, Pescovitz O H, *J Pediatr* 131: S8–12, 1997, with permission.)

mutant gene mosaicism in different tissues, and of different degrees of mutant gene expression in different tissues. For instance, peripheral blood leukocytes usually lack the mutant genes; probably, this reflects selection against those leukocyte precursor cells that carry the mutation mosaically.

Management.   Patients with this rare disorder will require elements of treatment shared with those who have only Albright's hereditary dystrophy, and other elements shared with those who have pure testotoxicosis.

Discussion.   It is remarkable that Arg201 is the precise amino acid residue in Gsα that, once ADP-ribosylated, inhibits GTPase activity; it is thereby responsible for the increased cAMP, culminating in the diarrhea produced by cholera toxin. Likewise, Arg201, or Gln227, is usually substituted in growth hormone–secreting adenomas of the anterior pituitary, whether these are isolated or part of the MAS (Dötsch et al., 1996). On the other hand, mutation of Gln227 has not occurred in MAS, presumably because it would yield a Gsα that is too active for normal cell survival.

The molecules that finally effect the clinical-pathologic consequences of mutant hyperactive Gsα proteins have just begun to be identified. Initial progress has revealed overexpression of the *c-fos* oncogene in fibrous dysplasia of the long bones of patients with MAS (Candeliere et al., 1995). The link between increased adenylate cyclase activity and increased c-fos expression in fibrous dysplasia of bone is as follows: increased cAMP promotes a series of phosphorylation steps, initiated by protein kinase A, and culminating in activation of a set of transcriptional regulatory proteins that bind to cAMP response elements in the promoter regions of selected target genes (Habener, 1990). One of these genes is human *c-fos* (Sassone-Corsi et al., 1988). Notably, about 4% of patients with MAS develop osteosarcoma (Yabut et al., 1988). Hyperexpression of *c-fos* may well be a contributing factor.

REFERENCES

Candeliere G A, Glorieux F H, Prud'homme J, St.-Arnaud R (1995). Increased expression of the *c-fos* proto-oncogene in bone from patients with fibrous dysplasia. *N Engl J Med* 332: 1546–1551.

D'Armiento M, Reda G, Camagna A, Rardella L (1983). McCune-Albright syndrome: evidence for autonomous multiendocrine hyperfunction. *J Pediatr* 102:584–586.

Dötsch J, Kiess W, Hänze J, Repp R, Lüdecke D, Blum W F, Rascher W (1996). G$_s$α mutation at codon 201 in pituitary adenoma causing gigantism in a 6-year-old boy with McCune-Albright syndrome. *J Clin Endocrinol Metab* 81:3839–3842.

Giovanelli G, Bernasconi S, Banchini G (1978). McCune-Albright syndrome in a male child: a clinical and endocrinologic enigma. *J Pediatr* 92:220–226.

Habener J F (1990). Cyclic AMP response element binding proteins: a cornucopia of transcription factors. *Mol Endocrinol* 4:1087–1094.

Sassone-Corsi P, Visvader J, Ferland L, Mellon P L, Verma I M (1988). Induction of proto-oncogene fos transcription through the adenylate cyclase pathway: characterization of a cAMP-responsive element. *Genes Dev* 2:1529–1538.

Weinstein L S, Shenker A, Gejman P V, Merino M J, Friedman E, Spiegel A M (1991). Activating mutations of the stimulatory G protein in the McCune-Albright syndrome. *N Engl J Med* 325:1688–1695.

Yabut S M Jr, Kenan S, Sissons H A, Lewis M M (1988). Malignant transformation of fibrous dysplasia: a case report and review of the literature. *Clin Orthop* 228:281–288.

Genetic Disorders of the Follicle-stimulating Hormone Receptor (FSHR)

HYPERGONADOTROPIC OVARIAN FAILURE AND VARIABLE IMPAIRMENT OF SPERMATOGENESIS DUE TO FSHR MUTATION THAT CAUSES RESISTANCE TO FSH

Clinical and Imaging Presentation (based on the Finnish mutation). In females, internal and external genital development is normal until puberty, when primary amenorrhea occurs and secondary sexual development is variably reduced. Ultrasound sometimes reveals streak ovaries akin to those in XO ovarian dysgenesis; however, in about half the patients it also reveals follicles of variable maturity. The reproductive phenotype in males has been delimited recently; expectedly, spermatogenesis may be impaired sufficiently to reduce fertility, but affected males do not have azoospermia (Tapanainen et al., 1997).

Laboratory Features. In affected females, the serum levels of FSH and LH are elevated because of impaired negative feedback in the hypothalamic-pituitary-gonad axis. On ovarian biopsy, nine of nine had primordial follicles, but only one had mature follicles. Four had primary follicles and two had preantral follicles (Aittomaki et al., 1996). Thus follicular maturation was qualitatively prepubertal, but follicles were few and fibrosis was substantial. Each of five affected men had elevated FSH, and low inhibin, levels, but the two with near-normal FSH levels also had normal LH levels and near-normal testicular volumes, and they were fertile.

Genotyping and Mutant Gene Expression. In Finland the condition is relatively frequent ($\sim 1/10^4$), and the mutant gene has been traced to a founder in an isolated subpopulation (Aittomäki, 1994). The Finnish mutation is a C-T transition at nucleotide 566 in exon 7 that yields Ala189Val in the extracellular (ligand-binding) domain (Fig. 11–9; Aittomäki et al., 1995). The patients are homozygous. The heterozygotes are normal. The mutation ablates a Bsml restriction site, facilitating mutation detection. When cultured Sertoli cells are transfected with a mutant FSHR plasmid, recombinant human FSH hardly stimulates cAMP production. With wild-type plasmid, the effect is three-to fourfold. The cells transfected with mutant plasmid had many fewer FSHRs than those transfected with the normal plasmid, but the mutant FSHR appeared to have the same affinity for FSH as normal FSHR. This proved the pathogenicity of the mutation but left its pathogenesis unclear.

Asn191Ile (Gromoll et al., 1996), near Ala189Val, and Phe591Ser in the sixth transmembrane helix (Kotlar et al., 1997) also inactivate the FSHR. Furthermore, FSHR with Ala189Val or Phe591Ser cause transfected cells to have several-fold reduced FSH binding without a change in its binding affinity (Kotlar et al., 1997).

Management. Genetic counseling is indicated to explain the risks of recurrence to relatives of various degrees of consanguinity, to indicate the availability of genetic testing (or screening), and to expose the option of ovum donation. Perhaps it will be possible to retrieve immature follicles and mature them *in vitro*.

Discussion. The FSHR gene contains 10 exons: the first nine encode the extracellular domain, the tenth encodes the transmembrane and intracellular domains. The hFSHR consists of 678 amino acids, and contains three or four glycosylation sites. Two of them are considered essential; and one must be glycosylated for FSH binding to occur (Davis et al., 1995). The mutation responsible for Finnish ovarian dysgenesis is in a region of the ligand-binding domain (LBD) that is highly conserved among its orthologous relatives in various mammals. Indeed, it is part of a 5-amino-acid sequence that is identical in the FSHR, LHR, and TSHR, and contains an "essential" N-linked glycosylation site. The identity of the sequence among all three receptors suggests that it may not contribute to ligand-binding affinity, notwithstanding its location in the LBD. Indeed, transfection studies indicate that the pri-

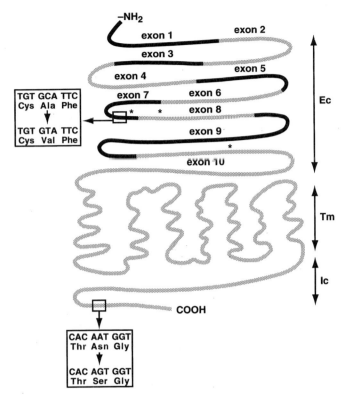

FIGURE 11–9. Ala 189Val in exon 7 reduces activity of the FSH receptor, prevents ovarian follicle maturation, and impairs spermatogenesis. Asn680Ser is a benign polymorphism. (Reproduced from Aittomäki K, et al., *Cell* 82:959–968, 1995, with permission.)

mary problem with the mutant Finnish receptor is a low B_{max}, attributable to decreased transcription/translation, increased turnover, or decreased movement of the receptor protein to the cell membrane, instead of a low affinity of the receptor for its ligand.

The initiation of follicular development is independent of FSH, but FSH is indispensable for maturation of follicles, and FSH deficiency is associated with accelerated follicular atresia. FSH binds to the FSHR on granulosa cells of immature follicles, and stimulates their growth as well as their production of estrogen. Estrogen, in turn, promotes follicular maturation, and eventually, ovulation.

FSH and testosterone contribute synergistically to the initiation and sustenance of spermatogenesis, partly by promoting Sertoli cell division and activity, but FSH is not indispensable for these purposes: testosterone, alone, can initiate (Bremner et al., 1981) and sustain substantive spermatogenesis (Zirkin et al., 1994; Kumar et al., 1997). Hence, it was predictable that homozygosity or compound heterozygosity for severe FSHR mutation may not always cause male infertility. This prediction has been confirmed by the recent report of Tapanainen and colleagues (1997) on men homozygous for the FSHR-resistance mutation.

The concept of a "resistant ovary syndrome" is nearly 30 years old (Jones and de Moraes-Ruehson, 1969). In fact, Kinch and colleagues (1965) alluded to it a few years earlier, when they distinguished between follicular and afollicular forms of premature (primary) ovarian failure. But relatively few additional patients have been described (Maxson and Wentz, 1983; Coulam, 1983), and their FSHR status has not been reported, except for one woman who appeared to develop antibodies against her FSHR (Scully, 1986). Indeed, autoimmune oophoritis, with or without other expressions of the polyglandular autoimmune syndrome, is important in the differential diagnosis of premature ovarian failure.

There have been several reports of familial 46,XX gonadal dysgenesis (see also Chapter 7); among these families, brothers of two affected females are described as having small testes, azoospermia, and normal testosterone but elevated FSH levels (Aleem, 1981; Purandare and Sathe, 1979; Youlton et al., 1982; Granat et al., 1983; Smith et al., 1979). The phenotypes of the individuals diagnosed as having familial XX ovarian dysgenesis (ODG) blend with those of patients labeled with a diagnosis of "premature ovarian failure" or "resistant ovary syndrome."

Transvaginal sonography has become a valuable diagnostic modality. Mehta and colleagues (1992) found follicles in seven of 17 patients younger than forty years of age who had hypergonadotropic ovarian failure. Aittomaki and colleagues (1996) systematically compared a group of 22 Finnish FSHR-mutant patients with a group of 30 Finnish ODG patients, only two of whom were sisters. The ODG patients were taller, their ovaries had follicles less often (by transvaginal sonography and biopsy), 30% had secondary amenorrhea, and their parental birthplaces differed from those of the FSHR-mutants.

It is important to rule out a dysfunctional mutant FSH (Chapter 10) as one cause of pseudoresistance to FSH. The frequency of FSHR resistance outside Finland, and the range of responsible FSHR mutations, both need systematic study.

REFERENCES

Aittomäki K (1994). The genetics of XX gonadal dysgenesis. *Am J Hum Genet* 54:844–851.

Aittomäki K, Lucena J L D, Pakarinen P, Sistonen P, Tapanainen J, Gromoll J, Kaskikari R, Sankila E M, Lehväslaiho H, Engel A R, Nieschlag E, Huhtaniemi I, de la Chapelle A (1995). Mutation in the follicle-stimulating hormone receptor gene causes hereditary hypergonadotropic ovarian failure. *Cell* 82:959–968.

Aittomäki K, Herva R, Stenman U H, Juntunen K, Ylöstalo P, Hovatta O, de la Chapelle A (1996). Clinical features of primary ovarian failure caused by a point mutation in the follicle-stimulating hormone receptor gene. *J Clin Endocrinol Metab* 81:3722–3726.

Aleem F A (1981). Familial 46,XX gonadal dysgenesis. *Fertil Steril* 35:317–320.

Bremner W R, Matsumoto A M, Sussman A M, Paulsen C A (1981) Follicle-stimulating hormone and human spermatogenesis. *J Clin Invest* 68:1044–1052.

Coulam C B (1983). The prevalence of autoimmune disorders among patients with primary ovarian failure. *Am J Reprod Immunol* 4:63–66.

Davis D, Liu X, Segaloff D L (1995). Identification of the sites of N-linked glycosylation on the follicle-stimulating hormone receptor and assessment of their role in FSH receptor function. *Mol Endocrinol* 9:159–170.

Granat M, Amar A, Mor-Yosef S, Brautbar C, Schenker J G (1983). Familial gonadal germinative failure: endocrine and human leukocyte antigen studies. *Fertil Steril* 40:215–219.

Gromoll J, Simmoni M, Nordhoff V, Behre H M, de Geyter C, Nieschlag E (1996). Functional and clinical consequences of mutations in the FSH receptor. *Mol Cell Endocrinol* 125:177–182.

Jones G S, de Moraes-Ruehsen M (1969). A new syndrome of amenorrhea in association with hypergonadotropism and apparently normal ovarian follicular apparatus. *Am J Obstet Gynecol* 104:597–600.

Kinch R A H, Plunkett E R, Smout M S, Carr D H (1965). Primary ovarian failure: a clinico-pathological and cytogenetic study. *Am J Obstet Gynecol* 91:630–644.

Kotlar T J, Young R H, Albanese C, Crowley W F Jr, Scully R E, Jameson J L (1997). A mutation in the follicle-stimulating hormone receptor occurs frequently in human ovarian sex cord tumors. *J Clin Endocrinol Metab* 82:1020–1026.

Kumar T R, Wang Y, Lu N, Matzuk M M (1997). Follicle stimulating hormone is required for ovarian follicle maturation but not for spermatogenesis. *Nat Genet* 15:201–204.

Maxson W S, Wentz A C (1983). The gonadotropin resistant ovary syndrome. *Semin Reprod Endocrinol* 1:147–160.

Metha A E, Matwijiw I, Lyons E A, Faiman C (1992). Noninvasive diagnosis of resistant ovary syndrome by ultrasonography. *Fertil Steril* 57:56–64.

Purandare V N, Sathe A (1979). Gonadal dysgenesis variants in sisters: a hitherto undescribed combination. *Int J Gynecol Obstet* 16:416–418.

Scully R E, Mark E J, McNeely B U (1986). Case records of the Massachusetts General Hospital. *N Engl J Med* 21:1336–1343.

Smith A, Fraser I S, Noel M (1979). Three siblings with premature gonadal failure. *Fertil Steril* 32:528–530.

Tapanainen J S, Aittomäki K, Min J, Vaskivuo T, Huhtaniemi I T (1997). Men homozygous for an inactivating mutation of the follicle-stimulating hormone (FSH) receptor gene present variable suppression of spermatogenesis and fertility. *Nat Genet* 15:205–206.

Youlton R, Michelsen H, Be C, Cruz-Coke R (1982). Pure XX gonadal dysgenesis in identical twins. *Clin Genet* 21:262–265.

Zirkin B R, Awonyi C, Griswold M D, Russell L D, Sharpe R M (1994). Is FSH required for adult spermatogenesis? *J Androl* 15:273–276.

SUSTAINED SPERMATOGENESIS DUE TO FSHR MUTATION THAT ACTIVATES THE RECEPTOR IN THE ABSENCE OF FSH

Clinical and Laboratory Presentation. A 20-year-old man required hypophysectomy for a pituitary tumor (Gromoll et al., 1996). Postoperatively, his serum gonadotropins were unmeasurable, even after GnRH stimulation. His sperm concentration and morphology remained substantially normal, even after testosterone replacement therapy was discontinued, and other signs of androgen deficiency became overt.

Genotyping and Gene Expression. An activating mutation in *FSHR* that induced autonomous (ligand-free) function of the FSHR was postulated to explain persistent spermatogenesis in the absence of FSH, and with severely deficient testosterone concentration. Genomic DNA was amplified with primer sequences for the *FSHR*, an aberrant fragment of exon 10 was detected by single strand conformation polymorphism (SSCP), and sequencing revealed an A → G transition at nt 1700 causing an Asp → Gly substitution in codon 567 of the third intracytoplasmic loop. When an expression plasmid containing a cDNA bearing the recreated mutation was transiently transfected into COS-7 cells, there was a 50% increase in constitutive (ligand-free) cAMP production. Furthermore, the normal and mutant FSHR reacted similarly to increasing doses of cAMP. These observations fortified the hypothesis of a gain-of-function mutation wherein the degree of gain is sufficient to be expressed heterozygously.

Management.   Despite the observation that this patient had near-normal sperm production when he was severely deficient in testosterone, and fully depleted of FSH, he did not demonstrate fertility until his testosterone replacement was resumed. This may simply reflect return of libido and augmented frequency of intercourse, or it may reflect unidentified androgenic determinants of male reproduction beyond the usual parameters of sperm and/or semen production.

Discussion.   As has become recognized universally, experiments of nature, such as the one provided by the need to remove this unique patient's tumorous pituitary gland, have proven very informative and/or raised important questions. First, the patient never received sufficiently high doses of testosterone to raise his intratesticular testosterone concentration to a physiologic level. It is apparent, therefore, that testosterone normally has a permissive (perhaps, synergistic) role in cooperating with FSH to promote spermatogenesis. Second, it would appear that a relatively low increment of functional constitutivity enables a mutant FSHR to contribute sufficiently to maintain spermatogenesis. Third, no male relatives of the index patient could be studied, and in a preliminary study, none of 13 patients with idiopathic macroorchidism had this activating mutation. Therefore, a phenotype of FSHR constitutivity may not exist in otherwise normal males, or females (the patient's mother and his only sister had normal reproductive histories). On the other hand, infertile males who seem to respond to LH or hCG therapy alone (Vicari et al., 1992) should be screened for FSHR constitutivity.

Certainly, the most interesting and constructive lesson of the unique patient discussed in this section is that his mutation, Asp567Gly, is precisely the same substitution that occurs germinally at homologous residue 564 of the LHR, and both somatically and germinally at homologous residue 619 of the TSHR (Fig. 11–10): the first leads to constitutional precocious male puberty (see this chapter), the second to acquired hyperfunctional thyroid adenomas (Parma et al., 1993) or diffuse

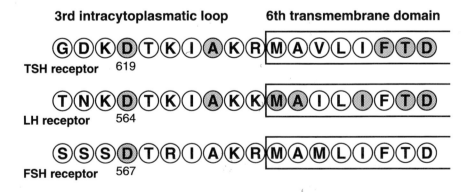

FIGURE 11–10. Asp567Gly at the junction between the third cytoplasmic loop and the sixth α-helix causes constitutive activation of the FSH receptor. Notice that substitution of the parologous Asp residue in the LH or TSH receptor is also activating. A variety of other amino acids that activate the LH receptor or the TSH receptor are identified by shaded circles. (Reproduced from Gromoll J, et al., *J Clin Endocrinol Metab* 81:1367–1370, 1996, with permission.)

thyroid hyperplasia, respectively (Duprez et al., 1994). Indeed, this mutation occurs in a region at the boundary of the third intracellular loop and the sixth transmembrane helix that is strongly conserved among the three glycoprotein hormone receptors.

REFERENCES

Duprez L, Parma J, Van Sande J, Allgeier A, Leclere J, Schwartz C, Delisle M J, Decoulx M, Oriazzi J, Dumont J. Vassart G (1994). Germline mutations in the thyrotropin receptor gene cause non-autoimmune autosomal dominant hyperthyroidism. *Nat Genet* 7:396–401.

Gromoll J, Simoni M, Nieschlag E (1996). An activating mutation of the follicle-stimulating hormone receptor autonomously sustains spermatogenesis in a hypophysectomized man. *J Clin Endocrinol Metab* 81:1367–1370.

Parma J, Duprez L, Van Sande J, Cochaux P, Gervy C, Mockel J, Dumont J, Vassart G. (1993). Somatic mutations in the thyrotropin receptor gene cause hyperfunctioning thyroid adenomas. *Nature* 365:649–651.

Vicari E, Mongioi A, Calogero A E, Moncada M L, Sidoti G, Polosa P, D'Agata R (1992). Therapy with human chorionic gonadotropin alone induces spermatogenesis in men with isolated hypogonadotrophic hypogonadism—long term follow-up study. *Int J Androl* 15: 320–329.

12

Genetic Disorders Expressed as Gonadotropin Excess

Gonadotropin excess may reflect (1) a response to excessive (perhaps premature) stimulation of the pituitary gonadotropes by GnRH, (2) autonomous over-production of LH, FSH, or both, by pituitary gonadotropes or, ectopically, as a paraendocrine expression of neoplasia, and (3) deficient production, or action, of inhibin or follistatin.

The most frequent clinical presentation of true gonadotropin excess is sporadic, idiopathic, central precocious isosexual puberty due to premature activation of pulsatility in the GnRH-gonadotrope-gonadal steroid axis. The female to male ratio is 4–8:1. A few families have been described in which like-sex or unlike-sex siblings have been affected with isosexual precocity. These cases are summarized immediately below. The most common cause of familial precocious puberty is a peripheral form in males due to constitutive activation of the LH receptor. It is described in Chapter 11.

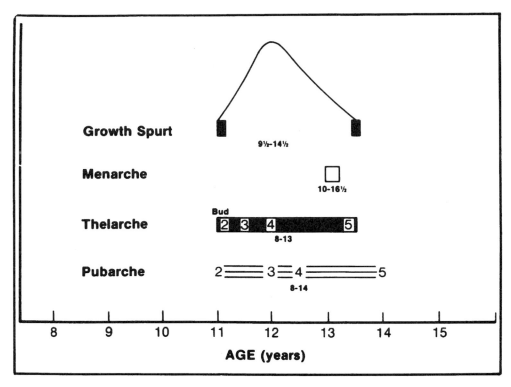

FIGURE 12–1. Chronology of somatic events during female puberty. (Reproduced from Spence, based on data from Marshall and Tanner, 1969, *Ann Roy Coll Phys Surg Can* 19:21–27, 1986, with permission.)

Familial Non-syndromal Sexual Precosity

FAMILIAL CENTRAL ISOSEXUAL PRECOCITY IN GIRLS

Clinical and Imaging Features.   The pair of sisters described by Rangasami and Grant (1992) started puberty with breast development (thelarche) at 4 and 5.3 years, respectively (Fig. 12–1). At 6.9 years, the first, 134 cm, had stage 3 breasts (Fig. 12–2), stage 2 pubic hair (Fig. 12–3), vaginal secretion, a bone age of 8 years, an adult-size uterus, and multicystic ovaries, 6 mL each. At 5.4 years, the second, 118 cm, had stage 2 breasts, stage 1 pubic hair, a small uterus, and prepubertal ovaries in size and follicular development. By 6 years, she had grown rapidly and puberty had progressed one more stage.

Laboratory Features.   Both sisters had brisk LH and FSH responses to a GnRH challenge test.

Management.   Both sisters responded well to long-acting GnRH agonist-analogues.

Discussion.   Rangasami and Grant (1992; references therein) refer to five previous case reports of familial central precocity in sisters. They wonder whether this ap-

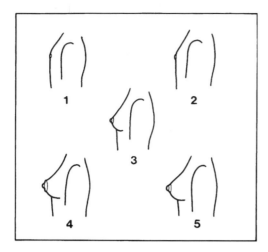

FIGURE 12–2. The stages of breast development (thelarche). Aside from size, stage 4 is distinctive in that the areola and papilla (nipple) form a secondary mound on the underlying breast. (Reproduced from Spence, based on data from Marshall and Tanner, 1969, *Ann Roy Coll Phys Surg Can* 19:21–27, 1986, with permission.)

parent rarity is due to underreporting, and they question whether familial "early" (but not formally precocious) female puberty may not form a continuum with true precocious puberty. Indeed, Rohn and Rousonelos (1986) found that 3 of 58 girls had positive family histories; in two of them, a mother, or a mother and maternal grandmother, had "early" but not formally "precocious" puberty.

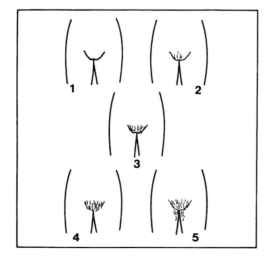

FIGURE 12–3. The stages of pubic hair development (pubarche). In stage 3, the hair is distributed triangularly but is still sparse. In stage 4, full density is achieved. In stage 5, there is extension of hair growth to upper inner thigh. (Reproduced from Spence, based on data from Marshall and Tanner, 1969, *Ann Roy Coll Phys Surg Can* 19:21–27, 1986, with permission.)

REFERENCES

Rangasami J J, Grant D B (1992). Familial precocious puberty in girls. *J R Soc Med* 85:499–500.

Rohn R, Rousonelos G (1986). Familial precocious puberty. *Am J Dis Child* 140:741–742.

FAMILIAL CENTRAL ISOSEXUAL PRECOCITY IN BOYS AND GIRLS

Clinical and Imaging Features. This condition can occur in two clinical contexts: primary or secondary. The most recent report of the primary form is a family described by Samuel and colleagues (1995) that had affected males and females in four generations, and contained one male-to-male transmission. The propositus was a male whose puberty began at 8.3 years when he was 137 cm tall. Ten months later, testis volumes were 8mL, pubic hair was stage 2, penile growth was prominent, and a growth spurt had occurred. His sister had breast development and a growth spurt at 8 years. Their father (33 years, 152 cm) started his puberty at 8 years; by 10 years he had mature male external genitalia. His precocious puberty caused school problems. Two paternal aunts had thelarche at 5 years and menarche at 8 years. The heights of the aunts were 145 cm and 138 cm. The paternal grandmother had thelarche at 8 years and menarche at 10.5 years. By history, a granduncle and a great grandmother of the father may also have been affected. Samuel and colleagues (1995; references therein) refer to only four previous examples of familial isosexual precocity in boys and girls.

In the family of Ruvalcaba (1985) a father and two daughters were affected. One daughter had breast buds and a growth spurt at 5.5 years, pubic hair at 6 years and axillary hair and menarche at 7.5 years when her height age and bone age were 11 and 11.5 years, respectively. Her sister had a similar course. Their father had pubic hair and large genitalia in kindergarten, shaved at 9 years, and reached adult height at 10 years.

In the family of Frasier and Brenner (1982), one girl and two brothers were affected, and their mother may have been affected partially; her menarche was at 9.5 to 10 years.

The family of Hopwood and colleagues (1981) involved a brother-sister pair and their father. Interestingly, all three achieved average adult heights.

Ferrier and colleagues (1961) apparently were the first to report a brother-sister pair.

Laboratory Features. The male propositus in the family of Samuel and colleagues (1995) had a brisk LH response but a feeble FSH response to GnRH stimulation. His sister had a brisk response of both LH and FSH. The same was true of the sister in the family of Hopwood and colleagues (1981).

Management. Affected boys and girls will respond to long-acting GnRH agonist-analogue therapy. This apparently paradoxical therapy works by down-regulating the GnRH receptor on pituitary gonadotropes.

Discussion. It has become well appreciated that familial central isosexual precocity, in girls mostly, but in boys as well, can develop *secondary to primary peripheral hyperandrogenic states.* The best known examples of this phenomenon are classic congenital adrenal hyperplasia (Pescovitz et al., 1984) and non-classic (late-onset)

21-hydroxylase deficiency (Kalter-Leibovici et al., 1989). A similar change from peripheral (gonadotropin-independent) to central (gonadotropin-dependent) sexual precocity has been observed in boys with LHR constitutivity (Laue et al., 1989). The conversion from peripheral to central precocity has also been observed in McCune-Albright syndrome (Chapter 11), and in children with androgenic tumors. The mechanism of the conversion is unclear; however, it is relevant to point out the polar phenomenon: delayed menarche is typical of females homozygous for 5α-reductase deficiency (Chapter 13), and it occurs in approximately 15% of those heterozygous for X-linked complete androgen insensitivity (Chapter 14).

To date, molecular-genetic analysis of the familial central forms of isosexual precocity has not been reported. Presumably, *cis*-regulatory elements of the GnRH gene, or the intrinsic and extrinsic factors that interact positively with these elements, perhaps indirectly, may be at fault. Alternative mechanisms would include constitutive activity of the GnRH receptor, and other forms of LH/FSH dysregulation.

REFERENCES

Ferrier P, Shepard T H, Knapp Smith E (1961). Growth disturbances and values for hormone excretion in various forms of precocious sexual development. *Pediatrics* 28:258–275.

Frasier S D, Brenner P F (1982). Familial complete precocious puberty affecting both sexes. *Am J Dis Child* 136:560–561.

Hopwood N J, Kelch R P, Helder L J (1981). Familial precocious puberty in a brother and sister. *Am J Dis Child* 135:78–79.

Kalter-Leibovici D, Dickerman Z, Zamir R, Weiss L, Kaufman H, Laron Z (1989). Late onset 21-hydroxylase deficiency in a girl mimicking true sexual precocity. *J Pediatr Endocrinol* 3:121–124.

Laue L, Kenigsberg D, Pescovitz O H, Hench K D, Barnes K M, Loriaux D L, Cutler G B Jr (1989). Treatment of familial male precocious puberty with spironolactone and testolactone. *N Engl J Med* 320:496–502.

Pescovitz O H, Comite F, Cassorla F, Dwyer A J, Poth M A, Sperling M A, Hench K, McNemar A, Skerda M, Loriaux D L, et al. (1984). True precocious puberty complicating congenital adrenal hyperplasia: treatment with a luteinizing hormone-releasing hormone analog. *J Clin Endocrinol Metab* 58:857–861.

Ruvalcaba R H A (1995). Familial sexual precocity. *Am. J. Dis. Child.* 140:741–742.

Samuel T J, Grant D B, Woodd-Walker R B (1995). An unusual family with precocious puberty. *B J Hosp Med* 54:48–49.

FAMILIAL ISOSEXUAL PRECOCITY IN A BOY AND HETEROSEXUAL PRECOCITY IN A GIRL ASSOCIATED WITH LH EXCESS

Clinical and Imaging Features (based on the sibling pair reported by Rosenfield et al., 1980).   The boy had a large penis at birth; pubic hair and macroorchidism were present at 1.5 years. At 5 years, his height was 124 cm, bone age was 10 years, pubic hair was stage 3 and penis was 8 cm. He did not have axillary hair or acne. The sister had pubic hair at 3 months. At 4 years, she was 110 cm tall, had stage 3 pubic hair and clitoral hypertrophy, no axillary hair or acne. The vaginal mucosa and uterus were prepubertal.

Laboratory Features.   The boy, at 5 years, had an LH level in the adult range, his FSH was well below it, and his T level was three-fold higher than the upper-normal level of prepubertal males. At 4 years, girl had an LH level in the adult female range, her FSH was below it, but her testosterone was well above the adult female range, and her estradiol was just at the lower-normal adult level. Both children had a brisk pubertal-type response of serum LH to GnRH challenge.

Discussion. The disparate premature secretion of LH but not of FSH in these two siblings raises the issue of the extent and manner in which LH and FSH secretion are controlled by GnRH itself, by the factors, in turn, that control GnRH positively or negatively, and by the possibility that LH and FSH are subject to separate inhibitory controls. The failure of high-dose estrogen to suppress the elevated LH levels in the children described by Rosenfield and colleagues (1980) supports the last idea. The clinical fate of these children is unknown but it is noteworthy that targetted overexpression of LH in female mice causes polycystic ovaries, infertility, and ovarian tumors (Risma et al. 1995). In contrast, it is remarkable that precocious puberty mediated by the LH receptor (hCG-producing tumors, LH receptor constitutivity) has no clinical effect on girls. This disparity awaits explanation.

REFERENCES

Risma K A, Clay C M, Nett T M, Wagner T, Yun J, Nilson J H. Targeted overexpression of luteining hormone in trnasgenic mice leads to infertility, polycystic ovaries, and ovarian tumors. *Proc Natl Acad Sci USA* 92:1322–1326. 1995.

Rosenfeld, R G, Reitz R E, King A B, Hintz R L (1980). Familial precocious puberty associated with isolated elevation of luteinizing hormone. *N Engl J Med* 303:859–862.

Precocious Puberty Associated with Various Genetic Syndromes or Birth Defects

PRIMARY HYPOTHYROIDISM

Clinical and Imaging Features. Primary hypothyroidism, whether or not of autoimmune origin, may be inherited. The literature has recognized the rare coexistence of so-called sexual precocity with various forms of primary hypothyroidism in children since Kendle (1905). Affected girls may develop breasts, galactorrhea, vaginal secretion, ovarian enlargement (occasionally massive) and menses, but premature pubarche is infrequent. In boys, the testes enlarge, usually without penile enlargement or other signs of virilization. Bone age and growth velocity are not usually increased (Castro-Magana et al., 1988; Anasti et al., 1995; Bruder et al., 1995).

Laboratory Features. In addition to elevated TSH levels, FSH, prolactin and α-subunit levels are all increased. However, LH and testosterone are not. Furthermore GnRH stimulation does not provoke a pubertal LH or FSH response. These facts indicate that the pathogenesis of the various expressions of premature puberty is GnRH-independent.

Management. Thyroxin replacement is necessary, but it also accelerates skeletal maturation and the risk of ultimate short stature. The addition of GnRH analogue to the treatment program delays gonadarche, prolongs the period of skeletal maturation, and increases ultimate stature.

Discussion. Several explanations have been proferred for this "asymmetrical" form of sexual pseudoprecocity in children of both sexes. First, feedback disinhibition on the hypothalamus results in increased TRH. This may stimulate gonadotropes to secrete FSH as well as TSH (Bruder et al., 1995). Second, the elevated TSH may promiscuously activate the FSH receptor (Anasti et al., 1995). Third, the hypothyroid gonad may have increased sensitivity to FSH stimulation (Jannini et al., 1995). Others have incriminated the elevated levels of prolactin (Slonim et al., 1982; Bruder et al., 1995). It is interesting that sexual precocity has been recorded in a child who developed hypothyroidism after treatment of her hyperthyroidism with propylthiouracil (Sadeghi-Nejad and Senior, 1971).

REFERENCES

Anasti J N, Flack M R, Froehlich J, Nelson L M, Nisula B C (1995). A potential novel mechanism for precocious puberty in juvenile hypothroidism. *J Clin Endocrinol Metab* 80:276–279.

Bruder J M, Samuels M H, Bremner W J, Ridgway E C, Wierman M E (1995). Hypothyroidism-induced macroorchidism: use of a gonadotropin-releasing hormone agonist to understand its mechanism and augment adult stature. *J Clin Endocrinol Metab* 80:11–16.

Castro-Magana M, Angulo M, Canas A, Sharp A, Fuentes B (1988). Hypothalamic-pituitary gonadal axis in boys with primary hypothroidism and macroorchidism. *J Pediatr* 112:397–402.

Jannini E A, Ulisse S, D'Armiento M (1995). Macroorchidism in juvenile hypothyroidism. *J Clin Endocrinol Metab* 80:2543–2544.

Kendle V W (1905). Case of precocious puberty in a female cretin. *Br Med J* 1:246.

Sadeghi-Nejad A, Senior B (1971). Sexual precocity: an unusual complication of propylthiouracil therapy. *J Pediatr* 79:833–837.

Slonim A E, Glick A D, Island D P, Kasselberg A G (1982). Hyperprolactinemia associated with advanced puberty in a male. *J Pediatr* 101:236–239.

NEUROFIBROMATOSIS, TYPE 1 (NF-1)

This is a good example of a genetic disorder that may be complicated by central sexual precocity in boys and girls (Riccardi et al., 1992). Habiby and colleagues (1995) recorded precocious puberty in 7 of 219 children with NF-1. All seven had optic pathway tumors involving the optic chiasm. On the other hand, 39% of NF-1 children with optic chiasm tumors had precocious puberty. This may be an underestimate because some subjects were still very young. Three quarters of the tumors were discovered in asymptomatic children by neuroimaging screening. In fact, screening by periodic LH assay, with or without GnRH challenge, and recognition of an early growth spurt may be equally effective.

REFERENCE

Habiby R, Silverman B, Listernick R, Charrow J (1995). Precocious puberty in children with neurofibromatosis type 1. *J Pediatr* 126:364–367.

Riccardi V M (1992). Type 1 neurofibromatosis and the pediatric patient. *Curr Probl Pediatr* 22:66–106.

HYPOTHALAMIC HAMARTOMAS

Hypothalamic hamartomas are a well-recognized cause of precocious puberty. The hamartomas produce GnRH autonomously and release it into portal-like blood vessels that communicate with the anterior pituitary gonadotropes (Judge et al., 1977). Hypothalamic hamartoblastoma is a major component of the Pallister-Hall syndrome (Chapter 15). Usually, this hypothalamic lesion is associated with hypopituitarism. A boy with precocious puberty as part of the *Pallister-Hall syndrome* has been reported by Topf and colleagues (1993). At 9 years, after a 1-year history of sexual precocity, he had stage 3 pubic hair and genitalia, and his bone age was 13.7 years. His father had polydactyly and a hypothalamic mass suggesting autosomal dominant transmission with variable expressivity.

REFERENCE

Topf K F, Kletter G B, Kelch R P, Brunberg J A, Biesecker L G (1993). Autosomal dominant transmission of the Pallister-Hall syndrome. *J Pediatr* 123:943–946.

KABUKI MAKEUP SYNDROME

This syndrome is composed of abnormal facies, mental retardation, postnatal growth failure, and skeletal anomalies. It occurs sporadically and affects boys more frequently than girls. Precocious puberty (vaginal mucosa changes, breast development) with increased basal and GnRH-stimulated gonadotropin secretion has been observed in affected infant girls (Kuroki et al., 1987). The frequency of precocious puberty in the syndrome is unknown.

REFERENCE

Kuroki Y, Katsumata N, Eguchi T, Fukushima Y, Suwa S, Kajii T (1987). Precocious puberty in Kabuki makeup syndrome. *J Pediatr* 110:750–752.

SEPTO-OPTIC DYSPLASIA

This refers to the association of optic nerve dysplasia with absence of the septum pellucidum and corpus callosum (see Chapter 15). Girls are affected more frequently than boys, and the affecteds are often the firstborn of young mothers. Abnormalities of the anterior hypothalamus, and multiple pituitary hormone deficiencies are common. In this setting, one does not expect sexual precocity; yet one of five girls reported by Huseman and colleagues (1978) did have it, and another had premature puberty as indicated by her hyperresponse to GnRH challenge.

REFERENCE

Huseman C A, Kelch R P, Hopwood N J, Zipf W B (1978). Sexual precocity in association with septo-optic dysplasia and hypothalamic hypopituitarism. *J Pediatr* 92:748–753.

COHEN SYNDROME

This is an autosomal recessive disorder of obesity, characteristic facies, narrow hands and feet, and mental retardation (Carey and Hall, 1978). A pair of identical female twins who had the appropriate facies, obesity, mental retardation, and retinal degeneration qualified for the appellation (North et al., 1995). Both twins had central precocious puberty. Apparently, this is the first report of such an occurrence; hence, it may be purely coincidental.

REFERENCES

Becker-Christensen F, Lund H T (1974). A family with Möbius syndrome. *J Pediatr* 84:115–117.

Pescovitz O H, Hench K D, Barnes K M, Loriaux D L, Cutler G B (1988). Premature thelarche and central precocious puberty: the relationship between clinical presentation and the gonadotropin response to luteinizing hormone-releasing hormone. *J Clin Endocrinol Metab* 67:474–479.

MÖBIUS SYNDROME

This is an etiologically heterogenous syndrome of facial nerve palsy, usually with other cranial nerve involvement, and facial and limb abnormalities. It may occur in families (Becker-Christensen and Lund, 1974). Hypogonadotropic hypogonadism has been reported in several cases. An affected infant with premature thelarche was reported by Ichiyama et al., 1995). She had a FSH-predominant response to GnRH stimulation, a pattern recognized by Pescovitz and colleagues (1988). It is probable that the vascular disruption(s) considered to be the basis of Möbius syndrome can sometimes result in hyperactivity of the hypothalamic-pituitary-gonadotrope axis.

REFERENCES

Carey J C, Hall B D (1978). Confirmation of Cohen syndrome. *J Pediatr* 93:239–244.

Ichiyama T, Handa S, Hayashi T, Furukawa S (1995). Premature thelarche in Möbius syndrome. *Clin Genet* 47:108–109.

Pescovitz O H, Hench K D, Barnes K M, Loriaux D L, Cutler G B (1988). Premature thelarche and central precocious puberty: the relationship between clinical presentation and the gonadotropin response to luteinizing hormone-releasing hormone. *J Clin Endocrinol Metab* 67:474–479.

FRAGILE X SYNDROME

Isosexual precocious puberty of the GnRH-dependent type has been reported in three females with the fragile X syndrome (Kowalczyk et al., 1996; Moore et al., 1990; Butler and Najjar, 1988). Only the latter subject had molecular-genetic diagnosis of 750 CGG repeats. CT and ultrasound examination of her pelvis revealed prominent cystic ovaries bilaterally. Interestingly, cystic ovarian enlargement in fragile X syndrome has been recorded previously (Turner et al., 1986). The macroorchidism of fragile X males is GnRH-independent; therefore, it is pathogenetically unrelated. It remains to be determined whether true precocious puberty in fragile X females is more common than expected by chance alone.

REFERENCES

Butler M G, Najjar J L (1988). Do some patients with fragile X syndrome have precocious puberty? *Am J Med Genet* 31:779–781.

Kowalczyk C L, Schroeder E, Pratt V, Conard J, Wright K, Feldman G L (1996). As association between precocious puberty and fragile X syndrome? *J Pediatr Adolesc Gynecol* 9:199–202.

Moore P S, Chudley A E, Winter J S (1990). True precocious puberty in a girl with the fragile X syndrome. *Am J Med Genet* 37:265–267.

North K N, Fulton A B, Whiteman D A H (1995). Identical twins with Cohen syndrome. *Am J Med Genet* 58:54–58.

Turner G, Opitz J M, Brown W T, et al. (1986) Conference report: Second International Workshop on the fragile X and X-linked mental retardation. *Am J Med Genet* 23:11–67.

TUBEROUS SCLEROSIS

This is a genetically heterogeneous, autosomal dominant disorder featuring a classic clinical triad of seizures, adenoma sebaceum, and mental retardation. Many patients have hypopigmented macules or Shagreen patches, and others have normal intelligence. Among their brain lesions are harmatomas called tubers. Isosexual precocity occurs rarely in tuberous sclerosis (Cummings et al., 1978); it is tacitly considered to originate centrally, in view of the variety of brain lesions that can occur in TS. However, Root and colleagues (1986) reported a boy with gonadotropin-independent isosexual precocity. At 4.2 years he had a 1-year history of penile enlargement, and a history of pubic hair development of several weeks. His height was above the 97th percentile and his height age was 5.2 years. He had a characteristic rash over his nose and cheeks, a macular hypopigmented patch on one thigh, and classic signs on computed tomography of the head. His basal LH and FSH levels were low, and they responded poorly to GnRH stimulation, yet his testosterone levels were in the pubertal range, and they responded briskly to hCG stimulation. The patient's precocious puberty responded poorly to spironolactone, but well to ketoconazole, an inhibitor of both 17α-hydroxylase and 17, 20-desmolase activities in the pathway of androgen biosynthesis.

REFERENCES

Chaussain J-L, Lemerle J, Roger M, Canlorbe P, Job J-C (1980). Klinefelter syndrome, tumor, and sexual precocity. *J Pediatr* 97:607–609.
Kahn A, Rappaport R (1982). Endocrine aspects and tumoral markers in intracranial germinoma: an attempt to delineate the diagnostic procedure in 14 patients. *J Pediatr* 101:374–378.

KLINEFELTER SYNDROME

This syndrome (Chapter 6) has been repeatedly associated with sexual precocity due to mediastinal teratoma (thoracic polyembryoma) (Job and Chaussain, 1978) and, rarely, with intracranial seminoma in the floor of the third ventricle (Chaussain et al., 1980). The mediastinal tumors secrete chorionic gonadotropin (CG) or a CG-like molecule that stimulates Leydig cell production of testosterone. The intracranial lesion presumably causes a central form of precocious puberty. The relatively small size of the testes in these particular patients with sexual precocity is a strong clue to their underlying Klinefelter syndrome. Indeed, the male patient with an hCG-secreting intracranial germinoma and sexual precocity mentioned by Pomarede and colleagues (1982) also had small testes, suggesting the diagnosis of Klinefelter syndrome (KS).

It is important to appreciate that germ cell tumors can be responsible for precocious puberty even in patients who have mosaic KS (Derenoncourt et al., 1995; Leschek et al., 1996). Moreover, the germ cell tumor may secrete excessive CG even when it is too small to be visible by modern imaging procedures (von Mühlendahl et al., 1994; Leschek et al., 1996). In these cases, multisite venous sampling is necessary to localize the CG-secreting cells. Obviously, karyotype analysis shouold be performed on all males with LHRH-independent precocious puberty.

REFERENCES

Cummings J L, Oppenheimer E Y, Hochman H I (1978). Tuberous sclerosis. *Am J Dis Child* 132:1215.

Derenoncourt A N, Castro-Magana M, Jones K L (1995). Mediastinal teratoma and precocious puberty in a boy with mosaic Klinefelter syndrome. *Am J Med Genet* 55:38–42.

Job J C, Chaussain J L (1978). Sexual precocity due to thoracic polyembryoma. *J Pediatr* 93: 895.

Pomarede R, Czernichow P, Finidori J, Pfister A, Roger M, Kalifa C, Zucker J M, Pierre-Kahn A, Rappaport R (1982). Endocrine aspects and tumoral markers in intracranial germinoma: an attempt to delineate the diagnostic procedure in 14 patients. *J Pediatr* 101:374–378.

Root A W, Zamanillo J, Duckett G, Sweetland M (1986). Gonadotropin-independent isosexual precocity in a boy with tuberous sclerosis: effect of ketoconazole. *J Pediatr* 109:1012–1015.

von Mühlendahl K E, Heinrich U (1994). Sexual precocity in Klinefelter syndrome: report on two new cases with idiopathic central precocious puberty. *Eur J Pediat* 153:322–324.

THE PEUTZ-JEGHERS SYNDROME

The Peutz-Jeghers syndrome (Chapter 13) of oral melanosis and GI polyposis is well known to be associated with feminizing tumors of the testis or ovary (Solh et al., 1983) that cause isosexual precocity in females and heterosexual precocity in males.

REFERENCE

Solh H M, Azoury R S, Najjar S S (1983). Peutz-Jeghers syndrome associated with precocious puberty. *J Pediatr* 103:593–593.

THE CARNEY COMPLEX

This is an autosomal dominant multisystem tumor syndrome composed of mesenchymal, endocrine, and peripheral nerve tumors with pigmented skin lesions (Carney et al., 1986). Sexual precocity in boys (Carney et al., 1985) arises from three types of testicular tumors: Sertoli cell, Leydig cell, or adrenocortical rest.

REFERENCES

Carney J A, Gordon H, Carpenter P C, Shenoy B V, Go V L (1985). The complex of myxomas, spotty pigmentation and endocrine overactivity. *Medicine* 64:270–283.

Carney J A, Hruska L S, Beauchamp G D, Gordon H (1986). Dominant inheritance of the complex of myxomas, spotty pigmentation, and endocrine overactivity. *Mayo Clin Proc* 61:165–172.

GLUCOCORTICOID RESISTANCE

This is a rare autosomal recessive disorder caused by mutation of the glucocorticoid receptor gene (Malchoff et al., 1993). It is characterized by excessive serum cortisol without clinical expression of cortisol excess. ACTH production is increased because of impaired negative feedback of the hypothalamic-pituitary axis by glucocorticoid.

The adrenal glands respond to increased ACTH by overproducing androgen, as well as gluco-and mineralocorticoid. In a male, the excess androgen can cause precocious isosexual puberty (Malchoff et al., 1994).

REFERENCES

Malchoff D M, Brufsky A, Reardon G, McDermott P, Javier E C, Bergh C H, Rowe D, Malchoff C D (1993). A point mutation of the human glucocorticoid receptor in primary cortisol resistance. *J Clin Invest* 91:1918–1925.

Malchoff C D, Reardon G, Javier E C, Rogol A D, McDermott P, Loriaux D L, Malchoff D M (1994) Dexamethasone therapy for isosexual precocious pseudodopuberty caused by generalized glucocorticoid resistance. *J Clin Endocrinol Metab* 79:1632–1636.

13

Genetic Disorders of Steroidogenesis

Steroid hormones are made or transformed in the gonads, the adrenal cortex, and in various "peripheral" organs (skin, fat, brain, placenta). Sex steroid hormones include androgens, estrogens, and progestins. The progestins can be considered intermediates in the biosynthetic pathways leading to the other steroid hormones. Specifically, in the gonads and the post-pubertal adrenal cortex, the 17,20-lyase activity of P450c17 preferentially transforms 17OH-pregnenolone to dehydro-epiandrosterone (DHEA), and DHEA is converted to androstendione by the enzyme known as 3β-hydroxysteroid dehydrogenase/$\Delta^5 \rightarrow \Delta^4$-ene isomerase (Fig. 13–1). Likewise, androgens can be considered precursors to estrogens by virtue of aromatase activity.

The genetic disorders of steroidogenesis could have been discussed in two large groups: those that involve adrenocortical and sex steroidogenesis in combination, and those that involve androgens or estrogens exclusively. We chose to extract disorders of aromatase from the latter group, largely to emphasize their recent clinical and heuristic prominence. On the other hand, we did not segregate the

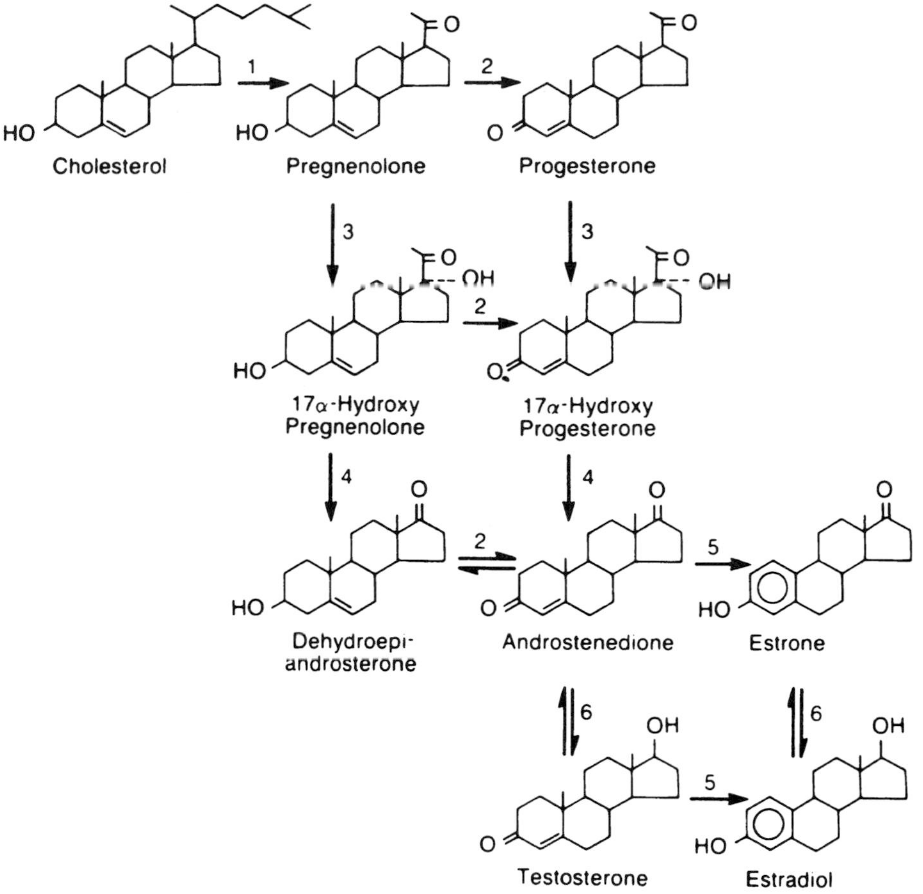

FIGURE 13–1. Biosynthesis of sex steroids. (1) Cholesterol side-chain cleavage enzyme complex; (2) 3β-hydroxysteroid dehydrogenase; (3) 17α-hydroxylase; (4) 17,20-lyase; (5) aromatase; (6) 17β-hydroxysteroid dehydrogenase.

"combined" disorders into those that stem from early biosynthetic defects common to both, and those that affect adrenocortical steroidogenesis primarily and sex steroidogenesis secondarily.

Genetic Disorders of Sex Steroidogenesis

MALE PSEUDOHERMAPHRODITISM DUE TO 17β-HYDROXYSTEROID DEHYDROGENASE TYPE 3 DEFICIENCY

17β-hydroxysteroid dehydrogenases (also known as 17-ketosteroid reductases; Fig. 13–2)catalyze the interconversion of active 17β-hydroxysteroids and relatively inactive 17-ketosteroids (Andersson et al., 1995). There are at least five different isoenzymes of 17β-HSD in humans. Each is encoded by a different gene that has been cloned. The type 1 enzyme is cytosolic and its preferred substrate is estrone (E$_1$),

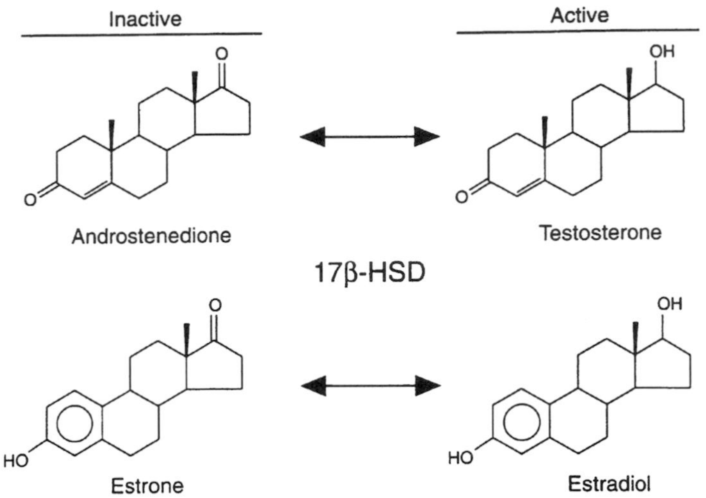

FIGURE 13–2. The reactions catalyzed by 17β-hydroxysteroid dehydrogenase in the oxidative direction. The same enzyme may catalyze the reductive reaction, hence its alternative name, 17-ketosteroid reductase.

which it reduces to 17β-estradiol (E_2), using NADPH as cofactor. Its gene is at 17q11–12, and it is expressed chiefly in the ovary, placenta, and breast (Poutanen et al., 1995). The type 2 17β-HSD is microsomal; it oxidizes testosterone (T) to androstenedione (Δ^4) and E_2 to E_1 using NAD as cofactor. Its gene is at 16q24, and it is expressed predominantly in the liver, endometrium, and placenta. Type 3 17β-HSD, a component of the endoplasmic reticulum, catalyzes the reduction of Δ^4 to T, androstanedione to 5α-dihydrotestosterone (DHT), E_1 to E_2, and dehydroepiandrosterone (DHEA) to 5-androstenediol, using NADPH as cofactor. Its gene is at 9q22 and it is expressed only in testes. Mutations in type 3 17β-HSD are the most frequent cause of male pseudohermaphroditism due to defective testosterone biosynthesis. Still, it is relatively rare: more than twice as many families with 5α-testosterone reductase deficiency have been described (Andersson et al., 1996). Type 4 17β-HSD is a peroxisomal isoenzyme that is distributed ubiquitously. It is exclusively oxidative and prefers estrogens as substrates (Adamski et al., 1995). Information about type 5 17β-HSD is limited to a recent abstract (Zhang et al., 1995). The enzyme is preferentially reductive using NADPH as cofactor. Its gene is located at 10p14–15. The degree of identity and similarity among the members of the 17β-HSD enzyme family points to convergent evolution of their respective genes.

Clinical and Imaging Features.   17β-HSD 3 deficiency was originally described by Saez and colleagues in 1971 and 1972. The 46,XY affected individuals had female external genitalia despite the presence of testes and of typically male derivatives of the wolffian ducts: epididymes, vasa deferentia, seminal vesicles, and ejaculatory ducts. These subjects, and those described later, were reared as females, but many of them experienced marked virilization at puberty, coincident with rises to normal male levels of plasma testosterone. In the most comprehensive report of this enzyme deficiency to date (Andersson et al., 1996) 11 new cases were added to six that have been reported previously in one degree or another. The majority of affected individuals have female external genitalia at birth, sometimes with a mass (a testis) in one labium majus/inguinal canal or in both. At puberty, appreciable virilization occurs (one or more of deepening voice, clitoral enlargement, hirsutism, and male muscularity) with coincident breast enlargement in about one half of the patients (Andersson et al., 1996). Menarche is absent. The vagina is blind. A minority have ambiguous external genitalia at birth and, in some families, variable expressivity encompasses affected individuals with female or ambiguous external genitalia (Andersson et al., 1996; Rösler et al., 1996). The pronounced virilization that occurs at puberty is accompanied, in some individuals, by the acquisition of a male gender identity and role, despite a female sex-of-rearing (Andersson et al., 1996).

Laboratory Features.   Plasma androstenedione and/or estrone levels exceed those of testosterone or estradiol, respectively, both before puberty (with stimulation by hCG or by GnRH) and after puberty. At puberty, testis biopsy usually reveals Leydig cell hyperplasia and seminiferous tubules containing Sertoli cells but no germ cells that have matured past the spermatocyte stage. In adult patients, the Δ^4 levels are elevated at least 10-fold; T or DHT levels are usually low but may be low-normal. LH is elevated and FSH may be as well. Occasionally, plasma estradiol is increased compared to normal male standards. Andersson and colleagues (1996) found 15-to 20-fold elevations of Δ^4, but 15-to 70-fold decreased levels of T in spermatic venous blood. The ratio of T to Δ^4 in these subjects was well below 1; the normal ratio is well above 20. When testis biopsies were incubated with pregnenolone, the predominant product was Δ^4. Its conversion to T was reduced consistently, whereas the conversion of E_1 to E_2 was inconstantly reduced. Ultrasonography reveals absent uterus.

Genotyping and Gene Expression.   To mid-1998, 16 different mutations in type 3 17β-HSD gene had been identified (Moghrabi et al., 1998; Andersson et al., 1996; Geissler et al., 1994) in 17 unrelated individuals/families. All have been point mutations or small rearrangements that are distributed through nearly the entire breadth of the 17β-HSD 3 gene. Of its 11 exons, only exons 1, and 5–7 have been spared mutation to date. The mutations were detected by single strand conformation polymorphism (SSCP) and identified by direct sequencing. Three of the mutations have occurred in more than one family. Four of the affected individuals are compound heterozygotes; a fifth probably is. Eleven of the missense mutations have been recreated in cDNA vectors and transfected into human embryonic kidney cells that are natively enzyme-free. All 11 cDNAs were expressed as judged by reactivity against antibodies to 17β-HSD 3, but only four of these mutant proteins (A56T, R80Q N130S, Q176P) had appreciable ($\sim$ 20%) residual catalytic activity as measured by the conversion of Δ^4 to T (Moghrabi et al., 1998).

Ethnic Considerations.   With one exception, the various mutations have been found in subjects of diverse ethnicity. The R80Q mutation in exon 3 is particularly frequent among the highly inbred Arab population in the Gaza Strip. Rösler and colleagues (1996) have recently reported it in nine such families. Interestingly, in the two largest of their families, individuals with female and ambiguous external genitalia were about equally numerous. Importantly, however, in the study of Andersson and colleagues (1996), subjects with ambiguous external genitalia had missense mutations, other than R80Q, that expressed no residual activity in transfected cells.

Management.   Subjects with female external genitalia are treated with orchidectomy, female hormone replacement therapy, and, if necessary, clitoral recession and vaginal elongation. Subjects with ambiguous external genitalia are managed surgically according to prevailing practices, taking into account anatomic and social considerations. If the female sex-of-rearing is chosen, the individuals are supported by hormone replacement therapy at the expected time of puberty. Prenatal diagnosis and selective termination are possible for those who wish to exercise this option.

Discussion and Speculation.   The interconversion reaction catalyzed by the family of 17β-HSDs is a major determinant of gonadal steroid balance. 17-keto reduction is the last step in the biosynthetic sequence leading to testosterone in Leydig cells and estradiol in granulosa cells. 17-keto oxidation, predominantly extraglandular, is the balancing force.

Two phenomena associated with 17β-HSD 3 deficiency have been more or less vexatious. The first is preservation of androgen-dependent differentiation of the wolffian ducts into several or all of its normal derivatives, despite complete or major impairment of external genital masculinization. The second is the appearance of appreciable androgen-dependent virilization at puberty in those subjects whose testes are preserved. The maintenance of internal genital masculinization despite faulty external genital masculinization implies different modes of androgenization between the internal and external genitalia. Either the wolffian ducts have a better extratesticular reserve system for converting Δ^4 to T than the external genital primordia, or their ARs respond better to Δ^4 as a ligand than can the ARs in the external genitalia primordia. Two explanations have been proffered for the greater pubertal virilization than prenatal masculinization in subjects with 17β-HSD 3 deficiency. The first is a puberty-dependent restitution of some testicular 17β-HSD 3 activity under the impetus of increased LH levels. The other is more efficient conversion of increased pubertal levels of circulating Δ^4 to T by one or more of the extratesticular isozymes of 17β-HSD. Such a protective mechanism may be nullified in fetal life because of the large capacity of the placenta to aromatize androgens, including Δ^4 to E_1.

Andersson and colleagues (1996) found that the testicular venous blood of two subjects with missense mutations that inactivate 17β-HSD 3 had only 5% as much T as normal, thereby supporting the proposed extratesticular origin of the raised plasma T at the time of puberty. Contrarily, it is provocative that several related subjects with the R80Q mutation that preserves residual 17β-HSD 3 function had appreciable testicular secretion of T. This may account, in part, for the relatively high frequency of congenital external genital ambiguity among subjects with the R80Q mutation. Clearly, however, stochastic or constitutional genetic factors must intervene to determine which of those with the R80Q mutation have female or ambiguous external genitalia at birth. Likewise, similar factors must determine whether subjects with apparently inactivating mutations of 17β-HSD 3 are born with ambiguous external genitalia.

The appearance of breast development in juxtaposition to predominant signs of virilization at the time of puberty presumably reflects relatively efficient peripheral aromatization of Δ^4 to E_1, and the subsequent peripheral reduction of E_1 to circulating E_2 levels that are elevated for pubertal males (Goebelsmann et al., 1973).

The lack of spermatogenesis in subjects with classical 17β-HSD 3 deficiency is not due to cryptorchidism, for it has been observed even in testes that have been treated by early orchidopexy. Rather, it stems from the need by the process of spermatogenesis for high intratesticular concentrations of testosterone.

REFERENCES

Adamski J, Normand T, Leenders F, Monte D, Begue A, Stephelin D, Jungblut P W, De Launoit Y (1995). Molecular cloning of a novel widely expressed human 80 kDa 17β-hydroxysteroid dehydrogenase IV. *Biochem J* 311:437–443.

Andersson S, Geissler W M, Patel S, Wu L (1995). The molecular biology of androgenic 17β-hydroxysteroid dehydrogenases. *J Steroid Biochem Mol Biol* 53:37–39.

Andersson S, Geissler W M, Wu L, Davis S L, Grumbach M M, New M I, Schwarz H P, Blethen S L, Mendonca B B, Bloise W, Witchel S F, Cutler Jr G B, Griffin J E, Wilson J D, Russell D W (1996). Molecular genetics and pathophysiology of 17β-hydroxysteroid dehydrogenase 3 deficiency. *J Clin Endocrinol Metab* 81:130–136.

Andersson S, Russell D W, Wilson J D (1996). 17β-hydroxysteroid dehydrogenase 3 deficiency. *Trends Endocrinol Metab* 81:130–136.

Geissler W M, Davis D L, Wu L, Bradshaw K D, Patel S, Mendonca B B, Elliston K O, Wilson J D, Russell D W, Andersson S (1994). Male pseudohermaphroditism caused by mutations of testicular 17β-hydroxysteroid dehydrogenase 3. *Nat Genet* 7:34–40.

Goebelsmann U, Horton R, Mestman J H, Arce J J, Nagata Y, Nakamura R M, Thorneycroft I H, Mishell D R Jr (1973). Male pseudohermaphroditism due to testicular 17β-hydroxysteroid dehydrogenase deficiency. *J Clin Endocrinol Metab* 36:867–879.

Moghrabi N, Hughes I A, Dunaif A, Andersson S (1998). Deleterious missense mutations and silent polymorphism in the human 17β-hydroxysteroid dehydrogenase 3 gene (HSD17B3). *J Clin Endocrinol Metab* 83:2855–2860.

Poutanen M (1995). Role of 17β-hydroxysteroid dehydrogenase type 1 in endocrine and intracrine estadiol biosynthesis. *J Steroid Biochem Mol Biol* 55:525–532.

Rösler A, Silverstein S, Abeliovich D (1996). A (R80Q) mutation in 17β-hydroxysteroid dehydrogenase type 3 gene among Arabs of Israel is associated with pseudohermaphroditism in males and normal asymptomatic females. *J Clin Endocrinol Metab* 81:1827–1831.

Zhang Y, Dufort I, Soucy P, Labrie F, Luu-The V (1995). Isolation and characterization of human type 5 17β-hydroxysteroid dehydrogenase. *Clin Invest Med* 18: B40.

GYNECOMASTIA (WITH OR WITHOUT IMPOTENCE OR DECREASED LIBIDO) POSSIBLY DUE TO LATE-ONSET TESTICULAR 17β-HSD TYPE 3 DEFICIENCY

There have been only two reports (Rogers et al., 1985; Castro-Magana et al., 1993) of boys with normal external genitalia who develop severe, persistent gynecomastia in their teenage years in the presence of high circulating levels of Δ^4 and E_1, both basally and in response to hCG challenge. The three unrelated subjects described by Castro-Magana and colleagues were among 48 with idiopathic pubertal gynecomastia. They also had decreased libido and impotence. The coding sequence of the 17β-HSD 3 gene in one of these patients is normal. Whether a mutation outside the coding sequence of this gene is involved or whether another member of the 17β-HSD enzyme family is at fault is not yet known. Castro-Magana and colleagues postulated increased testicular aromatase activity to explain the high level of estrogens in spermatic venous blood, and estrogen-mediated suppression of LH and FSH serum levels in the three subjects.

REFERENCES

Castro-Magana M, Angulo M, Uy J (1993). Male hypogonadism with gynecomastia caused by late-onset deficiency of testicular 17-ketosteroid reductase. *N Engl J Med* 328:1297–1301.

Rogers D G, Chasalow F I, Blethen S L (1985). Partial deficiency in 17-ketosteroid reductase presenting as gynecomastia. *Steroids* 45:195–200.

POLYCYSTIC OVARY DISEASE POSSIBLY DUE TO OVARIAN 17β-HSD TYPE 1 DEFICIENCY

In 1987, Pang and colleagues described an 18-year-old woman with hirsutism, acne, clitoromegaly, amenorrhea, and apparent polycystic ovary disease. Excessive Δ^4 was secreted by her ovaries, and elevated plasma levels of Δ^4, E_1, and T were regulated by gonadotropin. The patient had two younger sisters with signs of androgen excess who also had elevated plasma levels of Δ^4. The authors suggested a genetic deficiency of ovarian (type 1) 17β-HSD deficiency due to homozygosity in the proband and possibly to heterozygosity in her two sisters.

In 1990, Toscano and colleagues reported ovarian 17β-HSD deficiency in two of 43 patients with polycystic ovary disease. Two of three brothers of one patient had persistent pubertal gynecomastia, and one also had oligospermia. Both had elevated Δ^4/T and E_1/E_2 ratios, suggestive of testicular 17β-HSD 3 deficiency. The familial distribution of 17β-HSD deficiency in this family is provocative, but is not easily explained at this time. A mechanism for coordinate regulation of multiple 17β-HSD isozymes is implied, but none is known.

REFERENCES

Pang S, Softness B, Sweeney III W J, New M I (1987). Hirsutism, polycystic ovarian disease, and ovarian 17-ketosteroid reductase deficiency. *N Engl J Med* 316:1295–1301.

Toscano V, Balducci R, Bianchi P, Mangiantini A, Sciarra F (1990). Ovarian 17-ketosteroid reductase deficiency as a possible cause of polycystic ovarian disease. *J Clin Endocrinol Metab* 71:288–292.

MALE PSEUDOHERMAPHRODITISM DUE TO STEROID 5α-REDUCTASE, TYPE 2 (5α-R2) DEFICIENCY

Steroid 5α-reductase reduces the double bond at the C_4-C_5 position of testosterone and adds a hydrogen atom to C_5 in the alpha plane (Fig. 13–3) to produce 5α-dihydrotestosterone (DHT). There are two isozymes of steroid 5α-reductase, types 1 and 2. Type 1 has an alkaline pH optimum and is expressed apparently only after birth, primarily in liver and nongenital skin. Type 2 has an acidic pH optimum and is expressed before and after birth, predominantly in prostate, internal genital structures derived from the wolffian ducts, genital skin, and liver.

The type 1 gene (*SRD5A1*) is at 5p15. The type 2 gene is at 2p23. Both have five exons (Labrie et al., 1992), and similar intronic positions, suggesting that they are

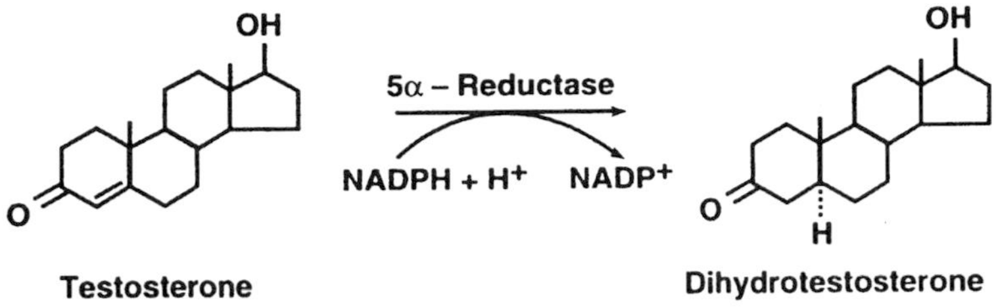

FIGURE 13–3. The reaction catalyzed by steroid 5α-reductase. The double bond between C4 and C5 of testosterone is reduced, and the H is bonded to C5 in the alpha configuration, as signified by the dashed line. In contrast, the hydroxyl bond at C17 is in the β configuration, as signified by the solid line.

duplicates. The type 2 gene yields a protein of 254 amino acids. A pseudogene, derived from the type 1 gene, maps to Xq24-qter. The type 1 gene has three biallelic polymorphisms. The type 2 gene has a microsatellite polymorphism on 4% of its chromosomes in the portion of exon 5 encoding the 3' UTR, a Val → Leu substitution at position 89, and a silent C → T substitution early in intron 1.

The ontogeny of 5α-R 2 activity is striking: it appears in the urogenital sinus and the external genital primordia before their differentiation into prostate, and penis and scrotum, respectively. Conversely, it appears in the wolffian duct derivatives only after they have differentiated. Predictably, therefore, steroid 5α-R2 deficiency typically results in an autosomal recessive form of male pseudohermaphroditism featuring severe undermasculinization of the external genitalia and undergrowth of the prostate gland while the wolffian ducts differentiate normally into the epididymes, vasa deferentia, seminal vesicles, and the ejaculatory ducts. The latter communicate with a pseudovagina, or with the vaginal outpouching from a urogenital sinus with a single perineal orifice. The disorder used to be known as pseudovaginal perineoscotal hypospadias.

Clinical and Imaging Features. The external genitalia of affected males usually have the overall appearance of being female. There is perineoscrotal hypospadias, meaning that the phallus is small and hypospadic and the scrotum is bifid, and there is a blind vaginal pouch. About 40 % of patients have a single urethral/vaginal opening (urogenital sinus); the remainder have separate openings. The testes are always extraabdominal, and usually inguinal, but scrotal location is not rare.

In some parts of the world it was common to rear typically affected males as females, and to make the diagnosis of 5α-R2 deficiency at or after puberty. Thus, the natural history of this condition has been documented. Temporal hair recession, facial and chest hair are much reduced and gynecomastia is rare, but skeletal muscularity can be impressive, as can phallic and testicular growth, scrotal rugosity and pigmentation. Strikingly, a high proportion of affected males reared as females choose to adopt a male gender identity and role by the time of puberty. In some, the change seems to be expressed in childhood, before the pubertal surge of androgens. These changes at puberty are a fascinating aspect of 5α-R2 deficiency that is treated further in the Discussion section below.

Notwithstanding this prototypic phenotype, it is crucial to appreciate that the actual phenotype can vary considerably. For instance, the external genitalia may have a predominantly male appearance with hypospadias of the penis and bifid scrotum, and rarely there is simply micropenis without hypospadias. Indeed, variability may be substantial not only among unrelated individuals with the same mutation, but even among affected siblings (Ng et al., 1990; Sinnecker et al., 1996). In addition to the variation described above, there may be normospermia or azoospermia, perhaps related to the degree of testicular maldescent, and to the volume of semen produced by hypoplastic prostate glands and seminal vesicles (Cai et al., 1994). Sperm motility and morphology may be normal (Katz et al., 1997).

Retrograde contrast radiography through a single perineal orifice will reveal a urogenital sinus; vaginography through a separate orifice will disclose a blind vaginal pouch. Ultrasonography will demonstrate prostatic hypoplasia.

Laboratory Features.   The diagnosis of 5α-R2 deficiency can be strongly suspected when the T blood level is normal but the T:DHT ratio is elevated either without Leydig cell stimulation during the first 3 months of life or after puberty, or after T treatment, or after hCG stimulation before puberty. The suspicion can be strengthened by elevated ratios of 5β-:5α-reduced versions of androgens and other steroids in the urine. The condition can also be suspected by demonstrating deficient 5α-R2 activity in cultured genital skin fibroblasts (GSF). However, some normal GSF also have negligible 5α-R2 activity, so a GSF diagnosis must remain tentative until any residual enzyme activity is demonstrated to be qualitatively defective, or until the 5α-R2 gene is examined directly for mutations in its coding sequences or its regulatory regions.

The Phenotype in Homozygous Females.   The clinical phenotype of 46,XX females homozygous for the Dominican Republic mutation was defined in three subjects by Katz and colleagues (1995). The external genitalia are normal female. At puberty, breast development is normal, limb hair is absent, pubic hair is reduced moderately, and axillary hair slightly. Sebum production is normal. Menarche is delayed, but fertility is normal (or supranormal). Their biochemical phenotype is like that of affected males.

Genotyping, Ethnic Considerations, and Gene Expression.   Expectedly, for a locus with relatively rare muations, the rate of consanguinity is high and more than two thirds of the families have homozygous mutations. On the other hand, the relatively high frequency of compound heterozygosity suggests that the carrier frequency is more common than appreciated heretofore. 5α-R2 gene mutations have been found in more than 50 families representing more than 22 ethnic groups. The greatest concentrations of cases have occurred in large inbred, geographically or socially isolated families in the Dominican Republic (Thigpen et al., 1992), Turkey (Imperato-McGinley, et al., 1987), and Papua, New Guinea (Mendonca et al., 1996). A founder mutation (Q126R) is relatively common among Brazilian families of Portuguese ancestry (Mendonca et al., 1996).

The mutations are distributed throughout all five exons, are mostly of the "point" variety, and are largely missense in character. Atypically, the New Guinea cluster is deleted for the full coding sequence.

Many of the mutations have been recreated, expressed, and characterized in reporter cells.

Of the first 22 missense mutations studied, 12 yielded no 5α-R2 activity, and 10 had low activity (Russell and Wilson, 1994). Two of the 10 had a low affinity for substrate and a normal half-life. The others had low affinity for the cofactor, NADPH, and a short half-life. None had decreased affinity for substrate and cofactor. Interestingly, the two with low substrate affinity are two missense substitutions at opposite ends of the molecule. Notwithstanding these substantive results, it does not appear possible to understand *in vivo* variability of the 5α-R2 deficiency phenotype by such relatively simple *in vitro* studies on overexpressing reporter cells.

Management.   The management of subjects with predominantly female external genitalia who are reared as females should include gonadectomy before mid-childhood (see Discussion below), clitoral resection, if necessary, vaginoplasty, and estrogen replacement. Clitoral resection and vaginoplasty can have appreciable emotional and physical sequelae that require long-term support. Those subjects with predominantly male external genitalia who are reared as males need staged repair of their hypospadias, and orchiopexy (if necessary). The use of supraphysiologic intramuscular doses of mixed testosterone esters to achieve normal circulating levels of DHT (largely by the intervention of 5α-R1) and the daily application of 1.5 mg of 2.5 % DHT cream to the abdominal skin and thighs will increase penis and prostate size, muscle bulk, facial and chest hair, temporal recession, and, perhaps, libido. It is important to note that in subjects treated after puberty, penis size did not continue to increase after 6 months of therapy. Interestingly, prepubertal subjects had a somewhat greater response than the postpubertal subjects. Whether their ultimate penis size will be greater having started prepubertal treatment remains to be seen. However, therapy did not affect their bone age. One patient with highly viscous, low-volume ejaculates and post-surgical urethroscrotal fistulas did achieve paternity by intrauterine insemination of his sperm (Katz et al., 1997).

Discussion and Speculation.   The clinical and laboratory investigation of 5α-R2 deficiency has generated much new knowledge, and has raised or resurrected many new questions, particularly in regard to the high frequency of gender reversal in subjects reared as females. For instance, it seems clear now that the normal or near-normal circulating levels of DHT in many pubertal subjects is a result of DHT that is produced in the liver and skin by the activity of the 5α-R1 isoenzyme. This also indicates that DHT can serve as a true endocrine hormone, in addition to its autocrine or paracrine roles in cells and tissues endowed with 5α-R2 activity. This "endocrine" version of DHT must be responsible for the impressive, but variable, degree of pubertal virilization in many subjects. On the other hand, although 5α-R1 is the predominant isozyme in scalp, subjects have reduced temporal hair recession. This suggests that expression of the two isozymes is regulated reciprocally by a mechanism yet to be discovered. Likewise, subjects have less male-pattern baldness and severe acne, suggesting that these are dependent on DHT produced locally by 5α-R2.

The failure of pubertal subjects to sustain penile growth beyond 6 months of therapeutic androgen may represent, to some extent, down-regulation of the AR by the physiologically high levels of androgen attained at puberty (Takane et al., 1990). In this event, androgen therapy before puberty might be more effective, as intimated by the greater early response recently reported in a set of three boys (Mendonca et al., 1996). If the limiting factor in sustaining penile growth is impaired penile development per se, then early prenatal therapy may be the only way to intervene successfully.

Despite rearing as females, an appreciable fraction of XY subjects with 5α-R2 deficiency experience a change in gender identity and wish to adopt a male gender role at puberty (Wilson et al., 1993). In a few, the expression of change begins prepubertally at 7 or 8 years of age. This chronological fact suggests that androgenization of certain portions of the central and/or peripheral nervous system can occur in embryonic life or in early infancy, the two other times besides puberty when androgen levels may be elevated, however transiently. The phenomenon of gender reversal is evidently contrary to the dictum that gender-of-rearing is the overwhelming influence in the development of gender identity and role. Gender switch has also been described, less commonly, in those forms of male pseudohermaphroditism caused by decreased T biosynthesis due to deficiency of 17β-HSD 3 or 3β-HSD deficiency. However, it is not seen in individuals with external genital ambiguity due to partial androgen resistance resulting from androgen receptor mutation. This implies that if gender reversal at puberty depends on a form of androgen imprinting during embryonic or neonatal life, then that process is AR-mediated.

The distribution of reduced body hair in homozygous XX females, despite their normal to elevated levels of serum testosterone (T), indicates that peripheral reduction of T to 5α-DHT is differentially necessary for normal female body hair. Their normal sebum production is probably due to the fact that, at puberty, skin and scalp only express 5α-R1 activity. Delayed menarche is unexplained; but it is also observed in about 15 % of females heterozygous for androgen receptor mutations causing severe androgen insensitivity. Hence, decreased or defective DHT-androgen receptor complexes appear to influence resetting of the gonadostat at puberty. Finally, two of the three homozygous females had nonidentical twin offspring; this has raised the suspicion that a low level of DHT in the ovary may promote FSH induction of LH in granulosa cells, facilitate follicle maturation, and ultimately increase ovulation.

REFERENCES

Cai L Q, Fratianni C F, Gautier T, Imperato-McGinley J (1994). Dihydrotestosterone regulation of semen in male psuedohermaphrodites with 5α-reductase-2 deficiency. *J Clin Endocrinol Metab* 79:409–414.

Imperato-McGinley J, Akgun S, Ertel N H, Sayli B, Shackleton C (1987). The coexistence of male pseudohermaphrodites with 17-ketosteroid reductase deficiency and 5α-reductase deficiency within a Turkish kindred. *Clin Endocrinol (Oxf)* 27:135–143.

Katz M D, Cai L Q, Zhu Y S, Herrera C, DeFillo-Ricart M, Shackleton C H L, Imperato-McGinley J (1995). The biochemical and phenotypic characterization of females homozygous for 5α-reductase-2 deficiency. *J Clin Endocrinol Metab* 80:3160–3167.

Katz M D, Kligman L, Cai L Q, Zhu Y S, Fratianni C M, Zervoudakis I, Rosenwaks Z, Imperato-McGinley J (1997). Paternity by intrauterine insemination with sperm from a man with 5α-reductase-2 deficiency. *N Engl J Med* 336:994–997.

Labrie F, Sugimoto Y, Luu-The V, Simard J, Lachance Y, Bachvarov D, Leblanc G, Durocher

F, Paquet N (1992). Structure of human type II 5α-reductase gene. *Endocrinology* 131:1571–1573.

Mendonca B B, Inacio M, Costa E M F, Arnhold I J P, Silva F A Q, Nicolau W, Bloise W, Russell D W, Wilson J D (1996). Male pseudohermaphoditism due to steroid 5α-reductase 2 deficiency. *Medicine* 75:64–76.

Ng W K, Taylor N F, Hughes I A, Taylor J, Ransley P G, Grant D B (1990). 5α-reductase deficiency without hypospadias. *Arch Dis Child* 65:1166–1167.

Russell D W, Wilson J D (1994). Steroid 5α-reductase: two genes/two enzymes. *Annu Rev Biochem* 63:25–61.

Sinnecker G H G, Hiort O, Dibbelt L, Albers N, Dörr H G, Hauss H, Heinrich K, Hemminghaus M, Hoepffner W, Holder M, Schnabel D, Kruse K (1996). Phenotypic classification of male pseudohermaphroditism due to steroid 5α-reductase 2 deficiency. *Am J Med Genet* 63:223–230.

Takane K K, George F W, Wilson J D (1990). Androgen receptor of rat penis is downregulated by androgen. *Am J Physiol* 258: E46–E50.

Thigpen A E, Davis D L, Gautier T, Imperato-McGinley J, Russell D W (1992). The molecular basis of steroid 5α-reductase deficiency in a large Dominican kindred. *N Engl J Med* 327: 1216–1219. (1993).

Wilson J D, Griffin J E, Russell D W. Steroid 5α-reductase 2 deficiency. *Endocrine Rev* 14:577–593.

Genetic Disorders of Aromatase Activity

Aromatase is the short name for the enzyme cytochrome P450-aromatase, which catalyzes the aromatization of various androgens to their respective estrogenic derivatives. The gene for P450arom (*CYP19*; 15q21.1) has 10 exons and is more than 70 kb long (Fig. 13–4). The heme-binding region is encoded by exon 10, and it has two polyadenylation sites. In addition to the ovary and testis, aromatase is found in skin, fat, brain, and placenta. P450arom expression depends partly on the use of tissue-specific promoters (Fig. 13–5) within various 5'-untranslated varsions of exon 1 that are generated by alternative splicing (Fig. 13–5)). All versions have the same

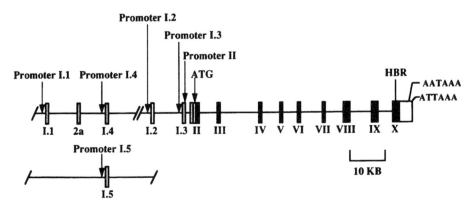

FIGURE 13–4. A schema for the human CYP19 gene. Solid bars are translated exons. Open bars are untranslated portions of exon 1. Portion 1.5 was not yet mapped. The arrows locate promoters, proven or putative. (Reproduced from Simpson et al., *Endocr Rev* 15:342–355, 1994, with permission.)

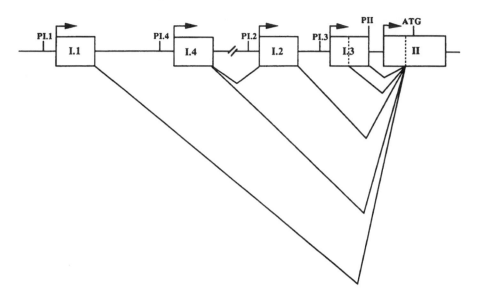

FIGURE 13–5. Alternative splicing patterns of exon 1 *CYP19* that presumably underlie the genesis of tissue-specific promoters. (Reproduced from Simpson et al., *Endocr Rev* 15:342–355, 1994, with permission.)

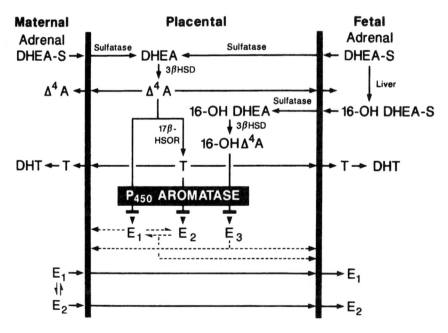

FIGURE 13–6. The maternal and fetal consequences of placental aromatase deficiency. 17βHSOR, 17β-hydroxysteroid oxidoreductase is otherwise known as 17β-hydroxysteroid dehydrogenase (17βHSD). (Reproduced from Conte et al., *J Clin Endocrinol Metab* 78:1287–1292, 1994, with permission.)

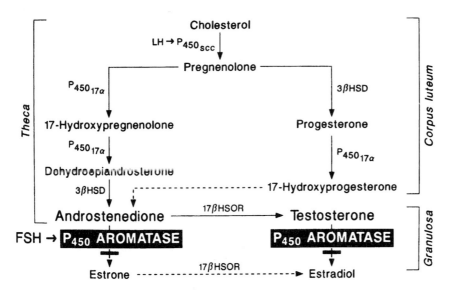

FIGURE 13–7. The consequences of aromatase deficiency in ovarian follicular cells. (Reproduced from Conte et al., *J Clin Endocrinol Metab* 78:1287–1292, 1994, with permission.)

translation start site (ATG) in exon 2. In ovarian granulosa cells, P450arom is induced by FSH and cAMP, and repressed by phorbol esters. In adipose fibroblasts, P450arom is induced by glucocorticoids in the presence of certain lymphokines. Appropriately, one of the three promoters that can be used in these cells (1.4) has both a glucocorticoid response element (GRE), and a γ-interferon activation sequence (GAS) element. The latter binds to a STAT (signal transducer and activator of transcription) protein after it has been phosphorylated by a JAK (Janus kinase). The other two promoters are differentially induced by cAMP in a manner that is phorbol ester–stimulated. Placental expression of *CYP*19 is controlled at a constitutively high level by promoter I.1. Pathogenic mutations that alter the coding portion of the *CYP*19 gene should impair or increase P450 aromatase activity in all its normal sites of expression, whereas those in its 5'-regulatory region might well express themselves in a tissue (organ)-selective pattern of aromatase excess or deficiency.

AROMATASE DEFICIENCY: A CAUSE OF FEMALE PSEUDOHERMAPHRODITISM WITH MATERNAL VIRILIZATION

Aromatase deficiency (Figs. 13–6 and 13–7)could be pathogenic because of androgen accumulation behind the block, or because of estrogen depletion beyond the block. Androgen excess could masculinize the external genitalia during the critical period of fetal development in a female, could prematurely virilize the external genitalia of an affected male fetus, or could virilize a woman during the pregnancy of an affected fetus of either sex (Bulun et al., 1996). The first and third of these scenarios have been observed, so far, in only five families.

Clinical and Imaging Presentation. In the first family (Shozu et al., 1991) the pregnant woman began to have various signs of virilization (acne, low voice pitch, clitoral hypertrophy) at about 30 weeks. From 24 to 35 weeks, she had frequent uterine contractions treated with bed rest and tocolytic agents. At near full-term, a baby of appropriate weight was born vaginally. Her external genitalia were frankly ambiguous: there was a single urogenital meatus at the base of an enlarged phallus; the labioscrotal folds, lacking gonads, were rugose and fused posteriorly. The baby developed normally and the maternal virilization disappeared. There has been no long-term follow-up.

In the second family (Conte et al., 1994), maternal virilization was not noted during a normal full-term pregnancy, but the newborn had ambiguous external genitalia essentially like those in the baby described above. Ultrasonography revealed normal kidneys, uterus, oviducts, and vagina, thereby making so-called non-specific female pseudohermaphroditism (Chapter 16) very unlikely. At 14 years, she had a bone age of only 10 years, and multiple cysts (~5 cm) in both ovaries were noted by sonography and magnetic resonance imaging. She had not yet had breast development, a growth spurt, or menarche; however, she did have normal pubic and axillary hair, clitoromegaly, and mild acne.

In the third family, affected XX and XY siblings were born to consanguineous parents (Morishima et al., 1995). Their mother had severe acne and hirsutism from the middle of each pregnancy till after delivery. At birth the female infant was considered to be a male with penoscrotal hypospadias and bilateral cryptorchidism. She grew normally during childhood. At puberty (about 12.5 years), she developed acne but not breasts or menses. Ultrasonography revealed bilateral polycystic ovaries, and her bone age was 12 years. Following appropriate therapy (see below), she developed breasts, menses and a growth spurt. Her hand and wrist epiphyses fused by 18 years, and her final height is more than three standard deviations above the mean.

The affected male infant in the third family was normal at birth, and grew normally during childhood, but he was still growing, with eunuchoid proportions, at 24 years when he was already 204 cm tall. At that time, his bone age was only 14 years, his wrists were osteopenic, and densitometry of his distal radii and lumbar spine indicated osteoporosis. Aside from his abnormal growth pattern and macroorchidism, the onset and course of his puberty were unremarkable.

The male propositus in the fourth family (Carani et al., 1997) had a clinical course very similar to the affected male in the third family, except that he had small testes. At 18 years, his height was 170 cm, and he continued to grow. When he was 28, incidental x-rays of one arm revealed unfused epiphyses and osteoporosis. At 30, he had severe oligospermia with 100 % immotility. By age 31, he was 187 cm tall, arm span was 204 cm and upper to lower segment ratio was 0.85. Bone age was only 15 years, osteoporosis was diffuse, and bone pain appeared. Penis, pubic hair, potency, libido, and sexual identity and orientation were all normal.

The female proposita in the fifth family (Mullis et al., 1997) was born with male external genitalia after a pregnancy that was remarkable only by progressive maternal virilization starting at 12 weeks: the mother had facial acne, hyperpigmentation, low-pitched voice, and clitoral hypertrophy. Except for some voice change, all these signs disappeared within 6 months after delivery.

When the infant was 6 months of age, ultrasonography exposed slightly enlarged ovaries and a urogenital sinus. At 2 years, laparoscopy revealed clearly enlarged, cystic ovaries. At 3.5 years, and again at 4 years, bone age was delayed to 2.5 years, despite a 50-day course of estradiol treatment that increased bone mineral density "drastically."

Laboratory Features.   Classical congenital adrenal hyperplasia was ruled out early during the course of all four infants with ambiguous or male external genitalia and a 46,XX karyotype. In the infant of the second family, an "XX-male" condition due to exaggerated testicular production of androgen by Leydig cells was ruled out by the lack of a testosterone response to a 3-day challenge of 1500U hCG per day. In her 35th week of pregnancy, the mother of the first family was challenged with 100 mg of DHEAS. There was a less than normal increase of blood and urine estrogens, and a more than normal increase of desulfated androgens (Fig. 13–6). This indicated that placental sulfatase activity was normal, whereas that of aromatase was low. Near term, the virilized mother in the second family had markedly decreased serum levels of estrone (E_1), estradiol (E_2), and estriol (E_3); those of the corresponding androgens were markedly high. The cord blood of her fetus yielded a comparable profile. Aromatase activity in placental homogenate was decreased. Strikingly, the infant had normal plasma E_2 levels when she was between 2 and 6 months of age, suggesting adventitious or residual aromatase activity in organs other than placenta.

In the second family, the affected infant at 17 months, and again at 14 years, had increased basal and GnRH-induced plasma FSH levels. At the later age, various tests continued to reveal androgen excess and estrogen deficiency. Thus, this patient, unlike the first, had persistent systemic aromatase deficiency, indicating the involvement of extraplacental isoforms of aromatase.

At about 12.5 years, the affected female sibling of the third family had elevated serum levels of androstenedione (Δ^4A), T, LH and FSH, while those of E_1 and E_2 were low. Fluid from her ovarian follicular cysts also had high concentrations of T and low concentrations of E (Fig. 13–7). The mother pregnant with the affected male sibling in the third family had high urinary excretion of 17-ketosteroids and 17-ketogenic steroids. At about 24 years, the affected male sibling of the third family had high serum androgens, LH, and FSH levels, whereas those of E_1 and E_2 were low. Additionally, he had hyperinsulinism associated with an abnormal blood lipid profile.

The propositus in the fourth family had very low serum estradiol but normal testosterone, upper-normal LH, and slightly high FSH levels. The latter two increased appropriately upon GnRH challenge. Total cholesterol and triglyceride levels were high; HDL cholesterol was low. Testis biopsy disclosed spermatogenic arrest at the stage of primary spermatocytes.

After testicular and adrenal causes of female pseudohermaphroditism were ruled out, the affected 46,XX infant in the fifth family was found, at 1 year, to have markedly elevated levels of FSH, both basally and after GnRH stimulation, and ovary biopsy revealed mature, preovulatory follicles. When the patient was 3.5

years, GnRH induced "striking" rises in FSH and LH; however, a 50-day course of "low-dose" E_2 normalized the basal level of LH and FSH and markedly reduced their peak levels after GnRH challenge.

In the mother, immediate prepartum assays revealed very low E_2 and E_3 levels, but very high androgen levels.

Genotyping and Gene Expression. The first infant is homozygous for a gt to gc transversion mutation at the 5' splice-donor site of intron 6 (Harada et al., 1992a). The consequent use of a cryptic splice site further upstream leads to the incorporation of 87 in-frame bases and the insertion of 29 amino acids. Expectedly, in view of the rarity of severe aromatase deficiency, the heterozygous parents were consanguineous (Harada et al., 1992b).

The second infant is heterozygous for each of two missense mutations, Arg435Cys and Cys437Tyr, in the heme-binding region of the enzyme (Ito et al., 1993). Laboratory expression of each mutated enzyme revealed 1% or less of normal enzyme activity. The patient's mother is a carrier of the first mutation; the origin of the second one could not be ascertained, because her father had died and there are no siblings.

In view of parental consanguinity, it is not surprising that the affected siblings of the third family (Morishima et al., 1995) are homozygous for a simple transition in exon 9 of the *CYP*19 gene that leads to R375C in a region that is highly conserved among members of the P_{450} enzyme family. The same applies to the homozygosity for Arg365Gln in the propositus of a fourth family (Carani et al., 1997); the pathogenicity of this mutation was confirmed by expression studies.

The affected female infant in the fifth family was born to nonconsanguineous Swiss parents. She is a compound heterozygote for two inherited point mutations that predict the production of markedly truncated versions of aromatase.

Management. When the second patient reached 14 years, her persistent aromatase deficiency was treated, orally, with 20 µg of ethinyl estradiol daily and 5 mg of medroxyprogesterone acetate for 10 days per month with the following benefits: plasma levels of LH, FSH, and androgens decreased markedly; a growth spurt occurred; the breasts enlarged; menses began; and ovarian cysts regressed. Surgery would be used as necessary to normalize the external genitalia in the female direction. Genetic counseling would disclose a 25% recurrence risk for this autosomal recessive disorder, and the possibility of recurrent maternal virilization in a subsequent pregnancy. The theoretical use of anti-androgen during the course of an affected pregnancy to prevent female masculinization and/or maternal virilization is considered below.

After ovarian cystectomy, the affected female sibling of the third family was treated with cyclic oral conjugated estrogen and medroxyprogesterone acetate. This regimen normalized the serum concentration of T, Δ^4A, LH, and FSH; initiated menses; suppressed ovarian cyst recurrence; promoted breast development; and precipitated a growth spurt. The patient has had staged corrective surgery to create female external genitalia. Her male sibling was treated with oral conjugated estrogen in an effort to correct his disturbed bone growth, hyperinsulinism, and dyslipidemia. The successful outcome of that treatment has recently been recorded (Bilezikian et al., 1998), in accord with the dramatic response of the male propositus in the fourth family. With 50 µg of transdermal estradiol twice weekly initially (maintenance dose, 25 µg) his bone pain disappeared; serum LH, FSH, T, and LDL cholesterol decreased; and HDL cholesterol decreased; and HDL cholesterol increased. Additionally, osteoporosis decreased, and epiphyseal fusion occurred. Interestingly, testicular volume and sperm parameters did not improve, and he was not hyperinsulimemic, although the insulin level had not been determined before treatment.

The experience with a 50-day course of "low-dose" (0.4 mg/day) estradiol in the 4-year-old girl of the fifth family supports the projection that appropriate manipulation of exogenous E_2 can permit near-normal bone and extraosseous sexual development, despite severe aromatase deficiency.

Discussion. Aromatase deficiency is a rare disorder. Yet there is no reason to believe that the *CYP*19 gene is protected against ordinary mutagenicity. Initially, its clinical rarity was thought to reflect blastocyst lethality at the time of implantation, because of estrogen deficiency. This hypothesis is negated by the several subjects described above, and by the recent reports of mice (Lubahn et al., 1993) and a man (Smith et al., 1994) with severe estrogen resistance because of experimental or natural estrogen receptor (ER) mutation, respectively. Mild or moderate systemic aromatase deficiency, in a heterozygote perhaps, may be subclinical except for accelerated follicular atresia, and organ-restricted aromatase deficiency has not yet been sought. The latter is not improbable, however, given that different organs use different *CYP*19 promoters and different patterns of splicing noncoding exon 1 (Simpson et al., 1994). For instance, ovary-restricted aromatase deficiency and resultant intraovarian androgen excess might be one cause of polycystic ovary disease.

The severe degree of external genital ambiguity in both 46,XX infants described above proves that the large amount of androgen, and androgenic precursor, normally secreted by the fetal adrenal cortex would always be teratogenic if it was not nullified by placental aromatase-catalyzed conversion of androgen to estrogen on a massive scale (Fig. 13–6). On the other hand, it seems equally clear that the large amount of estrogen so produced is not essential for the initiation or progress of labor at or near term. A similar conclusion was reached from studies on placental steroid sulfatase deficiency (France and Liggins, 1969). This deficiency results in severely compromised estrogen production because sulfated C-19 androgenic precursors cannot be aromatized.

Delayed epiphyseal maturation before treatment, and the growth spurt generated in the female patients by E_2 replacement, indicate that in addition to normal bone mineralization, estrogen is essential for normal bone growth and maturation, even with androgen excess. This notion is supported by the absence of eunuchoidism and the ability of estrogen to promote bone growth and maturation in the androgen insensitivity syndrome (Zachmann et al., 1986), and by the need for aromatase inhibitor to prevent premature epiphyseal closure, and ultimate short stature, in one strategy for treating boys with testotoxicosis (Laue et al., 1993), or girls with McCune-Albright syndrome (Feuillan-Philbrick et al., 1993).

During fetal life, androgen accumulation behind the block might be expected to produce precocity of the male external genitalia. However, even males with classic virilizing CAH do not have this sign. On the other hand, estrogen deficiency can retard epiphyseal closure, cause osteoporosis, and promote ultimate height, as also seen in the male with severe estrogen resistance due to homozygosity for an ER mutation (Smith et al., 1994).

In rodents, androgens have a masculine-imprinting effect on certain forms of sex-dimorphic behavior and gonadotropin regulation; paradoxically, this effect is mediated by estrogens derived from these androgens by virtue of aromatase activity. Androgens also influence certain forms of sex-dimorphic behavior in humans (Money et al., 1984). Judging from affected adult males and females, aromatase deficiency does not modify the latter influence; yet estrogens do contribute importantly to gonadotropin feedback regulation even in the adult human male with a high serum T level. For example, estrogen treatment of the affected male in the fourth family suppressed both gonadotropins dramatically; in contrast, androgen depressed them slightly. Furthermore, 5α-dihydrotestosterone, non-aromatizable, does not suppress gonadotropins (Bagatell et al., 1994).

Impaired spermatogenesis may not be a consequence of human aromatase deficiency: a brother in the fourth family was azoospermic but not aromatase-deficient, and estrogen therapy did not improve spermatogenesis in his aromatase-deficient sibling. On the other hand, male mice homozygous for estrogen receptor "knockouts" have microorchidism and are infertile.

Female spotted hyenas are born with fused labia (a pseudoscrotum) and a penile phallus, and as adults they are heavier and more aggressive than males (Yalcinkaya et al., 1993). The plasma concentration of Δ^4A in these adult females exceeds those in adult males. Recently, it has been shown, using Δ^4A as a precursor, that placental homogenates of pregnant female spotted hyenas have about 5 % as much aromatase activity as the same preparation from humans (Yalcinkaya et al., 1993). Yet these two sources have equal activities of 17-ketosteroid reductase, the enzyme that converts Δ^4A to testosterone (T). Thus, it seems that female spotted hyenas have excessive T because their relative aromatase deficiency consumes little Δ^4A by conversion to estrone, leaving a lot for conversion to T. They are also born with a paucity of ovarian follicles, presumably because of androgenic follicular atresia and, as adults, their ovaries are histologically similar to those of women with polycystic ovary syndrome. Female spotted hyenas can be considered a natural model of aromatase deficiency in human females. As such, they may help to support the hypothesis of reduced fertility to explain the rarity of human aromatase deficiency. They may also be useful for testing the use of antiandrogens to prevent external genital virilization of affected female fetuses with aromatase deficiency.

REFERENCES

Bagatell C J, Dahl K K, Brenner W J (1994). The direct pituitary effect of testosterone to inhibit gonadotropin secretion in men is partially mediated by aromatization to estradiol. *J Androl* 15:15–21.

Bilezikian JP, Morishima K, Bell J, Grumbach MM (1998). Increased bone mass as a result of estrogen therapy in a man with aromatase deficiency. *N Engl J Med* 339: 599–603.

Bulun S E (1996). Aromatase deficiency in women and men: would you have predicted the phenotypes? *J Clin Endocrinol Metab* 81:867–871.

Carani C, Quin K, Simoni M, Faustini-Fustini M, Serpente S, Boyd J, Korach K S, Simpson

E R (1997). Effect of testosterone and estradiol in a man with aromatase deficiency. *N Engl J Med* 337:91–95.

Conte F A, Grumbach M M, Ito Y, Fisher C R, Simpson E R (1994). A syndrome of female pseudohermaphrodism, hypergonadotropic hypogonadism, and multicystic ovaries associated with missense mutations in the gene encoding aromatase (P450arom). *J Clin Endocrinol Metab* 78:1287–1292.

Feuillan-Philbrick P, Jones J, Cutler G B (1993). Long-term testolactone therapy for precocious puberty in girls with the McCune-Albright syndrome. *J Clin Edocrinol Metab* 77:647–651.

France J T, Liggins G C (1969). Placental sulfatase deficiency. *J Clin Endocrinol Metab* 29:138–144.

Harada N, Ogawa H, Shozu M, Yamada K, Suhara K, Nishida E, Takagi Y (1992a). Biochemical and molecular genetic analyses of placental aromatase (P-450 arom) deficiency. *J Biol Chem* 267:4781–4785.

Harada N, Ogawa H, Shozu M, Yamada K (1992b). Genetic studies to characterize the origin of the mutation in placental aromatase deficiency. *Am J Hum Genet* 51:666–672.

Ito Y, Fisher C R, Conte F A, Grumbach M M, Simpson E R (1993). Molecular basis of aromatase deficiency in an adult female with sexual infantilism and polycystic ovaries. *Proc Natl Acad Sci USA* 90:11673–11677.

Laue L, Jones J, Barnes K, Cutler Jr G B (1993). Treatment of familial male precocious puberty with spironolactone, testolactone, and deslorelin. *J Clin Endocrinol Metab* 76:151–155.

Lubahn D B, Moyer J S, Golding T S, Couse J F, Korach K S, Smithies O (1993). Alteration of reproductive function but not prenatal sexual development after insertional disruption of the mouse estrogen receptor gene. *Proc Natl Acud Sci USA* 90:11162–11166.

Money J, Schwartz M, Lewis V G (1984). Adult erotosexual status and fetal hormonal masculinization and demasculiniation: 46,XX congenital virilizing adrenal hyperplasia and 4,XY androgen insensitivity compared. *Psychoneuroendocrinology* 9:405–414. 1984.

Morishima A, Grumbach M M, Simpson E R, Fisher C, Qin K (1995). Aromatase deficiency in male and female siblings caused by a novel mutation and the physiological role of estrogens. *J Clin Endocrinol Metab* 80:3689–3697.

Mullis P E, Yoshimura N, Kuhlmann B, Lippuner K, Jaeger P, Harada H (1997). Aromatase deficiency in a female who is compound heterozygote for two new point mutations in the P450$_{arom}$ gene: impact of estrogens on hypergonadotropic hypogonadism, multicystic ovaries, and bone densitometry in childhood. *J Clin Endocrinol Metab* 82:1739–1745.

Shozu M, Akasofu K, Harada T, Kubota Y (1991). A new cause of female pseudohermaphroditism: placental aromatase deficiency. *J Clin Endocrinol Metab* 72:560–566.

Simpson E R, Mahendroo M S, Means G D, Kilgore M W, Hinshelwood M M, Graham-Lorence S, Amarneh B, Ito Y, Fisher C R, Michael M D, Mendelson C R, Bulun S E (1994). Aromatase cytochrome P450, the enzyme responsible for estrogen biosynthesis. *Endocr Rev* 15:342–355.

Smith E P, Boyd J, Frank G R, Takahashi H, Cohen R M, Specker B, Williams T C, Lubahn D B, Korach K S (1994). Estrogen resistance caused by a mutation in the estrogen-receptor gene in a man. *N Engl J Med* 331:1056–1061.

Yalcinkaya T M, Siiteri P K, Vigne J L, Licht P, Pavgi S, Frank L G, Glickman S E (1993). A mechanism for virilization of female spotted hyenas *in utero*. *Science* 260:1929–1931.

Zachmann M, Prader A, Sobel E H, Crigler Jr J F, Ritzén E M, Atarés M, Ferrandez A (1986). Pubertal growth in patients with androgen insensitivity: indirect evidence for the importance of estrogens in pubertal growth of girls. *J Pediatr* 108:694–697.

PRIMARY ISOLATED AROMATASE EXCESS: A CAUSE OF GYNECOMASTIA IN MALES AND OF ISOSEXUAL PRECOCITY IN FEMALES

Gynecomastia (enlargement of the male breast) is common in early pubertal boys. Usually, it regresses within 18 months. Uncommonly, gynecomastia is persistent and progressive. This occurs in some boys with Klinefelter syndrome (Chapter 6), partial (mixed) gonadal dysgenesis (Chapter 6), partial 17-ketosteroid reductase deficiency (this chapter), or mild androgen insensitivity (Chapter 14). In each of these situations, increased estrogenicity is relative to a concomitant androgen deficit of one origin or another. Rarely, progressive prepubertal gynecomastia results from a primary increase of aromatase activity that is not part of a syndrome and that is mendelian, or apparently so. The latter type is discussed here. The syndromal type is discussed next. Isosexual precocity in a female refers to puberty before 8 years in a girl.

Clinical and Imaging Presentation. In one family (Wallace and Garcia, 1962) two brothers, their father, and their father's brother had gynecomastia without any other expression of male hypogonadism. In one sporadic subject (Hemsell et al., 1977), gynecomastia appeared at 8.5 years, but the first and only other signs of puberty were sparse axillary hair and Tanner III pubic hair at 10.5 years. At that age, the patient's bone age was about 15 years, and he was taller than his peers. In a second family (Berkovitz et al., 1985), three brothers, a maternal cousin, and a maternal uncle were affected. Their gynecomastia appeared at about the same time as their pubic hair, but the overall pace of their puberty was slower than normal. When two of the three affected siblings were 11.5 and about 12 years, respectively, their bone ages were more than two standard deviations above normal.

A third kindred with aromatase excess has recently been reported by Stratakis and colleagues (1996). At 9 years, the male propositus had gynecomastia, a bone age of 13.5 years, and the height of an average 13-year-old. At 7.5 years, his sister had breast development, pubic hair, and a height age of 9.5 years. Their father, only 165 cm tall, had severe gynecomastia at 15 years that required bilateral cosmetic mastectomy. Testicular volumes were decreased; otherwise, virilization was normal. Their mother was normal, but their paternal grandmother had massive macromastia.

Laboratory Features. In the affected family members related maternally, the fractional extraglandular conversion rate of androstenedione to estrone was ten times normal; in the sporadic subject, it was 50 times normal, and only 6 % of it was hepatic. In two members of the maternally related family, serum LH rose normally after LHRH stimulation; after hCG stimulation, there was a normal rise in blood T with a supranormal rise of E_2, as expected in a state of hyperaromatization.

In the three-generation third kindred, both siblings and their father had elevated serum estrogens (estrone; estradiol) levels and one can assume that their paternal grandmother did also. The father's testosterone level was low normal. Skin fibroblasts and transformed lymphoblasts from the affected individuals had markedly increased aromatase activity, measured by conversion of androstenedione to estrone.

Genotyping and Gene Expression. Definitive molecular-genetic analysis of constitutionally increased aromatase activity as an isolated finding has just appeared. Apparent paternal inheritance in one family suggests an autosomal dominant mutation; apparent maternal inheritance in a second family is compatible with autosomal dominant sex-limited inheritance, or X-linkage. In the third kindred (Stratakis et al., 1996, 1998) an intragenic microsatellite marker of the aromatase gene cosegregated with each affected individual. Rapid amplification of cDNA ends (RACE) revealed that only the patients had a novel promoter, and a novel form of exon 1 as by-products of alternative splicing in relation to exon 2 (Fig. 13–5).

Management.   Patients should be treated with an aromatase inhibitor and, perhaps, with a long-acting GnRH analogue to suppress gonadotropic stimulation of gonadal steroid production.

Discussion.   From the recent report of the three-generation family, it is apparent that aromatase hyperactivity can be transmitted as an autosomal dominant and can be expressed as isosexual pseudoprecocity in females and as heterosexual pseudoprecocity in males. Autosomal dominance is perfectly compatible with the gain-of-function nature of the mutant phenotype. Interestingly, the father in that family was fertile despite increased estrogen, low-normal testosterone, and reduced testicular volumes. The latter two result from increased estrogen feedback on the hypothalamic-pituitary axis. The consequences of aromatase hyperactivity for bone development are opposite to those of aromatase deficiency or estrogen resistance. In the latter two, epiphyseal closure is delayed and adult stature is increased.

It remains to be confirmed whether aromatase hyperactivity in humans is genetically heterogenous and, if so, to what extent. The family described by Bercovitz and colleagues (1985) suggested X-linked or sex-limited autosomal dominant inheritance. The family studied by Stratakis and colleagues (1996) is not compatible with X-linkage, and the autosomal dominance is not sex-limited. Furthermore, there is strong reason to presume that different constitutional alterations in the P450arom promoter may cause aromatase excess that is restricted to different cell types or organs.

REFERENCES

Berkovitz G D, Guerami A, Brown T R, MacDonald P C, Migeon C J (1985). Familial gynecomastia with increased extraglandular aromatization of plasma carbon$_{19-}$ steroids. *J Clin Invest* 75:1763–1769.

Hemsell D L, Edman C D, Marks J F, Siiteri P K, MacDonald P C (1977). Massive estraglandular aromatization of plasma androstenedione resulting in feminization of a prepubertal boy. *J Clin Invest* 60:455–464.

Stratakis C A, Vottero A, Brodie A, Kirschner S, DeAtkine D, Lu Q, Yue W, Mitsiades C S, Flor A W, Chrousos G P (1998). The aromatase excess syndrome is associated with feminization of both sexes and autosomal dominant transmission of aberrant P450arom gene transcription. *J Clin Endocrinol Metab* 83:1348–1357.

Stratakis C A, Vottero A, Brodie A, DeArkine D, Lu O, Mitsiades C S, Yue W, Flor A W, Garnica A, Mitsiades C S, Chrousos G P (1996). Biochemical and molecular genetics of the syndrome of increased aromatase activity: segregation with a marker from within the P450arom gene and evidence for aberrant alternative splicing of its 5'-end mRNA. *Am J Hum Genet* 59:A43.

Wallace E E, Garcia C R (1962). Hereditary gynecomastia without hypogonadism. *J Clin Endocrinol* 22:1201–1206.

PRIMARY SYNDROMAL AROMATASE EXCESS: OVARY OR TESTIS TUMORS IN PEUTZ-JEGHERS SYNDROME

Clinical and Imaging Presentation.   The Peutz-Jeghers (P-J) syndrome is an autosomal dominant condition of mucocutaneous pigmented macules, gastrointestinal hamartomatous polyposis, and a variety of other neoplasms, some malignant (Giardiello et al., 1987). Those in the gonads are, typically, multifocal "sex cord tumors with annular tubules" (SCTAT) that occur in the ovary or testis, often bilaterally (Young et al., 1982), and, less often, "sex cord-stromal tumors" of the ovary (Young et al., 1983). Usually the syndrome first presents in adolescence as intermittent abdominal pain ("colic") due to recurrent intussusception. Expressivity is variable in age and character: pigmentation or a sign of aromatase excess may be the initial sign early in infancy (Young et al., 1995). Although P-J syndrome affects males and females equally, ovarian tumors are much more frequent (5%) than testicular. Excessive estrogen synthesis by the ovarian tumor will cause menstrual disturbance postpubertally or isosexual precocity prepubertally. In a boy, the estrogen-secreting tumor will cause prepubertal gynecomastia and accelerate epiphyseal maturation. For instance, the patient reported by Coen and colleagues (1991) had gynecomastia from 3 years, and a bone age of 10 years when he was 4.25 years. Over the next 9 months he grew nearly 7 cm and his breast size reached Tanner stage III. Palpation of his testes was unremarkable, but repeated ultrasonography revealed mild bilateral enlargement with heterogeneous echogenicity. The boy described by Dubois and colleagues (1982) presented at 19 months with gynecomastia since birth, and unilateral testis enlargement for 5 months. Pubic hair was Tanner II, height was above the 96th percentile, and bone age was above 5 years. A similar picture, overall, has been described in five other boys (Young et al., 1995; Bulun et al., 1993a; Wilson et al., 1986; Cantu et al., 1980)

Solh and colleagues (1983) reported a pair of sisters with P-J syndrome and precocious puberty. The older presented at 4 years with Tanner III breasts, Tanner II pubic hair, estrogenized vaginal mucosa, and a unilateral adnexal mass. Ultrasonography revealed an enlarged ovary and uteromegaly. Her height was above the 90th percentile. The younger sister was first seen at 3.3 years with Tanner II breasts for 1 month and estrogenized vaginal mucosa. Ultrasonography revealed an enlarged ovary.

Laboratory Features.   One boy (Coen et al., 1991) had "barely detectable" levels of serum estrogens at the initial clinical presentation. Eventually, however, he was found to have prepubertal levels of gonadotropins, high 17β-estradiol (E_2) levels in testicular venous blood, high E_2 to T ratio in peripheral venous blood, and high aromatase activity in testicular homogenate. Testicular biopsy revealed the characteristic histology of SCTAT. Immunoreactive aromatase activity was restricted to the cytoplasm of some tumorous Sertoli cells.

At the time of presentation, the second, 19-month-old boy had blood E_2 and testosterone levels 40 and two-times normal, respectively; LH and FSH were prepubertal. Microscopy of the orchiectomized testis revealed typical SCTAT with occasional nests of Leydig-like cells. Possibly these accounted for the boy's mildly elevated testosterone level.

The older of the two sisters had a blood E_2 concentration 10-times normal despite prepubertal levels of LH and FSH basally, and prepubertal responses of them to LHRH stimulation. The histology of the mass in the ovary of each sister was that of SCTAT.

Genotyping.   The gene (*STK11*) that is responsible for P-J syndrome when it is mutated has recently been identified as encoding a novel serine threonine kinase that is composed of 433 amino acids (Jenne et al., 1998). Each of the first five un-related patients examined had a mutation that would be expected to truncate the kinase domain. *STK11* appears to act as a tumor-suppressor gene: germline muta-tions impose a pre-neoplastic (hamartomatous) state that is magnified by subse-quent somatic mutation(s) to one or more fully neoplastic conditions. The signaling pathway in which STK11 participates is unknown; hence, the manner in which its heterozygous deficiency causes the formation of benign harmartomas is also un-known (Jenne et al., 1998).

It has been determined that the Sertoli-like and granulosa-like cells, respectively, in the SCTAT of testes and ovaries of three boys and one girl with P-J syndrome use the regular (proximal) gonadal promoter (PII) for regulating the expression of the *CYP19* gene (Bulun et al., 1993a) (Fig 13–4). The neoplastic state is presumed to activate, or to prevent inhibition of, the PII promoter.

Management.   The oral aromatase inhibitor, testolactone, in a dose of 150 mg, three times a day, slows premature epiphyseal maturation and linear growth and, therefore, preserves ultimate height. Because of suboptimal response to this thera-peutic strategy, GnRH analogue has been used to achieve a more uniform inhibition of sex steroid production. Nonetheless, several affected boys required bilateral or-chiectomy for definitive control, in addition to mammoplasty for esthetic purposes (Bulun et al., 1993a). Likewise, affected girls have required bilateral ovariectomy (Sohl et al., 1983).

Discussion.   Mutant genes whose products cause disease by a "gain of function" are much less common than those that are pathogenic by a loss of function. Among all gain-of-function mutations, those due to the acquisition of a new function by the mutant product are much more common than those due simply to a gain in the amount of a normal function. Inherited aromatase excess, sufficient to cause isosexual precocity in girls or prepubertal gynecomastia in boys, falls into the last category. The apparent rarity of extraglandular aromatase excess may be largely a matter of suboptimal clinical recognition. For instance, women with complete an-drogen insensitivity who are castrated prepubertally for prophylactic purposes sometimes develop breasts. The normal levels of circulating estrogens in one such patient (Andler and Zachman, 1979) were not dexamethasone-suppressible, indi-cating their nonadrenal origin. This suggests that some normal women have mod-erate extraglandular aromatase excess that remains subclinical. In the context of androgen insensitivity, however, that same degree of aromatase excess becomes evident clinically. Similarly some aging men may develop more pronounced gy-necomastia than others because their lifelong state of aromatase excess is ultimately uncovered by the physiologic onset of androgen insufficiency.

Notwithstanding the apparent rarity of inherited aromatase excess, patients with it stimulate important suggestions about the dysregulation of aromatase expression, particularly in view of organ-specific differences in the promoters used for regu-lation. One suggestion is that a local, organ (skin or fat)-restricted form of aromatase excess may sometimes be responsible for gynecomastia that appears at the usual time during early puberty, but that is persistent rather than transient. Indeed, there is a single report of increased aromatase activity in the pubic skin fibroblasts of such men (Bulard et al., 1987). It is provocative to consider whether somatic or germinal mutations causing aromatase excess that is restricted to the female breast may sometimes be responsible for initiating or promoting breast cancer (Bulun et al., 1993b). Another suggestion is that testis-restricted aromatase excess may sometimes cause human male infertility.

The henny feathering trait of Sebright Bantam chickens is a genuine animal model of inherited extraglandular aromatase excess (George and Wilson, 1980). It is an autosomal dominant disorder in which aromatase excess is associated with the accumulation of aromatase mRNA in many organs, but primarily skin (and skin fibroblasts). The affected males develop a female feathering pattern; often they are infertile, thereby supporting the suggestion of a similar problem in some infertile men. The aberration of aromatase gene expression in mutant chickens is attributable to the use of a novel promoter, derived from a retroviral long terminal repeat, that is far upstream of the usual (proximal) promoter used by the gonads (Matsumine et al., 1991). The machanism(s) by which this particular promoter accomplishes aromatase gene expression in multiple organs (tissues), including the ovary, remains to be defined.

It is disputed whether the clinical expression of estrogen excess may derive, in part, from a direct androgen antagonist action at the peripheral target level and/ or from suppression of T secretion by a primary feedback effect on LH (Veldhuis et al., 1985). It is conceivable that the extreme sensitivity of prepubertal males to relatively small excesses of estrogen may be due to its multiple levels of action. The appropriate investigation of subjects with inherited aromatase excess may help to resolve this dispute.

Sertoli cells of the testis and granulosa cells of the ovary are considered to have homologous origins. Granulosa cells are prominently steroidogenic and estrogenic. Normal Sertoli cells are nonsteroidogenic and nonestrogenic. SCTAT shares histologic features with granulosa cell tumor and Sertoli cell tumor (Young et al., 1982). Neoplastic Sertoli cells are well known to be estrogenic, so it is not surprising that they are estrogenic when they are components of SCTAT. The regulatory mechanism that switches estrogenesis "on" in neoplastic Sertoli cells and "up" in neoplastic granulosa cells deserves attention.

REFERENCES

Andler W, Zachman M (1979). Spontaneous breast development in an adolescent girl with testicular feminization after castration in early childhood. *J Pediatr* 94:304–305.

Bulard J, Mowszowicz I, Schaison G (1987). Increased aromatase activity in pubic skin fibroblasts from patients with isolated gynecomastia. *J Clin Endocrinol Metab* 64:618–623.

Bulun S E, Rosenhal I M, Brodie A M H, Inkster S E, Zeller W P, DiGeorge A M, Frasier D, Kilgore M W, Simpson E R (1993). Use of tissue-specific promoters in the regulation of aromatase cytochrome P450 gene expression in human testicular and ovarian sex cord tumors, as well as in normal fetal and adult gonads. *J Clin Endocrinol Metab* 77:1616–1621.

Bulun S E, Price T M, Aitken J, Mahendross M S, Simpson E R (1993b). A link between breast cancer and local estrogen biosynthesis suggested by quantification of breast adipose tissue aromatase cytochrome P450 transcripts using competitive polymerase chain reaction after reverse transcription. *J Clin Endocrinol Metab* 77:1622–1628.

Cantu J M, Rivera H, Ocampo-Campos R, Bedolla N, Cortes-Gallegos V, Gonzalez-Mendoza

A, Diaz M, Hernandez A (1980). Peutz-Jeghers syndrome with feminizing Sertoli cell tumor. *Cancer* 46:223–228.

Coen P, Kulin H, Ballantine T, Zaino R, Frauenhoffer E, Boal D, Inkster S, Brodie A, Santen R (1991). An aromatase-producing sex-cord tumor resulting in prepubertal gynecomastia. *N Engl J Med* 324:317–322.

Dubois R S, Hoffman W H, Krishman T H, Rising J A, Tolia V K, Sy D A, Chang C H (1982). Feminizing sex cord tumor with annular tubules in a boy with Peutz-Jeghers syndrome. *J Pediatr* 101:568–571.

George F W, Wilson J D (1980). Pathogenesis of the henny feathering trait in the Sebright bantam chicken. *J Clin Invest* 66:57–65.

Giardiello F M, Welsh S B, Hamilton S R, Offerhaus G J A, Gittelsohn A M, Booker S V, Krush A J, Yardley J H, Luk G D (1987). Increased risk of cancer in the Peutz-Jeghers syndrome. *N Engl J Med* 316:1511–1514.

Jenne D E, Reimann H, Nezu J-i, Friedel W, Loff S, Jeschke R, Müller O, Back W, Zimmer M (1998). Peutz-Jeghers syndrome is caused by mutations in a novel serine threonine kinase. *Nat Genet* 18:38–43.

Matsumine H, Herbst M A, Ou S H I, Wilson J D, McPhaul M J (1991). Aromatase mRNA in the extragonadal tissues of chickens with the henny-feathering trait is derived from a distinctive promoter structure that contains a segment of a retroviral long terminal repeat. *J Biol Chem* 266:19900–19907.

Solh H M, Azoury R S, Najjar S S (1983). Peutz-Jeghers syndrome associated with precocious puberty. *J Pediatr* 103:593–595.

Stratakis C A, Vottero A, Brodie A, Kirschner S, DeAtkine D, Lu Q, Yue W, Mitsiades C S, Flor A W, Chrousos G P. The aromatase excess syndrome is associated with feminization of both sexes and autosomal dominant transmission of aberrant P450arom gene transcription. *J Clin Endocrinol Metab* 83:1348–1357, 1998.

Stratakis C A, Vottero A, Brodie A, DeArkine D, Lu O, Mitsiades C S, Yue W, Flor A W, Garnica A, Mitsiades C S, Chrousos G P. Biochemical and molecular genetics of the syndrome of increased aromatase activity: segregation with a marker from within the P450arom gene and evidence for aberrant alternative splicing of its 5'-end mRNA. *Am J Human Genet* 59: A43, 1996.

Veldhuis J D, Sowers J R, Rogol A D, Klein F A, Miller N, Dufau M M L (1985). Pathophysiology of male hypogonadism associated with endogenous hyperestrogenism. *N Engl J Med* 312:1371–1375.

Wallace E E, Garcia C R. Hereditary gynecomastia without hypogonadism. *J Clin Endocrinol* 22:1201–1206, 1962.

Wilson D M, Pitts W C, Hintz R L, Rosenfeld R G (1986). Testicular tumors with Peutz-Jeghers syndrome. *Cancer* 57:2238–2240.

Young R H, Welch W R, Dickersin G R, Scully R E (1982). Ovarian sex cord tumor with annular tubules. *Cancer* 50:1384–1402.

Young R H, Dickersin G R, Scully R E (1983). A distinctive ovarian sex cord-stromal tumor causing sexual precocity in the Peutz-Jeghers syndrome. *Am J Surg Pathol* 7:233–243.

Young S, Gooneratne S, Straus F H, Zeller W P, Bulun S E, Rosenthal I M (1995). Feminizing Sertoli cell tumors in boys with Peutz-Jeghers syndrome. *Am J Surg Pathol* 19:50–58.

Genetic Disorders of Combined Adrenocortical and Sex Steroidogenesis

In this important category, two classes of disorder can affect sexual development: in the first, both pathways of steroidogenesis are involved primarily, because the impairment occurs at one or another of the several biosynthetic steps common to

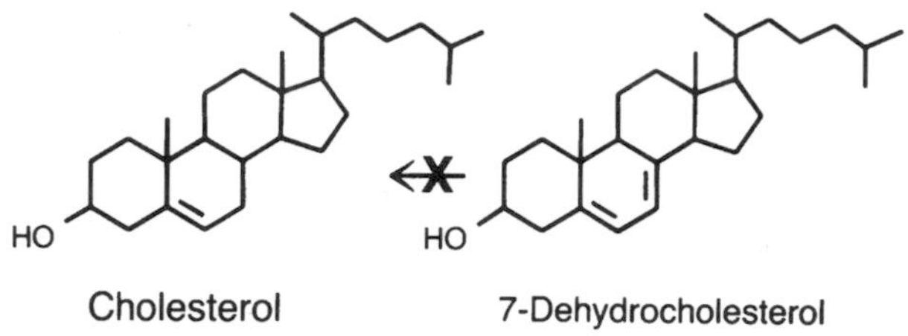

Cholesterol 7-Dehydrocholesterol

FIGURE 13–8. Deficiency of 7-dehydrocholesterol reductase in the Smith-Lemli-Opitz syndrome.

both; in the second, adrenocortical steroidogenesis is involved primarily, and gonadal steroidogenesis secondarily (for example, classical congenital adrenal hyperplasia due to 21-hydroxylase deficiency).

The first class includes deficiency of 7-dehydrocholesterol reductase, the enzyme responsible for the last step in the synthesis of cholesterol, and disorders of the following three complex enzyme systems (Fig. 13–1): one—mitochondrial—responsible for cleavage of the side chain between carbon atoms (C)-20 and-22 so that cholesterol can become pregnenolone; a second—microsomal—responsible, successively, for α-hydroxylation of C-17 and cleavage between C-17 and C-20, so that Δ^5-pregnenolone and Δ^4-progesterone can become 17α-hydroxylated before conversion to Δ^5-dehydroepiandrosterone (DHEA) and Δ^4-androstenedione, respectively; and, a third, also microsomal and bifunctional, responsible for Δ^5(double bond C-5, C-6) $\rightarrow \Delta^4$ (double bond C-3, C-4) isomerization and 3β-hydroxysteroid dehydrogenation, enabling the three Δ^5 compounds to become their respective Δ^4 versions.

We now consider each of the four disorders in sequence.

THE SMITH-LEMLI-OPITZ SYNDROME: A PROBABLE EXAMPLE OF COMBINED DEFECTIVE STEROIDOGENESIS DUE TO DEFICIENT SYNTHESIS OF CHOLESTEROL DE NOVO

The SLO syndrome is considered in this section of the book on the supposition that deficient steroid hormone production is likely to be a consequence of its basic biochemical defect. The SLO syndrome is an excellent example of an extremely variable autosomal recessive syndrome of congenital anomalies in which 46,XY males may be born with all degrees of external genital submasculinization: from micropenis and/or coronal hypospadias through frank ambiguity to unambiguous female external genitalia. Tint and colleagues (1994) found that patients had low plasma cholesterol but a high level of its biosynthetic precursor, 7-dehydrocholesterol (7-dC), implying a deficiency of the responsible enzyme, 3β-hydroxysteroid Δ^7-reductase (Fig. 13–8). They concluded that cholesterol insufficiency in cell membranes may be the ubiquitous dysmorphogenetic agent in SLO syndrome, but they did not question whether cell membranes might be injured by excessive cholesterol precursors. They predicted that prenatal diagnosis might be possible by measuring 7-dC in amniotic fluid, and they suggested that heterozygotes might be identifiable by a provocative test that challenged their reduced level of Δ^7-reductase activity. Interestingly, Tint and colleagues (1994) did not speculate on the possibility that cholesterol deficiency could lead to deficient steroid hormone synthesis, thereby contributing both to failure to thrive on the one hand and to external genital submasculinization on the other.

Clinical and Imaging Features.   Patients with SLO syndrome have a classical craniofacies that coarsens with age: it includes microcephaly, blepharoptosis, flat nasal bridge, anteverted nares, broad maxillary alveolus, and micrognathia. Mental retardation and failure to thrive are constant. Postaxial polydactyly, second-third toe syndactyly, cleft palate, and cataract are typical. Serious brain, cardiac, great vessel, and visceral anomalies are more likely if polydactyly and cleft palate are present and the external genitalia are female (Bialer et al., 1987). Imaging analysis will help to reveal various brain dysplasias (Trasimeni et al., 1997), cardiac and great vessel defects, urinary tract anomalies, and gastrointestinal defects such as Hirschsprung disease and malrotation. Ultrasonography will usually reveal absence of müllerian duct–derived structures, even in those XY males with completely female external genitalia.

Laboratory Features.   Excess 7-dC has also been found in red blood cells, lens, cultured skin fibroblasts, cerebrospinal fluid (van Rooij et al., 1997), and feces. Bile acids are severely decreased in fecal samples, reflecting a deficiency of cholesterol, their obligate precursor, and a 7α-hydroxylase, the rate-limiting enzyme in bile acid synthesis. Second-trimester amniotic fluid analysis of 7-dC and cholesterol by gas chromatography–mass spectrometry can yield a prenatal diagnosis (McGaughran et al., 1994). Prenatal diagnosis can also be made by first-trimester analysis of chorionic villi (Mills et al., 1996). The 7-dC:C ratio in plasma can suggest heterozygosity; it can be proven with skin fibroblasts (Shefer et al., 1997). Rapid screening for plasma 7-dC can be done by ultraviolet spectrometry (Honda et al., 1997). Thrombocytopenia and acanthocytosis responsive to cholesterol therapy have been observed in children around 10 years of age. Their neutrophil function was normal (Elias et al., 1997a).

Epidemiology.   The distribution of the SLO syndrome is panethnic. Its frequency is estimated to be between 1 in 20,000 to 40,000; in the Czech Republic, it may be as high as 1 in 9000 (Kelley, 1997).

Management.   Substantial biochemical improvement is noted when patients are treated with enteral cholesterol and bile acids (Tint et al., 1997). The bile acids are meant to help absorb cholesterol from the intestine. The results of two single-center (Elias et al. 1997b; Nwokoro and Mulvihill, 1997) and one multicenter (Irons et al. 1997) treatment trials have been reported recently. Because the developmental pathology is likely to begin in early prenatal life, dramatic amelioration would not be expected from the initiation of cholesterol replacement after birth. Nevertheless, it is gratifying to record that all three trials have, at least, noted improved growth and development. And the two single-center trials have revealed fewer behavioral and gastrointestinal problems, fewer and less severe injections, less skin rash, and reduced photosensitivity, among other benefits, such as pubertal progression and better socialization in older patients. To try a different treatment strategy, Jira and colleagues (1997) have used exchange transfusion and a HMG CoA reductase inhibitor in order to reduce cholesterol precursor concentration in one patient. The donor blood also raised the patient's plasma and erythrocyte membrane cholesterol, and there was clinical improvement. The long-term benefit of this approach needs to be assessed in a formal clinical trial.

Discussion and Speculation. The extreme clinical variability of the SLO syndrome led Curry and colleagues (1987) to suggest that there were two types based on severity. Indeed, the biochemical defect is the same, but more severe, in more severely affected type II patients (Tint et al., 1997). The breadth of the expressivity has prompted others to suggest that the SLO appellation be applied to various patients with external genital submasculinization together with nonsexual anomalies, including some otherwise considered to have the genito-palato-cardiac syndrome (Opitz et al., 1987). The validity of this suggestion will become clear once 7dC:C ratios have been done, and the SLO gene(s) has been cloned. The concurrence of the syndrome with certain translocations incriminates 7q32 as the candidate region (Alley et al., 1997).

To our knowledge, the question of adrenocorticosteroid deficiency in patients with SLO syndrome has been raised rarely (McKeever and Young, 1990), despite the fact that "large adrenals" are included among the "less common" abnormalities in SLO, type II (Curry et al., 1987). Yet the external genital undermasculinization of SLO males may, indeed, reflect deficient synthesis of androgenic steroids. In fact, Greene and colleagues (1984) reported an unusually low level of testosterone and a meager response to stimulation with human chorionic gonadotropin in one XY SLO infant with female external genitalia. The apparent discrepancy between adrenocorticosteroid and androgenic steroid production suggests that Leydig cell synthesis of androgenic steroids is more dependent on cholesterol synthesized *de novo* than is adrenal synthesis of corticosteroids. Other sources of cholesterol for steroid hormone synthesis include plasma cholesterol transported as part of low density lipoproteins, and storage forms of cholesterol esters from which cholesterol is released by the enzyme cholesterol esterase.

Experiments with cholesterol-deficient mice fed a cholesterol-synthesis inhibitor on days 4 to 7 of pregnancy have yielded offspring with malformations akin to those of the SLO syndrome. These results have been interpreted entirely in the context that cholesterol contributes importantly to the function of the sonic hedgehog morphogenetic protein (Lanoue et al., 1997).

A detailed review of the cholesterol synthesis defect in the SLO syndrome has appeared recently (Tint et al., 1997). Likewise, Ryan and colleagues (1998) have reviewed the clinical phenotype based on all known cases in the United Kingdom.

REFERENCES

Alley T L, Scherer S W, Huizenga J J, Tsui L-C, Wallace M R (1997). Physical mapping of the chromosome 7 breakpoint region in an SLOS patient with t(7;20)(q32.1;q13.2). *Am J Med Genet* 68:279–281.

Bialer M G, Penchaszadeh V B, Kahn E, Libes R, Kirgsman G, Lesser M L (1987). Female external genitalia and Müllerian duct derivatives in a 46,XY infant with the Smith-Lemli-Opitz syndrome. *Am J Med Genet* 28:723–731.

Curry C J R, Carey J C, Holland J S, Chopra D, Fineman R, Golabi M, Sherman S, Pagon R A,

Allanson J, Shulman S, et al. (1987). Smith-Lemli-Opitz syndrome-type II: multiple congenital anomalies with male pseudohermaphroditism and frequent early lethality. *Am J Med Genet* 26:45–57.

Elias E R, Irons M, Wolfe L C, Klempner M (1997a). Effect of cholesterol deficiency on erythrocytes and neutrophils in children with Smith-Lemli-Opitz syndrome (SLOS). *Am J Hum Genet* 61:A250, Abstract 1453.

Elias E R, Irons M B, Hurley A D, Tint S G, Salen G (1997b). Clinical effects of cholesterol supplementation in six patients with the Smith-Lemli-Opitz syndrome (SLOS). *Am J Med Genet* 68:305–310.

Greene C, Pitts W, Rosenfold R, Luzzatti I, (1984). Smith-Lemli-Opitz syndrome in two 46, XY infants with female external genitalia. *Clin Genet* 25:366–372.

Honda A, Batta A K, Salen G, Tint G S, Chen T S, Shefer S (1997). Screening for abnormal cholesterol biosynthesis in the Smith-Lemli-Opitz syndrome: rapid determination of plasms 7-dehydroxholesterol by ultraviolet spectrometry. *Am J Med Genet* 68:288–293.

Irons M, Elias E R, Abuelo D, Bull M J, Greene C L, Johnson V P, Keppen L, Schanen C, Tint G S, Salen G (1997). Treatment of Smith-Lemli-Opitz syndrome: results of a multicenter trial. *Am J Med Genet* 68:311–314.

Jira P, Wevers R, de Jong J, Rubio-Gozalbo E, Smeitink J (1997). New treatment strategy for Smith-Lemli-Opitz syndrome. *Lancet* 349:1222.

Kelley R I (1997). Editorial: A new face for an old syndrome. *Am J Med Genet* 68:251–256,

Lanoue L, Dehart D B, Hinsdale M E, Maeda N, Tint S, Sulik K K (1997). Limb, genital, CNS, and facial malformations result from gene/environment-induced cholesterol deficiency: further evidence for a link to sonic hedgehog. *Am J Med Genet* 73:24–31.

McGaughran J, Clayton P (1994). Diagnosis of Smith-Lemli-Opitz syndrome. *N Engl J Med* 330:1685–1686.

McKeever P A, Young I D (1990). Smith-Lemli-Opitz Syndrome II: a disorder of the fetal adrenals? *J Med Genet* 27:465–466.

Mills K, Mandel H, Montemagno R, Soothhill P, Gershoni-Baruch R, Clayton P T (1996). First trimester prenatal diagnosis of Smith-Lemli-Opitz syndrome (7-dehydrocholesterol reductase deficiency). *Pediatr Res* 39:816–819.

Nwokoro N A, Mulvihill J J (1997). Cholesterol and bile acid replacement therapy in children and adults with Smith-Lemli-Opitz (SLO/RSH) syndrome. *Am J Med Genet* 68:315–321.

Opitz J M, Penchaszadeh V C, Holt M C, Spano L M (1987). Smith-Lemli-Opitz (RSH) syndrome bibliography. *Am J Med Genet* 28:745–750.

Ryan A K, Bartlett K, Clayton P, Eaton S, Mills L, Donnai D, Winter R M, Burn J (1998). Smith-Lemli-Opitz syndrome: a variable clinical and biochemical phenotype. *J Med Genet* 35:558–565.

Shefer S, Salen G, Honda A, Batta A, Hauser S, Tint G S, Honda M, Chen T, Holick M F, Nguyen L B (1997). Rapid identification of Smith-Lemli-Opitz syndrome homozygotes and heterozygotes (carriers) by measurement of deficient 7-dehydrocholesterol-delta-7-reductase activity in fibroblasts. *Metabolism* 46:844–850.

Tint G S, Batta A K, Xu G, Shefer S, Honda A, Irons M, Elias E R, Salen G (1997). The Smith-Lemli-Opitz syndrome: a potentially fatal birth defect caused by a block in the last enzymatic step in cholesterol biosynthesis. *In*: Subcellular Biochemistry: Volume 28: Cholesterol: Its Functions and Metabolism in Biology and Medicine, Bittman R (ed), Plenum Press, New York, 117–144.

Tint G S, Irons M, Elias E R, Batta A K, Frieden R, Chen T S, Salen G. (1994). Defective cholesterol synthesis associated with the Smith-Lemli-Opitz syndrome. *N Engl J Med* 330: 107–113.

Trasimeni G, Di Biasi C, Iannilli M, Orlandi L, Boscherini B, Balducci R, Gualdi G F (1987). MRI in Smith-Lemli-Opitz syndrome type 1. *Childs Nerv Syst* 13:47–49.

van Rooij A, Nijenhuis A A, Wijburg F A, Schutgens R B (1997). Highly increased CSF concentrations of cholesterol precursors in Smith-Lemli-Opitz syndrome. *J Inherit Metab Dis* 20:578–580.

CONGENITAL LIPOID ADRENAL HYPERPLASIA (CLAH): DEFICIENT
CYTOCHROME P450 SIDE CHAIN CLEAVAGE (P450scc) ACTIVITY
DUE TO MUTATION IN THE STEROIDOGENIC ACUTE REGULATORY
(StAR) PROTEIN AS A CAUSE OF MALE PSEUDOHERMAPHRODITISM

CLAH is a severe autosomal recessive impairment of combined steroidogenesis.
The adrenal cortex and Leydig cells become loaded with cholesterol and with lipid
droplets containing cholesterol esters. Functionally, adrenal or gonadal mitochondria from patients have a cholesterol → pregnenolone block (Hauffa et al., 1985).
This suggested a defect in one of the three components of the cholesterol scc enzyme
system: two components form a chain to transfer electrons to P450scc. The latter
binds cholesterol and uses the electrons to convert it to Δ^5-pregnenolone. The electron transfer proteins are normal in CLAH, and in several patients no mutations
were found in CYP11A, the chromosome 15–linked gene encoding P450scc (Sakai
et al., 1994). In contrast, P450scc deletions have been found in the rabbit model of
CLAH (Yang et al., 1993). Recently, the search for a mutant gene product in human
CLAH turned, successfully, to a protein, StAR, that is evidently crucial for the
transport of cholesterol from the outer mitochondrial membrane to the matrix surface of the inner one, where P450scc resides (Fig. 13–9; Sugawara et al., 1995a).

Clinical and Imaging Presentation. Male or female infants affected by CLAH
may die neonatally if the pathophysiologic consequences of severe absolute mineralocorticoid and glucocorticoid deficiency are not recognized. Others can remain
well for months. The inability to make sufficient androgenic steroids means that all
affected males are born with unambiguous female external genitalia. Surprisingly,
these levels of androgenic steroid may permit wolffian duct differentiation into a
vas deferens and/or epididymis, occasionally in a vestigial form. There are no müllerian duct derivatives because müllerian regression by the anti-müllerian hormone
is essentially androgen-independent. The testes may be palpable in the inguinal
canals. At birth, hypermelanotic pigmentation of the skin creases, scars, the skin
over the knuckles, and the lips, labia, and nipples is common; this indicates fetal
glucocorticoid deficiency resulting in hypersecretion of ACTH. About one third of
the newborns have hypoglycemia and/or immature lung development (Bose et al.,
1996) despite normal birth weights and gestational lengths. At puberty, some affected females feminize and have ovulatory cycles that culminate in premature
ovarian failure. Ultrasonography will reveal adrenomegaly in both sexes and uterine absence, inguinal testes in affected males.

Laboratory Features. Maternal estriol levels are low. The secretion of various
adrenocortical and gonadal steroids into the blood will be unmeasurable, or barely
detectable (Hauffa et al., 1985), and the presence of various representative urinary
excretion products will be undetectable, or inappropriately low after stimulation
with ACTH or hCG. Hyponatremia and hyperkalemia vary appreciably, just as
symptomatic age-of-onset varies. ACTH and plasma renin activity are elevated, as
are LH and FSH at puberty.

Genotyping and Ethnic Considerations. The gene for StAR protein is at 8p11.2
It has seven exons, and its analysis may be complicated by an expressed pseudo-

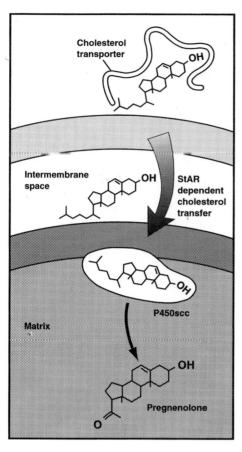

Cholesterol
transporter

OH

Intermembrane
space

OH

StAR
dependent
cholesterol
transfer

P450scc

Matrix

OH

Pregnenolone

O

FIGURE 13–9. A scheme of StAR action in promoting cholesterol transfer to the matrix surface of the inner mitochondrial membrane. (Reproduced from Root A W, *Growth Genet Horm* 4:7, 1995, with permission.)

gene on chromosome 13 (Sugawara et al., 1995b). To date, mendelian mutations have been detected in the StAR gene of 20 patients with CLAH (Lin et al., 1995; Tee et al., 1995; Bose et al., 1996). These patients are derived from several genetically distinct populations. Among five Korean and Japanese patients, eight of 10 affected alleles carried the same premature translation termination mutation at the codon for Gln258. Among six patients of Palestinian origin, seven of nine mutant alleles carried an Arg182Leu substitution. Each of these ethnically predominant mutations ablates or creates a recognition sequence for a restriction enzyme, thereby affording a simple PCR-based diagnostic test. A Caucasian patient is homozygous for a premature translation termination mutation at the codon for Arg193. A Vietnamese patient is homozygous for a single-base transversion 11bp from the splice-acceptor site of intron 4 in the StAR gene (Tee et al., 1995). The ethnic backgrounds of these particular 13 patients are not surprising in view of the fact that 18 of the first 32 reported patients with CLAH were of Japanese ancestry (Hauffa et al., 1985). Interestingly, a large fraction of the remaining 14 came from either Switzerland or southern Germany, an observation not borne out by the patients genotyped to date

(Bose et al., 1996). Importantly, among the 33 affected alleles, only two of 15 different mutations did not involve the C-terminal exons 5-7. The significance of this distribution is discussed in the section below.

Gene Expression.   StAR protein is synthesized as a 285-amino acid, 37-kd precursor that is processed to a 32.5-kd mature protein by removal of an N-terminal mitochondrial import sequence. It was assumed that the ability of the StAR protein to promote the mitochondrial import of cholesterol was dependent on its own mitochondrial import. But N-terminal deletion mutants of StAR protein still facilitate the transport of cholesterol to the inner mitochondrial membrane (Arakane et al., 1996). This suggests that StAR protein is active while still on the mitochondrial surface, and it implies that the C-terminal portion of the molecule is necessary and sufficient for its activity. This implication is supported by the great predominance of mutations affecting exons 5–7 of the StAR gene, and by the fact that some inactive missense mutations affecting exons 5–7 are, nevertheless, processed normally by mitochondria.

When COS-1 cells are transfected with a vector expressing the P450scc system, they secrete pregnenolone (synthesized from endogenous cholesterol) at a rate equal to 15% of that secreted by cells cotransfected with a vector expressing the StAR protein. This rate can be said to represent the StAR protein–independent level of steroidogenesis by COS-1 cells. Pregnenolone secretion by cells transfected with the vectors carrying Gln258X or Arg182Leu were indistinguishable from the basal level; those carrying Ala216Val or Leu275Pro were 50% to 60% higher. Of the two missense mutations discovered by Nakae and colleagues (1997), Ala218Val was inactive, but Met225Thr was partly functional, and the patient had a late-onset disorder.

Management   Appropriate hormone replacement together with skilled fluid and electrolyte support permits recovery from the initial acute episodes. Compliance with chronic therapy can lead to survival into adulthood. Female puberty can be initiated and maintained by serial combinations of estrogen and progesterone replacement. Notably, estrogen replacement at 12 years 10 months in one patient produced an adequate growth spurt, in the absence of androgens. The proper pubertal management of affected males includes adequate replacement of glucocorticoid, mineralocorticoid, and androgen. Genetic counseling would convey a 25% risk of recurrence in subsequent children, and the possibility of prenatal diagnosis (Saenger et al., 1995) would be entertained.

Discussion and Speculation.   The conversion of cholesterol to pregnenolone is the first committed step in steroid hormone biosynthesis; appropriately, it is the step that is stimulated by LH in the gonads or by ACTH in the adrenal cortex. The acute effect of these tropins is cAMP-mediated and is rate-limited by cholesterol transport into mitochondria. The chronic effect of the trophic hormones is also cAMP-mediated, but it depends on transactivation of genes that encode steroidogenic enzymes (Lin et al., 1995). The way in which the StAR protein promotes the transfer of cholesterol into mitochondria is not known. There is good evidence, however, that StAR protein does not "drag" cholesterol into mitochondria during its own import into this organelle. Indeed, it may be that StAR protein achieves its effect by acting on the outer mitochondrial membrane, and that its transport across that membrane serves to terminate its action (Arakane et al., 1996).

The StAR gene is not expressed in the placenta; expectedly, the placenta of fetuses affected by *StAR* mutations produces progesterone normally (Saenger et al., 1995). This suggests that the placenta uses a molecule other than StAR to promote cholesterol transport into or within its mitochondria. The same reasoning applies to brain (Lin et al., 1995).

The existence of mitochondrial cholesterol-transport proteins other than StAR (Yamamoto et al., 1991), makes it possible that mutations of genes other than *StAR* will be found to be responsible for some patients with phenocopies of CLAH. Contrarily, Miller (1998) has recently explained why mutations of the P450 side chain cleavage (SCC) system are very unlikely to be found in humans. In rabbits, progesterone is secreted by the corpus luteum throughout pregnancy; in humans, placental progesterone, made by fetal syncytiotrophoblasts, supervenes at about 6 weeks gestation, when corpus luteum progesterone shuts down. Anything that severely impairs placental progesterone production, including a defective P450scc system, will cause spontaneous miscarriage.

Bose and colleagues (1996) have offered interesting interpretations of various sex-specific features in the organismal expression of human CLAH. Thus, the testis is normally actively steroidogenic in early fetal life, so one would expect severe autotoxicity due to cholesterol ester accumulation in the testis of affected males. Such autotoxicity would eliminate the basal level of StAR-independent steroidogenesis in such testes and would explain why affected males never have even slight evidence of partial external genital masculinization, such as clitoromegaly or posterior labial fusion.

Likewise, the fetal adrenal cortex of both sexes normally secretes large amounts of dehydroepiandrosterone that are converted to estriol placentally. Autotoxicity for the reasons defined above culminates in low plasma estriol levels in women with affected fetuses.

In contrast, the ovary is steroidogenically inert until puberty, and even then it is active only inconstantly during the cyclic recruitment of cohorts of follicles for possible ovulation. Hence, the affected ovary remains sufficiently active steroidogenically to account for the initiation of menstruation and some features of feminization in some affected females.

The sex ratio of human CLAH is apparently highly skewed toward males. Only three of 21 patients studied by Bose and colleagues (1996) were 46,XX females, and of 63 Japanese patients surveyed by Matsuo and colleagues (1994) only 16 were. Among the possible reasons for this sex bias are (1) disadvantaged 23,X sperm, (2) loss of 46,XX fetuses in early pregnancy, and (3) a higher rate of underdiagnosis in female than in male infants.

REFERENCES

Arakane F, Sugawara T, Nishino H, Liu Z, Holt J A, Pains K, Stocco D M, Miller W L, Strauss J F III (1996). Steroidogenic acute regulatory protein (StAR) retains activity in absence of its mitochondrial import sequence: implications for the mechanism of StAR action. *Proc Natl Acad Sci USA* 93:13731–13736.

Bose H S, Sugawara T, Strauss III J F Miller W L (1996). The pathophysiology and genetics of congenital lipoid adrenal hyperplasia. *N Engl J Med* 335:1870–1878, 1996.

Hauffa B P, Miller W L, Grumbach M M, Conte F A, Kaplan S L (1985). Congenital adrenal hyperplasia due to deficient cholesterol side-chain cleavage activity (20, 22 desmolase) in a patient treated for 18 years. *Clin Endocrinol* 23:481–493.

Lin D, Sagawara T, Strauss III J F Clark B J, Stocco D M, Saenger P, Rogol A, Miller W L (1995). Role of steroidogenic acute regulatory protein in adrenal and gonadal steroidogenesis. *Science* 267:1828–1831.

Matsuo N, Tsuzaki S, Anzo M, Ogata T, Sato S (1994). The phenotypic definition of congenital lipoid adrenal hyperplasi: analysis of the 67 Japanese patients. *Horm Res* 41: suppl: 106. Abstract.

Miller W L (1998). Why nobody has P450scc (20, 22 desmolase) deficiency. *J Clin Endocrinol Metab* 83:1399–1400.

Nakae J, Tajima T, Sugawara T, Arakane F, Hanaki K, Hotsubo T, Igarashi N, Igarashi Y, Ishii T, Koda N, Kondo T, Kohno H, Nakagawa Y, Tachibana K, Takeshima Y, Tsubouchi K, Strauss J F III, Fujieda K (1997). Analysis of the steroidogenic acute regulatory protein (StAR) gene in Japanese patients with congenital lipoid adrenal hyperplasia. *Hum Mol Genet* 6:571–576.

Saenger P, Klonari Z, Black S M, Compagnone N, Mellon S H, Fleischer A, Abrams C A L, Shackleton C H L, Miller W L (1995). Prenatal diagnosis of congenital lipoid adrenal hyperplasia. *J Clin Endocrinol Metab* 80:200–205.

Sakai Y, Yanase T, Okabe Y, Hara T, Waterman M R, Takayanagi R, Haji M, Nawata H (1994). No mutation in cytochrome P450 side chain cleavage in a patient with congenital lipoid adrenal hyperplasia. *J Clin Endocrinol Metab* 79:1198–1201.

Sugawara T, Lin D, Holt J A, Martin K O, Javitt N B, Miller W L, Strauss J F III (1995a). The structure of the human steroidogenic acute regulatory (StAR) protein gene: StAR stimulates mitochondrial cholesterol 27-hydroxylase. *Biochemistry* 34:12506–12512.

Sugawara T, Holt J A, Driscoll D, Strauss J F III, Lin D, Miller W L, Patterson D, Clancy K P, Hart I M, Clark B J, Stocco D M (1995b). Human steroidogenic acute regulatory protein (StAR): functional activity in COS cells, tissue-expression, mapping of the structural gene to 8p11.2 and an expressed pseudogene to chromosome 13. *Proc Natl Acad Sci. USA* 92: 4778–4782.

Tee M K, Lin D, Sugawara T, Holt J A, Guiguen Y, Buckingham B, Strauss J F III (1995). T → A transversion 11 bp from a splice acceptor site in the gene for steroidogenic acute regulatory protein causes congenital lipoid adrenal hyperplasia. *Hum Mol Genet* 4:2299–2305.

Yamamoto R, Calen C B, Bahalola G O, Rennert H, Bilheimer J T, Strauss J F III (1991). Cloning and expression of a cDNA encoding human sterol carrier protein 2. *Proc Natl Acad Sci USA* 88:463–467.

Yang X, Iwamoto K, Wang M, Artwohl J, Mason J L, Pang S (1993). Inherited congenital adrenal hyperplasia in the rabbit is caused by a deletion in the gene encoding cytochrome P450 cholesterol side-chain cleavage enzyme. *Endocrinology* 132:1977–1982.

P450c17 DEFICIENCY

P450c17 is a bifunctional enzyme responsible for sequential 17α-hydroxylase and 17,20-lyase activities in the pathways of steroidogenesis (Fig. 13–1, 13–10,). Mutations that impair both activities reduce the production of cortisol, androgen, and estrogen, but increase production of certain mineralocorticoids. Both activities may be lost nearly completely (85%) or significant residual activities (15%) may be expressed (Yanase, 1995). About 130 cases have been reported, and approximately 10% seem to have a selective form of 17,20-lyase deficiency that spares adrenocortical steroidogenesis but impairs gonadal steroidogenesis (Yanase et al., 1991).

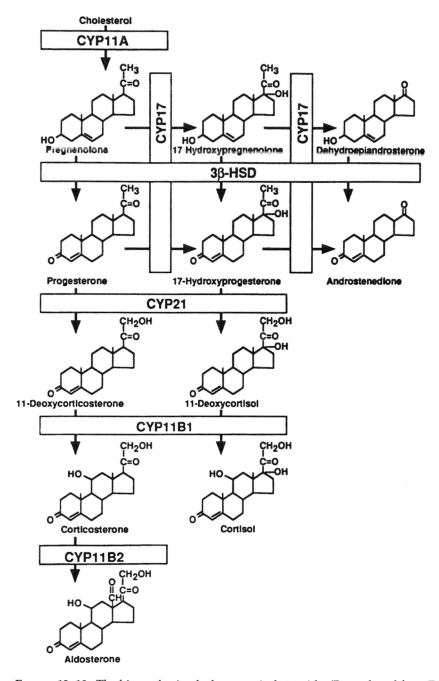

FIGURE 13–10. The biosynthesis of adrenocortical steroids. (Reproduced from Donohoue P A, Parker K, Migeon C J (1995). Congenital adrenal hyperplasia. Scriver C R, Beaudet A L, Sly W S, Valle D (eds). *Metabolic and Molecular Bases of Inherited Disease*, 7th ed., New York, McGraw-Hill, pp. 2929–2966.)

Recently, Geller and colleagues (1997) have reported a genetic and functional basis for "isolated" 17,20-lyase deficiency. The *CYP17* gene is located at 10q24.3 (Fan et al., 1992). It has eight exons encoding 508 amino acids. The sequence between residues 435 and 455 in exon 8 constitutes the heme-binding portion of the enzyme, and Cys442, specifically, binds to the heme iron (Yanase, 1995).

Clinical and Imaging Features.   The severe deficiency of P450c17 impairs androgen production sufficiently to cause the appearance of female external genitalia in XY males and sexual infantilism in 46,XX females at puberty. Deficient cortisol synthesis causes a compensatory elevation of ACTH levels with consequent excess of mineralocorticoid production. This causes hypertension and hypokalemia. *CYP17* mutations that are less severe permit some degree of external genital masculinization in 46,XY males and may permit some degree of pubertal feminization with menstruation in 46,XX females (Oshiro et al., 1995). Ultrasonography reveals no uterus in males, and uterine hypoplasia in females. Adrenomegaly is detectable by computed tomography.

Laboratory Features.   Expectedly, the plasma levels of precursors to the P450c17 block, such as pregnenolone and progesterone, are elevated, while the levels of their respective products are depressed. Despite overproduction of corticosterone and 11-deoxycorticosterone by the mineralocorticoid pathway, plasma levels of aldosterone are usually low because the renin-angiotensin system is, in turn, suppressed. Hypokalemia and hypertension are not always seen, even when the levels of these mineralocorticoid precursors are clearly elevated (Laflamme et al., 1996). Occasionally, plasma aldosterone is inexplicably high (Yanase et al., 1991).

Genotyping and Gene Expression.   To mid-1995, 18 different mutations had been described in 27 individuals with deficient P450c17 activity. Four different single missense mutations have been described that completely eliminate both P450c17 activities. These mutations extend from Tyr64Ser to Arg496Cys. A fine structure-function map of P450c17 will be necessary to interpret the functional significance of particular point mutations in the *CYP17* gene. Nevertheless, some inferences have already been drawn from a model of the human enzyme based on the three-dimensional state of a bacterial P450 enzyme. Thus, Ser106Pro may impair substrate binding (Lin et al., 1994), and His 273Leu and Arg440His (close to Cys442) likely affect heme (heme iron) binding. None of these mutants, nor Arg96Trp, had appreciable residual activity, whereas Tyr64Ser had 15% residual activity when expressed in *E. coli*. Likewise, Pro342Thr had 20% residual activity in transfected COS-1 cells.

In rat P450c17, experimental mutagenesis of Arg346Ala causes selective loss of 17,20-lyase activity; Arg357Ala loses twice as much lyase as hydroxylase activity (Kitamura et al., 1991). In this context, it is striking to learn that homozygosity for Arg347His (rat Arg346) was recently found in one XY patient with ambiguous external genitalia due to selective 17,20-lyase activity (Geller et al, 1997). His parents were consanguineous. A second male patient with the same enzyme defect, and a similar clinical phenotype of external genitalia ambiguity, was homozygous for Arg358Gln (rat 357). In coexpression studies performed on COS-1 cells, Geller and colleagues (1997) determined that these two human mutations cause isolated 17,20-lyase deficiency, not by impaired substrate or cofactor binding, but by impaired electron transfer (or electron coupling). This interpretation is supported by computer-graphic modeling studies indicating that Arg347His and Arg358Gln change the surface electrostatic charge distribution in the portion of human P450c17 that contains the P450 reductase-binding site.

Gene expression studies have revealed that 46,XY individuals with about 20% residual 17,20-lyase activity may have sufficient masculinization to be born with ambiguous external genitalia (Yanase et al., 1992; Ahlgren et al., 1992). Similarly, in 46,XX females about 5% of residual activity is sufficient to support irregular menstruation (Yanase, 1995).

Ethnic Considerations. A four-base-pair duplication starting at codon 480 has been found in seven different families in Holland and in two different Canadian families belonging to the Mennonite religious sect.

Both patients with isolated 17,20-lyase activity studied by Geller and colleagues (1997) came from the same rural village in Brazil. They were unrelated. Homozygosity for different mutations in a single gene has been reported in various population isolates (see Geller et al., 1997), and it has been suggested that the phenomenon may be common (Zlotogora et al., 1996).

Discussion and Speculation. One XY patient with a female phenotype who was thought to have selective lyase deficiency at age 15 evolved into a state of combined hydroxylase-lyase deficiency by age 25 (Yanase et al., 1992). In fact, he is a compound heterozygote for two point mutations, and expression studies have revealed very little of either activity, in conformity with his adult phenotype. The reason for the temporal change is enigmatic. However, Zhang and colleagues (1995) have made the interesting observations that the 17,20-lyase activity of P450c17 in adrenal cortex is age-dependent by a mechanism that depends on hormonal regulation of serine-threonine phosphorylation. On the basis of this observation, they have postulated that adrenarche results from IGF-1 stimulation of a cAMP-dependent kinase that mediates such phosphorylation.

So far, studies on the regulation of *CYP17* expression have been limited to the porcine (Zhang et al., 1996) and bovine (Bakke and Lund, 1995) genes. Both have cAMP-responsive elements. The bovine gene has two such elements, and the SF-1 or COUP transcription factors bind to a part of one of them in a way that excludes the binding of the other. SF-1 promotes expression, and cAMP is complementary, whereas COUP is inhibitory (Bakke and Lund, 1995).

REFERENCES

Ahlgren R, Yanase T, Simpson E R, Winter J, Waterman M R (1992). Compound heterozygous mutations (Arg 239 → stop, Pro 342 → Thr) in the CYP17 (P45017α) gene lead to ambiguous external genitalia in male patient with partial combined 17α-hydroxylase/17,20-lyase deficiency. *J Clin Endocrinol Metab* 74:667–672.

Bakke M, Lund J (1995). Mutually exclusive interactions of two nuclear orphan receptors determine activity of a cyclic adenosine 3', 5'-monophosphate-responsive sequence in the bovine *CYP17* gene. *Mol Endocrinol* 9:327–339.

Fan Y S, Sasi R, Lee C, Winter J S D, Waterman M R, Lin C C (1992). Localisation of the human CYP17 gene (cytochrome P450 17α) to 10q24.3 by fluorescence *in situ* hybridization and simultaneous chromosome banding. *Genomics* 14:1110–1111.

Geller D H, Auchus R J, Mendonça B B, Miller W L (1997). The genetic and functional basis of isolated 17,20-lyase deficiency. *Nat Genet.* 17:201–205.

Kitamura M, Buczko E, Dufau M L (1991). Dissociation of hydroxylase and lyase activities by site-directed mutagenesis of the rat P450-17α. *Mol Endocrinol* 5:1373–1380.

Laflamme N, Leblanc J-F, Mailloux J, Faure N, Labrie F, Simard J (1996). Mutation R96W in cytochrome P450c17 gene causes combined 17α-hydroxylase/17-20-lyase deficiency in two French Canadian patients. *J Clin Endocrinol Metab* 81:264–268.

Lin D, Zhang L-H, Chiao E, Miller W L (1994). Modeling and mutagenesis of the active site of human P450c17. *Mol Endocrinol* 8:392–402.

Oshiro C, Takasu N, Wakugami T, Komiya I, Yamada T, Eguchi Y, Takei H (1995). Seventeen α-hydroxylase deficiency with one base pair deletion of the cytochrome P450c17 (*CYP17*) gene. *J Clin Endocrinol Metab* 80:2526–2529.

Yanase T (1995). 17α-hydroxylase/17,20-lyase defects. *J Steroid Biochem Mol Biol* 53:153–157.

Yanase T, Imai T, Simpson E R, Waterman M R (1992). Molecular basis of 17α-hydroxylase/17,20 lyase deficiency. *J Steriod Biochem Mol Biol* 43:973–979.

Yanase T, Simpson E R, Waterman M R (1991). 17α-hydroxylase/17,20-lyase deficiency: from clinical investigation to molecular definition. *Endoc Rev* 12:91–108.

Zhang P, Han X G, Mellon S H, Hall P F (1996). Expression of the gene for cytochrome P-450 17 alpha-hydroxylase/C17-20 lyase (CYP17) in porcine Leydig cells: identification of a DNA sequence that mediates cAMP response. *Biochim. Biophys. Acta* 1307:73–82.

Zhang L-H, Rodriguez H, Ohno S, Miller W L (1995). Serine phosphorylation of human P450c17 increases 17,20-lyase activity: implications for adrenarche and the polycystic ovary syndrome. *Proc Natl Acad Sci USA* 92:10619–10623.

Zlotogora J, Gieselmann V, Bach G (1996). Multiple mutations in a specific gene in a small geographic area: a common phenomenon? *Am J Hum Genet* 58:241–243.

Genetic Disorders of 3β-Hydroxysteroid Dehydrogenase/$\Delta^5 \rightarrow \Delta^4$-ene Isomerase (3β-HSD)

Humans have two highly homologous 3β-HSD genes (types I and II) and three pseudogenes. The five genes form a gene family that is located tandemly in the region of 1p13.1, near the centromeric marker D1Z5 (Simard et al., 1995a). Not surprisingly, the comparable mouse genes are linked on a portion of chromosome 3 that is orthologous with human chromosome 1 (Payne et al., 1995). The type I (*HSD* 3B1) and type II (*HSD* 3B2) genes each have four exons. They share 77% to 94% homology exonically, and 74% to 84% intronically and in the 5' flanking region. The type I gene occupies 7.8 kb and encodes 372 amino acids; the type II occupies 7.7 kb and encodes 371 amino acids. The types I and II isoenzymes each catalyze the oxidative conversion of all Δ^5-ene-3β-hydroxysteroids into their respective Δ^4-ene-3-ketosteroids (Figs. 13–1 and 13–10). NAD$^+$ is the preferred cofactor for the 3β-HSD activity. Type I gene expression predominates in the placenta and diverse peripheral tissues (skin, mammary gland). The type II gene is expressed predominantly in the adrenal glands and gonads. Expectedly, mutations in the type II gene interfere with the synthesis of mineralocorticoids, glucocorticoids, progesterone, androgens, and estrogens. Severe mutations cause congenital adrenal hyperplasia with salt-losing crises, markedly undermasculinized external genitalia in 46,XY males and, occasionally, clitoromegaly at birth in 46,XX females. Milder mutations may not cause salt loss despite pseudohermaphroditism in 46,XY males, and premature pubarche, acne (Medonça et al., 1994), hirsutism, or clitoromegaly in affected 46,XX women (Rhéaume et al., 1994; Russell et al., 1994; Mébarki et al., 1995). The diverse distribution of the type I isoenzyme explains a biochemical paradox in the diagnosis of these mutations: the absolute levels of the Δ^4-ene compounds may be elevated, even when the ratio of Δ^5-ene to Δ^4-ene compounds is also elevated. Likewise, the activity of the type I isoenzyme presumably explains the masculinization/virilization of some affected 46,XX females.

Clinical and Imaging Features. This disorder was originally described by Bongiovanni in 1962. In the absence of a premonitory family history, the severe form is diagnosed in 46,XX females within a few weeks to months because of circulatory collapse due to salt loss. In 46,XY males, the diagnosis should be sought even earlier in the course of pursuing an explanation for incomplete masculinization of the external genitalia extending to third-degree perineoscrotal hypospadias. If the diagnosis is not made in that context, then it should be stimulated by premature pubarche with or without a early growth spurt. In 46,XX females not affected by salt loss, diagnosis is occasionally precipitated by congenital clitoromegaly or posterior labial fusion. It is usually held up until premature pubarche occurs with or without signs of premature, excessive virilization (acne, hirsutism, clitoromegaly) and a early growth spurt. Ultimately delayed menarche (primary amenorrhea) will bring the 46,XX female to diagnostic attention. Internal male wolffian duct derivatives may be seen in 46,XY affected males (Russell et al., 1994). Polycystic ovaries may be visible by ultrasound examination.

Laboratory Features. An elevated plasma ratio of Δ^5-ene to Δ^4-ene steroids, representing depressed isomerase activity, is the most sensitive measurement for the diagnosis of 3β-HSD deficiency. However, the absolute levels of plasma 17-hydroxyprogesterone and Δ^4-androstenedione may also be elevated. Presumably, the latter elevations represent the action of the type I isoenzyme on Δ^5-ene precursors produced in the adrenal cortex and gonads and released into the circulation for peripheral conversion to their Δ^4-ene counterparts.

Genotyping, Ethnic Considerations, and Gene Expression. Simard and colleagues (1995a,b) and Tajima and colleagues (1995) summarized data on 11 different point mutations among 11 families with severe (classic) 3β-HSD deficiency. Interestingly, Trp171 stop was found in four families (two Swiss, two American), Arg249 stop in two Japanese families, and the frameshift deletion due to deletion of two adenines at codon 273 was reported in three Afghan/Pakistani families; it has since been reported in a fourth Pakistani family (Zhang et al., 1996). Appropriately, very little residual enzyme activity was measurable in intact COS-1 cells transfected with cDNA expression vectors carrying any of the clinically severe mutations. Interestingly, the Gly15Asp mutant enzyme had appreciably more activity in COS-1 cell homogenates than in intact cells, suggesting that intracellular compartmentation is an important determinant of its biological activity.

Simard and colleagues (1995b) also summarized seven different point mutations in *HSD3B2* among six families with the non-salt-losing form of 3β-HSD deficiency. The Ala82Thr mutation was found in two Brazilian families. Strikingly, in one of the Brazilian families, a 46,XY female was affected cryptically; in a second family, another 46,XX female had Tanner III pubic hair and acne at 5 years of age (Mendonça et al., 1994). The residual activity of the Ala82Thr mutation was 12% of normal in intact transfected cells or glycerol-treated cell homogenates, but was much less in untreated homogenates, suggesting a problem in the binding of enzyme to intracellular membranes. On the other hand, the analysis of other mutants in the non-salt-losing category revealed that the absence of salt-losing crises could be correlated with very little enzyme activity, if the limited capacity to synthesize aldosterone was compensated by a high level of plasma renin.

Management. Salt losers require glucocorticoid and mineralocorticoid replacement therapy throughout life. The glucocorticoid not only fulfills the need for itself as an end product, but it serves to restore normal feedback regulation on the pituitary-adrenal axis, so that the generation of androgenic precursors is limited. Males with external genital undermasculinization may require staged reconstructive surgery before and after androgen replacement. Females with external genital masculinization may also require reconstructive surgery, as well as estrogen replacement at the time of puberty.

Discussion and Speculation. The paradoxical juxtaposition of impaired external genital undermasculinization in males with a tendency to congenital overmasculinization in females is explained by the fact that the 3β-HSD type II deficiency causes insufficient gonadal androgen synthesis for normal male development, but permits sufficient conversion of androgen precursors to androgens by extraglandular tissue to produce masculinization of females. Likewise, the relatively normal wolffian duct development into internal male genitalia must mean that this process is relatively less dependent on testicular androgens, or that wolffian duct tissue can make its own androgens, or that androgenic precursors can somehow bind to the androgen receptor in wolffian duct tissue. The fact that the type I 3β-HSD has a 10-fold higher affinity than the type II isoenzyme for the same substrates is commensurate with the likelihood that the type I must normally deal with lower levels of substrate. Conversely, the higher affinity can explain the efficiency with which it converts precursors that accumulate behind the type II block into active androgens.

The dysfunctional properties of particular missense mutations have begun to help illuminate the structure-function attributes of the 3β-HSD type II isozyme. Thus, the L108W and P186L mutants have decreased affinity both for the substrate, pregnenolone, and the cofactor, NAD^+ (Sanchez et al., 1994).

Some girls with premature pubarche and some women with hirsutism have modestly or moderately increased Δ^5-steroid levels, and Δ^5 to Δ^4 steroid ratios. By analogy with late-onset (non-classic) forms of 21-hydroxylase deficiency, these girls and women were assumed to have relatively mild mutations in the 3β-HSD type II gene. This assumption has been negated by several recent studies (Chang et al., 1995; Zerah et al., 1994).

REFERENCES

Bongiovanni A M (1962). The andrenogenital syndrome with deficiency of 3β-hydroxysteroid dehydrogenase. *J Clin Invest* 41:2086–2092.

Chang Y T, Zhang L, Alkaddour H S, Mason J I, Lin K, Yang X, Garibaldi L R, Bourdony C J, Dolan L M, Donaldson D L, Pang S (1995). Absence of molecular defect in the type II 3β-hydroxysteroid dehydrogenase (3β-HSD) gene in premature pubarche children and hirsute female patients with moderately decreased adrenal 3β-HSD activity. *Pediatr Res* 37: 820–824.

Mébarki F, Sanchez R, Rhéaume E, Laflamme N, Simard J, Forest M G, Bey-Omar F, David M, Labrie F, Morel Y (1995). Nonsalt-losing male pseudohermaphroditism due to the novel homozygous N100S mutation in the type II 3β-hydroxysteroid dehydrogenase gene. *J Clin Endocrinol Metab* 80:2127–2134.

Mendonça B B, Russell A J, Vasconcelos-Leite M, Arnhold I J P, Bloise W, Wajchenberg B L, Nicolau W, Sutcliffe R G, Wallace A M (1994). Mutation in 3β-hydroxysteroid dehydrogenase type II associated with pseudohermaphroditism in males and premature pubarche or cryptic expression in females. *J Mol Endocrinol* 12:119–122.

Payne A H, Clarke T R, Bain P A (1995). The murine 3β-hydroxysteroid dehydrogenase multigene family: structure, function and tissue-specific expression. *J Steroid Biochem Mol Biol* 53:111–118.

Rhéaume E, Sanchez R, Simard S, Chang Y T, Wang J, Pang S, Labrie F (1994). Molecular basis of congenital adrenal hyperplasia in two siblings with classical nonsalt-losing 3β-hydroxysteroid dehydrogenase deficiency. *J. Clin Endocrinol Metab* 79:1012–1018.

Russell A J, Wallace A M, Forest M G, Donaldson M D C, Edwards C R W, Sutcliffe R G (1994). Mutation in the human gene for 3β-hydroxysteroid dehydrogenase type II leading to male pseudohermaphroditism without salt loss. *J Mol Endocrinol* 12:225–237.

Sanchez R, Mébarki F, Rhéaume E, Laflamme N, Forest M G, Bey-Omard F, David M, Morel Y, Labrie F, Simard J (1994). Functional characterization of the novel L108W and P186L mutations detected in the type II 3β-hydroxysteroid dehydrogenase gene of a male pseudohermaphrodite with congenital adrenal hyperplasia. *Human Mol Genet* 3:1639–1645.

Simard J, Rheaume E, Mébarki F, Sanchez R, New M I, Morel Y, Labrie F (1995a). Molecular basis of human 3β-hydroxysteroid dehydrogenase deficiency. *J Steroid Biochem Mol Biol* 53:127–138.

Simard J, Sanchez R, Durocher F Rhéaume E, Turgeon C, Labrie Y, Luu-The V, Mébarki F, Morel Y, de Launoit Y, Labrie F (1995b). Structure-function relationships and molecular genetics of the 3β-hydroxysteroid dehydrogenase gene family. *J Steroid Biochem Mol Biol* 55:489–505.

Tajima T, Fujieda K, Nakae J, Shinohara N, Yoshimoto M, Baba T, Kinoshita E-I, Igarashi Y, Oomura T (1995). Molecular analysis of type II 3β-hydroxysteroid dehydrogenase gene in Japanese patients with classical 3β-hydroxysteroid dehydrogenase deficiency. *Hum Mol Genet* 4:969–971.

Zerah M, Rhéaume E, Mani P, Schram P, Simard J, Labrie F, New M I (1994). No evidence of mutations in the genes for type I and type II 3β-hydroxysteroid dehydrogenase (3βHSD) in nonclassical 3βHSD deficiency. *J Clin Endocrinol Metab* 79:1811–1817.

Zhang L, Sakkal-Alkaddour H, Chang Y T, Yang X, Pang S (1996). A new compound heterozygous frameshift mutation in the type II 3β-hydroxysteroid dehydrogenase (3β-HSD) gene causes salt-wasting 3β-HSD deficiency congenital adrenal hyperplasia. *J Clin Endocrinol Metab* 81:291–295.

CLASSIC (C; CONGENITAL) AND NONCLASSIC (NC; LATE-ONSET) ADRENAL HYPERPLASIA (AH) DUE TO 21-HYDROXYLASE (P450c21) DEFICIENCY

P450c21 is responsible for catalysis of progesterone (P) to deoxycorticosterone (DOC) in the aldosterone biosynthetic pathway, and for 17-OH-P to 11-deoxycortisol in the cortisol biosynthetic pathway (Fig. 13–10). The precursors and substrates that accumulate behind each of these blocks are detoured into the pathway of androgen biosynthesis. The resulting products are weak androgens them-

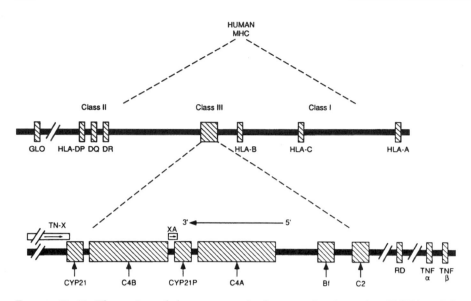

FIGURE 13–11. The region of chromosome 6p that contains the active *CYP21* and the *CYP21P* pseudogene. (Reproduced from Donohoue P A, Parker K, Migeon C J (1995). Congenital adrenal hyperplasia. Scriver C R, Beaudet A L, Sly W S, Valle D (eds). *Metabolic and Molecular Bases of Inherited Disease*, 7th ed., New York, McGraw-Hill, pp. 2929–2966.) The CYP21 and C4 (fourth component of complement) genes are duplicated in tandem.

selves, but are converted to potent androgens extra-adrenally. The gene for P450c21, *CYP21*, lies in the HLA complex of loci on 6p (Fig. 13–11). It is part of a group of genes that is duplicated in tandem: the other genes are *C4A* and *C4B* (for the fourth complement component), and *XA* and *XB* (for tenascin-X), an extracellular matrix protein (Bristow et al., 1993). Both C4 genes are expressed. The *CYP21P* and *XA* genes lack open reading frames. The region of 6p housing the HLA complex is also the site of frequent recombination. This is mirrored in the unusual array of mutations in *CYP21* that cause P450c21 deficiency.

Clinical and Imaging Features. P450c21 deficiency is responsible for at least 95% of cases of CAH. About two thirds of affected patients have the "salt-losing" (SL) form because they are seriously deficient in aldosterone as well as cortisol. Untreated, these infants will die in early infancy of hyponatremia, hyperkalemia, hypovolemia, and acidosis. This is less likely to happen in 46,XX females, who are more likely to be diagnosed and treated early because their external genitalia are more or less masculinized at birth. They may have simple clitoromegaly, labioscrotal fusion with a phallic urethra or, rarely, a penis and a nonhypospadic scrotum with bilateral cryptorchidism. Pelvic ultrasonography will reveal a uterus.

One third of the patients with apparently normal aldosterone biosynthesis are said to have the "simple virilizing" (SV) form. Interestingly, affected males do not have macropenis at birth. Postnatally, untreated males and females may grow rapidly, close their epiphyses early, have short stature, and express a form of androgenic pseudoprecocity. At puberty, females have absent or irregular menses, a small uterus and polycystic ovaries (Salardi et al., 1988). Males, at puberty, have a form of isosexual pseudoprecocity. Importantly, however, their testes remain relatively small compared to males with true (central) precocious puberty. Males with CAH may develop intratesticular masses representing hyperplastic ectopic adrenal tissue. These are detectable by gray-scale and color Doppler ultrasonography (Avila et al., 1996).

Nonclassic P450c21 deficiency is typically expressed in females at puberty by hirsutism, acne, and oligomenorrhea or amenorrhea (Azziz et al., 1994). It is particularly difficult to distinguish the SV from the NC form in males. In fact, there is a clinical continuum between the SV and NC forms in both sexes. This is a reflection of the appreciable mutational diversity in the CYP21 gene.

Laboratory Features. Baseline 17-OH-P levels and those of other precursors are elevated to different extents in the blood of patients with all three clinical forms of P450c21 deficiency. In the SV form, cortisol secretion is normal or nearly so: this represents the successful compensatory response of increased ACTH stimulation to overcome the relatively mild enzyme deficiency. Furthermore, plasma aldosterone may actually be increased. This, likewise, represents the successful compensatory response of increased aldosterone secretion to the stimulus of increased plasma renin activity that, in turn, is due to the salt loss caused by the excess concentrations of 17-OH-P. With ACTH stimulation, the ratio of stimulated to baseline 17-OH-P can be used to discriminate most patients with the SV and NC forms from heterozygotes, normal individuals, or those with acquired adrenocortical disease (White et al., 1987). Large amounts of pregnanetriol, a metabolite of 17-OH-P, are excreted in the urine, as are 17-ketosteroids, the metabolites of adrenal androgens.

In the SL form, P450c21 deficiency is more severe. Hence, feedback disinhibition leading to increased ACTH cannot stimulate sufficient cortisol production, and the salt loss caused by increased 17-OH-P cannot be compensated by increased renin-stimulated aldosterone secretion. In addition, the extremely high production of ACTH causes a major detour of precursors into the androgen biosynthetic pathway, leading to severe external genital masculinization in females.

Management. The essential principle in the medical management of the SV form of P450c21 deficiency is to replace the cortisol that the patients cannot make for themselves; this prevents a compensatory increase of ACTH, and the concomitant cost of hyperandrogenism. The replacement is usually in the form of some long-acting pharmaceutical glucocorticoid. The medical management of the NC form is similar to that of the SV form. For the SL form, it is necessary to prevent or treat salt-losing crises, and to maintain the patients on glucocorticoid plus mineralocorticoid replacement.

Surgical correction of masculinized external genitalia in the SV or SL forms should be started in infants aged between 2 and 4 months and continue, in stages, thereafter. The medical management must be tailored to the stress of surgery.

Prenatal Diagnosis (PND) and Management. PND is usually done to allow parents to make informed decisions leading either to pregnancy termination or early postnatal treatment. In the case of classic P450c21 deficiency, PND may be used for the purpose of preventing virilization of an affected female fetus by treating the mother with sufficient glucocorticoid (specifically, dexamethasone) in order to protect her female fetus from serious masculinization of the external genitalia (Miller, 1994). For this purpose, therapy must ideally begin before 6 weeks of gestation; yet DNA diagnosis by chorionic villus sampling can only be done at approximately 10 weeks. Nonetheless, it has been suggested that until a definitive prenatal diagnosis can be made, it is worth starting treatment blindly, knowing that seven of eight fetuses will be treated unnecessarily in order to benefit one. This proposal has stimulated hope and controversy. One important consideration is that even early vigorous glucocorticoid replacement still leaves two thirds of the patients with the neeed for at least one surgical procedure. Second, there are maternal complications of dexamethasone therapy. Finally, and most important, long-term studies must be done on developmental outcome of treated fetuses—both genetically affected and unaffected—before this form of prenatal therapy can be recommended universally.

Epidemiology and ethnic considerations.   The classic SV and SL forms of P450c21 deficiency have an incidence of 1 in 5000 to 15,000 in various Caucasian populations. In the Yupik Inuit of Alaska, it is 1 in 700. NC P450c21 deficiency is more common: 3 in 1000 in Caucasians generally, and perhaps as high as 3 in 100 among Ashkenazi Jews (Miller, 1994). In the latter group, it may be a frequent cause of female infertility.

Affected females are recognized more frequently than are males because of their external genital masculinization. Indeed, affected males may die in a SL crisis before they are formally diagnosed. This is the rationale for newborn screening programs based on 17-OH-P measurements of filter-paper blood spots (Witchel et al., 1997).

Genotyping and Gene Expression.   Most patients are compound heterozygotes for different mutant alleles of *CYP21*. There is strong linkage disequilibrium (haplotype association) between particular mutant alleles of *CYP21* and particular combinations of alleles at the class I, II, and III loci of the HLA gene complex. For instance, SL adrenal hyperplasia is associated with HLA-Bw60 and with HLA-A3; Bw47; DR7, the SV form with HLA-Bw51, and the NC form with HLA-B14; DR1 (White et al., 1987).

The tandem arrangement of two sets of highly homologous genes (Fig. 13–12) facilitates meiotic mispairing and unequal crossing over between sister chromatids. This yields duplications and deletions. About 20% of *CYP21* mutants originate deletionally. There are 10 exons in *CYP21*. Its most frequent deletion boundary is between exons 3 and 8. Thus, the 5' end of the fusion gene contains *CYP21P* sequences that have nonsense or missense regions. Most of them are "microconversions" in which a small region of nonsense or missense *CYP21P* replaces a corresponding region of the active gene. These events probably involve meiotic mismatch followed by mismatch repair. The remainder (about 10%) are "macroconversions": an entire *CYP21* is replaced by an entire *CYP21P*.

Despite the complexity of gene conversion as a form of mutagenesis, its very nature limits the variety of mutations responsible for adrenal hyperplasia. This facilitates molecular-genetic diagnosis. For instance, both mutant *CYP21* alleles were identified in 12 of 15 infants initially ascertained in a newborn screening program (Witchel et al., 1997). Eleven of the 12 were microconversions, and eight of the 11

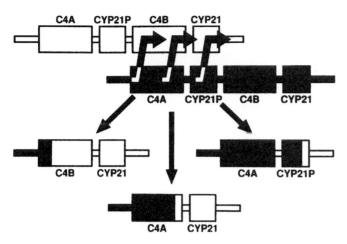

FIGURE 13–12. Types of unequal crossing over that may occur because of homologous pairing between unequal but parologous portions of the CYP21 and C4 genes. (Reproduced from Donohoue P A, Parker K, Migeon C J (1995). Congenital adrenal hyperplasia. Scriver C R, Beaudet A L, Sly W S, Valle D (eds). *Metabolic and Molecular Bases of Inherited Disease*, 7th ed., New York, McGraw-Hill, pp. 2929–2966.)

were the highly frequent intron 2 splicing mutation. Allele "dropout" during PCR amplification of the *CYP21* locus may yield false homozygosity (Day et al., 1996). So, microsatellite haplotyping should complement *CYP21* genotyping in prenatal diagnosis.

Because compound heterozygosity is frequent, much clinical experience has generated the rule that the severity of disease in compound heterozygotes is determined by that of the less severely affected allele.

When one spouse is an obligate carrier, or is identified as a carrier in a family with affected individuals, it may be necessary to seek heterozygosity in a second spouse. This can be done by determining the ratio of progesterone or 17-OH-P to their respective products after ACTH stimulation. The test must be done very early in the menstrual cycle to avoid the consequences of the large amounts of 17-OH-P and P produced by the ovaries later in the menstrual cycle. Unfortunately, this test does not discriminate completely between heterozygotes and normal individuals.

Discussion.   Because of its life-threatening complications, CAH should be the first diagnostic consideration for any newborn with ambiguous external genitalia. This is particularly true in the presence of cryptorchidism: it is not possible to distinguish, clinically, between an overmasculinized female and an undermasculinized cryptorchid male. Similarly, CAH should be the first diagnostic consideration in any young male infant who has diarrhea and vomiting, dehydration, decreased sodium, increased potassium and acidosis. The failure to diagnose such male infants is responsible for the apparent excess of affected females in all series. Indeed, the diagnosis of CAH must be considered prominently in all rapidly growing and/or virilizing boys, and in all rapidly growing adolescent females with or without hirsutism and menstrual irregularity.

It has been long recognized that polycystic ovary syndrome and related hyperandrogenic states are etiologically and pathogenetically heterogeneous, The NC form of P450c21 deficiency is one appreciable source of this heterogeneity, with minor contributions by the NC forms of 3β-HSD and (see below) P450c11 B1 deficiency.

Recent studies support the notion that some form of androgenic imprinting of the brain occurs in female fetuses with CAH. This is another rationale for prenatal therapy. However, attendant issues steming from sex assignment, parental attitudes, and the remote sequelae of genital surgery need further evaluation.

Two aspects of management deserve emphasis. First, it is advocated by some that mineralocorticoid be added to the therapy of the SV form. The rationale, in part, is that this will lower the requirement for glucocorticoid, and it will reduce dependency on PRA and angiotensin for maintenance of aldosterone secretion. The benefit of this reduction is avoidance of other undersirable side effects attributable to increased PRA and increased angiotensin. Second, a patient may appear to improve with age because extra-adrenal 21-hydroxylases become active, reducing the requirement for mineralocorticoid replacement.

REFERENCES

Avila N A, Premkumar A, Shawker T H, Jones J V, Laue L, Cutler Jr G B (1996). Testicular adrenal rest tissue in congenital adrenal hyperplasia: findings at gray-scale and color Doppler US. *Radiology* 198:99–104.

Azziz R, Dewailly D, Owerbach D (1994). Nonclassic adrenal hyperplasia: current concepts. *J Clin Endocrinol Metab* 78:810–815.

Bristow J, Tee M K, Gitelman S E, Mellon S H, Miller W L (1993). Tenascin-X: a novel extracellular matrix protein encoded by the human Xβ gene overlapping P450c21B. *J Cell Biol* 122:265–278.

Day D J, Speiser P W, Schulze E, Bettendord M, Fitness J, Barany F, White P C (1986). Identification of non-amplifying CYP21 genes when using PCR-based diagnosis of 21-hydroxylase deficiency in congenital adrenal hyperplasia (CAH) affected pedigrees. *Hum Mol Genet* 5:2039–2048.

Miller W L (1994). Genetics, diagnosis, and management of 21-hydroxylase deficiency. *J Clin Endocrinol Metab* 78:241–246.

Salardi S, Orsini L F, Cacciari E, Partesotti S, Brondelli L, Cicognani A, Frejaville E, Pluchinotta V, Tonioli S, Bovicelli L (1988). Pelvic ultrasonography in girls with precocious puberty, congenital adrenal hyperplasia, obesity, or hirsutism. *J Pediatr* 112:880–887.

Witchel S E, Nayak S, Suda-Hartman M, Lee P A (1997). Newborn screening for 21-hydroxylase deficiency: results of CYP21 molecular genetic analysis. *J Pediatr* 131:328–331.

White P C, New M I, Dupont B (1987). Congenital adrenal hyperplasia. *N Engl J Med* 316:1519–1524.

11β-HYDROXYLASE DEFICIENCY

The gene encoding 11β-hydroxylase, *CYP11B1*, is at 8q21–22. It has nine exons. It lies adjacent to highly homologous gene (*CYP11B2*) that encodes another enzyme responsible for the terminal two steps in aldosterone biosynthesis (Mornet et al., 1989; Domalik et al., 1991). 11β-hydroxylase deficiency accounts for approximately 5% of all CAH. A late-onset form has been recognized (Gabrilove et al., 1965).

Clinical and Imaging Features. 11β-hydroxylase deficiency results in a block of the conversion of 11-deoxycortisol to cortisol, and in a block of the conversion of deoxycorticosterone (DOC) to corticosterone (Fig. 13–10). DOC is a salt-retaining steroid that provokes a low-renin form of hypertension. By decreased feedback inhibition, cortisol deficiency leads to a compensatory increase in ACTH and, consequently, increased production of precursors that are diverted into the pathway of adrenal androgen biosynthesis. Hence, affected females are born with more-or-less masculinized external genitalia and, untreated, virilize further during infancy and childhood (Rösler et al., 1982). As in 21-hydroxylase deficiency, males have normal genitalia at birth but then proceed to virilize prematurely in childhood (Zachman et al., 1983). They also may have palpable or sonographically visible adrenal rests; these are nodules of ectopic hyperplastic adrenal tissue in or around the testes.

Laboratory Features.   DOC and 11-deoxycortisol levels are increased in blood, and their tetrahydro derivatives are increased in urine.

Management.   Cortisol replacement nullifies the compensatory increase in ACTH, the consequent accumulation of DOC and 11-deoxycortisol, and the diversion of their precursors into androgens. Because the patients can synthesize DOC, they don't need a mineralocorticoid replacement.

Genotyping, Gene Expression, Ethnic Considerations.   11β-hydroxylase deficiency is frequent among Jews from Morocco (Rösler et al., 1992). In six Moroccan Jewish families, 11 of 12 mutant alleles had R448H in exon 8 (White et al., 1991). A variety of 10 other point mutations has been reported: one half are nonsense or frameshift in type. All of these are predicted to interfere with synthesis of essential functional regions of CYP450 proteins (Curnow et al., 1993). When the missense mutations are recreated and expressed in the laboratory, all abolish enzyme activity. Two of them, V441G and R448H, are close to Cys450, which helps to coordinate the heme iron in all CYP450 enzymes. Heterozygotes for the R448 mutation may have elevated responses of plasma 11-deoxycortisol and 11-deoxycorticosterone to ACTH stimulation (Peter and Sippell, 1997). If a mutant genotype has not been identified, prenatal diagnosis is possible by measuring maternal urinary tetrahydro-11-deoxycortisol (Rösler et al., 1988).

REFERENCES

Curnow K C, Slutsker L, Vitek J, Cole T, Speiser P W, New M I, White P C, Pascoe L (1993). Mutations in the *CYP11B1* gene causing congenital adrenal hyperplasia and hypertension cluster in exons 6, 7 and 8. *Proc. Natl. Acad. Sci. USA* 90:4552.

Domalik L J, Chaplin D D, Kirkman M S, Wu R C, Liu W, Howard T A, Sedlin M F, Parker K L (1991). Different isozymes of mouse 11β-hydroxylase produce mineraolcorticoids and glucocorticoids. *Mol Endocrinol* 5:1853–1861.

Gabrilove J L, Sharma D C, Dorfman R I (1965). Adrenocortical 11β-hydroxylase deficiency and virilism first manifest in the adult woman. *N Engl J Med* 72:1189.

Mornet E, Dupont J, Vitek A, White P C (1989). Characterization of two genes encoding human steroid 11β-hydroxylase (P-45011β). *J Biol Chem* 264:20961–20967.

Peter M, Sippell W G (1997). Evidence for endocrinological abnormalities in heterozygotes for adrenal 11 beta-hydroxylase deficiency of a family with the R448H mutation in the CYP11B1 gene. *J Clin Endocrinol Metab* 82:3506–3508.

Rösler A, Leiberman E, Cohen T (1992). High frequency of congenital adrenal hyperplasia (classic 11β-hydroxylase deficiency) among Jews from Morocco. *Am J Med Genet* 42:827–834.

Rösler A, Leiberman E, Sack J, Landau H, Benderly A, Moses S W, Cohen T (1982). Clinical variability of congenital adrenal hyperplasia due to 11β-hydroxylase deficiency. *Horm Res* 16:133–141.

Rösler A, Weshler N, Lieberman E, Hochberg Z, Weidenfeld J, Sack J, Chemke J (1988). 11β-hydroxylase deficiency congenital adrenal hyperplasia: update of prenatal diagnosis. *J Clin Endocrinol Metab* 66:830–838.

White P C, Dupont J, New M I, Lieberman E, Hochberg Z, Rösler A (1991). A mutation in CYP11B1 (Arg448His) associated with steroid 11β-hydroxylase deficiency in Jews of Moroccan origin. *J Clin Invest* 87:1664–1667.

Zachmann M, Tassinari D, Prader A (1983). Clinical and biochemical variability of congenital adrenal hyperplasia due to 11β-hydroxylase deficiency: a study of 25 patients. *J Clin Endocrinol Metab* 56:222–229.

14

Genetic Disorders of Sex Hormone Sensitivity

It is astonishing to consider that only 30 years ago essentially nothing was known about estrogen or androgen receptors (ER or AR). It was appreciated then that certain cells, tissues, organs had the capacity to "concentrate" estrogens or androgens. However, the idea that the same molecules serving as "concentrators" would also turn out to be direct regulators of gene transcription could hardly be imagined.

In the sections below, much more space is devoted to genetic disorders of the AR than of the ER. This is largely because the AR gene is X-linked, so that only one mutation is necessary to yield an affected (XY) hemizygote. In contrast, the ER gene is autosomal, so two mutations are usually necessary for pathogenicity, either by homozygosity or by compound heterozygosity. Three other reasons for the great excess of knowledge about AR mutations are that (1) they do not impair organismal viability, (2) they almost always cause infertility (genetic lethality), and (3) there are relatively few functionally silent areas in the AR, so benign polymorphisms are relatively uncommon, apart from the one involving the $(CAG)_n$ tract that encodes a polyglutamine stretch in the N-terminal portion of the AR.

Pathogenic mutation of the human progesterone receptor has not been described, presumably because it causes infertility by virtue of early embryolethality. The possibility of such mutation has, however, been considered in the form of a local defect of progesterone action on endometrial stroma (Keller et al., 1979).

There has been a great explosion of interest in the role of nonreceptor proteins that serve to coregulate the action of steroid receptors, including the AR and ER (Kamei et al., 1996; Horowitz, et al. 1996; Jenster et al., 1997; McEwan et al., 1997). Some of these coregulators collaborate with multiple steroid receptors, so one or more forms of generalized resistance to steroid hormones can be predicted. It is also predictable that forms of steroid resistance, of a more-or-less local nature, may result from mutations in certain nonreceptor coregulatory proteins that have a restricted cell or tissue distribution.

Recently, a new form of ER, the β form, has been discovered. It is encoded by a different autosomal gene than the one for ERα. ERβ is found in places where ERα is not; for instance, in developing spermatids (Enmark et al., 1997). The role of ERβ mutation in human disease remains to be determined.

GENETIC DISORDERS OF THE ANDROGEN RECEPTOR (AR)

The AR is an exemplary "nuclear receptor" protein, encoded by a eight-exon gene at Xq11-12. It serves to bind androgen, and once androgen-bound, the AR [the androgen-receptor (A-R) complex] becomes a transcription factor that dimerizes and binds to certain regulatory sequences of DNA (androgen response elements; ARE) in order to regulate the expression of androgen target genes that are controlled by nearby promoters (Fig. 14–1). An AR does not work alone: it collaborates with a variety of transcriptional coregulatory factors (coactivators, corepressors), some themselves DNA-binding, in order to achieve vectorial (positive or negative) control over a given target gene. The AR has a typical structure-function organization (Fig. 14–2): a C-terminal, approximately 270-amino-acid androgen-binding domain (ABD; exons 4–8) that contributes to nuclear localization, dimerization, and transactivation; a central 67-amino-acid DNA-binding domain (DBD; exons 2,3) that contributes to dimerization and nuclear localization (Fig. 14–3); and a 560-amino-acid N-terminal domain (exon 1; containing several polyamino acid tracts) that modulates the amplitude and specificity of target gene regulation, presumably by its ability to interact with promoter-or cell-specific transcriptional coregulators. A consensus ARE is an imperfectly inverted hexanucleotide repeat with a spacer of 3 nucleotides (Fig. 14–4): for example, 5' GGA/TACANNNTGTTCT-3' (Roche et al., 1992). Such an ARE has limited specificity; for instance, it can react with the DBD of the glucocorticoid receptor. To achieve full specificity, a typical ARE must collaborate with additional protein-binding DNA sequences that form *cis* components of composite AREs (Kasper et al., 1994) and/or, once bound, its androgen-receptor complexes must interact with promoter-or cell-specific coregulators (Scheller et al., 1996). An evolutionary analysis of all parts of the androgen receptor has led to the recognition of amino acids that are fully conserved among the ARs and not shared with other steroid receptors (Thornton and Kelley, 1998). It has been predicted that these residues can explain the specificity of the AR in its affinity for androgens, and for androgen response elements.

A sufficient amount of normal AR must be available, *at the correct times*, in order

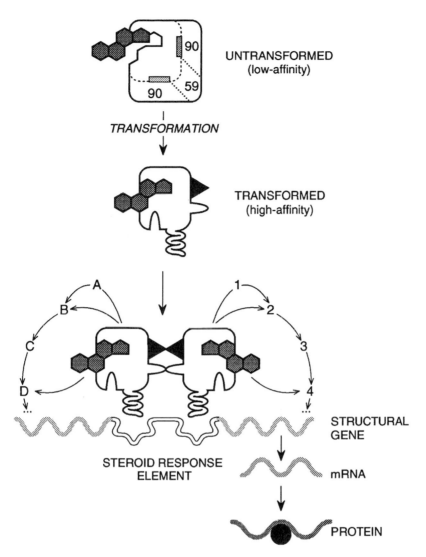

FIGURE 14–1. The *untransformed* androgen receptor (AR) associates with several heat shock proteins as chaperones, and binds androgens with "low" affinity. the *transformed* AR dissociates from its chaperones, binds androgen with "higher" affinity, enters the nucleus, dimerizes, and binds, as a dimer, to a bipartite androgen response element (ARE). The net rate of transcription of a structural gene under the control of a nearby promoter depends on the "positive" and "negative" interactions that occur between the AR and coregulatory proteins, some upstream of the ARE, some downstream, some DNA-binding, others not. This sequence of events is shared, more or less, with other steroid hormones and their cognate receptors.

for androgen(s) to turn on (or off) the expression of those genes whose products effect normal masculinization of male fetuses before birth and normal virilization of boys at puberty. A defective AR or a deficient amount of AR, *during a critical period of development*, will cause one or another degree (or phenotype) of androgen insensitivity (resistance).

Clinical and Imaging Features. Androgen insensitivity (AI) comes in three major classes of severity according to the external genital phenotype: *complete*, the phe-

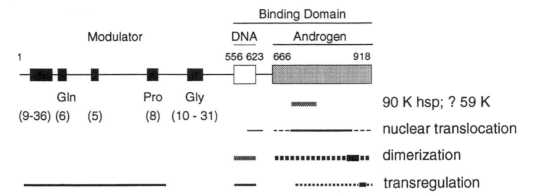

FIGURE 14–2. The N-terminal transcriptional modulatory domain of the AR contains several homopolyamino acid tracts, two of them polymorphic. The principal "binding" domains, and the subfunctions embedded within each, are indicated. It has recently been proposed that the N-terminal domain also contributes to dimerization by interacting intermolecularly with the C-terminal domain of another monomer (Langley et al., 1998).

notype is normal or near-normal female, whether or not the testes are visible; *partial*, the phenotype is frankly ambiguous, with a phallic urethra or penoscrotal hypospadias, and the testes are usually undescended; *mild*, the phenotype is normal or near-normal male (the penis and scrotum may be small; there may be coronal hypospadias; the testes are usually descended). Typically, there is no uterus or cervix, because müllerian duct regression is independant of androgen. Rarely, a vestigial uterus or a müllerian duct remnant will be found by ultrasonography; probably, this is no more frequent than in a population of normal males. In theory, the upper one third of the vagina is of müllerian origin and should be absent in those with the "complete" form; however, the vagina is not always clinically short. Examined by urethrogenitography, ultrasonography, or magnetic resonance imaging, devel-

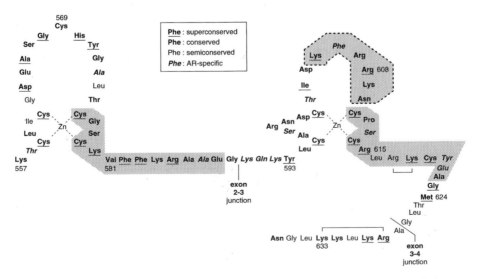

FIGURE 14–3. The amino acid compositions of the zinc fingers, putative α-helices (shaded), and the bipartite nuclear localization signal (bracketed) of the AR.

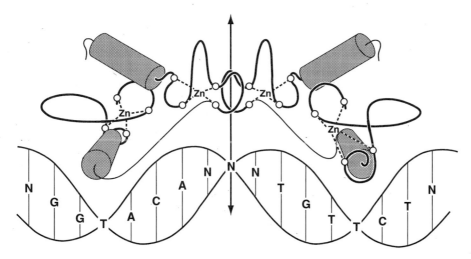

FIGURE 14–4. A schematic illustration of (AR)$_2$ dimer-ARE interaction as deduced from studies on the glucocorticoid receptor. Note that the N-terminal α-helices (cylinders) of each other monomer interact with the major groove of the ARE, and that the C-terminal zinc fingers of each monomer contribute to dimerization.

opment of the internal genital structures—the prostate (from the urogenital sinus), the seminal vesicles, epididymes, and vasa deferentia (from the wolffian ducts)—is usually coordinate with the status of the external genitalia. However, one (or more) wolffian duct derivatives is sometimes found even in those with complete AI, suggesting that their development is not fully androgen-dependent.

At puberty, subjects with complete AI develop breasts and female fat deposition; the voice remains feminine. Pubic and axillary hair are absent or scant (because these are androgen-dependent) and menses do not appear. Subjects tend to be taller than average but do not become eunuchoidal. Hence, if the testes are visibly undescended, until definitive diagnosis, the overall phenotype is that of incoordinate puberty in an otherwise normal pubertal female.

At puberty, subjects with partial AI have various degrees of feminization and virilization, depending on the quality and/or quality of the mutant AR, on the action of auxiliary (coregulatory) factors, and on stochastic factors. This variation may be expressed in different degrees of post-pubertal gynecomastia; facial, axillary, truncal, and pubic hair; feminine fat deposition; high-pitched voice; subnormal skeletal muscularity; impotence; and impaired spermatogenesis.

Subjects with mild AI may or may not have various degrees of gynecomastia; decreased ejaculate volume; impaired spermatogenesis; high-pitched voice; subnormal skeletal muscularity; impotence; and facial, axillary, body, or pubic hair (in a female distribution). In other words, it is reasonable to expect that someone with mild AI due to a mildly deficient or defective AR could present with any one of the foregoing signs (or a combination of them). In particular, infertility due to impaired spermatogenesis may be the only or nearly the only sign of mild AI (Migeon et al., 1984; Yong et al., 1994, 1996), yet it is not an obligate expression of mild AI (Grino et al., 1988; Tsukada et al., 1994).

Sometimes, intrafamilial expressivity can vary appreciably (Rodien et al., 1996;

Evans et al., 1997); it is rare, however, for it to encompass the phenotypes of complete AI at one extreme and mild AI at the other. Nonetheless, because of variable expressivity, a sophisticated family history is an essential component in differential diagnosis. For instance, an affected maternal uncle may simply have impaired spermatogenesis and infertility as the sole presenting sign of his mild AI, whereas his affected nephew may have been born with cryptorchidism and a marked degree of penoscrotal hypospadias that required multiple, staged, corrective surgical procedures. Furthermore, heterozygous females may have reduced, asymmetric, or delayed public and/or axillary hair development and, occasionally, delayed menarche. Indeed, in some families the diagnosis of complete AI in a hemizygote is delayed because delayed menarche has occurred in a heterozygous mother or sister and is, therefore, assumed to be a benign familial trait.

There is a special form of mild AI that is a component of spinobulbar muscular atrophy [SBMA; Kennedy disease (Fischbeck 1997)]. This is due to a unique mutation of the AR [expansion of the polymorphic (n = 11-35) polyglutamine tract (CAG_n) in exon 1 to n >36]. In addition to a mild loss of AR function, the expansion also causes a motor neuronopathy by a gain of function that is yet to be explained. Typically, there is slowly progressive atrophy and weakness of the pelvic and shoulder girdle muscles starting in the third to fourth decades. This is followed by limb muscle involvement, and those muscles served by certain cranial nerves yielding dysphonia, dysarthria, and dysphagia. Fasciculation (twitching) is common, especially of the tongue and perioral muscles. A fine rapid hand tremor may precede muscle atrophy. Gynecomastia is the single most common, and usually the first, sign of mild AI in SBMA. Reduced libido, and impotence may appear next. Impaired spermatogenesis appears late, so that infertility is not usually a major issue.

Laboratory Features. The serum levels of testosterone (T), 5α-dihydrotestosterone (DHT) should be normal or elevated, and the T:DHT ratio should be normal *without* hCG challenge in the first 3 months of life, when the hypothalamic-pituitary gonadotrope axis is active, and should respond appropriately to hCG challenge from that time in infancy until puberty has been well established. If the T level is increased, so may be the E_2 level, because T is aromatizable. A high T to DHT ratio would suggest 5α-reductase, type 2 deficiency. A low T level would suggest deficient testosterone synthesis with accumulation of androgen precursor (a biosynthetic defect; Chapter 13) or without such accumulation (Leydig cell defect or deficiency; Chapter 11). Because of defective androgen feedback on an active hypothalamic-pituitary gonadotrope axis, random LH levels are likely to be high, and so may testosterone levels, in response to elevated LH. However, because of circadian pulsatility, elevated LH and T (and/or androstenedione) levels may only be observed by frequent periodic sampling in order to assess pulse frequency and amplitude, and to calculate mean levels during the day. Likewise, defective androgen feedback may permit GnRH stimulation to cause an exaggerated LH response in amplitutide and/or in duration.

The most frequent diagnostic problem in AI is to sustain the presumptive diagnosis in prepubertal subjects whose T biosynthetic activity is normal, and whose phenotypes are compatible with partial or mild AI. The problem is to distinguish those with genuine AI from those who simply had a delay in the acquisition of normal T biosynthesis or normal androgen sensitivity beyond a critical period(s) in external and/or internal genital morphogenesis. Delayed acquisition of androgen sensitivity may indeed reflect mutation in a regulatory portion of the AR gene. But, to date, very little is known about those portions, or about the regulatory "factors" that interact with those portions.

The differential diagnosis of mild AI in a postpubertal subject with SBMA is not usually problematic, unless the signs of subnormal virilization precede those of the motor neuronopathy by a long interval.

Two in vivo tests have been proffered to deal with the differential diagnosis of partial AI in a subject with ambiguous genitalia. The Stanozolol test (Sinnecker et al., 1997) measures the ability of this synthetic androgenic-anabolic steroid to depress the blood level of the sex hormone–binding globulin, a protein produced in the liver. The validity of the test depends on the assumption that the liver is affected in all cases of partial AI. The latest results indicate that the degree of depression is about 15% in subjects with partial AI whose external genitalia are predominantly female, and about 30% in subjects with partial AI whose external genitalia are predominantly male. Whether the test can recognize at least some subjects with mild AI is unknown.

The anti-müllerian hormone (AMH) test (Rey et al., 1994) measures the ability of endogenous androgen to suppress the Sertoli cell synthesis and secretion of AMH. Elevated levels of AMH are observed in subjects with complete AI during the first year of life, and in puberty. In the interval, the levels of AMH in patients with complete AI remain within normal limits. The preliminary results on subjects with partial AI are less decisive. No patient with mild AI has been tested.

Failing the performance of these in vivo tests, it would be logical to assess suspect GSF for some physiologic response to androgen. Unfortunately, no such response has been identified. Instead, an equally powerful in vitro method for substantiating the presumption of AI is to infect a GSF line with a recombinant adenovirus vector containing an androgen-responsive reporter gene. Incubation with androgen should then provoke less reporter-gene expression in the mutant than in the normal cells (McPhaul et al., 1997). This test can easily discriminate subjects with complete AI, and it can do so with impressive efficiency even for subjects with partial AI, or those with the mild AI that is a component of SBMA. Most important, the test assesses overall transactivational competence of the suspect AR, without a priori knowledge whether the mutation affects quantity of quality of the AR. And, if the latter, whether the mutation affects the ABD, the DBD, or the N-terminal transcriptional modulatory domain.

The in vitro biochemical diagnosis of AI due to aberrant androgen binding of a mutant AR depends on the analysis of GSF or public skin fibroblasts (PSF) derived from subjects with the presumptive diagnosis of AI. GSF and PSF have, on average, about three and two times more specific androgen-binding activity than nongenital skin fibroblasts. Therefore, it is best to use GSF to quantitate deficient androgen binding, or to recognize qualitative abnormalities of androgen binding even when androgen binding is not deficient.

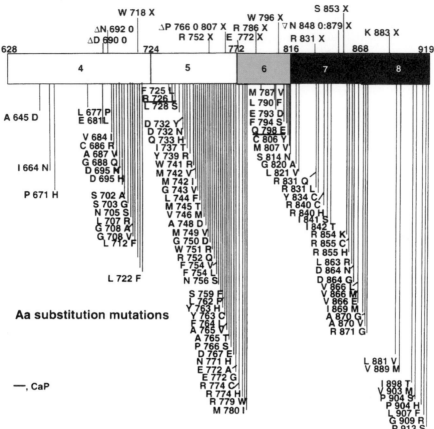

FIGURE 14–5. Constitutional *AR* mutations affecting the exons encoding its LBD. The two underlined missense mutations were first discovered somatically in prostatic cancer DNA from the subjects. (Adapted from *Nucleic Acids Res* 26:234–238, 1998.)

Replicate monolayers from a control and the subject are used to measure maximum androgen-binding capacity, the equilibrium affinity constant (a ratio of the rates at which androgen binds to the AR and dissociates from it at equilibrium), and the nonequilibrium dissociation rate. Both measurements of androgen-receptor avidity should be made because for some mutations, only one of the two is abnormal (Beitel et al., 1994). They should also be performed at various temperatures in order to seek thermolability as an expression of mutant phenotype. Furthermore, synthetic androgens (mibolerone, methyltrienolone) and natural androgens (T and DHT) should be used in these assays to look for androgen-restricted expressions of mutant phenotype. Normal, deficient, or defective androgen binding has been reported in the GSF or PSF of subjects with SBMA. Whatever the explanation for this disparity, it is clear that expansion of the polyglutamine tract in the AR is associated with decreased transactivational potency.

Over 150 different constitutional point mutations have been discovered in the

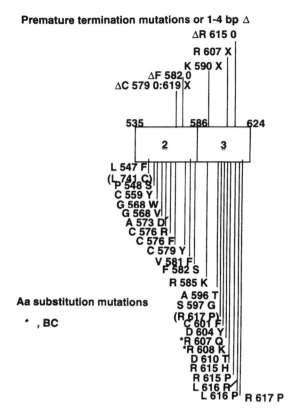

FIGURE 14–6. Constitutional *AR* mutations affecting the exons encoding the DBD of the AR. The asterisked missense mutations occurred in individuals who developed breast cancer. The missense mutations in parentheses coexisted with the missense mutation listed just above each.

coding portion of the *AR* (Gottlieb et al., 1998). Most of the mutations in the ABD (Fig. 14–5) and DBD (Fig. 14–6) are of the missense type. About half are responsible for complete AI, another half for partial AI, and a small number (only five, to date) are associated with mild AI.

There is a strong correlation between the degree of deficient or defective androgen-binding activity due to ABD mutations and the severity of the AI phenotype. Thus, subjects with ABD mutations that yield very low B_{max} values or very low affinity constants and very high dissociation rates with all four ligands are very likely to have complete AI. Those with lesser degrees of all these defects, or with fewer of them, are likely to have partial AI. Those that yield normal parameters for most of these androgen-binding assays are likely subjects with mild AI. However, there is appreciable scatter of the data, so it is difficult to predict individual clinial phenotype from these data alone. Indeed, intrafamilial expressivity can vary sufficiently so that one person affected may have partial AI, and another may have complete (Rodien et al., 1996) or mild AI. Nor is it rare for members of one family to be raised as boys or girls depending on the predominant appearance of their ambiguous external genitalia (Evans et al., 1997). It is rare, however, for the expressivity to enclose the entire range of phenotype from complete to mild AI.

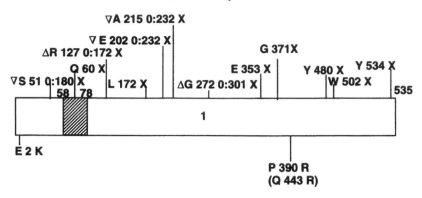

Aa substitution mutations

FIGURE 14–7. Constitutional *AR* mutations affecting exon 1. The abundance of primary and secondary (frameshift) nonsense mutations is striking. This suggests that the precise amino acid sequence of this domain is not crucial to its functions.

There are no facile tests available for measuring the ability of a DBD to bind to an ARE. An estimate of the ability of the DBD to bind to an ARE may be obtained by evaluating the nuclear-cytoplasmic distribution of mutant androgen-receptor complexes.

Genotyping and Gene Expression. There are two approaches to the identification of *AR* mutation in subjects with strong clinical-endocrine suspicion of AI. One is to screen the coding portion of the *AR* by SSCP or DGGE, recognizing that the sensitivity of either technique is likely to be suboptimal, at least for certain portions of the gene; another is to first identify an androgen-binding abnormality in GSF. If such an abnormality is found, then one should proceed directly to sequencing of exons 4–8 that encode the ABD of the AR protein. Mutations in the DBD are not usually associated with androgen-binding abnormalities; however, there have been exceptions (Beitel et al., 1994). In any event, exons 2 and 3 are small and easily sequenced. Likewise, exon 1 mutations may sometimes affect androgen binding (Chong et al., 1996), and ABD mutation may sometimes impair DBD binding, without any apparent effect on androgen binding (Yong et al., 1996). Exon 1, by far the largest in the *AR* gene and the least conserved compared to other steroid receptor genes, is seldom the site of point mutations causing constitutional AI; the great majority of them are of the nonsense or frameshift variety (Fig. 14–7). Hence, it is wise to screen exon 1 for mutations when there is strong presumptive evidence of AI from the family history, or from the result of *in vivo* or *in vitro* testing.

A decreased amount of androgen-binding activity can be an expression of a missense or nonsense mutation, attributable to a decreased amount of immuno-reactive AR protein, or to a decreased amount of *AR* mRNA as quantitated by RT-PCR. The remainder probably reflect mutations in regulatory portions of the *AR* gene, but little is known of these portions.

Intronic mutations close to exons are detectable by primers designed for exonic PCR. However, deep intronic mutations may be overlooked, unless RT-PCR is done in order to size, and sequence, the fragments produced.

Recreation of particular mutations and their expression in AR-free transfected cells has been useful in proving their pathogenicity by observing new functional AR abnormalities, or by reproducing one previously observed in skin fibroblast lines. Occasionally, the failure of a cotransfected androgen-responsive reporter gene to be expressed normally has been the first indication of pathogenicity for a given point mutation (Bevan et al., 1996; Yong et al., 1996).

Recently, it has been appreciated that variable expressivity of a particular point mutation may simply reflect somatic mosaicism for the mutation (Boehmer et al., 1997; Holterhus et al., 1997), rather than the modifying influence of "background" genetic factors.

The issue of somatic mosaicism also relates to two aspects of genetic counseling for sporadic (isolated) cases of AIS. First, somatic/germ cell mosaicism may explain recurrence to a mother whose extragonadal genotype is apparently normal; hence, the "never say never" rule applies, at least until two methods of mutation detection have been used to rule out maternal heterozygosity (Boehmer et al., 1997). Second, the finding of somatic mosaicism in a sporadic case substantially decreases the likelihood that the mother is a covert (somatic/germ cell mosaic) heterozygote (Holterhus et al., 1997), but it does not eliminate that possibility.

Finally, it is important to record that, in a recent study, 8 of 30 mothers with an androgen-insensitive child did not carry the child's *AR* mutation in her blood lymphocytes (Hiort et al., 1998). Five of the 8 patients presumably inherited a new germline mutation from their mothers. In the remaining 3 there was evidence of somatic mosaicism, suggesting a post-zygotic origin of their mutations.

Management. Subjects with normal or near-normal female external genitalia ("complete"), and those with normal or near-normal male external genitalia ("mild") may require relatively minor external genital surgery: in the female, to correct posterior labial fusion or clitoromegaly; in the male, to correct hypospadias or cryptorchidism. However, in females with short vaginas that cause dyspareunia, surgical lengthening and repeated insertion of dilators may be necessary, not always with entirely satisfactory results. The testes should be removed from the females either before puberty or shortly thereafter, to minimize the risk of neoplasia associated with any dystopic testis. Estrogen replacement therapy, perhaps with androgen supplementation, will be necessary for the females. Subjects with frankly ambiguous external genitalia ("partial") are problematic: sex assignment must be conditional on surgical correctability in one direction or another, on parental attitudes, and on the influence of social and temporal factors.

The earlier sex assignment is made the better; but overall outcome, whether toward maleness or femaleness, is seldom fully satisfactory. One important consideration in choosing a sex-of-rearing would be the ability to predict the degree of androgen responsiveness at puberty in an infant with partial AI. The underlying assumption is that a deficient amount of an otherwise normal AR, or defective AR with a particular mutation in the ABD might be "corrected" by provision of extra androgenic ligand. There is abundant experimental precedent (Marcelli et al., 1994; Bevan et al., 1994) and some clinical support for this concept (Price et al., 1984; Grino et al., 1988, 1989; McPhaul et al., 1991; Hiort et al., 1993; Yong et al., 1994). One approach to this question is to judge the infant's response to a course of androgen therapy in pharmacologic doses. Some infants do seem to respond sufficiently to facilitate surgical correction toward maleness. However, no long-term studies have been done to relate infantile with pubertal responsiveness in such infants. Another approach would be to assess androgen responsiveness *in vitro*, after infecting the patient's GSF with an androgen-responsive reporter gene (McPhaul et al., 1997). This approach will require much more experience before it can be used routinely.

Weidemann and colleagues (1998) recently reported an impressive virilization response in a 19-year-old man after 3.5 years of treatment with testosterone enanthate (250 mg, intramuscularly, weekly). He was born with perineoscrotal hypospadias due to a Arg607GIn mutation in the DBD. This observation is the first of its kind. It has two possible explanations, both based on the fact that normal ABD function is required for normal DBD function: either the pharmacologic doses of androgen can act on a normal ABD to partially overcome DBD dysfunction due to the mutation, or the DBD mutation has a detrimental effect on ABD function that is partially overcome by excess androgen. The latter explanation assumes that the SSCP procedure used to look for muationas in the ABD portion of the patient's AR gene was 100% sensitive.

There is a tendency, at least in Western cultures, to choose a female sex-of-rearing for infants with partial AI: the rationale is that for the purpose of sexual intercourse, it is easier to create a vagina than a penis. This seems, often, to be an oversimplified view judging from the frequency and vehemence of complaints registered in the Newsletter of the AIS Support Group. In other words, "easier" technically does not necessarily mean "better" functionally. Furthermore, despite the fact that many women, even those with complete AI, adjust well to biological knowledge of their special form of infertility, many others do not. Hence, the decision of when to tell, and how much to tell, must be individualized, taking into consideration the views of other family members, possible effects of disclosure on them, and the availability of support from other affected individuals in the family or from the AIS Support Group.

REFERENCES

Beitel L K, Kasemi-Esfarjani P, Kaufman M, Lumbroso R, DiGeorge A M, Killinger D W, Trifiro M A, Pinsky L (1994). Substitution of arginine-839 by cysteine or histidine in the androgen receptor causes different receptor phenotypes in cultured cells and coordinate degrees of clinical androgen resistance. *J Clin Invest* 94:546–554.

Bevan C L, Brown B B, Davies H R, Evans B A J, Hughes I A, Patterson M N (1996). Functional analysis of six androgen receptor mutations identified in patients with partial androgen insensitivity syndrome. *Hum Mol Genet* 5:265–273.

Boehmer A L M, Brinkmann A O, Niermeijer M F, Bakker L, Halley D J J, Drops S L S (1997). Germline and somatic mosaicism in the androgen insensitivity syndrome: implications for genetic counseling. *Am J Hum Genet* 60:1003–1006.

Choong C S, Quigley C A, French F S, Wilson E M (1996). Novel missense mutation in the amino-terminal domain of the human androgen receptor gene in a family with partial androgen insensitivity syndrome causes reduced efficiency of protein translation. *J Clin Invest* 98:1423–1431.

Enmark E, Pelto-Huikko M, Grandien K, Lagercrantz S, Lagercrantz J, Fried G, Nordenskjold M, Gustafsson J A (1997). Human estrogen receptor beta-gene structure, chromosomal localization, and expression pattern. *J Clin Endocrinol Metab* 82:4258–4265.

Evans B A J, Hughes I A, Bavan C L, Patterson M N, Gregory J W (1997). Phenotypic diversity in siblings with partial androgen insensitivity syndrome. *Arch Dis Childhood* 76:529–531.

Fischbeck K H (1997). Kennedy disease. *J Inher Metab Dis* 20:152–158.

Gottlieb B, Lehvaslaiho H, Beitel L K, Trifiro M, Lumbroso R, Pinsky L (1998). The androgen receptor gene mutations database. *Nucleic Acids Res* 26:234–238.

Grino P B, Griffin J E, Cushard W G, Wilson J D. (1988). A mutation of the androgen receptor associated with partial androgen resistance, familial gynecomastia, and fertility. *J Clin Endocrinol Metab* 66:754–761.

Grino P B, Isidro-Gutierrez F, Griffin J E, Wilson J D (1989). Androgen resistance associated with a qualitative abnormality of the androgen receptor and responsive to high dose androgen therapy. *J Clin Endocrinol Metab* 68:578–584.

Hiort O, Huang Q, Sinnecker H G, Sadeghi-Nejad A B, Kruse K, Wolfe H J, Yandell D W (1993). Single strand conformation polymorphism analysis of androgen receptor gene mutations in patients with androgen insensitivity syndromes: application for diagnosis, genetic counseling, and therapy. *J Clin Endocrinol Metab* 77:262–266.

Hiort O, Sinnecker G H G, Holterhus P-M, Nitsche E M, Kruse K (1998). Inherited and de novo androgen receptor gene mutations: investigation of single-case families. *J Pediatr* 131:939–943.

Holterhus P-M, Brüggenwirth H T, Hiort O, Kleinkauf-Houcken A, Kruse K, Sinnecker G H G, Brinkmann A O (1997). Mosaicism due to a somatic mutation of the androgen receptor gene determines phenotype in androgen insensitivity syndrome. *J Clin Endocrinol Metab* 82:3584–3589.

Horowitz K B, Jackson T A, Bain D L, Richer J K, Takimoto G S, Tung L (1996). Nuclear receptor coactivators and corepressors. *Mol Endocrinol* 10:1167–1177.

Jenster G, Spencer T E, Burcin M M, Tsai S Y, Tsai M-J, O'Malley B W (1997). Steroid receptor induction of gene transcription: a two-step model. *Proc Natl Acad Sci USA* 94:7879–7884.

Kamei Y, Xu L, Heinzel T et al. (1996). A CBP integrator complex mediates transcriptional activation and AP-1 inhibition by nuclear receptors. *Cell* 85:403–414.

Kasper S, Rennie P S, Bruchovsky N, Sheppard P C, Cheng H, Lin L, Shiu R P C, Snoek R, Matusik R J (1994). Cooperative binding of androgen receptors to two DNA sequences is required for androgen induction of the probasin gene. *J Biol Chem* 269:31763–31769.

Keller D W, Wiest W G, Askin F B, Johnson L W, Strickler R C (1979). Pseudocorpus luteum insufficiency: a local defect of progesterone action on endometrial stroma. *J Clin Endocrinol Metab* 48:127–132.

Marcelli M, Zoppi S, Wilson C M, Griffin J E, McPhaul M J (1994). Amino acid substitutions in the hormone-binding domain of the human androgen receptor alter the stability of the hormone receptor complex. *J Clin Invest* 94:1642–1650.

McEwan J J, Gustafsson J-A (1997). Interaction of the human androgen receptor transactivation function with the general transcription factor TFIIF. *Proc Natl Acad Sci USA* 94: 8485–8490.

McPhaul M J, Marcelli M, Tilley W D, Griffin J E, Isidro-Gutierrez F, Wilson J D (1991). Molecular basis of androgen resistance in a family with a qualitative abnormality of the androgen receptor and responsive to high-dose androgen therapy. *J Clin Invest* 87:1413–1421.

McPhaul M J, Schweikert H-U, Allman D R (1997). Assessment of androgen receptor function in genital skin fibroblasts using a recombinant adenovirus to deliver an androgen-responsive reporter gene. *J Clin Endocrinol Metab* 82:1944–1948.

Migeon C J, Brown T R, Lanes R, Palacios A, Amrhein J A, Schoen E J (1984). A clinical syndrome of mild androgen insensitivity. *J Clin Endocrinol Metab* 59:672–678.

Price P, Wass J A H, Griffin J W, Leshin M, Savage M O, Largo D M, Bu'Lock D E, Anderson D C, Wilson J D, Besser G M (1984). High dose androgen therapy in male pseudohermaphroditism due to 5α-reductase deficiency and disorders of the androgen receptor. *J Clin Invest* 74:1496–1508.

Rey R, Mebarki F, Forest M G, Mowszowicz I, Cate R L Morel Y, Chaussain J-L, Josso N. (1994). Anti-Müllerian hormone in children with androgen insensitivity. *J Clin Endocrinol Metab* 79:960–964.

Roche P J, Hoare S A, Parker M G (1992). A consensus DNA-binding site for the androgen receptor. *Mol Endocrinol* 6:2229–2235.

Rodien P, Mebarki F, Mowszowicz I, Chaussain J-L, Young J, Morel Y, Schaison G (1996). Different phenotypes in a family with androgen insensitivity caused by the same M7801 point mutation in the androgen receptor gene. *J Clin Endocrinol Metab* 81:2994–2998.

Scheller A, Scheinman R I, Thompson E, Scarlett C O, Robins D M (1996). Contextual dependence of steroid receptor function on an androgen-responsive enhancer. *Mol Cell Endocrinol* 121:75–86.

Sinnecker G H G, Hiort O, Nitsche E M, Holterhus P-M, Kruse K (1997). Functional assessment and clinical classification of androgen sensitivity in patients with mutations of the androgen receptor gene. *Eur J Pediatr* 156:7–14.

Thornton J W, Kelley D B (1998). Evolution of the androgen receptor: structure-function implications. *Bio Essays* 20:860–869.

Tsukada T, Inoue M, Tachibana S, Nakai Y, Takebe H (1994). An androgen receptor mutation causing androgen resistance in undervirilized male syndrome. *J Clin Endocrinol Metab* 79:1202–1207.

Yong E L, Abdullah A A R, Choo C K, Lim J, Tut T G, Lumbroso R, Trifiro M A, Pinsky L (1996). Mild androgen insensitivity and male infertility: substitution in the ligand-binding domain of the androgen receptor that impairs transactivation but not androgen binding. *Am J Hum Genet* 59:A43. Abstract 217.

Yong E L, Ng S C, Roy A C, Yun G, Ratnam S S (1994). Pregnancy after hormonal correction of severe spermatogenic defect due to mutation in androgen receptor gene. *Lancet* 344:826–827.

Weidemann W, Peters B, Romalo G, Spindler K-D, Schweikert H-U (1998). Response to androgen treatment in a patient with partial androgen insensitivity and a mutation in the deoxyribonucleic acid-binding domain of the androgen receptor. *J Clin Endocrinol Metab* 83:1173–1176.

GENETIC DISORDERS OF THE ESTROGEN RECEPTOR (ER)

The ER belongs to a distinct branch of the ligand-modulated transcriptional regulatory factor superfamily, but it is most closely related to the subfamily composed of the androgen, progesterone, glucocorticoid, and mineralocorticoid receptors. It is encoded by a gene on 6q. It has the typical structure-function organization of these so-called "nuclear receptors": its C-terminal ligand-binding domain is able to recognize both estrogens and anti-estrogens, and to change its conformation appropriately; its central DNA-binding domain is able to recognize regulatory sequences of nucleotides (estrogen resonse elements) located around the promoter elements of estrogen-regulated target genes; and the N-terminal domain modulates the agonist or antagonistic action of a particular ligand-ER complex by its interaction with a host of collaborative transcriptional regulatory cofactors that determine the net effect (positive or negative) on the expression of a given target gene.

The rarity of estrogen resistance, compared to other autosomally determined syndromes of resistance to steroids, thyroid hormone, and vitamin D hormone, compelled the view that ER mutation leading to moderate or severe ER dysfunction is embryonically lethal, perhaps by impairing placental implantation. This view was supported by the fact that blastocysts express ER mRNA (Hou and Gorski, 1993). Recently, however, male and female mice with insertionally disrupted ER genes have been well studied (Lubahn et al., 1993), and a single very tall, young adult man, of consanguineous parentage, has been discovered to be estrogen-resistant because of homozygosity for a premature *ER* stop codon (Smith et al., 1994). The remainder of this section summarizes descriptions of this man and of estrogen-resistant mice.

Clinical and Imaging Features.   At 28 years of age, the patient had a normal beard, incipient temporal recession, a normal prostate gland, and normal male genitalia. He had bilateral axillary acanthosis nigricans, was 204 cm tall, his upper segment to lower segment ratio was 0.88, his arm span was 213 cm, and his epiphyses were unfused. The bone age of his left hand was 15 years, his lumbar spine was markedly undermineralized, and he had progressive genu valgum. He grew normally until adolescence, did not have a marked growth spurt during adolescence, and did not stop growing after adolescence.

Laboratory Findings.   The patient had normal sperm density but reduced viability; serum T level was normal but E_1, E_2, FSH, and LH levels were all high. He was insulin-resistant: an abnormal glucose tolerance test result was accompanied by hyperinsulinemia.

Genotyping.   After PCR amplification of all eight exons in the ER gene, a variant SSCP pattern was identified in exon 2. Direct sequencing revealed a C-T transition leading to a Arg-Stop mutation at a position preceding the DNA-binding domain. Both parents were heterozygous and so were three of his four sisters. Gene expression studies were not performed *in vitro*. However, the patient was given high doses of estrogen by dermal patch for 6 months without response by any clinical, biochemical, or imaging parameter. Classically, the homozygous stop mutation carried by the patient would produce, at best, a physically and functionally truncated protein that might be very unstable. It is likely, moreover, that mRNA instability, as described for other relatively N-terminal stop mutations, would interdict the translation of an appreciable amount of protein, whatever its truncation. On the other hand, "read-through" across a stop mutation may permit appreciable synthesis of full-length product. This possibility deserves exploration in the case of the subject's mutation.

Discussion and Speculation.   It is apparent that a human carrying a mutant ER that causes full resistance to estrogen, as measured in male adulthood, is not inviable in early embryonic life. It remains to be seen whether heterozygous females have decreased fertility and whether "read-through" across the premature stop mutation might account for appreciable functional ER in the subject; nevertheless, it now becomes likely that other cases of estrogen resistance will be found among adults of both sexes who are tall, who have unfused epiphyses and osteoporosis, and who are hyperestrogenemic with elevated gonadotropins. Contrarily, relatively mild mutations may be able to generate a compensatory hyperestrogenemia that normalizes the phenotype. So, the penetrance or expressivity of some ER mutations may be much reduced.

It has long been assumed that the adolescent growth spurt and epiphyseal maturation are the primary responsibility of androgen in males and estrogen in females. The data from the "experiment of nature" in this one mutant subject indicate that, by collaborating with androgens, estrogens contribute to these processes in males as well as in females. Such collaboration is also evinced by the need to combine an aromatase inhibitor with an anti-androgen in order to retard skeletal growth and epiphyseal maturation in boys with testotoxicosis due to gain-of-function mutations in the LH receptor (Laue et al., 1989). It is further supported by the normal pubertal growth spurt that occurs in 46,XY females as the result of complete androgen insensitivity (Zachman et al., 1986). Another lesson on androgen-estrogen complementarity from this one estrogen-resistant man lies in his elevated levels of LH, FSH, and estradiol. LH and FSH elevation reflect deficient estrogen-mediated feedback on the hypothalamic-pituitary axis and, in turn, LH elevation stimulates the synthesis of more androgen precursor for aromatization to estrogen. The elevated estradiol may be viewed as a vain attempt to compensate for estrogen resistance, but it does explain the subject's normal androgen levels despite elevated LH.

Acanthosis nigricans is a classical sign of insulin resistance, particularly in hyperandrogenic situations (Barbieri and Ryan, 1993). The subject had normoandrogenemia in the face of estrogen resistance, probably explaining his acanthosis nigricans.

Observations on mice heterozygous or homozygous for insertionally disrupted ER genes have been informative (Korach, 1994). The heterozygous animals are fertile and the sex ratio of their offspring is unremarkable. However, homozygous ER mutant mice of both sexes are infertile, and the females have cystic ovaries, possibly reflecting feedback dysinhibition and excessive gonadotropin stimulation. Granulosa and theca cells are present, but follicle development is interrupted before the formation of ovulatory follicles. Estrogen resistance causes a secondary decrease in progesterone receptor concentration. So, some of the ovarian effects of estrogen resistance may represent deficient progesterone action. Surprisingly, homozygous mutant male mice have seminiferous tubular dysgenesis and severe oligospermia. Hence, estrogen resistance may be a cause of male infertility in humans. Interestingly, as is true in humans, estrogen-resistant mice of both sexes have decreased bone density. Finally, the "early responses" of the uterus to estrogen (water imbibition and hyperemia) are also missing from estrogen-resistant mice. Thus, the ER also mediates at least some of those estrogen responses that do not depend on transcriptional regulation.

An intriguing rationale for the pharmacology of estrogen resistance due to ER mutation lies in the possibility that estrogen analogues may be able to bind to a receptor other than the classic ER and yet achieve estrogenic action that is therapeutically desirable.

REFERENCES

Barbieri RL, Ryan KJ (1993). Hyperandrogenism, insulin resistance, and acanthosis nigricans syndrome: a common endocrinopathy with distinct pathophysiologic features. *Am J Obstet Gynecol* 147:90–101.

Hou Q, Gorski J (1993). Estrogen receptor and progesterone receptor genes are expressed differentially in mouse embryos during preimplantation development. *Proc Natl Acad Sci USA* 90:9460–9464.

Korach KS (1994). Insights from the study of animals lacking functional estrogen receptor. *Science* 266:1524–1527.

Laue L, Kenigsberg D, Pescovitz OH, Hench KD, Barnes KM, Loriaux DL, Cutler Jr GB (1989). Treatment of familial male precocious puberty with spironolactone and testolactone. *N Engl J Med* 320:496–502.

Lubahn DB, Moyer JS, Golding TS, Couse JF, Korach KS, Smithies O (1993). Alteration of reproductive function but not prenatal sexual development after insertional disruption of the mouse estrogen receptor gene. *Proc Natl Acad Sci USA* 90:11162–11166.

Smith EP, Boyd J, Frank GR, Takahashi H, Cohen RM, Specker B, Williams TC, Lubahn DB, Korach KS (1994). Estrogen resistance caused by a mutation in the estrogen-receptor gene in a man. *N Engl J Med* 331:1056–1061.

Zachmann M, Prader A, Sobel EH, Crigler JF Jr, Ritzen EM, Atares M, Ferrandez A (1986). Pubertal growth in patients with androgen insensitivity: indirect evidence for the importance of estrogens in pubertal growth of girls. *J Pediatr* 108:694–697.

15

Syndromes with Sexual Maldevelopment

A host of syndromes involve genital abnormalities in one or both sexes. In many of these conditions, hypogonadism also has been established, often on the basis of a central or hypothalamic-pituitary deficit (secondary hypogonadism, Table 15–1). In other cases, the gonadal failure is thought to be primary or the functional and anatomical status of the gonad is not known because of age or inaccessibility or simply lack of study.

Some of the conditions in this chapter were found in apparently unique families or in a series of unrelated, phenotypically similar patients, and are included to stimulate discussion of possible etiologic factors that may be important in patho-genesis. Considerable license has been taken in the naming of these conditions and eponyms, often new, have been used in an attempt to avoid an even more cumbersome nomenclature. The emphasis is obviously on genital/gonadal defects, and the reader desiring more detail outside this area must go to the original articles. Undoubtedly, experienced "syndromologists" will detect oversights; the authors welcome their input.

TABLE 15–1. Some Syndromes with
Hypogonadotropic Hypogonadism

Alopecia-anosmia-deafness
Alström
Anophthalmia-esophageal-genital
Ataxia-hypogonadism
Bardet-Biedl
Belgian mental retardation
Biemond
Bird-headed dwarf*
Börjeson-Forssman-Lehman*
Chudley
Jennings
Laurence-Moon*
LEOPARD
Lissencephaly
Micro
Möbius-peripheral neuropathy
Neurofibromatosis
Pallister-Hall
Prader-Willi
Retinitis pigmentosa–hypogonadism
Septo-optic dysplasia
Urban-Rogers-Meyer
Walker-Warburg
Werner*
X-linked MR-hypogonadism

*In some families, the hypogonadism was considered to be
primary, perhaps indicating genetic heterogeneity.

AARSKOG-SCOTT SYNDROME (FACIOGENITAL DYSPLASIA)

This syndrome comprises short stature, unusual facies, brachydactyly with occasional interdigital webbing, ligamentous laxity, and a rather unusual penoscrotal relationship, the so-called saddlebag or shawl scrotum (Aarskog, 1970). Retractile or cryptorchid tests are commonly seen. The short stature is not marked. The scrotal abnormality tends to disappear after puberty and affected individuals are usually fertile (Fryns, 1992), although an acrosomal sperm defect has been identified in one patient (Meschede et al., 1996).

The original pedigrees were compatible with X-linked inheritance. The gene, which maps to Xp11.21, a region that escapes X-inactivation (Miller and Willard, 1998), has been isolated and characterized (Pasteris et al., 1994). It codes for a putative Rho/Rac guanine nucleotide exchange factor that likely is involved in signal transduction. The condition is genetically heterogeneous—an autosomal recessive (Teebi et al., 1988) and dominant form (Grier et al., 1983) have also been described.

REFERENCES

Aarskog D (1970). A familial syndrome of short stature associated with facial dysplasia and genital abnormalities. *J Pediatr* 77:856–871.

Fryns J P (1992). Aarskog syndrome: the changing phenotype with age. *Am J Med Genet* 43: 420–427.

Grier R E, Farrington F H, Kendig R, et al. (1983). Autosomal dominant inheritance of the Aarskog syndrome. *Am J Med Genet* 15:39–46.

Meschede D, Rolf C, Neugebauer D C, et al. (1996). Sperm acrosomal defects in a patient with Aarskog-Scott syndrome. *Am J Med Genet* 66:340–342.

Miller A P, Willard H F (1998) Chromosomal basis of X chromosome inactivation: identification of 2 multigene domain in Xp11.21-p11.22 that escapes inactivation. *Proc Nat Acad Sci USA* 95:8709–8714.

Pasteris N G, Cadle A, Logie L J, et al. (1994). Isolation and characterization of the faciogenital dysplasia (Aarskog-Scott syndrome) gene: a putative Rho/Rac guanine nucleotide exchange factor. *Cell* 79:669–678.

Teebi A S, Naguilo K K, Al-Awadi S A, et al. (1988). New autosomal recessive faciodigito-genital syndrome. *J Med Genet* 25:400–406.

ABLEPHARON-MACROSTOMIA

The most striking feature of this condition is the absence or marked hypoplasia of eyelids, eyebrows, and eyelashes, along with thin, sparse hair, a triangular face, macrostomia, syncamptodactyly, absent or hypoplastic nipples, and umbilical hernia or omphalocele (McCarthy and West, 1977; Hornblass and Reifler, 1985). All affected children have been male and have exhibited a posteriorly displaced micropenis, absent scrotum, and cryptorchidism. No genetic basis for this unusual condition is evident at this time.

REFERENCES

Hornblass A, Reifler D M (1985). Ablepharon macrostomia syndrome. *Am J Ophthal* 99:552–556.

McCarthy G T, West C M (1977). Ablepharon macrostomia syndrome. *Dev Med Child Neurol* 19:659–672.

ABRUZZO-ERICKSON SYNDROME

Abruzzo and Erickson (1977) described male sibs and their maternal uncle who had ocular colobomas, cleft palate, incomplete nerve deafness, short stature, radial synostoses, and hypospadias. The mother of the sibs had a high-arched palate and mild nonbony hand anomalies. This family was cited as being a familial example of the CHARGE association (Metlay et al., 1987) but longitudinal information suggests the condition is a distinct, probably X-linked disorder (Abruzzo and Erickson, 1989).

Colobomas of various parts of the eye are a feature of a variety of different syndromes—mendelian, chromosomal, teteratogenic, and of unknown genesis. Some feature genital anomalies, but the other aspects of the disorders usually define the etiology. For example, Halal and Farsky (1981) described a family in which a boy had bilateral colobomas and hypospadias, his brother had unilateral coloboma, and the father had hypospadias alone. This condition is probably a separate autosomal dominant trait.

REFERENCES

Abruzzo M A, Erickson R P (1977). A new syndrome of cleft palate associated with coloboma, hypospadias, deafness, short stature and radial synostosis. *J Med Genet* 14:76–80.

Abruzzo M A, Erickson R P (1989). Re-evaluation of new X-linked syndrome for evidence of CHARGE syndrome or association. *Am J Med Genet* 34:397–400.

Halal R, Farsky K (1981). Coloboma-hypospadias. *Am J Med Genet* 8:53–56.

Metlay L A, Smythe P S, Miller M E (1987). Familial CHARGE syndrome: clinical report with autopsy findings. *Am J Med Genet* 26:577–581.

ACRODYSOSTOSIS

These patients are short, with short, stubby hands and feet; they exhibit brachycephaly, maxillary hypoplasia, and a up-tilted nose (Robinow et al., 1971). Underdeveloped external genitalia are common in both sexes, and males frequently have hypogonadism. Menses are commonly irregular in females.

The condition is inherited as an autosomal dominant trait. Many workers feel that acrodysostosis is simply a limited form of pseudohypoparathyroidism (Albright's hereditary osteodystrophy), which appears in the main to be due to a defect in the guanine nucleotide-binding stimulatory protein (Gs), a critical factor in the intracellular signaling pathway (Davies and Hughes, 1992; see also Chapter 11).

REFERENCES

Davies S J, Hughes H E. Familial acrodysostosis: can it be distinguished from Albright's hereditary osteodystrophy? *Clin Dysmorphol* 1:207–210, 1992.

Robinow M, Pfeiffer R A, Gorlin R J, et al. (1971). Acrodysostosis: a syndrome of peripheral dysostosis, nasal hypoplasia and mental retardation. *Am J Dis Child* 121:195–203.

ACRO-RENAL-MANDIBULAR SYNDROME

Limb deficiency and renal anomalies appear to be significantly associated, and in some instances genital defects occur as well, although the causal pathogenesis is unknown and/or complex in most cases (Johnson and Munson, 1990; Evans et al., 1992). Some syndromes are familial as exemplified by the report of Halal and colleagues (1980), who recorded two females, the offspring of consanguineous French-Canadian parents, who had severe ectrodactyly and mandibular hypoplasia; one sib had renal agenesis, the other had cystic dysplastic kidneys. A unicornuate uterus was found at autopsy in one sib whereas her sister had a uterus didelphys. In a third surviving female sib, intravenous urography revealed unilateral ureteral duplication and normal kidneys. The mother had a separate uterus, but neither she nor the surviving sib had extremity malformations. The authors postulated autosomal recessive inheritance for the lethal disease in the sibs.

Other syndromes with associated renal and/or urinary tract abnormalities are shown in Table 15–2.

REFERENCES

Evans J A, Vitez M, Czeizel A (1992). Patterns of acrorenal malformation associations. *Am J Med Genet* 44:413–419.

Halal F, Desgranges M F, Leduc B, et al. (1980). Acro-renal-mandibular syndromes. *Am J Med Genet* 5:227–284.

Johnson V P, Munson D P (1990). A new syndrome of aphalangy, hemivertabrae, and urogenital-intestinal dysgenesis. *Clin Genet* 78:346–352.

TABLE 15–2. Some Syndromes of Hypogonadism
with Renal and/or Urinary Tract Anomalies

Acro-renal-mandibular
Beckwith-Wiedemann*
Brosnan
Cerebrohepatorenal
EEC
Femoral hypoplasia–unusual facies
Fryns
Goeminne
Hand-foot-genital
Lawrence-Moon
Lenz microphthalmia
LEOPARD
Miller-Diecker
Meckel
Oculocerebrorenal
Opitz G/BBB
Pallister-Hall
Perlmann*
Renal dysplasia–limb defects
Roberts
Rüdiger
Simpson-Golabi-Behmel*
Wiedemann
Winter

*Nephroblastomatosis and/or Wilms tumor.

AL-AWADI ALOPECIA-HYPOGONADISM SYNDROME

A rather unusual syndrome was described by Al-Awadi and colleagues (1985) in three sibs who were the children of a couple related as first cousins once removed. They had unusual alopecia in that all the remaining hair was confined to the central scalp. The two female sibs had absent ovaries and streak gonads, respectively, with hypoplasia of müllerian derivatives, whereas their brother had germ cell aplasia. No similar cases have been reported.

REFERENCE
Al-Awadi, S A, Farag T I, Teebi A S, et al. (1985). Primary hypogonadism and partial alopecia in three sibs with müllerian hypoplasia in the affected females. *Am J Med Genet* 22:619–622.

ALOPECIA-ANOSMIA-DEAFNESS SYNDROME (JOHNSON NEUROECTODERMAL SYNDROME, OTHERS)

Johnson and colleagues (1983) reported a three-generation family whose affected members showed varying degrees of total body alopecia, anosmia, ear anomalies with conductive deafness, and hypogonadotropic hypogonadism. Other occasional features included cleft palate, facial asymmetry, and congenital heart disease. There was no consistent relationship between the presence or absence of the secondary hypogonadism and the severity of the other malformations. Other cases have been

Table 15–3. Some Syndromes of Hypogonadism
with Deafness

Abruzzo-Erickson
Alopecia-anosmia-deafness
Alström
Branchial arch
Cockayne
Cogenital deafness with pinna malformations
Congenital sensory mixed hearing loss
Edwards
Gorlin-Chaudhry-Moss
Ieshima
Johanson-Blizzad
LEOPARD
N
Oto-facio-osseous-gonadal
Oto-palatal-digital II
Winter

since reported (Johnson et al., 1987; Hennekam and Holtus, 1993). The original authors postulated that the gene defect resulted in aberrant development of certain neuroectodermal derivatives of the superior brachial arches. Autosomal dominant inheritance is likely.

The combination of alopecia, deafness, and hypogonadism, is clinically and genetically heterogeneous. Crandall and colleagues (1973) reported three sibs with secondary hypogonadism, deafness, and alopecia, with the hair exhibiting pili torti. In two consanguineous Arab families, Woodhouse and Sakati (1983) found seven individuals with thin scalp and eyebrow hair, diabetes mellitus, mental retardation, mild sensory deafness, and hypogonadism, the latter ranging from mild to severe, and most likely primary in type. The family described by Oerter and colleagues (1992) probably fits into this same category as well. Salti and Salem (1979) recorded a family in which both female and male sibs from a consanguineous marriage had frontoparietal alopecia and hypogonadotropic hypogonadism. No mention was made of hearing or ability to smell. (See also Al-Awadi hypogonadism syndrome. Some syndromes that feature hypogonadism with deafness are listed in Table 15–3.

REFERENCES

Crandall B F, Samec L, Sparkes R S, et al. (1973). A familial syndrome of deafness, alopecia and hypogonadism. *J Pediatr* 8:461–465.

Hennekam R C M, Holtus F J A M (1993). Johnson-McMillin syndrome: report of another family. *Am J Med Genet* 47:714–716.

Johnson V P, McMillin J M, Aceto T (1983). A newly recognized neuroectodermal syndrome of familial alopecia, anosmia, deafness and hypogonadism. *Am J Med Genet* 15:497–506.

Johnston K, Golabi M, Hall B, et al. (1987). Alopecia-anosmia-deafness-hypogonadism syndrome revisited: report of a new case. *Am J Med Genet* 26:925–927.

Oerter K E, Friedman T C, Anderson H C, et al. (1992). Familial syndrome of endocrine and neuroectodermal abnormalities. *Am J Med Genet* 44:487–491.

Salti IS, Salem Z (1979). Familial hypogonadotropic hypogonadism and alopecia. *Can Med Assn J* 121:428–434.

Woodhouse NJY, Sakati NA (1983). A syndrome of hypogonadism, diabetes mellitus, mental retardation, deafness and ECG abnormalities. *J Med Genet* 20:216–219.

ALSTRÖM SYNDROME

In 1959, Alström and coworkers (1959) described two sibs and a distant cousin with atypical retinitis pigmentosa, neurosensory deafness, obesity, and diabetes mellitus. The proband had secondary hypogonadism and a testicular histology similar to that seen in the Klinefelter syndrome. The diabetes mellitus is of the insulin-resistant type and is accompanied by acanthosis nigricans (Goldstein and Fialkow, 1973). Female patients have had oligomenorrhea and polycystic ovary disease, in retrospect likely due to the obesity and hyperinsulinism. Intelligence is normal. Inheritance is autosomal recessive.

Other occasional features include a chronic nephropathy (Goldstein and Fialkow, 1973), chronic hepatitis (Connolly, 1991), and secondary hypothyroidism (Charles et al., 1990). Whether or not the patients reported by Weinstein and colleagues (1969) had the same condition is problematic. Those patients later developed dilated cardiomyopathy, which was felt to be a distinguishing feature (Warren et al., 1987). However, longstanding diabetes may also be associated with dilated cardiomyopathy without significant coronary disease, so the status of these patients remains diagnostically uncertain. By the same token, the sibs described by Edwards and colleagues (1976) were felt to be distinct based on the fact that they had mental retardation (see p. 515). The gene for Alström syndrome has been mapped to chromosome 2p (Collin et al., 1997). Other syndromes that feature hypogonadism and significant obesity are listed in Table 15–4. Obesity is usually multifactorial and as such is hardly syndrome-specific (However, see Leptin Deficiency and Hypogonadism in Chapter 17)

REFERENCES

Alström C H, Hallgren B, Nilsson L B, et al. (1959). Retinal degeneration combined with obesity, diabetes mellitus and neurogenous deafness: a specific syndrome (not hitherto

TABLE 15–4. Syndromes of Hypogonadism with Obesity

Alström
Bardet-Biedl
Biemond
Börjeson-Forssman-Lehmann
Chudley MR
Cohen
Edwards
Prader-Willi
Urban-Rogers-Meyer
Vasquez
X-linked mental retardation, gynecomastia, and hypogonadism

described) distinct from the Laurence-Moon-Bardet-Biedl Syndrome: a clinical, endocrinological and genetic examination based on a large pedigree. *Acta Psychiat Neurol Scand* 34:1–35.

Charles S J, Moore A T, Yates J R W, et al. (1990). Alström's syndrome: further evidence of autosomal recessive inheritance and endocrinologic dysfunction. *J Med Genet* 27:590–592.

Collin G B, Marshall J O, Cardon L R et al. (1997). Homozygosity mapping of Alström syndrome to chromosome 2p. *Hum Mol Genet* 6:213–219.

Connolly M B, Jan J E, Couch R M, et al. (1991). Hepatic dysfunction in Alström's disease. *Am J Med Genet* 40:421–424.

Edwards J A, Sethi P K, Scoma A J, et al. (1976). A new familial syndrome characterized by pigmentary retinopathy, hypogonadism, mental retardation, nerve deafness and glucose intolerance. *Am J Med* 60:23–32.

Goldstein J L, Fialkow, P J (1973). The Alström syndrome. *Medicine* 52:53–71.

Warren S E, Schnitt S J, Bauman A J, et al. (1987). Late onset dilated cardiomyopathy in a unique family syndrome of hypogonadism and metabolic abnormalities. *Am Heart J* 114: 1522–1524.

Weinstein R L, Kliman B, Scully R E (1969). Familial syndrome of primary testicular insufficiency with normal virilization, blindness, deafness and metabolic abnormalities. *N Engl J Med* 281:969–977.

Anophthalmia-Esophageal-Genital Syndrome

Shah and colleagues (1997) reported one case and reviewed three other similar reports of individuals with anophthalmia or microphthalmia, esophageal atresia, and cryptorchidism and micropenis in males. One patient had olfactory hypoplasia, leading to the suggestion that the hypogonadism was central. The one affected female had no obvious genital anomaly. All cases were sporadic.

REFERENCE

Shah D, Jones R, Porter H, et al. (1997). Bilateral microphthalmia, esophageal atresia and cryptorchidism: the anophthalmia-esophageal-genital syndrome. *Am J Med Genet* 70:171–173.

Ataxia-Hypogonadism Syndrome

Spinocerebellar ataxia with central hypogonadism has been reported on a number of occasions. When the combination is seen with choroidal dystrophy, the triad is referred to as the Boucher-Neuhäuser syndrome (Boucher and Gibberd, 1969; Neuhäuser and Opitz, 1975; Limber et al., 1989; Baroncini et al., 1991). The hypogonadism appears at puberty, whereas the ataxia and retinal degeneration often do not appear until early adult life or later. Fok and colleagues (1989) and Erdem and colleagues (1994) suggested that the hypogonadism originates in the pituitary. Others have suggested that the hypogonadism is due to a defect in gonadotropin-releasing hormone secretion (Berciano et al., 1982).

Other patients with ataxia and hypogonadism have been reported without the retinal change (Volpé et al., 1963; Matthews and Rundle, 1964; Abs et al., 1990), but in view of the fact that the choroidal dystrophy may be subtle and not appear until the sixth decade, the families may all harbor mutations in the same gene. Because the central hypogonadism may have different origins, the ataxia-hypogonadism combination also may be genetically heterogeneous. For example, Fryns and colleagues (1998) described mentally retarded female sibs with ataxia and choroidal atrophy whose hypogonadism was primary. In most instances, the pedigrees are compatible with autosomal recessive inheritance, although in the family reported by Volpé and colleagues (1963) male sibs had a maternal uncle historically affected, perhaps indicating extra X-linked recessive or male-limited dominant inheritance. Moreover, retinal, cerebellar, and endocrine dysfunction may occur as a result of mitochondrial mutations.

REFERENCES

Abs R, Van Vleyman E, Parizel P M, et al. (1990). Congenital cerebellar hypoplasia and hypogonadotropic hypogonadism. *J Neurol Sci* 98:259–265.

Baroncini A, Franco N, Forobosco A (1991). A new family with chorioretinal dystrophy, spinocerebellar ataxia and hypogonadotropic hypogonadism (Boucher-Neuhäuser syndrome). *Clin Genet* 39:274–277.

Berciano J, Amado J A, Freijanes J, et al. (1982). Familial cerebellar ataxia and hypogonadotropic hypogonadism: evidence for hypothalamic LHRH deficiency. *J Neurol Neurosurg Psychiatry* 45:747–751.

Boucher B J, Gibbert F B (1969). Familial ataxia, hypogonadism and retinal deterioration. *Acta Neurol Scand* 45:507–510.

Erdem E, Kirath H, Erbas T, et al. (1994). Cerebellar ataxia associated with hypogonadotropic hypogonadism and chorioretinopathy: a poorly recognized association. *Clin Neurol Neurosurg* 96:86–91.

Fok A C K, Wong M C, Cheah J S (1989). Syndrome of cerebellar ataxia and hypogonadotropic hypogonadism: evidence for pituitary gonadotropin deficiency. *J Neurol Neurosurg Psychiatry* 52:407–409.

Fryns J-P, VanLingen C, Devriendtk K, et al. (1998). Two adult females with a distinct mental retardation syndrome: non-progressive neurologic symptoms with ataxia, hypotonia, similar facial appearance, hypergonadotropic hypogonadism and retinal dystrophy. *J Med Genet* 35:333–335.

Limber E R, Brosnick G H, Lebovitz R M, et al. (1989). Cerebellar ataxia, hypogonadotropic hypogonadism, and choroidal dystrophy (Boucher-Neuhäuser syndrome). *Am J Med Genet* 33:409–414.

Matthews W B, Rundle A T (1964). Familial cerebellar ataxia and hypogonadism, *Brain* 87: 463–468.

Neuhäuser G, Opitz JM (1975). Autosomal recessive syndrome of cerebellar ataxia and hypogonadotropic hypogonadism. *Clin Genet* 7:426–434.

Volpé R, Metzler WS, Johnson MS (1963). Familial hypogonadotropic eunuchoidism with cerebellar ataxia. *J Clin Endocrinol* 23:107–115.

ATAXIA-TELANGIECTASIA

This multisystem autosomal recessive disorder generally comes to medical attention in childhood because of progressive cerebellar ataxia. The telangiectasia, most notably involving the eyes, external ears, and flexor surfaces of the extremities, may not be evident until later. Immunologic deficiency, premature aging, growth retardation, chromosome instability with *in vitro* hypersensitivity to ionizing radiation and radiomimetic drugs, and an increased incidence of malignancy, especially of the lymphoreticular system, are other features (Boder, 1985).

Primary hypogonadism is common in both sexes, and affected males may have cryptorchidism and females have hypoplastic external genitalia. Ovarian pathology is variable, ranging from complete absence of both ovaries to dysgenesis with absence of primary follicles (Zadik et al., 1978; Waldmann et al., 1983). In older females, both gonadoblastomas and dysgerminomas have been described. About 1% of the U.S. white population may be heterozygotes, and there is roughly a fourfold increased relative risk of all types of cancer in these individuals, but most particularly of the female breast (Swift et al., 1991). In the mouse homologue, male spermatogenesis is blocked at the zygotene/pachytene stage (Xu et al., 1996)

The gene (ATM), previously mapped to 11q, has been sequenced (Savitsky et al., 1995). The putative protein has at least two domains, one of which may regulate cellular growth; the other bears responsibility for DNA repair (Rotman and Shiloh, 1998).

REFERENCES

Boder E (1985). Ataxia-telangiectasia: an overview. In Gatti RA, Swift M, eds. Ataxia-telangiectasia: Genetics, Neuropathology and Immunology of a Degenerative Disease of Childhood. New York: Alan R. Liss, pp 1–63.

Rotman G, Shiloh Y (1998). ATM: from gene to function. *Hum Mol Genet* 7:555–1563.

Savitsky K, Bar-Shiru A, Gilad S, et al. (1995). A single ataxia-telangiectasia gene with a product similar to Pl-3 kinase. *Science* 268:1749–1753.

Swift M, Morrell D, Massey R B, et al. (1991). Incidence of cancer in 161 females affected by ataxia-telangiectasia. *N Engl J Med* 325:1831–1836.

Waldmann TA, Misiti J, Nelson DL, et al. (1983). Ataxia-telangiectasia: a multisystem heredity disease with immunodeficiency, impaired organ maturation, x-ray sensitivity, and a high incidence of neoplasia. *Ann Intern Med* 99:367–379.

Xu Y, Ashley T, Brainerd E E, et al. (1996). Targeted disruption of ATM leads to growth retardation, chromosomal fragmentation during meiosis, immune defects, and thymic lymphoma. *Genes Dev* 10:2411–2422.

Zadik Z, Levin S, Prager-Lewin R, et al. (1978). Gonadal dysfunction in patients with ataxia-telangiectasia. *Acta Paediat Scand* 67:477–479.

BARDET-BIEDL SYNDROME

This condition, previously eponymously linked to the Laurence-Moon syndrome (this chapter) is now considered to be distinct. The syndrome is characterized by mental retardation, pigmentary retinopathy, polydactyly, obesity, and hypogenitalism (Green et al., 1989). Hypogonadism is primary and progressive in some cases (Toledo et al., 1977) but may be hypogonadotropic in others (Chang et al., 1981). The latter is not surprising, because locus heterogeneity has been demonstrated (Carmi et al., 1995; Beales et al. 1997), although all forms appear to be inherited as autosomal recessive traits. Hypoplastic external genitalia are well recognized in males, but less well known are genital anomalies in affected females—uterine, tubal, and ovarian hypoplasia, duplex uterus, and atretic or septate vagina—most of which are not discovered until early adult life (Stoler et al., 1995). However, one affected female infant presented with hydrometroculpos (Mehrotra et al., 1997). Adult-onset hirsutism and ovarian hyperthecosis have been described in other women (Haning et al., 1980). Obesity-related, and presumably insulin-resistant, diabetes mellitus is often present; thus, it is possible the hirsutism is a secondary phenomenon in these patients (Ehrmann et al., 1995).

REFERENCES

Beales P L, Warner A M, Hitman G A, et al. (1997). Bardet-Biedl syndrome; a molecular and phenotypic study of 18 families. *J Med Genet* 34:92–98.

Carmi R, Elbedour K, Stone E M (1995). Phenotypic differences among patients with Bardet-Biedl syndrome linked to three different chromosome loci. *Am J Hum Genet* 59:199–203.

Chang R J, Davidson B J, Carlson H E, et al. (1981). Hypogonadotropic hypogonadism associated with retinitis pigmentosa in a female sibship: evidence for gonadotropin deficiency. *J Clin Endocrinol Metab* 53:1179–1185.

Ehrmann D A, Barnes R B, Rosenfield R L (1995). Polycystic ovary syndrome as a form of functional ovarian hyperandrogenism due to dysregulation of androgen secretion. *Endocr Rev* 16:322–353.

Green J S, Parfrey P S, Harnett J D et al. (1989). The cardinal manifestations of Bardet-Biedl syndrome, a form of Laurence-Moon-Biedl syndrome. *N Engl J Med* 321:1002–1009.

Haning R V, Carlson I H, Gilbert E F, et al. (1980). Virilism as a late manifestation in the Bardet-Biedl syndrome. *Am J Med Genet* 7:279–292.

Mehrotra N, Taub S, Covert R F (1997). Hydrometrocolpos as a neonatal manifestation of the Bardet-Biedl syndrome. *Am J Med Genet* 69:220–222.

Stoler J M, Herrin J T, Holmes L B (1995). Genital abnormalities in females with Bardet-Biedl syndrome. *Am J Med Genet* 55:276–278.

Toledo S P A, Medieros-Nefo G A, Knobel M, et al. (1977). Evaluation of hypothalamic-pituitary-gonadal function in the Bardet-Biedl syndrome. *Metabolism* 26:1277–1291.

BECKWITH-WIEDEMANN SYNDROME (EMG SYNDROME)

The cardinal features of this disorder at birth are exomphalos, macroglossia, and gigantism, hence the alternative designation as the EMG syndrome (Filippi and McKusick, 1970). Hypoglycemia, visceromegaly, and hemihypertrophy may also be seen and embryonal malignancies are relatively common (Niikawa et al., 1986; Wiedemann, 1983).

A variety of confusing genital and gonadal alterations have been noted (Flippi and McKusick, 1970; Kosseff et al., 1976; Niikawa et al., 1986). For example, affected males may show cryptorchidism, hypospadias, and a small penis, whereas others may have genital enlargement at birth with interstitial cell hyperplasia of the testes. Similarly, large ovaries and uterus, clitoromegaly, and bicornuate uterus have been recorded in affected females.

Early somatic growth is excessive, but growth velocity normalizes after the first 6 years (Sippell et al., 1989). The enlarged tongue and hemihypertrophy become less exaggerated with time such that the syndrome may not be immediately recognizable in adult life.

The condition has been documented in pedigrees consistent with autosomal dominant inheritance with sex limitation, and mutations in p57[kip2] have been identified in some of these families (Hatada et al., 1997). It may also result from partial trisomy of 11p15.5, which may also be heritable (Slavotinek et al., 1997) and from paternal disomy (Kubota et al., 1994) The syndrome may be due to disruption of maternal imprinting of the insulin-like growth factor 2 gene in the 11p15.5 region (Weksberg et al., 1993), although alternative explanations have been offered (Kubota et al., 1993.) Somatic mosaicism for paternal isodisomy has been seen (Henry et al., 1993) and possibly could account for some cases of discordant monozygotic twins (Olney et al., 1988) or those in whom the characteristic features have developed after birth (Chitayat et al., 1990).

REFERENCES

Chitayat D, Rothchild A, Ling E, et al. (1990). Apparent postnatal onset of some manifestations of the Wiedemann-Beckwith syndrome. *Am J Med Genet* 36:434–485.

Filippi G, McKusick V A 1970. The Beckwith-Wiedemann syndrome (the exomphalos-macroglossia-gigantism syndrome): report of two cases and review of the literature. *Medicine* 49:279–298.

Hatada I, Naketani A, Morisaki H, et al. (1997). New p57^{kip2} mutations in Beckwith-Wiedeman syndrome. *Hum Genet* 100:681–683.

Henry I, Puech A, Riesewijk A, et al. (1993). Somatic mosaicism for partial paternal isodisomy in Wiedeman-Beckwith syndrome: a postfertilization event. *Eur J Hum Genet* 1:19–29.

Kosseff A L, Herrman J, Gilbert E F, et al. (1996). Study of malformation syndromes in man XXIX: The Wiedemann-Beckwith syndrome: clinical, genetic and pathogenic studies of 12 cases. *Eur J Pediatr* 123.139–166.

Kubota T, Saitoh S, Matsumoto T, et al. (1994). Excess functional copy of allele at chromosome region 11p15 may cause Wiedemann-Beckwith (EMG) syndrome. *Am J Med Genet* 49:378–383.

Niikawa N, Ishikiriyama S, Takahashi S. et al, (1986). The Wiedemann-Beckwith syndrome: pedigree studies on five females with evidence for autosomal dominant inheritance with variable expressivity. *Am J Med Genet* 24:41–55.

Olney A H, Buehler B A, Waziri M (1988). Wiedemann-Beckwith syndrome in apparently discordant monozygotic twins. *Am J Med Genet* 29:491–499.

Sippell W G, Partsch C-J, Wiedemann H R (1989). Growth, bone maturation and pubertal development in children with the EMG syndrome. *Clin Genet* 35:20–28.

Slavotinek A, Gaunt L, Donnai D (1997). Paternally inherited duplications of 11p15.5 and Beckwith-Wiedemann syndrome. *J Med Genet* 34:819–826.

Weksberg R, Shen D R, Fei Y L et al. (1993). Disruption of insulin-like growth factor 2 imprinting in Beckwith-Wiedemann syndrome. *Nat Genet* 5:143–150.

Wiedemann H R (1983). Tumours and hemihypertrophy associated with Wiedemann-Beckwith syndrome. *Eur J Pediatr* 141:129.

BEEMER LETHAL MALFORMATION SYNDROME

Beemer and van Ertbruggen (1984) described 46,XY sibs of consanguineous parents who had unusual facies, cyanotic congenital heart disease, radiographically dense bones, and CNS and genital anomalies. The latter consisted, in sib 1, of an enlarged clitoris with a ventral urethral groove and undescended, presumably histologically normal, testes; and in sib 2, a normal penis but with hypoplastic scrotum and no palpable testes. However, no autopsy was performed on sib 2, so the gonadal status is uncertain.

There are similarities between this condition and the genito-palato cardiac and the Smith-Lemli-Opitz syndromes.

REFERENCE
Beemer F A, van Ertbruggen I (1984). Peculiar facial appearance, hydrocephalus, double outlet ventricle, genital anomalies, and dense bones with lethal outcome. *Am J Med Genet* 19: 391–394.

BELGIAN MENTAL RETARDATION SYNDROME

Fryns and colleagues (1990) reported four siblings, three male and one female, with mental retardation, craniofacial dysmorphism (long face with broad nose and coloboma of alae nasi, deep-set eyes, and mandibular prognathism), diabetes mellitus, and seizures. The males were adequately virilized but had small testes and moderately elevated serum gonadotropin levels. The female sibling exhibited poor development of secondary sex characteristics with menopausal gonadotropin levels. The authors felt the syndrome was a unique autosomal recessive trait.

REFERENCE

Fryns J P, Vogels A, van der Berghe H (1990). Mental retardation, craniofacial dysmorphism, hypogonadism, diabetes mellitus and epilepsy in four siblings: a "new" mental retardation syndrome. *Clin Genet* 37:111–116.

BIEMOND SYNDROME

The Biemond syndrome closely resembles and must be distinguished from a number of syndromes involving the eye and the gonads. It is characterized by hypogenitalism secondary to hypogonadotropic hypogonadism, mental retardation, iris colobomata, postaxial polydactyly, and obesity (Biemond, 1934). Kindreds with affected sibs have been reported, suggesting autosomal recessive inheritance. However, a partial manifestation of the syndrome such as colobomas alone or polydactyly alone has been found in some relatives, suggesting autosomal dominant inheritance with incomplete penetrance and variable expressivity; hence the genetics of the disorder is in some doubt (Grebe, 1953). Some families recorded as having Bardet-Biedl syndrome (p. 478) may actually have had the Biemond syndrome. To add to the confusion, the Biemond eponym has been used in conjunction with another syndrome involving neurologic dysfunction, but without genital or known endocrine abnormalities (Verloes et al., 1997)

REFERENCES

Biemond A (1934). Het syndrome van Laurence-Biedl en een aanverwant, nieuw syndroom. *Nederl T Geneesk* 78:1801–1814.

Grebe H (1953). Contribution au diagnostic differential du syndrome de Bardet-Biedl. *J Hum Genet* 2:127–144.

Verloes A, Temple I K, Bennet S, et al. (1997). Coloboma, mental retardation, hypogonadism, and obesity: critical review of the so-called Biemond syndrome type 2, updated nosology, and delineation of three "new" syndromes. *Am J Med Genet* 69:379–379.

BIRD-HEADED DWARFISM SYNDROMES
(SECKEL SYNDROME AND OTHERS)

This appellation is perjorative but unfortunately pervades the literature. It was offered by Seckel (1960) in a monograph in which he described a number of individuals with similar facial features as well as other anomalies. Majewski and Goecke (1982) noted that Seckel's original cases were not identical and proposed that the Seckel syndrome include severe intrauterine and postnatal growth retardation with proportionate short stature, severe microcephaly with typical receding forehead and prominently curved nose, together giving rise to the "bird-headed" appellation. Severe mental retardation, antimongoloid obliquity of the orbits, high arched palate, hirsutism, fifth finger chondactyly, dislocation of radial head, and dysharmonic retardation of ossification without generalized skeletal abnormalities present in the majority of patients. Of the cases from the literature these workers would accept as examples of the syndrome were some males with cryptorchidism and females with clitoromegaly. The Seckel syndrome is inherited as an autosomal recessive trait with males and females being equally severely affected.

Other bird-headed dwarfs with somewhat different features were described by Fitch and colleagues (1970) who described a male with premature senility and cryptorchidism. Bangstad and colleagues (1989) reported a family in which a male and female sib pair had the typical facial features, progressive ataxia, goiter, insulin-resistant diabetes mellitus, and primary hypogonadism. Fryns and colleagues (1997) reported three sibs with associated eye anomalies (microphthalmia, colobomas, cloudy cornea) with urogenital defects: the males had hypospadias. These bird-headed dwarf syndromes are probably also autosomal recessive traits.

References

Bangstad H J, Beck-Nielsen H, Hother-Nielsen O, et al. (1989). Primordial bird-headed dwarfism associated with progressive ataxia, early onset insulin-resistant diabetes, goiter and primary gonadal insufficiency. *Acta Paediat Search* 78:488–493.

Fitch N, Pinsky L, Lechance LC (1970). A form of bird-headed dwarfism with features of premature senility. *Am J Dis Child* 120:260–264.

Fryns J-P, Verresen H, Van der Berghe H (1997). Prenatal growth retardation, microphthalmia/iris coloboma, cloudy cornea, urogenital anomalies and microcephaly: a possible new sublethal syndrome. *Clin Genet* 51:164–166.

Majewski F, Goecke T (1982). Studies of microcephalic primordial dwarfism I: Approach to a delineation of the Seckel syndrome. *Am J Med Genet* 12:7–21, 1982.

Seckel H P G (1960). Bird-headed dwarfs. Charles C. Thomas, Springfield, IL, 1960.

Blepharochalasis Syndrome

Blepharochalasis refers to a condition where the upper eyelid is redundant and pendulous. As an isolated entity it is inherited as an autosomal dominant trait. Collins and colleagues (1990) described a mother and two daughters with blepharochalasis plus valvular heart disease, postnatal-onset short stature, and small hands. Wilson and colleagues (1996) found hypospadias and undescended testes in another similar family and suggested these features should also be considered part of the symptom complex.

References

Collins F A, Partington M W, Mulcahy D, et al. (1990). A new syndrome of familial short stature, small hands, valvular heart disease and a characteristic facies. *Clin Genet* 37:18–23.

Wilson L, Kerr B, Super M (1996). A new autosomal dominant syndrome of blepharochalasis, short statue, joint laxity, cardiac and urogenital defects. *J Med Genet* 33 (Suppl): 530.

Blepharophimosis-Ptosis-Epicanthus Inversus Syndrome (BPES)

Ostensibly there are two variants of this condition, one with, the other without, female infertility, the latter due to primary gonadal failure of unknown etiology (Zlotogora et al., 1983). The syndrome is inherited as a sex-limited autosomal dominant trait. The ocular findings can be reproduced by deletions in 3q22, prompting the suggestion that BPES plus ovarian failure is a contiguous gene syndrome (Smith et al., 1989). Given the likelihood that a gene important for ocular development resides in 3q22, allelic variation is equally possible. Compounding the situation still further are the findings of unilateral BPES (ovarian status unknown) with partial trisomy for distal 3q (Cai et al., 1997), and a report of an Indian family in which the combination of anomalies have been linked to chromosome 7p (Maw et al., 1996).

REFERENCES

Cai T, Tagle D A, Xia X, et al. (1997). A novel case of unilateral blepharophimosis syndrome and mental retardation associated with *de novo* trisomy 8 for chromosome 3q. *J Med Genet* 34:772–776.

Maw M, Kar B, Biswas J, et al. (1996). Linkage of blepharophimosis syndrome in a large Indian pedigree to chromosome 7p. *Hum Mol Genet* 5:2045–2054.

Smith A, Fraser I S, Shearma R P, et al. (1989). Blepharophimosis plus ovarian failure: a likely candidate for a contiguous gene syndrome. *J Med Genet* 26:434–438.

Zlotogora J, Sagi M, Cohen T (1983). The blepharophimosis, ptosis and epicanthus inversus syndrome: delineation of two types. *Am J Hum Genet* 35:1020–1027.

BLOOM SYNDROME

The Bloom syndrome comprises proportional short stature, dolicocephaly, a characteristic facies, sun-sensitive telangiectatic erythema of exposed areas, and increased sister-chromatoid exchange in a variety of different types of cells in culture (Bloom, 1966; German, 1992). The gene, mapped to 15q26.1 codes for a DNA helicase (Ellis et al., 1995). There is an established increased incidence of cancer as with other chromosome instability syndromes (German, 1992).

Primary hypogonadism of mild to moderate degree is present in all males and cryptorchidism may be present (Kauli et al., 1977; Vanderscheuren-Lodeweyckx et al., 1984). Sterility may be universal. Whether this is due to a hormonal deficiency or meiotic chromosome instability requires further study. Secondary sex characteristics may be reasonably well preserved even in the face of sterility. Infrequent or irregular menses are common in affected females. The condition is an autosomal recessive trait.

REFERENCES

Bloom D (1966). The syndrome of congenital telangiectatic erythema and stunted growth: observations and studies. *J Pediat* 68:103–113.

Ellis N A, Groden J, Ye T-Z, et al. (1995). The Bloom's syndrome gene product is homologous to Rec Q helicases. *Cell* 83:655–666.

German J (1992). Bloom's syndrome: incidence, age of onset, and types of leukemia in the Bloom's syndrome registry. In: Bartsocas C S, Loukopoulos (eds). *Genetics of Hematologic Disorders*. Washington, D.C., Hemisphere Publ., pp. 241–258.

Kauli R, Prager-Lewis R, Kaufman H, et al. (1977). Gonadal function in Bloom's syndrome. *Clin Endocrinol* 6:285–289.

Vanderschueren-Lodeweyckx M, Fryns J P, et al. (1984). Bloom's syndrome. *Am J Dis Child* 138:812–816.

BÖRJESON-FORSSMAN-LEHMANN SYNDROME

Börjeson, Forssman, and Lehmann (1962) described a kindred in which three males had a similar disorder consisting of severe mental retardation, obesity, grotesque facies, dwarfism, knock-knees, a large space between the first and second toes, hypometabolism with normal thyroid function, and hypogonadism. Two of the three suffered from seizures. All had small genitalia and either cryptorchidism or small, soft scrotal testes. Secondary sexual development did not take place, and sexual hair was absent. The prostate was small but otherwise normal. Testicular histology in one patient showed prepubertal testicular tissue with absence of germinal cells, and interstitial fibrosis. Laboratory evaluation revealed a normal karyotype and low urinary gonadotropin and 17-ketosteroid excretion. In one of the original cases and in a sporadic case described later, the pituitary was small, suggesting hypogonadotropism as the cause of the hypogonadism (Brun et al., 1974; Barr and Galindo, 1965). However, there is also evidence suggesting that central and peripheral hypogonadism may coexist, and variation within a family has been seen, such that the issue remains in doubt (Robinson et al., 1983; Ardinger et al., 1984).

The constellation of anomalies appears to represent a distinct recessive syndrome. The gene has been localized to Xq26–27 (Turner et al., 1989). This region also contains SOX 3, deletion of which resulted in partial testicular failure in a patient who had no other features of the syndrome (Rousseau et al., 1991).

Other patients who had a phenotype similar to the Börjeson-Forssman-Lehmann syndrome were reported in an extended family by Wilson and colleagues (1991). However, the gene in the latter family mapped to the pericentromeric region of the X chromosome, and affected males additionally had gynecomastia. The family described by Vasquez and colleagues (1972) probably had one of the two syndromes.

REFERENCES

Ardinger H H, Hanson J W, Zellweger H W (1984). Börjeson-Forssman-Lehmann syndrome: further delineation in five cases. *Am J Med Genet* 19:653–664.

Barr H S, Galindo J (1965). The Börjeson-Forssman-Lehmann syndrome. *J Ment Def Res* 9: 125–130.

Börjeson M, Forssman H, Lehmann O (1962). An X-linked recessively inherited syndrome characterized by grave mental deficiency, epilepsy and endocrine disorder. *Acta Med Scand* 171:13–21.

Brun A, Börjeson M, Forssman H (1974). An inherited syndrome with mental deficiency and endocrine disorder. *J Ment Def Res* 18:317–325.

Robinson L K, Jones K L, Culler F, et al. (1983). The Börjeson-Forssman-Lehmann syndrome. *Am J Med Genet* 15:457–468.

Rousseau F, Vincent A, Rivella S, et al. (1991). Four chromosomal breakpoints and four new probes mark out a 10-cM region encompassing the fragile-X locus (FRAXA). *Am J Med Genet* 48:108–116.

Turner G, Gedeon A, Mulley J, et al. (1989). Börjeson-Forssman-Lehmann syndrome: clinical manifestations and gene localization to Xq26–27. *Am J Med Genet* 34:463–496.

Vasquez S B, Hurst D L, Sotos J F (1972). X-linked hypogonadism, gynecomastia, mental retardation, short stature, and obesity—a new syndrome. *J Pediatr* 94:56–60.

Wilson M, Mulley J, Gedeon A, et al. (1991). New X-linked syndrome of mental retardation, gynecomastia, and obesity is linked to DXS255. *Am J Med Genet* 40:406–413.

BRACHIO-SKELETAL-GENITAL SYNDROME
(ELSAHY-WATERS SYNDROME)

Elsahy and Waters (1971) described three male sibs, whose parents were first cousins, with unusual facies (brachycephaly, marked midface hypoplasia, hypertelorism, ptosis, cleft palate, and relative mandibular prognathism), fused second and third cervical vertebrae, and hypospadias of varying degrees. Autosomal recessive inheritance is likely.

REFERENCE

Elsahy N I, Waters W R (1971). The brachio-skeletal-genital syndrome. *Plast Reconstr Surg* 48: 542–550.

BRANCHIAL ARCH SYNDROME

There are a number of different disorders that feature defective branchial arch development, with and without anomalies outside the head and neck. Toriello and colleagues (1985) described two male sibs and their male cousin with maxillofacial dysostosis, microcephaly, mild mental retardation, protuberant ears with mixed hearing loss, and cryptorchidism. One of these children also had subvalvar pulmonary stenosis. The condition appears to be X-linked.

REFERENCE

Toriello H V, Higgins J V, Abrahamson J, Waterman D F, Moore W D (1985). X-linked syndrome of branchial arch and other defects. *Am J Med Genet* 21:137–142.

BROSNAN SYNDROME

Brosnan and coworkers (1980) noted heterogeneity in the 46,XY pure gonadal dysgenesis group when they described two phenotypic female sibs, both of whom had short stature, facial anomalies, rather peculiar punched-out ectodermal scalp defects and displaced hair whorls, VSD, renal anomalies, bicornuate uterus, and streak gonads. No endocrine tissue could be identified in the gonads, which essentially were composed of dense fibroelastic tissue. The fallopian tubes were immature and contained no cilia.

The condition could be either an autosomal or an X-linked recessive trait.

REFERENCE

Brosnan P G, Lewandowski R C, Toguri A G, et al. (1980). A new familial syndrome of 46,XY gonadal dysgenesis with anomalies of ectodermal and mesodermal structures. *J Pediatr* 97:586–590.

C SYNDROME (OPITZ TRIGONOCEPHALY SYNDROME)

Trigonocephaly is a nonspecific malformation that may be a component of a variety of conditions. However, Opitz and colleagues (1969) described this condition in sibs who also had mental retardation, unusual facies, polydactyly, cardiac defects, and, in the boy, cryptorchidism. Other similar patients were described by Antley and colleagues (1981), Sargent and colleagues (1985), and Schaap and colleagues (1992). Additional genital anomalies included male hypospadias and clitoral hypertrophy. Most described individuals were infants, so gonadal status is uncertain, although at least one female apparently had normal pubertal development (Sargent et al., 1985). The syndrome is inherited as an autosomal recessive trait (Haaf et al., 1991).

REFERENCES

Antley R M, Hwang D S, Theopold W, et al. (1981). Further delineation of the C (trigono-cephaly) syndrome. *Am J Med Genet* 9:147–163.

Haaf T, Hofmann R, Schmid M (1991). Opitz trigonocephaly syndrome. *Am J Med Genet* 40: 444–446.

Opitz J M, Johnson R C, McCreadie S R, et al. (1969). The C syndrome of multiple congenital anomalies. *Birth Defects Orig Art Ser* 5(2):161–166.

Sargent C, Dunn J, Baraitser M, et al. (1985). Trigonocephaly and the Opitz C syndrome. *J Med Genet* 22:39–45.

Schaap C, Schrander-Stumpel C T, Fryns J P (1992). Opitz-C syndrome: on the nosology of mental retardation and trigonocephaly. *Genet Couns* 3:209–215.

Camptobrachydactyly (Edwards-Gale syndrome)

Edwards and Gale (1972) described a kindred in which multiple members had brachydactyly of the hands and feet and flexion contractures of the fingers. Syndactyly and polydactyly were present in some members as well. Septate vagina was seen in a few affected females. The condition is an autosomal dominant trait.

REFERENCE

Edwards J A, Gale R P (1972). Camptobrachydactyly: a new autosomal dominant trait with two probable homozygotes. *Am J Hum Genet* 24:464–474.

Cardiomyopathy-Hypogonadism Syndrome

The association of dilated cardiomyopathy with hypoplastic external genitalia was first reported in three brothers by Najjar and colleagues (1973). Other sib pairs, both male and female, were subsequently described (Najjar et al., 1984; Malouf et al., 1985; Thomas et al., 1993). The hypogonadism is hypergonadotropic in type. It is conceivable the condition is heterogeneous. For example, in the first family described by Najjar and colleagues (1973), the boys were retarded. In the female sibs reported by Malouf and colleagues, ptosis was present and the cardiomyopathy pursued a less relentless course. This latter feature was also noted in a single female patient with ovarian dysgenesis recorded by Narahara and colleagues (1992). In any case, autosomal recessive inheritance is likely.

Whether the family reported by Sachs and colleagues (1980) had the same condition is uncertain. These authors described congestive cardiomyopathy, primary hypogonadism, and peculiar scalp tumors, histologically defined as collagenomas, in male sibs. Their father died of congestive heart failure, etiology uncertain, but did have historically similar scalp lesions. A variably expressed autosomal dominant trait is the most plausible explanation for the findings, but other alternatives are possible.

REFERENCES

Malouf J, Alam S., Kanj H, et al. (1985). Hypergonadotropic hypogonadism with congestive cardiomyopathy: an autosomal recessive disorder? *Am J Med Genet* 20:483–485.

Narahara K, Kamada M, Takahashi Y, et al. (1992). Case of ovarian dysgenesis and dilated cardiomyopathy supports existence of Malouf syndrome. *Am J Med Genet* 44:364–373.

Najjar S S, Der Kaloustian V M, Nassif S I (1973). Genital anomaly, mental retardation, and cardiomyopathy: a new syndrome? *J Pediatr* 83:286–288.

Najjar S S, De Kaloustian V M, Ardati K O (1984). Genital anomaly and cardiomyopathy: a new syndrome. *Clin Genet* 26:371–373.
Sachs H N, Crawley I S, Ward J M, et al. (1980). Familial cardiomyopathy, hypogonadism, and collagenoma. *Ann Intern Med* 93:813–817.
Thomas I T, Jewett T, Lantz P, et al. (1993). Najjar syndrome revisited. *Am J Med Genet* 47: 1151–1152.

CARDIO-PULMONARY-GENITAL SYNDROME

Two unrelated patients were described by Meacham and colleagues (1991), with complex cyanotic heart disease, diaphragm defects with attendant lung hypoplasia, genital ambiguity, and a 46,XY karyotype. Both had small but histologically normal testes capable of secreting testosterone, an epididymis, vas deferens, and prostate. The phallus was small, and in both cases, a true double vagina, not a septate vagina, was present. A uterus and fallopian tubes were evident as well. Although no biochemical or molecular studies of MIF were done, a defect in this protein or its receptor are not likely, given the complexity of the genital anomalies. Perturbations in steroid metabolism are also not likely. Moreover, the vagina is never a paired structure under any circumstances. Toriello and Higgins (1992) reported another patient.

A somewhat similar patient was described by Maaswinkel-Mooij and Stokuis-Brantsma (1992). However, in the latter patient, the uterus was bicornuate with no mention of the condition of the vagina.

REFERENCES

Meacham L R, Winn K J, Culler F L, et al. (1991). Double vagina, cardiac, pulmonary, and other genital malformations with 46,XY karyotype. *Am J Med Genet* 41:445–451.
Maaswinkel-Mooij P D, Stokuis-Brantsma W W (1992). Phenotypically normal girl with male pseudohermaphroditism, hypoplastic left ventricle, lung aplasia, horseshoe kidney, and diaphragmatic hernia. *Am J Med Genet* 42:647–648.
Toriello H V, Higgins J V (1992). Report of another child with sex reversal and cardiac, pulmonary, and diaphragm defects. *Am J Med Genet* 44:252.

CATARACTS AND HYPOGONADISM (BASSÖE-LUBINSKY SYNDROME)

Lubinsky (1983) described three brothers with primary hypogonadism and cataracts, the latter becoming symptomatic in adolescence. Earlier, Bassöe (1956) had reported an affected male and female sib pair from a Norwegian isolate. The sibs also had a congenital, apparently stable form of muscular dystrophy. However, other family members had the myopathy without the endocrine disease, so the combination was likely coincidental. In the affected female the hypogonadism was clearly hypergonadotropic in type.

REFERENCES

Bassöe H H (1956). Familial congenital muscular dystrophy with gonadal dysgenesis. *J Clin Endocrinol Metab* 16:1614–1621.
Lubinsky M S (1983). Cataracts and testicular failure in three brothers. *Am J Med Genet* 16: 149–152.

CEREBROHEPATORENAL SYNDROME (ZELLWEGER SYNDROME)

This complex syndrome features craniofacial defects—macrocephaly, high fore-head, and a mid-face reminiscent of trisomy 21, along with ocular abnormalities such as optic atrophy and retinitis pigmentosa; cerebral dysgenesis with hypotonia, retardation, and seizures; hepatic dysfunction and multicystic kidneys (Lazarow and Moser, 1995).

Other abnormalities such as the Di George developmental field complex, cardiac defects, and skeletal anomalies are variable features. Affected males usually have cryptorchidism and micropenis, and females often have clitoromegaly (Wanders et al., 1988). Excessive quantities of very long chain saturated fatty acids (C26) have been found in plasma, cultured skin fibroblasts, and cultured amniocytes, and are useful in diagnosis (Wanders et al., 1990).

The cause of the syndrome is a failure of peroxisomes to import newly synthe-sized proteins. There are a number of complementation groups, and clinical features overlap. Because peroxisomes are vital, multiorgan dysfunction is the rule in gen-eralized peroxisomal disorders; early lethality is common, and it is likely that hypothalamic-pituitary-gonadal dysfunction occurs regularly, although no specific studies have been reported.

REFERENCES

Lazarow P B, Moser H W (1995). Disorders of peroxisome biogenesis. In: Scriver C R, et al. (eds.). *The Metabolic and Molecular Basis of Inherited Disease*, McGraw-Hill, New York, 7th ed., pp. 2287–2324.
Wanders R J A, Heymans H S A, Schutgens R B H, et al. (1988). Peroxisomal disorders in neurology. *J Neurol Sci* 88:1–39.
Wanders R J A, van Roermund C W T, Schutgens R B H, et al. (190). The inborn errors of peroxisomal beta-oxidation: a review. *J Inherit Metab Dis* 13:4–36.

CHUDLEY MENTAL RETARDATION SYNDROME

Chudley and colleagues (1988) described a 3-year-old boy and two maternal uncles with mental retardation, short stature, mild obesity, unusual facies, and small or undescended testes. Affected individuals superficially resembled patients with Prader-Willi syndrome: they had bitemporal narrowing, almond-shaped eyes, de-pressed nasal bridge, anteverted nares, a short and everted upper lip, and macros-tomia. Two other males in the family who died in infancy had similar facial anomalies. X-linked inheritance is likely.

REFERENCE

Chudley A E, Lowry R B, Hoar D I (1988). Mental retardation, distinct facial changes, short stature, obesity and hypogonadism: a new X-linked mental retardation syndrome. *Am J Med Genet* 31:741–751.

CHUDLEY SYNDROME

Distinct from the Chudley mental retardation syndrome, discussed above, is an-other disorder described by the author and other coworkers in which a male-female adult sib pair had congenital multicore myopathy, severe mental retardation, short stature, a small pituitary fossa, and hypoplastic external genitalia, the latter on the basis of hypogonadotropic hypogonadism (Chudley et al., 1985). In the male the testes were undescended. The parents were consanguineous, indicating autosomal recessive inheritance.

REFERENCE

Chudley A E, Rozdelsky B, Houston C S, et al. (1985). Multicore disease in sib with severe mental retardation, short stature, facial anomalies, hypoplasia of the pituitary fossa, and hypogonadotropic hypogonadism. *Am J Med Genet* 20:145–158.

COCKAYNE SYNDROME

Dwarfism, microcephaly, premature senility, mental retardation, deafness, pigmentary retinopathy, and extreme photosensitivity characterize this rare autosomal recessive disorder (Nance and Berry, 1992). Affected males are frequently cryptorchid and the testes, if descended, are small. Females have developed menses, but they are usually irregular. Ovarian atrophy and fibrosis have been reported in one case (Sugarman et al., 1977). The pathogenesis and extent of the hypogonadism is not precisely known.

Cultured skin fibroblasts show an extreme sensitivity to UV light (Lehmann et al., 1993). Cell-fusion studies are compatible with genetic heterogeneity, with at least three and possibly more complementation groups. These groups likely represent specific defects in the DNA repair mechanism after exposure to UV light. There appears to be some molecular overlap with various genes that are responsible for xeroderma pigmentosa, especially those involving helicase proteins (Troelstra et al., 1992). However, unlike other disorders involving DNA repair, malignancy is not a major feature of the Cockayne syndrome. Although classically affected individuals rarely live beyond age 20, longer survival has been seen. Autosomal recessive inheritance of all forms seems assured.

REFERENCES

Lehmann A R, Thompson A F, Harcourt S A, et al. (1993). Cockayne's syndrome: correlation of clinical features with cellular sensitivity of RNA synthesis to UV irradiation. *J Med Genet* 30:679–682.

Nance M A, Berry S A (1992). Cockayne syndrome: review of 140 cases. *Am J Med Genet* 42: 68–84.

Sugarman G I, Landing B H, Reed W B (1977). Cockayne syndrome: clinical study of two patients and neuropathologic findings in one. *Clin Pediatr* 16:225–232.

Troelstra C, van Gool A, deWit J, et al., (1992). ERCC6, a member of subfamily of putative helicases is involved in Cockayne's syndrome and preferential repair of active genes. *Cell* 71:939–953.

COHEN SYNDROME

Mental retardation, obesity, and long narrow fingers and toes characterize the Cohen syndrome (North et al., 1985). Additionally, affected individuals have mild microcephaly, down-slanting palpebral fissures, short stature, and open mouth with prominent central incisors. The obesity is mild to moderate and develops in mid-childhood. Congenital heart disease occurs in some patients and most are short as adults. Delayed or absent puberty is common in both sexes, but isosexual precocity was noted on one occasion (Chapter 12). Roughly one third of males are cryptorchid (Sack and Friedman, 1986). The syndrome seems to be unusually frequent in Finland and Israel, and it has been suggested that the condition in each country is different, the Finnish patients showing the additional feature of pigmentary retinopathy (Kondo et al., 1990). All evidence supports autosomal recessive inheritance. The gene for the Finnish form has been localized to chromosome 8 (Tahvanainen et al., 1994).

REFERENCES

Kondo I, Nagataki S, Miyaga N (1990). The Cohen syndrome: does mottled retina separate a Finnish and Jewish type? *Am J Med Genet* 37:109–113.

North C, Patton M A, Baraitser M, et al. (1985). The clinical features of the Cohen syndrome: further case reports. *J Med Genet* 22:131–134.

Sack J, Friedman E (1986). The Cohen syndrome in Israel. *Israel J Med Sci* 22:766–770.

Tahvanainen E, Norio R, Karila E, et al. (1994). Cohen syndrome gene assigned to the long arm of chromosome 8 by linkage analysis. *Nat Genet* 7:201–204.

CONDUCTIVE DEAFNESS, WITH PINNA MALFORMATIONS AND HYPOGONADISM

Mengel and colleagues (1969) noted conductive hearing loss, probably due to abnormal ossicles, in conjunction with low-set, malformed external ears in an inbred Mennonite kindred. Some of the affected males had cryptorchidism, and hypogonadism was present in an additional male. The gonadal status of the affected females was not described. A similar family was reported by Cantu and colleagues (1978). A rare recessive trait is the logical genetic basis of the syndrome.

REFERENCES

Cantu M, Ruenes R, Garcia-Cruz D (1978). Autosomal recessive sensorineural-conductive deafness and pinna abnormalities. *Hum Genet* 40:231–234.

Mengel M C, Konigsmark B W, Berlin C I, et al. (1969). Conductive hearing loss and malformed low-set ears, as a possible recessive syndrome. *J Med Genet* 6:14–21.

CONGENITAL SEVERE MIXED DEAFNESS AND HYPOGONADISM

The combination of deafness of various etiologies and hypogonadism has been recorded as partial components of a number of syndromes (Table 15–3). Myhre and colleagues (1982) described six males in two pedigrees all with congenital mixed hearing loss and primary hypogonadism. At operation, one patient was found to have fixation of the stapes. X-rays revealed striking thickness of the bones of the calvarium and the authors postulated that the sensory component of the deafness could have been due to eighth nerve compression. Plasma testosterone levels were low and responded only marginally to HCG. LH and FSH levels were mildly elevated and did not respond to clomiphene. However, the two patients so tested were teenagers and were at a Tanner stage I developmental state, a situation where unresponsiveness to clomiphene is the rule; that is, no definite decision can be made about the hypothalamic-pituitary axis. A testicular biopsy obtained on a 15-year-

TABLE 15–5. Some Craniosynostosis Syndromes With Genital Anomalies

Syndrome	Genital Abnormality	References
Saethre-Chotzen	Cryptorchidism	Bartsocas et al., 1970
Carpenter	Cryptorchidism, hypogonadism	Gorlin et al., 1990; Palacios and Schimke, 1969
Antley-Bixler	Hypoplastic labia majora, clitoral enlargement, fused labia minora	Escobar, 1988
Gomez-Lopez-Hernandez	Hypoplastic labia	Gomez, 1987
Herrmann-Opitz	Cryptorchidism	Hermann and Opitz, 1969
Lowry	Cryptorchidism	Lowry, 1972
Sprintzen-Goldberg	Cryptorchidism, small genitalia	Cohen, 1986
Pfeiffer	Suprarenal cryptorchidism	Goldfisher and Cromie, 1997
Pfeiffer cardiocranial	Cryptorchidism, hypospadias	Williamson-Kruge and Biesecker, 1995
Sakati	Cryptorchidism, micropenis	Sakati, 1971
Lin-Gettig	Cryptorchidism, hypospadias	Lin and Gettig, 1990
SCARF	Cryptorchidism, hypospadias, micropenis	Koppe et al., 1989
Baller-Gerold	Peristence of cloaca	Lin et al., 1993

old patient revealed seminiferous tubule dysgenesis, primitive germ cells, and decreased Leydig cells. No biopsy was obtained on any older patient. The pedigrees were compatible with X-linked inheritance of the trait. However, evidence has since been presented that the combination is in reality a contiguous gene syndrome (Bach et al., 1992).

REFERENCES

Bach I, Brunner H G, Beighton P, et al. (1992). Microdeletions in patients with Gusher-associated X-linked mixed deafness (DFN3). *Am J Hum Genet* 50:38–44.
Myhre S A, Ruvalcaba R H, Kelley V C (1982). Congenital deafness and hypogonadism: a new X-linked recessive disorder. *Clin Genet* 22:299–307.

CRANIOSYNOSTOSIS

Premature closure of the various cranial sutures may be isolated or syndromic. The latter feature a variety of extracranial abnormalities occasionally, including those of the genitalia (Table 15–5). The inheritance pattern is variable and some syndromes arise from specific chromosome alterations that disrupt causative genes. For the most part, the genital findings are of micropenis, hypospadias, and/or cryptochidism in males and hypoplastic labia in females. However, bicornuate uterus, vaginal atresia, and clitoromegaly have been seen on occasion—for example, in the Apert syndrome (Cohen and Kreiborg, 1993). Functional gonadal status is often unknown in individuals with craniosynostosis. Many of these syndromes are sporadic cases, others have been reported in only one or two families, so the genital abnormalities are neither consistent nor consistently present. These syndromes have been extensively reviewed (Cohen, 1986, 1988; Gorlin et al., 1990).

In actuality many of these syndromes may represent variations on a theme (see review by Wilkie, 1997). For example, mutations in the same exon of the fibroblast growth factor receptor 2 (FGFR2) have been found in the Crouzon, Jackson-Weiss, and Pfeiffer syndromes (Meyers et al., 1996). Mutations elsewhere in the same gene also present with a common phenotype—for example, Crouzon syndrome with mutations either in exon IIIa or in IIIc. In other words, both inter-and intrafamilial variability characterize mutations in this gene and these various conditions are not necessarily unique, but represent a spectrum of related craniosynostotic disorders. Other craniosynostosis syndromes result from mutations in a homeobox gene (Boston type; Jabs et al., 1993), and in a helix-loop-helix transcription factor (TWIST) in some cases of the Saethre-Chotzen syndrome (Howard et al., 1997). Others, like the Baller-Gerold syndrome, may not be true entities.

REFERENCES

Bartsocas C S, Weber A L, Crawford J D (1970) Acrocephalosyndactyly III Chotzen's syndrome.*J Pediatr* 77:267–272.

Cohen M M Jr (1986). *Craniosynostosis: Diagnosis, Evaluation and Management.* New York: Raven Press.

Cohen M M Jr (1988). Craniosynostosis update 1987. *Am J Med Genet Suppl* 4:99–148.

Cohen M M Jr, Kreiborg S (1993). Visceral anomalies in the Apert syndrome. *Am J Med Genet* 45:758–760.

Escobar L F, Bixler D, Sadove M, et al. (1988). Antley-Bixler syndrome from a prognostic perspective. *Am J Med Genet* 29:829–836.

Goldfischer E R, Cromie W F (1997). Bilateral suprarenal cryptorchidism with Pfeiffer syndrome. *J Urol* 158:597–598.

Gomez M R (1987). Cerebello-trigemino-dermal dysplasia. In *Neurocutaneous Disease I.*, Gomez M R (ed). Raven Press, New York, pp. 145–438.

Gorlin R J, Cohen M M Jr, Levin L S (1990). *Syndromes of the Head and Neck.* Oxford, New York, 3rd ed., pp. 519–465.

Herrmann J, Opitz J (1969). An unusual form of acrocephalosyndactyly. *Birth Defects* 5:39.

Howard T D, Paznekas W A, Green E D, et al. (1997). Mutations in TWIST, a basic helix-loop-helix transcription factor in Saethre-Chotzen syndrome. *Nat Genet* 15:42–46.

Lin A E, Gettig E (1990). Craniosynostosis, agenesis of corpus callosum, severe mental retardation, distinctive facies, camptodactyly and hypogonadism. *Am J Med Genet* 35:582–585.

Lin A E, McPherson E, Nwokoro N A, et al. (1993). Further delineation of the Baller-Gerold syndrome. *Am J Med Genet* 45:591–524.

Jabs E W, Miller V, Li X (1993). A mutation in the homeodomain of the human MSX2 gene in a family affected with autosomal dominant craniosynostosis. *Cell* 75:443–450.

Koppe, Kaplan P, Hunter A, et al (1989). Ambiguous genitalia with skeletal abnormalities, cutis laxa, craniosynostosis, psychomotor retardation and facial abnormalities (SCARF syndrome). *Am J Med Genet* 34:305–312

Lowry R B (1972). Congenital absence of the fibula and craniosynostosis in sibs. *J Med Genet* 9:227–229.

Palacios E, Schimke R (1969). Craniosynostosis-syndactylism. *Am J Roentgenol* 106:144–155.

Sakati N (1971). A new syndrome with acrocephalopolysyndactyly, cardiac disease, and distinctive defects of the ear, skin and lower limbs. *J Pediatr* 79:104–109.

Wilkie A O (1997). Cranosynostosis: genes on mechanisms. *Human Mol Genet* 6:1647–1656.
Williamson-Kruse L, Biesecker L G (1995). Pfeiffer type cardiocranial syndrome: a third case
report. *J Med Genet* 32:901–903.

CRYPTOPHTHALMOS SYNDROME (FRASER SYNDROME)

Cryptophthalmos is a developmental malformation of the eyelids in which the skin
is continuous over the globe. It may be uni-or bilateral, but even when unilateral
the opposite eye and lid are usually malformed. As an isolated finding it may be
sporadic or genetic, but it may also be part of a syndrome in which other anomalies
occur, including abnormal hairline, coloboma of the alae nasae, hypertelorism, often
with midface or palatal cleft, ear malformations with frequent hearing loss, laryn-
geal stenosis and uni-or bilateral renal agenesis (Thomas et al., 1986). The males
are usually cryptorchid and may have hypospadias and micropenis. Affected females have varying degrees of clitoral hypertrophy, labial fusion, bicornuate uterus,
malformed fallopian tubes and vaginal atresia. In one instance, an affected female
had gonadal dysgenesis and a gonadoblastoma in situ (Greenberg et al., 1986).
Because cryptophthalmos may be absent, many prefer the eponymic designation of
the Fraser syndrome (Gattuso et al., 1987). The condition has been reported only in
sibs, often with a background of consanguinity, so that autosomal recessive inheritance seems assured.

REFERENCES

Gattuso J, Patton M A, Baraitser M (1987). The clinical spectrum of the Fraser syndrome:
report of three new cases and review. *J Med Genet* 24:549–555.
Greenberg F, Keenan B, DeYanis V, et al (1986). Gonadal dysgenesis and gonadoblastoma in
situ in a female with Fraser (cryptophthalmos) syndrome. *J Pediatr* 108:952–954.
Thomas I T, Frias J L, Felix V, et al (1986): Isolated and syndromic cryptophthalmos. *Am J
Med Genet* 25:85–98.

DE LANGE SYNDROME

Affected children have primordial growth deficiency, mental retardation, a peculiar
facies consisting of microbrachycephaly, bushy eyebrows with synophrys, a small
nose with anteverted nostrils, and various abnormalities of the limbs including
micromelia and phocomelia, flexion contractures, and clindactyly and syndactyly.
Affected males commonly have hypoplastic genitalia and undescended testes (Jackson et al., 1993). Females may have bicornuate or septate uterus (Vischer, 1965).

Most cases of the condition are sporadic but some familial aggregation has been
seen (Finegold and Lin, 1993; Kozma, 1996). Partial duplication of the long arm of
chromosome 3 can produce somewhat similar features (Wilson et al., 1985), and it
is possible that at least some familial cases of the de Lange syndrome might have
had translocations with dup 3q not detected by older cytogenetic techniques. A
milder form of the condition may exist as well (Smith et al., 1993). The recurrence
risk for the nonchromosomal de Lange phenotype is probably less than 5%.

REFERENCES

Finegold M, Lin A E (1993). Brief clinical report: familial Brachmann-de Lange syndrome: further evidence for autosomal dominant inheritance and review of the literature. *Am J Med Genet* 47:1064–1069.

Jackson L, Kline A D, Barr M A, et al. (1993). de Lange syndrome: a clinical review of 310 individuals. *Am J Med Genet* 47:940–946.

Kozma C (1996). Autosomal dominant inheritance of Brachmann-de Lange syndrome. *Am J Med Genet* 66:445–448.

Smith C R, Magee J F, Ritchie S, et al. (1993). Clinical variability within Brachmann-de Lange syndrome: a proposed classification system. *Am J Med Genet* 47:947–958.

Vischer D (1965). Typus degenerativus Amstelodamensis (Cornelia de Lange Syndrom). *Helv Pediat Acta* 20:415–445.

Wilson G N, Dasouki M, Barr M (1985). Further delineation of the dup (3q) syndrome. *Am J Med Genet* 22:117–123.

DEVRIENDT-LEGIUS-FRYNS SYNDROME

In addition to the Al-Awadi syndrome (this chapter) another alopecia-hypogonadism syndrome was described in a male-female sib pair by Devriendt and coworkers (1996). The alopecia became evident in the second decade and was not appreciably influenced by sex hormone replacement. The hypogonadism was primary. The sibs also developed progressive neurologic dysfunction, also in the second decade, characterized initially by spasticity and later by dystonia and choreoathetosis. The syndrome is likely autosomal recessive and appears to be distinct from other alopecia-hypogonadism syndromes.

REFERENCE

Devriendt K, Legius E, Fryns J P (1996). Progressive extrapyramidal disorder with primary hypogonadism and alopecia in sibs: a new syndrome? *Am J Med Genet* 62:54–57.

DUBOWITZ SYNDROME

This is a form of low-birth-weight proportionate short stature in which the children have unusual facies, an eczema-like skin disorder, and borderline intelligence (Dubowitz, 1965). Aplastic anemia and leukemia may also occur (Emami et al., 1997). Cryptorchidism and hypospadias are common in affected males, and females may have genital hypoplasia. The adult gonadal status in either sex has not been reported. The syndrome is inherited as an autosomal recessive trait (Tsukahara and Opitz, 1996).

REFERENCES

Dubowitz V (1965). Familial low birth weight dwarfism with an unusual facies and a skin eruption. *J Med Genet* 2:12–17.

Emami A, Vats T S, Schimke R N, et al. (1997). Bone marrow failure followed by acute myelocytic leukemia in a patient with Dubowitz syndrome. *Int J Pediat Hematology/Oncology* 4:187–193.

Tsukahara M, Opitz J M (1996). Dubowitz syndrome: review of 141 cases including 36 previously unreported patients. *Am J Med Genet* 63:268–276.

DYSKERATOSIS CONGENITA (ZINSSER-COLE-ENGMAN SYNDROME)

The clinical picture consists of cutaneous pigmentation, nail dystrophy, lacrimal duct atresia, testicular atrophy, often anemia and thrombocytopenia, and leukoplakia of the oral and anal mucosa (Davidson and Conner, 1988). Patients often succumb before the fourth decade because of pancytopenia or malignant transformation of the mucous membrane lesions. The reason for the testicular atrophy is unknown.

The condition superficially resembles Fanconi panmyelopathy (this chapter) but there are a number of differences, not the least of which is that the usual form of dyskeratosis congenita is X-linked (Xq28; Arngrimsson et al., 1993) whereas Fanconi panmyelopathy is an autosomal recessive trait. The gene for dyskeratosis congenita, DKC1, codes for a protein, dyskerin, that may exert control on rRNA and ribosome assembly (Heiss et al., 1998). However, a recessive variety of dyskeratosis may exist (Pai et al., 1989), and an autosomal dominant form (Scoggins type) has been described (Davidson and Conner, 1988). When females are affected, the spectrum of mucosal malignancy extends to the cervix and vagina.

REFERENCES

Arngrimsson R, Dokal I, Luzzato L et al. (1993). Dyskeratosis congenita: three additional families show linkage to a locus in Xq28. *J Med Genet* 30:615–619.

Davidson H R, Conner J M (1988). Dyskeratosis congenita. *J Med Genet* 25:843–846.

Heiss N S, Knight S W, Vulliamy T J et al. (1998). X-linked keratosis congenita is caused by mutations in a highly conserved gene with putative nucleolas function. *Nat Genet* 19:32–38.

Pai G S, Morgan S, Whetsell C (1989). Etiologic heterogeneity in dyskeratosis congenita. *Am J Med Genet* 32:63–66.

EEC (ECTRODACTYLY-ECTODERMAL DEFECTS-CLEFTING) SYNDROME

The constituent components of the syndrome include split hand/foot, thin hair, dysplastic or absent teeth, nails and nipples, hypohidrosis, and cleft lip with or without cleft palate. Less commonly reported features of the syndrome include urinary tract anomalies and, in males, occasional cryptorchidism, hypospadias, and micropenis (Mass et al., 1996). The EEC syndrome is inherited as a variably expressed autosomal dominant trait. The gene has been mapped to 7 q21-q22 (Scherer et al., 1994).

REFERENCES

Mass S M, de Jong T P V M, Buss P, et al. (1996). EEC syndrome and genitourinary anomalies: an update. *Am J Med Genet* 63:472–478.

Scherer S W, et al. (1994). Fine mapping of the autosomal dominant split hand/split foot locus on chromosome 7, band q21.3. *Am J Hum Genet* 55:12–20.

EDWARDS SYNDROME

Edwards and colleagues (1976) described three siblings with pigmentary retinopathy, mental retardation, nerve deafness, and either diabetes mellitus or hyperinsulinism or both, and acanthosis nigricans. The two male sibs had gynecomastia and small testes with elevated plasma gonadotropin levels. The affected female had oligomenorrhea. Although the features overlap those of other syndromes with obesity, hypogonadism, and ophthalmologic abnormalities (Table 15–2), the authors considered the syndrome to be a distinct autosomal recessive trait. Two additional sibs were reported by Boor and colleagues (1993), who noted impaired binding of insulin to its receptor with secondary hyperinsulinism and polycystic ovaries.

REFERENCES

Boor R., Herwig J, Schrezenmeir J, et al. (1993). Familial insulin resistant diabetes mellitus associated with acanthosis nigricans, polycystic ovaries, hypogonadism, pigmentary retinopathy, labyrinthine deafness, and mental retardation. *Am J Med Genet* 45:649–653.

Edwards J A, Sethi P K, Scoma A J, et al. (1976). A new familial syndrome characterized by pigmentary retinopathy, hypogonadism, mental retardation, nerve deafness and glucose intolerance. *Am J Med* 60:23–32.

ELLIS-VAN CREVELD SYNDROME (CHONDROECTODERMAL DYSPLASIA)

Prenatal-onset short stature, postaxial polydactyly, a peculiar short upper lip bound to the alveolar ridge ("partial lip tie"), and frequently large atrial septal defect characterize this disorder (Ellis and van Creveld, 1940). Males often have epispadias and cryptorchidism. Affected females have no consistent genital abnormalities, and both sexes are fertile. Extensive study of this syndrome in the Amish by McKusick and colleagues (1964) has established autosomal recessive inheritance. The gene has been mapped to 4p16 (Polymeropoulos et al., 1996).

REFERENCES

Ellis R W B, van Creveld S (1940). A syndrome characterized by ectodermal dysplasia, polydactyly, chondro-dysplasia and congenital morbis coidis. Report of three cases. *Arch Dis Child* 15:65–75.

McKusick V A, Egeland J A, Eldridge R, et al. (1964). Dwarfism in the Amish. I. The Ellis-van Creveld syndrome. *Bull Johns Hopkins Hosp.* 115:306–336.

Polymeropoulos M H, Ide S E, Wright M, et al. (1996). The gene for Ellis-van Creveld syndrome is located on chromosome 4p16. *Genomics* 35:1–5.

FANCONI PANMYELOPATHY

The Fanconi panmyelopathy syndrome classically features upper extremity malformations, hyperpigmentation, aplastic anemia, often leukemia, and enhanced chromosome breakage when cells from an affected individual are exposed in culture to either diepoxybutane (DEB) or mitomycin C (Chaganti and Holdsworth, 1991; Giampietro et al., 1993). Affected males commonly have small external genitalia and cryptorchidism. The hypogonadism appears to be primary (Berkovitz et al., 1984). Ovarian function may be preserved for some time in many females; others have irregular menses and early menopause.

The condition exhibits both allele and locus heterogeneity but all forms are inherited as autosomal recessive traits.

REFERENCES

Berkovitz G D, Zinkham W H, Migeon C J (1984). Gonadal function in two sibs with Fanconi's anemia. *Hormone Res* 19:137–141.

Chaganti R S K, Holdsworth J (1991). Fanconi anemia: a pleiotropic mutation with multiple cellular and developmental abnormalities. *Ann Genet* 34:206–211.

Giampietro P F, Adler-Brecher B, Verlander P C, et al. (1993). The need for more accurate and timely diagnosis in Fanconi anemia: a report from the International Fanconi Anemia Registry. *Pediatrics* 81:1116–1120.

FEMORAL HYPOPLASIA-UNUSUAL FACIES SYNDROME (FEMORAL-FACIES SYNDROME)

Based on two previous cases and their own experience, Daentl and colleagues (1975) described a new malformation syndrome consisting of absent or hypoplastic femurs, occasional similar shortening of the humeri, and facial anomalies—short nose with hypoplastic alae, long philtrum, thin upper lip, and micrognathia with or without cleft palate (Hurst and Johnson, 1980). Absent or polycystic kidneys have been noted. Small and/or cryptorchid testes and small penis have been seen in some males, and the labia majora may be hypoplastic in affected females. The syndrome is similar in many respects to milder variants of caudal dysplasia (Chapter 16) and like the latter has been reported in infants of diabetic mothers (Johnson et al., 1983).

Evidence that a possible genetic basis for the syndrome exists comes from one report of an affected father-daughter pair (Lampert, 1980) and another in which an infant and great-aunt were affected (Kelly, 1974). Because most cases are sporadic occurrences, the syndrome is quite likely causally heterogenous. A lethal variant has been described (Gillerot et al., 1997).

REFERENCES

Daentl D L, Smith D W, Scott C I et al., (1975). Femoral hypoplasia–unusual facies syndrome. *J Pediatr* 86:107–111.

Gillerot Y, Fourneau C, Willems T, et al. (1997). Lethal femoral-facial syndrome: a case with unusual manifestations. *J Med Genet* 34:518–519.

Hurst D, Johnson D F (1980). Femoral hypoplasia-unusual facies syndrome. *Am J Med Genet* 5:255–258.

Johnson J P, Carey J C, Gooch W M III (1983). Femoral hypoplasia–unusual facies syndrome in infants of diabetic mothers. *J Pediatr* 102:866–872.

Kelly T E (1974). Proximal focal femoral deficiency (familial). *Birth Defects Orig Art Ser X* (12): 508–509.

Lampert R P (1980). Dominant inheritance of femoral hypoplasia–unusual facies syndrome. *Clin Genet* 17:255–258.

FG SYNDROME (OPITZ-KAVEGGIA SYNDROME)

Opitz and Kaveggia (1974) initially described this condition (named by using the first letter of the surname of two branches of the family) in three brothers and their male cousins. It comprises mental retardation, agenesis of the corpus callosum, imperforate anus, hypotonia, relative macrocephaly, and a number of other abnormalities (Opitz et al., 1988). Thompson and Baraitser (1987) noted that nearly one third of males had cryptorchidism. The disorder is an X-linked recessive trait, with the gene provisionally mapped to Xq21–22 region (Zhu et al., 1991; Graham et al., 1998). However, localization in this region has been excluded in some families, indicating heterogeneity (Briauld et al., 1996).

REFERENCES

Briauld S, Hill R, Shrimpton A, et al. (1996). A gene for the FG syndrome maps in the proximal Xq region. *Eur J Hum Genet* 4 (Suppl 1):65.

Graham J M, Tackels D, Dibbern K, et al. (1998). FG Syndrome: report of three new families with linkage to Xq12-q22.1. *Am J Med Genet* 80:145–156.

Opitz, J M, Kaveggia E G (1974). The FG syndrome: an X-linked syndrome of multiple congenital anomalies and metal retardation. *Z Kinderheilk* 117:1–18.

Opitz J M, Richieri-da Costa A, Aase J M, et al. (1988). FG syndrome update 1988: note of 5 new patients and bibliography. *Am J Med Genet* 30:309–328.

Thompson E, Baraitser M (1987). FG syndrome. *J Med Genet* 24:139–143.

Zhu D, Mitchell T N, Maumanee I H (1991). Mapping the X-linked FG syndrome to Xq21.31-Xq22. *Cytogenet Cell Genet* 58:2091.

FLOATING-HARBOR SYNDROME

The rather whimsical title of this syndrome refers to the hospitals where the first cases were ascertained—Boston Floating Hospital and Harbor General Hospital (Pellitier and Feingold, 1973; Leisti et al., 1975). The patients have intrauterine and postnatal growth retardation, they also have unusual facies, short neck, and mild mental retardation, with significant speech delay. Affected males have a hypoplastic penis, sometimes with hypospadias. Most cases are sporadic (Majewski and Lenard, 1991), but affected sibs were described on one occasion (Fryns et al., 1996).

REFERENCES

Fryns J P, Kleczkowska A, Timmermans J, et al. (1996). The Floating-Harbor syndrome: two affected siblings in a family. *Clin Genet* 50:217–219.

Leisti J, Hollister D W, Rimoin D L (1975). The Floating-Harbor syndrome. *Birth Defects* 11 (5):305.

Majewski F, Lenard H-G (1991). Floating-Harbor syndrome. *Eur J Pediatr* 150:250–252.

Pellitier G, Feingold M (1973). Case report 1. *Syndrome Ident* I (1):8–9.

FRYNS SYNDROME

Fryns and colleagues (1979; Fryns, 1987) described a multiple congenital anomaly syndrome featuring coarse facies, cleft palate, distal digital hypoplasia, lung hypoplasia in some instances due to defects in the diaphragm, and urogenital anomalies; the latter consist of bicornuate uterus, duplex uterus/vagina, or uterine atresia in females, and hypospadias, cryptorchidism, and bifid scrotum in males. The condition is usually lethal, but prolonged survival has been seen, generally in patients whose diaphragmatic defect is not so severe (Bamforth et al., 1989). Survivors are mentally retarded (Hanssen et al., 1992). Affected sibs have been reported, indicating autosomal recessive inheritance (Moerman et al., 1988; Cunniff et al., 1990).

REFERENCES

Bamforth J S, Leonard C O, Chodirker B N, et al. (1989). Congenital diaphragmatic hernia, coarse facies, and acral hypoplasia: Fryns syndrome. *Am J Med Genet* 32:93–99.

Cunniff C, Jones K L, Sael H M, et al. (1990). Fryns syndrome: an autosomal recessive disorder associated with craniofacial anomalies, diaphragmatic hernia and distal digital hypoplasia. *Pediatrics* 85:499–504.

Fryns J P, Moerman F, Goddeeris P, et al. (1979). A new lethal syndrome with cloudy corneae,
diaphragmatic defects, and distal limb deformities. *Hum Genet* 50:65–70.

Fryns J P (1987). Fryns syndrome: a variable MCA syndrome with diaphragmatic defects,
coarse face, and distal limb hypoplasia. *J Med Genet* 24:271–274.

Hanssen A M N, Schrander-Stumpel C T R M, Thery P A E, et al. (1992). Fryns syndrome:
another example of non-lethal outcome with severe mental handicap. *Genet Counsel* 3:
187–193.

Moerman P, Fryns J P, Vandenberghe K, et al. (1988). The syndrome of diaphragmatic hernia,
abnormal facies and distal limb anomalies (Fryns syndrome): report of two sibs with
further delineation of this multiple congenital anomaly (MCA) syndrome. *Am J Med Genet*
31:805–814.

GENITO-PALATAL-CARDIAC SYNDROME (GARDNER-SILENGO-WACHTEL SYNDROME)

The term genito-palatal-cardiac syndrome was coined by Greenberg and colleagues (1987) to describe a condition comprising cleft lip/palate, micrognathia, other skeletal defects (flexion deformities of thumbs and great toes, campto-and polydactyly, dysplastic ribs), conotruncal cardiac defects, and usually female, but occasionally ambiguous, genitalia in 46,XY males. The authors summarized early reports of what they felt was the same entity by Gardner and colleagues (1970), Silengo and colleagues (1974), and Wachtel (1983), among others.

The two sibs reported by Greenberg and colleagues were discordant for genital development. One had female genitalia with normal uterus, ovaries, and fallopian tubes; the other had a penis with first-degree hypospadias and undescended testes.

The defect is likely either a rare autosomal or an X-linked recessive trait. It is conceivable that at least some of the patients reviewed had the Smith-Lemli-Opitz syndrome (Curry et al., 1987). Future patients with this phenotype should certainly be tested for 7-dehydrocholesterol reductase deficiency.

REFERENCES

Curry C J R, Carey J C, Holland J S, et al. (1987). Smith-Lemli-Opitz syndrome—type II: multiple congenital anomalies with male pseudohrmaphroditism and frequent early lethality.
Am J Med Genet 26:45–57.

Gardner L I, Assemany S R, Neu R L (1970). 46,XY female: anti-androgenic effect of oral
contraceptives? *Lancet* 2:667–668.

Greenberg F, Gresik M V, Carpenter R J, et al. (1987). The Gardner-Silengo-Wachtel or genito-
palatal-cardiac syndrome: male pseudohermaphroditism with micrognathia, cleft palate,
and conotruncal cardiac defect. *Am J Med Genet* 26:59–64.

Silengo M, Kaufman R L, Kissane J (1974). A 46,XY infant with uterus, dysgenetic gonads,
and multiple anomalies. *Humangenetik* 25:65–68.

Wachtel S S (1983). *H-Y Antigen and the Biology of Sex Determination.* New York, Grune and
Stratton, pp 224–225.

GOEMINNE SYNDROME

Goeminne (1968) described a family in which several individuals were affected with a syndrome consisting of congenital muscular torticollis, spontaneous multiple keloids, and uni-or bilateral cryptorchidism in the males. Renal dysplasia appeared in several affected members, as did multiple cutaneous nevae and varicose veins. The proband was infertile and was found to have seminiferous tubular failure with supposedly normal Leydig cell function. None of the affected males in this family had reproduced. Although several of the female relatives had partial manifestations of this syndrome, males were primarily affected, and the trait was transmitted by completely unaffected females, findings compatible with an X-linked trait. Zuffardi and Fraccaro (1982) mapped the gene to Xq28 distal to the G6PD locus.

REFERENCES

Goeminne L (1968). A new probably X-linked inherited syndrome (congenital torticollis, multiple keloids, cryptorchidism and renal dysplasia). *Acta Genet Med (Roma)* 17:439–467.

Zuffardi O, Fraccaro M (1982). Gene mapping and serendipity: the locus for torticollis, keloids, cryptorchidism and renal dysplasia (31430 McKusick) is at Xq28 distal to the G6PD locus. *Hum Genet* 62:280–281.

GORLIN SYNDROME (BASAL CELL NEVUS SYNDROME)

The diagnostic hallmarks of this disorder are nevoid basal cell carcinoma, jaw cysts, skeletal anomalies, and intracranial calcification (Gorlin, 1987; Evans et al., 1993). Affected females commonly have ovarian fibromas and cysts that may calcify but do not ordinarily impair fertility. Males may be normal, but primary hypogonadism, hypoplastic external genitalia, and cryptorchidism have been seen. The disorder is an autosomal dominant trait. The gene has been localized to the long arm of chromosome 9, and it behaves as a tumor suppressor gene, with malignant transformation of the basal cell nevi and lesions in other organs being significantly associated with allelic loss of heterozygosity, particularly in response to ultraviolet light and ionizing irradiation (Gailani et al., 1992). Some of the developmental anomalies, such as the jaw cysts, may also be due to a two-hit phenomenon (Levant et al., 1996). The gene appears to be the human homologue of the Drosophila gene *patched* whose protein product is a receptor that acts to suppress some functions of the sonic hedgehog protein in primary embryologic development (Johnson et al., 1996). A number of germline mutations have been identified (Leuch et al., 1997).

REFERENCES

Berlin N I, Van Scott E J, Clendening W E, et al. (1966). Basal cell nevus syndrome. *Ann Intern Med* 64:403–421.

Evans D G R, Ladusans E J, Rimmer S, et al. (1993). Complications of the naevoid basal cell carcinoma syndrome: results of a population based study. *J Med Genet* 30:460–464.

Gailani M R, Bales S J, Leffell D J, et al. (1992). Developmental defects in Gorlin syndrome related to a putative tumor suppressor gene on chromosome 9. *Cell* 69:111–117.

Gorlin R J (1987). Nevoid basal cell carcinoma syndrome. *Medicine* 66:99–109.

Johnson R L, Rothman A L, Xie J et al. (1996). Human homolog of *patched*, a candidate gene for the basal cell nevus syndrome. *Science* 272:1668–1671.

Leuch N J, Telford E A, High A S, et al. (1997). Characterization of human patched germline mutations in naevoid basal cell carcinoma syndrome. *Hum Genet* 100:497–502.

Levant S, Gorlin R J, Fallot S, et al. (1996). A two-hit model for developmental defects in Gorlin syndrome. *Nat Genet* 12:85–87.

GORLIN-CHAUDHRY-MOSS SYNDROME

Gorlin and colleagues (1960) described two sisters with craniofacial dysostosis, mid-face hypoplasia, eye and dental abnormalities, mild conductive deafness, hypertrichosis, patent ductus arteriosus, hypoplastic distal phalanges, and normal intelligence. Both sibs had hypoplastic labia and absent secondary sex characteristics when studied early. However, both menstruated although menopause occurred in the fourth decade of life (R. Gorlin, personal communication). Ippel and colleagues (1992) provided follow-up on the two original cases and added two sporadic patients.

REFERENCES
Gorlin R J, Chaudhry A P, Moss M L (1960). Craniofacial dysostosis, patent ductus arteriosus, hypertrichosis, hypoplasia of labia majora, dental and eye anomalies—a new syndrome? *J Pediatr* 56:778–785.
Ippel P F, Gorlin R J, Lenz W, et al. (1992). Craniofacial dysostosis, hypertrichosis, genital hypoplasia, ocular, dental and digital defects: confirmation of the Gorlin-Chaudhry-Moss syndrome. *Am J Med Genet* 44:518–522.

HALAL SYNDROME

The concordance of limb and renal anomalies is well known and is probably not uncommon (Froster-Iskenius and Baird, 1989; Evans et al., 1992). Anomalies of both male and female genitalia may be present as well, and the genital findings may help in differential diagnosis, although there may be considerable phenotypic overlap (Pinsky, 1974). Some of the better-defined syndromes are listed in Table 15–2. The distinguishing features of each entity are discussed elsewhere in this volume.

A seemingly unique family was reported by Halal (1986) in which severe abnormalities of the upper limb (shortened arms, split hand, polydactyly) were combined with uterine duplication and septate vagina in females and micropenis in males. No renal abnormalities were detected. The syndrome is inherited as an autosomal dominant trait.

REFERENCES
Evans J A, Vitez M, Czeizel A (1992). Patterns of acrorenal malformation associations. *Am J Med Genet* 44:414–419.
Froster-Istenius U G, Baird P A (1989). Limb reduction defects in over one million consecutive live births. *Teratology* 39:127–135.
Halal F (1986). A new syndrome of severe upper limb hypoplasia and Müllerian duct anomalies. *Am J Med Genet* 24:119–126.
Pinsky L (1974). A community of human malformation syndromes involving the Müllerian ducts, distal extremities, urinary tract and ears. *Teratology* 9:65–79.

HALLERMAN-STREIFF SYNDROME

The clinical features include bird-like facies with beaked nose and hypoplastic mandible, hypotrichosis, microphthalmia, congenital cataract, and proportionate short stature (Cohen, 1991). Males may have small genitalia and cryptorchidism. However, affected individuals have reproduced, so the overall gonadal status is uncertain and perhaps variable (Ponte, 1962; Guyard et al., 1962; Harrod and Friedman,

1991). Although autosomal recessive inheritance has been suggested, the evidence is not compelling (Cohen, 1991).

REFERENCES

Cohen M M Jr. (1991). Hallerman-Streiff syndrome: a review. *Am J Med Genet* 41:438–499.
Guyard M, Perdriel G, Ceruti F (1962). Sur deux cas de syndrome dyscéphalique à tête d'oiseau. *Bull Soc Fr Ophthal* 62:443–447.
Harrod M J, Friedman J M (1991). Congenital cataracts in mother, sister, and son of a patient with Hallerman-Streiff syndrome. *Am J Med Genet* 41:500–502.
Ponte F (1962). Further contributions to the study of the syndrome of Hallerman and Streiff (congenital cataract with "bird's face"). *Ophthalmologica* 143:399–408.

HAND-FOOT-GENITAL SYNDROME

This syndrome comprises characteristic changes in the hands and feet (short first metacarpals and metatarsals, carpal and tarsal fusion, fifth finger clinodactyly) with genital anomalies in both sexes (Stern et al., 1970; Donnenfeld et al., 1992). Both sexes may have vesicourethral reflux and recurrent urinary tract infections (Verp et al., 1983). Females have fusion defects of the uterus and vagina. If surgical correction of the uterine anomaly is possible, fertility is generally restored. Males exhibit hypospadias (Donnenfeld et al., 1992; Fryns et al., 1993). Autosomal dominant inheritance of the syndrome seems secure. Mortlock and Innis (1997) have defined a mutation in a homeobox gene (HOXA 13) in this syndrome. The nonsense mutation gives rise to a stop codon that truncates the protein and presumably interferes with DNA binding ability.

Interestingly, autosomal dominant polysyndactyly has been found to be due to a triplet repeat expansion (coding for polyalanine) in the HOXD 13 gene, and affected males with 14 alanine repeats not only have a more severe limb malformation but have hypospadias as well (Goodman et al., 1997).

REFERENCES

Donnenfeld A E, Schrager D S, Corson S L (1992). Update on a family with hand-foot-genital syndrome: hypospadias and urinary tract abnormalities in two boys from the fourth generation. *Am J Med Genet* 44:482–484.
Fryns J P, Vogel A, Decock P, et al. (1993). The hand-foot-genital syndrome: on the variable expression in affected males. *Clin Genet* 43:232–234.
Goodman F R, Mundlos S, Muragaki Y, et al. (1997). Synpolydactyly phenotypes correlate with size of expansions in HOXD13 polyalanine tract. *Proc Natl Acad Sci USA* 94:7458–7463.
Mortlock D P, Innis J W (1997). Mutation of HOXA13 in hand-foot-genital syndrome. *Nat Genet* 15:179–181.
Stern A M, Gall J C Jr, Perry B L, et al. (1970). The hand-foot-uterus syndrome: a new hereditary disorder characterized by hand and foot dysplasia, dermatoglyphic abnormalities, and partial duplication of the female genital tract. *J Pediatr* 77:109–116.
Verp M S, Simpson J L, Elias S, et al. (1983). Heritable aspects of uterine anomalies I. Three familial aggregates with Mullerian fusion anomalies. *Fertil Steril* 40:80–85.

HYDROLETHALUS SYNDROME

This is a lethal malformation syndrome found largely in Finland (Salonen and Herva, 1990). The cardinal features include severe CNS malformations (hydrocephalus, hydranencephaly, anencephaly), polydactyly, and micrognathia with or without cleft palate. The larynx, trachea, and bronchi are often malformed and the lungs are usually unilobar. Roughly half the cases have congenital heart disease.

Hypospadias may be present in males. Many females have duplication of the uterus occasionally with malformation of the vagina. There is convincing evidence for autosomal recessive inheritance.

REFERENCE
Salonen R, Herva R (1990). Hydrolethalus syndrome. *J Med Genet* 27:756–759.

IESHIMA SYNDROME

Ieshima and colleagues (1986) recorded a brother and sister with a peculiar face, deafness, cleft palate, short stature, and mental retardation. The male had hypospadias, micropenis, and cryptorchidism. The external genitalia in the female were normal. Nothing is known concerning the functional gonadal status. This is likely a rare autosomal recessive syndrome.

REFERENCE
Ieshima S, Koeda T, Inagaka M. (1986). Peculiar face, deafness, cleft palate, male pseudohermaphroditism and growth and psychomotor retardation: a new autosomal recessive syndrome. *Clin Genet* 30:136–141.

JARCHO-LEVIN SYNDROME

The spondylocostal dysplasias are a clinically and genetically heterogeneous group of disorders involving segmentation defects of the vertebrae with absence, fusion, or distortion of the ribs. In most instances, the genetic defect is confined to the skeleton. A severe variety with respiratory complications leading to early death was described by Jarcho and Levin (1938). Other authors noted similar skeletal changes in conjunction with other anomalies including congenital heart disease, anal atresia, abdominal and inguinal hernias, and genital anomalies such as undescended testes, absent external genitalia, and hypospadias in males and a bicornuate uterus in a female (Casamassima et al., 1981; Poor et al., 1983; Aurora et al., 1996). The severe form of disease is most likely an autosomal recessive trait and is probably also heterogeneous. As there is very little autopsy material available, the degree of extraskeletal involvement is difficult to assess.

REFERENCES
Aurora P, Wallis C E, Winter R M (1996). The Jarcho-Levin syndrome (spondylocostal dysplasia) and complex congenital heart disease: a case report. *Clin Dysmorph* 5:165–169.
Casamassima A C, Morton C C, Nance W E, et al. (1981). Spondylocostal dysostosis with anal and urogenital anomalies in a Mennonite sibship. *Am J Med Genet* 8:117–127.
Jarcho S, Levin P M (1938). Hereditary malformation of the vertebral bodies. *Bull Johns Hopkins Hosp* 62:216–226.
Poor M A, Alberti O, Griscom N T, et al. (1983). Nonskeletal malformations in one of three siblings with Jarcho-Levin syndrome of vertebral anomalies. *J Pediat* 102:270–272.

JENNINGS SYNDROME

Two brothers with endocardial fibroelastosis, unusual facies, and cryptorchidism with microphallus were described by Jennings and colleagues (1980). One boy succumbed to refractory congestive heart failure at 4 months of age. The surviving sib subsequently developed retardation, seizures, and apparent hypothalamic dysfunction. Serum cortisol, insulin, and HGH levels were normal. FSH and LH levels were within the low-normal range for a prepubescent child, and serum testosterone level was extremely low. Independent macrocephaly was also segregating in the family. Either a rare autosomal or an X-linked recessive defect in hypothalamic function is the probable basis for the syndrome.

REFERENCE

Jennings M T, Hall J G, Kukolich M (1980). Endocardial fibroelastosis, neurologic dysfunction and unusual facial appearances in two brothers, coincidentally associated with dominantly inherited macrocephaly. *Am J Med Genet* 5:271–276.

JOHANSON-BLIZZARD SYNDROME

Hypoplasia of the nasal alae, cutis aplasia of the scalp, microcephaly, deafness, exocrine pancreatic insufficiency, and growth failure are the chief features of this unusual syndrome (Johanson and Blizzard, 1971). Most patients have non-goitrous hypothyroidism and anorectal anomalies (Hurst and Baraitser, 1989). Clitoromegaly and septate uterus and/or vagina have been seen in affected females and micropenis and cryptorchidism in males (Gershoni-Bauch et al., 1990). Autosomal recessive inheritance is established.

REFERENCES

Gershoni-Baruch R, Lerner A, Braun J, et al. (1990). Johanson-Blizzard syndrome: clinical spectrum and further delineation of the syndrome. *Am J Med Genet* 35:546–551.

Hurst J A, Baraitser M (1989). Johanson-Blizzard syndrome. *J Med Genet* 26:45–48.

Johanson A, Blizzard R (1971). A syndrome of congenital aplasia of the alae nasi, deafness, hypothyroidism, dwarfism, absent permanent teeth, and malabsorption. *J Pediatr* 79:982–987.

KRAUS-RUPPERT SYNDROME

Kraus-Ruppert (1956) described three brothers, the offspring of a consanguineous mating, who had microcephaly, severe mental retardation, syndactyly of the second to fourth toes, and hypogonadism. There was no evidence of spermatogenesis, and the testicular interstitium was occupied primarily by connective tissue. Widespread hypoplasia of the hypothalamic nuclei was found on postmortem examination. This appears to be a distinct syndrome inherited as an autosomal recessive trait.

REFERENCE

Kraus-Ruppert R (1956). Zur Frage vererbter diencephaler Storungen; infantiler Eunochoidismus sowie Mikrocephalie bei recessivem Ergang. *Z Menschl Vererb Konstitutionsl* 34:643–656.

LAURENCE-MOON SYNDROME

This condition is often considered together with the Bardet-Biedl syndrome as a single entity. There is considerable disagreement on this point, however, as most workers feel that the two conditions are distinct (Schacht and Maumenee, 1982). The Laurence-Moon syndrome consists of short stature, mental retardation, hypogenitalism, either pigmentary retinopathy or choroidal sclerosis, early ataxia and later spastic paraplegia, occasional polydactyly, and rather consistent obesity. Renal disease expressed as either severe interstitial nephritis or renal dysplasia is also part of the clinical spectrum (Churchill et al., 1981).

The hypogonadism is probably hypogonadotropic in type and occurs in a substantial proportion of both sexes. However, it has been suggested that primary hypogonadism may be present in some cases, largely on the basis of normal pituitary histomorphology (Whitaker et al., 1987). Vaginal atresia with hematocolpos was found in one female and a duplex uterus and septate vagina were noted in another, although these conceivably could be coincidental malformations (Churchill et al., 1981). The syndrome is inherited as an autosomal recessive trait.

REFERENCES
Churchill D N, McManamon P, Hurley R M (1981). Renal disease a sixth cardinal feature of the Laurence-Moon-Biedl syndrome. *Clin Nephrol* 16:151–154.
Schachat A P, Maumenee I H (1982). Bardet-Biedl syndrome and related disorders. *Arch Ophthalmol* 150:285–288.
Whitaker M D, Scheithauer B W, Kovacs K T, et al. (1987). The pituitary gland in the Laurence-Moon syndrome. *Mayo Clin Proc* 62:216–222.

LENZ-MAJEWSKI SYNDROME

A disproportionately large head, hypertelorism, atrophic lax skin, short extremities, and mental retardation characterize this condition (Robinow et al., 1977). The patients have a progerioid appearance. X-rays typically show sclerosis of the skull, facial bones and vertebrae, along with broad, undermodeled diaphyses.

Virtually all cases are sporadic. Cryptorchidism is universal in males, and hypospadias has been reported. No female genital anomalies have been noted.

REFERENCE
Robinow M, Johanson A J, Smith T H (1977). The Lenz-Majewski hyperostotic dwarfism: a syndrome of multiple congenital anomalies, mental retardation, and progressive skeletal sclerosis. *J Pediat* 91:417–421.

LENZ MICROPHTHALMIA SYNDROME

This syndrome was first described by Lenz (1955) as an X-linked form of microphthalmia associated with other malformations. Study of subsequent families has established that the eye changes may range from microphthalmia to anophthalmia, colobomas, and cataracts (Dinno et al., 1976; Goldberg and McKusick, 1991). The extraocular features are also variable, even in the same family, and include microcephaly, mental retardation, short stature, dental abnormalities, and dysplastic or absent kidneys. Varying degrees of hypospadias and cryptorchidism have been reported in affected males. Carrier females may show minor skeletal malformations and more subtle ocular pathology. The family described by Siber (1984) with the additional feature of spastic quadriplegia may have the same entity.

REFERENCES

Dinno N D, Lawwill T, Leggett A E, et al. (1976). Bilateral microsomia, coloboma, short stature and other skeletal anomalies—a new hereditary syndrome. *Birth Defects Orig Art Ser* 12(6):109–114.

Goldberg M F, McKusick V A (1971). An X-linked colobomatous microphalmos and other congenital anomalies: a disorder resembling Lenz's dysmorphogenetic syndrome. *Am J Ophthalmol* 71:1128–1133.

Lenz W (1955). Recessiv-geschlechtsgebundene Microphthalmie mit multiplen Misbil dungen. *Z Kinderheilk* 66:384–390.

Siber M (1984). X-linked recessive microencephaly, microphthalmia, with corneal opacities, spastic quadriplegia, hypospadia and cryptorchidism. *Clin Genet* 26:453–456.

LEOPARD Syndrome

The name of the syndrome is a mnemonic formed acrostically from the chief components: *l*entigenes, *E*KG defects, *o*cular hypertelorism, *p*ulmonary stenosis, *a*bnormalities of the genitalia, *r*etardation of growth, and sensorineural *d*eafness (Gorlin et al., 1969). The lentigenes are present at birth or appear shortly thereafter and occur all over the body. Various cardiac conduction abnormalities may be seen as well as pulmonary stenosis and hypertrophic cardiomyopathy (Voron et al., 1976). The gonads in both sexes may be hypoplastic, and affected males may have hypospadias and cryptorchidism, but these are not consistent features (Sevanez et al., 1976). The entire syndrome is quite variable, as would be expected in an autosomal dominant trait. Hypogonadism, when present, is most likely hypogonadotropic in type (Swanson et al., 1971), and, obviously, normal gonadal function is present in a great many individuals (Coppin and Temple, 1997).

REFERENCES

Coppin B D, Temple I K (1997). Multiple lentigenes syndrome (LEOPARD) syndrome) or progressive cardiomyopathic lentiginosis. *J Med Genet* 34:582–586.

Gorlin R J, Anderson R C, Blau M (1969). Multiple lentigenes syndrome. *Am J Dis Child* 117:652–662.

Sevanez H, Mane-Garzon F, Kolski R (1976). Cardiocutaneous syndrome (the 'LEOPARD' syndrome). Review of the literature and a new family. *Clin Genet* 9:266–276.

Swanson S L, Santen R J, Smith D W (1971). Multiple lentigenes syndrome: new findings of hypogonadotrophism, hyposmia, and unilateral renal agenesis. *J Pediatr* 78:1035–1037.

Voron D A, Hatfield H H, Kalkhoff R K (1976). Multiple lentigenes syndrome. *Am J Med* 60:447–456.

Limb/Pelvis-Hypoplasia/Aplasia Syndrome

Al-Awadi and colleagues (1985) described a male and female sibling pair of consanguineous parents who had absence to severe reduction deformities of all four limbs along with unusual facies and a normal thorax. Further sporadic and sibling cases with and without consanguinity were described from Brazil and Italy (Richieri-Costa, 1987; Camera et al., 1993). Bony pelvis deformities along with anteverted displaced, hypoplastic, or even absent external genitalia were also noted by others (Raas-Rothschild, 1988; Farag et al., 1993; Mollica et al., 1995). One male had cryptorchidism (Camera et al., 1993), whereas two affected females have had absence of the uterus (Farag et al., 1993; Teebi, 1993). In one of these females, secondary sex characteristics developed at age 15 and normal-appearing ovaries were seen by ultrasound (Teebi, 1993). Autosomal recessive inheritance seems assured. Some of the external genital deformities can be attributed to mechanical effects secondary to the deformed pelvis, but the müllerian aplasia or hypoplasia is less readily explained. It is possible the Schinzel-phocomelia syndrome (Schinzel, 1990; Chitayat et al., 1993) is the same entity (Lurie and Wolfsberg, 1993). There is also some clinical overlap with the Roberts-pseudothalidomide syndrome (this chapter).

REFERENCES

Al-Awadi S A, Teebi A S, Farag T I, et al. (1985). Profound limb deficiency, thoracic dystrophy, unusual facies and normal intelligence: a new syndrome. *J Med Genet* 22:36–38.

Camera G, Ferrailo G, Leo D, et al. (1993) Limb/pelvis-hypoplasia/aplasia syndrome (Al-Awadi-Raas-Rothschild syndrome): report of two Italian sibs and further confirmation of autosomal recessive inheritance. *J Med Genet* 30:65–69.

Chitayat D, Stalker H J, Vekemans M, et al. (1993). Phocomelia, oligodactyly, and acrania: The Schinzel-phocomelia syndrome. *Am J Med Genet* 45:297–299.

Farag T I, Al-Awadi S A, Marafie M J, et al. (1993). The newly recognized limb/pelvis–hypoplasia/aplasia syndrome: report of a Bedouin patient and review. *J Med Genet* 30:62–64.

Lurie I W, Wulfsberg E A (1993) On the nosology of the "Schinzel-phocomelia" and "Al-Awadi/Raas-Rothschild" syndromes. *Am J Med Genet* 47:1234.

Mollica, F, Mazzone D, Cimino G, et al. (1995). Severe case of Al-Awadi/Raas-Rothschild syndrome or new, possibly autosomal recessive facio-skeletal-genital syndrome. *Am J Med Genet* 56:168–192.

Raas-Rothschild A, Goodman R M, Meyers S, et al. (1988). Pathologic features and prenatal diagnosis in the newly recognized limb/pelvis-hypoplasia/aplasia syndrome. *J Med Genet* 25:687–99.

Richieri-Costa A (1987) Profound limb deficiency, thoracic anomalies, unusual facies and normal intelligence. The Al-Awadi syndrome—report of a Brazilian patient. *Rev Brasil Genet* 10:611–16.

Schinzel A (1990). Phocomelia and additional anomalies in two sisters. *Hum Genet* 84:539–541.

Teebi A (1993). Limb/pelvis/uterus-hypoplasia/aplasia syndrome. *J Med Genet* 30:797–800.

LISSENCEPHALY

Lissencephaly (smooth brain) is an etiologically nonspecific finding that has been reported in a number of syndromes (Dobyns and Truwit, 1995). One of the more familiar conditions with lissencephaly is the Miller-Diecker syndrome, a condition due to a deletion in the 17q13 region that features, in addition to loss of the brain morphogenesis gene LIS1 and lissencephaly, microcephaly, profound mental retardation, seizures, growth deficiency, congenital heart disease, and urogenital abnormalities, including cryptorchidism as a contiguous gene syndrome (Pilz and Quarrell, 1996). Point mutations in LIS1 have also been described (LoNigro et al., 1997). Another is the Walker-Warburg syndrome, in which lissencephaly occurs with other CNS malformations, eye abnormalities, congenital muscular dystrophy, occasionally cleft palate, and cryptorchidism and micropenis in males (this chapter). This syndrome is an autosomal recessive trait. It is quite likely that hypoplastic external genitalia with or without cryptorchidism could be associated with lissencephaly of any type, the reason being inadequacy of the hypothalamic-pituitary-gonadal axis. No specific gonadal or genital anomaly has been described in affected females.

REFERENCES

Dobyns W B, Truwit C L (1995). Lissencephaly and other malformations of cortical development: 1995 update. *Neuropaediatrics* 26:132–147.

LoNigro C, Chong S, Smith A C (1997). Point mutations and intragenic deletions in L1S1, the lissencephaly causative gene in isolated lissencephaly sequence and Miller-Diecker syndrome. *Hum Mol Genet* 6:157–164.

Pitz D B, Quarrell O W J (1996). Syndromes with lissencephaly. *J Med Genet* 33:319–323.

LUNDBERG SYNDROME

Lundberg (1997) reported three sibs, two females and one male, with a primary myopathy beginning at puberty, cataracts, minor skeletal abnormalities, mental retardation, and progressive gonadal failure. Curiously, the sibs had prominent long tract signs in childhood with pathologic reflexes. The author postulated that the progressive myopathy obscured the earlier findings. The hypogonadism was hypergonadotropic in type. The disorder is likely an autosomal recessive trait.

REFERENCE

Lundberg P O (1973). Hereditary myopathy, oligophrenia, cataract, skeletal abnormalities and hypergonadotropic hypogonadism: a new syndrome. *Eur Neurol* 10:261–280.

MARDEN-WALKER SYNDROME

The characteristic features of this syndrome include blepharophimosis, micrognathia, immobile facies, generalized hypotonia, multiple joint contractures, and mental retardation (Schrander-Stumple et al., 1993). Micropenis, hypospadias, and cryptorchidism are occasional features in affected males. Sib involvement and parental consanguinity support autosomal recessive inheritance.

REFERENCE

Schrander-Stumple C, Die-Smulders C, deKrom M, et al. (1993). Marden-Walker syndrome; case report, literature review and nosologic discussion. *Clin Genet* 43:303–308.

MARTSOLF SYNDROME

Martsolf and coworkers (1978) described two severely retarded brothers with short stature, microbrachycephaly, cataracts, mild maxillary hypoplasia with relative prognathism, minor digital anomalies, and primary hypogonadism. The parents were first cousins of Polish-Jewish extraction. Other cases have been described, including an opposite-sex sib pair, indicating autosomal recessive inheritance (Sanchez et al., 1985; Hennekam et al., 1988; Harbord et al., 1989). In one of these reports a male and female sib pair of consanguineous Pakistani parents had dilated cardiomyopathy, which may be an additional feature of the syndrome (Harbord et al., 1989).

REFERENCES

Harbord M G, Baraitser M, Wilson J (1989). Microcephaly, mental retardation, cataracts, and hypogonadism in sibs: Martsolf's syndrome. *J Med Genet* 26:397–406.

Hennekam R C M, Van de Meeberg A G, van Doorne J M, et al. (1988). Martsolf syndrome in a brother and sister: clinical features and pattern of inheritance. *Eur J Pediatr* 147:539–543.

Martsolf J T, Hunter A G W, Haworth J C (1978). Severe mental retardation, cataracts, short stature and primary hypogonadism in two brothers. *Am J Med Genet* 1:291–299.

Sanchez J M, Barreiro C, Freilij H (1985). Two brothers with Martsolf's syndrome. *J Med Genet* 22:308–310.

McKusick-Kaufman Syndrome

Hydrocolpos refers to the dilatation of the uterus and vagina with fluid. In the newborn the condition results from hypersecretion of the endocervical glands stimulated by maternal estrogens. If the patient is post-pubertal, menstrual blood accumulates and the condition is designated hydrometrocolpos. The usual reason is obstruction, most generally due to imperforate hymen, transverse vaginal septum or vaginal atresia. Transverse septa and partial vaginal atresia probably arise from failure of the respective urogenital sinus and müllerian duct derivatives to canalize, and the anomalies are usually sporadic. The McKusick-Kaufman syndrome is a disorder in which hydro(metro)colpos, usually due to either vaginal atresia or a transverse vaginal septum, is associated with postaxial polydactyly and congenital heart disease Robinow and Shaw, 1979; Goecke et al., 1981). Micropenis, glandular hypospadias, and prominent scrotal raphe with or without cryptorchidism have been seen in affected males (Goecke et al., 1981; Vince and Martin, 1989; Pul et al., 1994). The condition is an autosomal recessive trait.

REFERENCES

Goecke T, Dopfer R, Huenges R, et al (1981). Hydrometrocolpos, postaxial polydactyly, congenital heart disease, and anomalies of the gastrointestinal and genitourinary tracts: a rare autosomal recessive syndrome. *Eur J Pediatr* 136:297–305.

Pul N, Pul M, Gedik Y (1994). McKusick-Kaufman syndrome associated with esophageal atresia and distal tracheoesophageal fistula: a case report and review of the literature. *Am J Med Genet* 49:341–343.

Robinow M, Shaw A (1979). The McKusick-Kaufman syndrome: recessively inherited vaginal atresia, hydrometrocolpos, uterovaginal duplications, anorectal anomalies, postaxial polydactyly, and congenital heart disease. *J Pediatr* 94:776–778.

Vince J D, Martin N J (1989). McKusick-Kaufman syndrome: report of an instructive family. *Am J Med Genet* 32:174–177.

Meckel Syndrome

The primary components of this lethal malformation syndrome are posterior encephalocele, postaxial polydactyly and polycystic dysplastic kidneys (Salomen and Paavola, 1998). A host of other more inconsistent abnormalities also have been described. Genital abnormalities in the male range from simple hypospadias and cryptorchidism to sexual ambiguity. Septate vagina and/or bicornuate uterus in females have likewise been observed (Blankenberg et al., 1987; Rappola and Salonen 1985).

The syndrome has been reported in multiple affected sibs with parental consanguinity and in concordant monozygotic twins, indicating autosomal recessive inheritance. One responsible gene locus has been mapped to 17q21-q24 (Paavola et al., 1997) but there is evidence for locus heterogeneity.

REFERENCES

Blankenberg T A, Ruebner H, Ellis W G, et al. (1987). Pathology of renal and hepatic anomalies in Meckel syndrome. *Am J Med Genet* Suppl. 3:395–410.

Paavola P, Salonen R, Baumer A, et al. (1997). Clinical and genetic heterogeneity in Meckel's syndrome. *Hum Genet* 101:88–92.

Rappola J, Salonen R (1985). Visceral anomalies in the Meckel syndrome. *Teratology* 31:193–202.

Salonen R, Paavola P (1998). Meckel syndrome. *J Med Genet* 35:497–501.

Micro Syndrome

Warburg and colleagues (1993) described a male and female sibling and a male first cousin from a consanguineous Pakistani family who had microcephaly, microcornea with congenital cataracts, optic atrophy, mental retardation, diabetes, spasticity, and epilepsy. The males had crytorchidism, hypospadias, and a small phallus. The female had rudimentary secondary sex characteristics and absent menses. The available evidence was most compatible with secondary hypogonadism. The authors dubbed this constellation as the Micro syndrome on the basis of the cranial and ocular findings.

REFERENCE

Warburg M, Sjö O, Fledelius H C, et al. (1993). Autosomal recessive microcephaly, microcornea, congenital cataract, mental retardation, optic atrophy, and hypogenitalism: Micro syndrome. *Am J Dis Child* 147:1309–1312.

Microcephaly and Primary Hypogonadism

Microcephaly, mental retardation, and hypogonadism are components of a number of different syndromes. In most, however, the hypogonadism is secondary and presumably related to altered hypothalamic function. Mikati and colleagues (1985) described four affected sibs of consanguineous parents who had microcephaly, mental retardation, short stature, and an unusual facies consisting of a narrow forehead, synophrys, micrognathia, and abnormally shaped ears. Endocrine studies were consistent with primary gonadal failure. Gonadal histology in one patient showed decreased spermatogenesis and focal atrophy of seminiferous tubules. Autosomal recessive inheritance for this trait is likely.

REFERENCE

Mikati M A, Najjar S S, Sahli I F, et al (1985). Microcephaly, hypergonadotropic hypogonadism, short stature, and minor anomalies: a new syndrome. *Am J Med Genet* 22:599–608.

Möbius Sequence with Peripheral Neuropathy and Hypogonadism

Möbius sequence formally refers to patients with isolated bilateral paresis of the sixth and seventh cranial nerves, presumably due to disruption of the basilar artery system. Since the original description by Möbius (1888), the "syndrome" has been expanded to include involvement of other cranial nerves, oral defects, limb anomalies, and occasionally other structures to the extent that confusion reigns and no realistic genetic statement can be made. Hypogonadism is not a usual feature. However, central hypogonadism has been reported in four isolated patients who had Möbius sequence and peripheral neuropathy (Kawai et al., 1990; Baraitser and Rudge, 1996). Whether this triad represents a distinct entity is uncertain.

REFERENCES

Baraitser M, Rudge P (1996). Möbius syndrome, an axonal neuropathy and hypogonadism. *Clin Dysmorph* 5:351–355.
Kawai M, Momoi T, Fujii T, et al. (1990). The syndrome of Möbius sequence, peripheral neuropathy and hypogonadotropic hypogonadism. *Am J Med Genet* 37:578–582.
Möbius P J (1888). Über angeborene doppelseitige Abducens-Facialis Lähmung. *Münch Med Wsch* 35:91–94, 108–111.

Myotubular Myopathy (centronuclear myopathy)

This condition is named after the characteristic muscle histopathology, which resembles the myotubes of fetal muscle. Dominant, recessive, and X-linked varieties have been described; the X-linked form is often lethal in infancy. Males affected with the X-linked disease have an elongated myopathic facies and a large, often hydrocephalic head, extreme hypotonia, and absent deep tendon reflexes (Joseph et al., 1995). They do not survive without ventilatory support. Virtually all have cryptorchidism with an otherwise normal penis. The functional status of the gonads is unknown. The gene has been mapped to the Xq28 region, but there is some evidence for locus heterogeneity even on the X chromosome (Leichti-Gallati et al., 1991; Starr et al., 1990). Interestingly, one 46,XY patient with a deletion encompassing the myopathy gene also had ambiguous external genitalia. No mention was made of the histology of the gonads, which were presumably testes (Hu et al., 1996). Although the genital findings might have been unrelated, their presence may be indicative of an additional sex-determining gene in this chromosome region.

REFERENCES

Hu L-J, Laporte J, Kress W et al. (1996). Deletions in Xq28 in two boys with myotubular myopathy and abnormal genital development define a new contiguous gene syndrome in a 430 kb region. *Hum Genet* 5:139–143.
Joseph M, Pai G S, Holden K R, et al. (1995). X-linked myotubular myopathy: clinical observations in ten additional cases. *Am J Med Genet* 59:168–173.
Leichti-Gallati S, Wolff G, Ketelsen V, et al. (1991). X-linked centronuclear myopathy: mapping the gene to Xq28. *Neuromusc Disord* 1:239–245.
Starr S, Lamont M, Iselius L, et al. (1990). A linkage study of a large pedigree with X-linked centronuclear myopathy. *J Med Genet* 27:281–283.

Myotonic Dystrophy

Patients with myotonic dystrophy have cataracts as well as any number of associated endocrine abnormalities. Gonadal function is normal in childhood and young adult life; the majority of patients have normal secondary sex characteristics and evidence of fertility. With time, testicular atrophy ensues, accompanied by impotence and loss of libido (Harper, 1989). The histologic findings are of tubular degeneration with relative Leydig cell hyperplasia. Serum gonadotropic levels are slightly to moderately increased, whereas serum testosterone values may be only slightly reduced. Even when serum LH values are not increased, the response to GnRH infusion is supernormal. Affected females generally have little difficulty, although some may have menstrual irregularities or reduced fertility.

Myotonic dystrophy is inherited as an autosomal dominant trait. The molecular defect is an expanded trinucleotide repeat (CTG) in the 3' untranslated region of a protein kinase gene on chromosome 19 (Brook et al., 1992). More severe early-onset disease appears in children whose mother is affected, as the CTG repeat is expanded even further, a phenomenon called anticipation (Tsifidis, 1992).

REFERENCES

Brook J D, McCurrack M E, Harley H G, et al. (1992). Molecular basis of myotonic dystrophy: expansion of trinucleotide (CTG) repeat at the 3-prime-end of a transcript encoding a protein kinase family member. *Cell* 68:799–808.

Harper P S (1989). *Myotonic Dystrophy*. W. B. Saunders Co., Philadelphia, 2nd ed.

Tsilfidis C, McKenzie A E, Mettler G, et al. (1992). Correlation between CTG trinucleotide repeat length and frequency of severe congenital muscular dystrophy. *Nat Genet* 1:192–195.

N Syndrome

Hess and colleagues (1974) described two mentally retarded brothers with deafness, decreased vision, large corneas, peculiar overlap of the eyelids at their lateral margins, and spasticity. Both had cryptorchidism and hypospadias. Both boys and their mother later succumbed to leukemia (Hess et al., 1987). Increased chromosome breakage was induced by bleomycin, suggesting a deficit in DNA polymerase. X-linked inheritance is probable.

REFERENCES

Floy K M, Hess R O, Meisner L F (1990). DNA polymerase alpha defect in the N syndrome. *Am J Med Genet* 35:301–305.

Hess R O, Kaveggia E G, Opitz J M (1974). The N syndrome, a "new" multiple congenital anomaly-mental retardation syndrome. *Clin Genet* 6:237–246.

Hess R O, Hafez G R, Meisner L F (1987). Updating the N syndrome: occurrence of lymphoid malignancy and possible association with an increased role of chromosome breakage. *Am J Med Genet Suppl* 3:383–388.

Naguib-Richieri-Costa Syndrome
(Acrofrontonasal Dysostosis)

Naguib (1988) in Kuwait and Richieri-Costa and colleagues (1989) from Brazil independently described male and female sibs with microbrachycephaly, hypertelorism, broad nose with midline groove, broad thumbs and toes, with or without polysyndactyly, and hypospadias in the males. Both families were consanguineous, findings compatible with autosomal recessive inheritance (Teebi, 1992).

REFERENCES

Naguib K K (1988). Hypertelorism, proptosis, ptosis, polysyndactyly, hypospadias and normal height in three sibs: a new syndrome? *Am J Med Genet* 29:35–41.

Richieri-Costa A, Montagnoli L, Kamiya T Y (1989). Autosomal recessive acro-fronto-nasal dysosteous associated with genitourinary abnormalities. *Am J Med Genet* 33:121–124.

Teebi A S (1992). Neguib-Richieri-Costa syndrome: hypertelorism, hypospadias, polysyndactyly syndrome. *Am J Med Genet* 44:115–116.

NEU-LAXOVA SYNDROME

This syndrome consists of intrauterine growth retardation, microcephaly, exophthalmos, limb malformations, desquamating ichthyosis and hypoplastic genitalia in both sexes with cryptorchidism in the male (Fitch et al., 1982). The infants either are stillborn or die in the first few days of life. Autosomal recessive inheritance seems likely.

REFERENCE

Fitch N, Resch L, Rochon L (1982). The Neu-Laxova syndrome: comments on syndrome identification. *Am J Med Genet* 13:445–452.

NEUROFIBROMATOSIS (VON RECKLINGHAUSEN DISEASE)

Altered gonadal function is seen in neurofibromatosis but it is not common. Either precocious puberty or hypogonadism can develop and both are on a hypothalamic, usually—but not invariably—tumorous basis (Schimke, 1990). Enlarged external genitalia also may develop, probably as a consequence of production of local growth factors by the neurofibromatosis. Enlargement of the clitoris may be so severe as to cause confusion in sex assignment (Kaneti et al., 1988; Sutphen et al., 1995). Plexiform neuromas may distort pelvic anatomy in either sex. The condition is an autosomal dominant trait. The gene, located on chromosome 17, may act in part as a tumor suppressor (Basu et al., 1992).

REFERENCES

Basu T N, Gutmann D H, Fletcher J A (1992). Aberrant regulation of ras proteins in malignant tumor cells from Type I neurofibromatosis patients. *Nature* 356:713–715.

Kaneti J, Lieberman E, Mosha P, et al. (1988). A case of ambiguous genitalia owing to neurofibromatosis—review of the literature. *J Urol* 140:584–585.

Schimke R N (1990). The endocrine system, in *Neurofibromatosis: A Handbook for Patients, Families and Health Care Professionals*. Thieme, New York, p. 142–149. Rubenstein A F, Korf B R (eds).

Sutphen R, Galán-Gomés E, Kousseff B G (1995). Clitoromegaly in neurofibromatosis. *Am J Med Genet* 55:325–330.

NIJMEGEN BREAKAGE SYNDROME

This disorder resembles ataxia-telangiectasia at a cellular level in that affected individuals have chromosome hypersensitivity to ionizing radiation, common spontaneous rearrangement of chromosomes 7 and 14, and immunodeficiency (Weemaes et al., 1981; Taalman et al., 1989). These patients also have an increased incidence of lymphoreticular malignancy and, as expected, frequent infections. Clinically, however, the syndrome also features microcephaly, normal serum alpha fetoprotein levels, no ataxia, and no consistent skin changes, in contrast to ataxia-telangiectasia.

Primary ovarian failure has been described in some females (Conley et al., 1986; Chrzanowska et al., 1996), although the overall incidence is unknown. No information is available on sexual development in males affected with this autosomal recessive disorder.

REFERENCES

Chrzanowska K H, Krajewska-Walasek M, Biaecka M, et al. (1996). Ovarian failure in female patients with the Nimegen breakage syndrome. *Eur J Hum Genet* 4 (Suppl. 1):122.

Conley M E, Spinner N B, Emanuel B S, et al. (1986). A chromosome breakage syndrome with profound immunodeficiency. *Blood* 67:1251–1256.

Taalman R D, Hustinx T W, Weemaes C M et al. (1989). Further delineation of the Nimegen breakage syndrome. *Am J Med Genet* 32:425–431.

Weemaes C M, Hustinx T W, Scheres J M, et al. (1981). A new chromosomal instability disorder: the Nimegen breakage syndrome. *Acta Paediat Scand* 70:557–564.

NOONAN SYNDROME

This condition has been erroneously referred to as the male Turner syndrome. There are, however, no chromosome abnormalities, the physical resemblance of patients with the two syndromes is superficial at best, and both sexes may be affected. Individuals with the Noonan syndrome are usually short and may have ptosis, low-set ears, webbed neck, and pectus excavatum (Mendez and Opitz, 1985). Mental retardation is an inconsistent feature. The cardiovascular lesion is characteristically that of pulmonary stenosis, but septal defects may be present as well. Males may have small penis and/or cryptorchidism but normal fertility is not uncommon. Hypogonadism when present is generally, but not invariably, primary. Normal ovarian function characterizes affected females, but both primary and secondary amenorrhea may occur (Allanson, 1987).

The Noonan syndrome has until recently been considered genetically heterogeneous. Examination of a number of individuals spanning an age range from infancy to adult life has revealed a changing physiognomy such that there is less evidence of heterogeneity (Allanson et al., 1985). However, the Noonan phenotype may be a variable feature of neurofibromatosis (Watson syndrome, Tassabehji et al., 1993) and perhaps other independent syndromes (Seaver and Cassidy, 1991; Cohen and Gorlin, 1991). Some feel the cardio-facio-cutaneous syndrome also is, in reality, the Noonan syndrome (Leichtman, 1996). Evaluation of the Noonan syndrome gene now localized to chromosome 12q will help resolve the heterogeneity (Jamieson et al., 1994). The condition appears to be inherited as a variable autosomal dominant trait.

REFERENCES

Allanson J E, Hall J G, Hughes H E, et al. (1985). Noonan syndrome: the changing phenotype. *Am J Med Genet* 21:507–514.

Allanson J E (1987). Noonan syndrome. *J Med Genet* 24:9–13.

Cohen M M Jr, Gorlin R D (1991). Noonan-like/multiple giant cell lesion syndrome. *Am J Med Genet* 40:159–166.

Jamieson C R, Van der Burgt I, Brady A F, et al. (1994). Mapping a gene for Noonan syndrome to the long arm of chromosome 12. *Nat Genet* 8:357–360.

Leichtman L G (1996). Are cardio-facio-cutaneous syndrome and Noonan syndrome distinct? A case of CFC offspring of a mother with Noonan syndrome. *Clin Dysmorphol* 5:61–64.

Mendez H M M, Opitz J M (1985). Noonan syndrome: a review. *Am J Med Genet* 21:493–506.

Seaver L H, Cassidy S B (1991). New syndrome: mother and son with hypertelorism, downslanting palpebral fissures, malar hypoplasia, and apparently low-set ears associated with joint and scrotal anomalies. *Am J Med Genet* 41:405–409.

Tassabehji M, Strachan T, Sharland M, et al. (1993). Tandem duplication with a neurofibromatosis type I (NF1) gene exon in a family with features of Watson syndrome and Noonan syndrome. *Am J Med Genet* 53:90–95.

NORRIE DISEASE

The ocular features dominate the phenotype of Norrie disease: early retinal vascular proliferation, atrophy, corneal clouding, cataracts, and eventually phthises bulbi (Norrie, 1927). However, significant mental retardation is present in more than 50% of cases, microcephaly is common, and cryptorchidism with hypogonadism has been seen in some (Donnai et al., 1988) The condition is X-linked, and the gene (NDP), localized within or close to band Xp11.3 (Pettenati et al., 1993), codes for an extracellular matrix component called norrin (Chen et al., 1992)

REFERENCES

Chen Z-Y, Hendriks R W, Jobling M A et al. (1992) Isolation and characterization of a candidate gene for Norrie disease *Nat Genet* 1:204–208

Donnai D, Mountford R C, Read A P (1988). Norrie disease resulting from a gene deletion: clinical features and DNA studies. *J Med Genet* 25:73–78.

Norrie G (1927) Causes of blindness in children. *Acta Ophthalmol* 5:357–86.

Pettenati M J, Rao P N, Weaver R G, et al. (1993). Inversion (X) (p 11.4922) associated with Norrie disease in a four generation family. *Am J Med Genet* 45:577–80.

OCULOCEREBRAL SYNDROME (CROSS SYNDROME)

Cross and coworkers (1967) described a syndrome in three sibs from an inbred Amish community, composed of mental retardation, spastic diplegia, ocular anomalies, and cutaneous hypopigmentation resembling albinism. The ocular anomalies consist of microphthalmia, microcornea, corneal opacities, ectropion, hystagmus, and total blindness. Testes could not be palpated in the scrotum or inguinal canal in the two affected brothers. Abdominal exploration was not performed; therefore, it is not known whether this simply represented cryptorchidism or true anorchia. The one affected female was 12 years of age and had not menstruated. Genital abnormalities have not been consistent in subsequently described patients (Fryns et al., 1988). Autosomal recessive inheritance is likely.

REFERENCES

Cross H E, McKusick V A, Breen W (1967). A new oculocerebral syndrome with hypopigmentation. *J Pediatr* 70:398–406.

Fryns J P, Dereymaeker A M, Heremans G (1988). Oculocerebral syndrome with hypopigmentation (Cross syndrome). *Clin Genet* 34:81–84.

Oculocerebrorenal Syndromes

The X-linked oculocerebrorenal syndrome of Lowe (ORCL 1) is a well-recognized disorder associated with growth and mental retardation, hypotonia, metabolic acidosis, generalized aminoaciduria, proteinuria, vitamin D–resistant rickets, congenital cataracts, and glaucoma (Charnas and Nussbaum, 1995). Cryptorchidism has been described in a number of patients. Carrier females may have lens opacities. The ORCL 1 gene encodes a phosphotidylinositol 4,5 biphosphate-5-phosphatase, an enzyme loosely associated with the golgi apparatus (Suchy and Nussbaum, 1998; Attree et al., 1992).

McCance and associates (1960) have described a somewhat different oculocerebrorenal syndrome in two brothers who also had congenital absence of the testes. These brothers had failure to thrive, hypotonia, corneal opacities, mental retardation, severe hyperchloremic acidosis, and a defect in ammonia excretion. They differed from patients with the classic Lowe syndrome in having a very acid urine, structural abnormalities of the cerebrum and cerebellum, and a distinct type of renal lesion. On postmortem examination, in lieu of testes, only slight swellings on the spermatic cords near the attachment of the gubernaculum to the scrotum were found. Further heterogeneity within this category may well be present.

REFERENCES

Attree O, Olivos I M, Okabe I, et al. (1992). The Lowe's oculocerebrorenal syndrome gene encodes a protein highly homologous to inositol polyphosphate-5-phosphatase. *Nature* 358:239–242.

Charnas L R, Nussbaum R L (1995). The oculocerebrorenal syndrome of Lowe (Lowe syndrome). In Scriver C R, et al. (eds.), *The Metabolic and Molecular Bases of Inherited Disease*, 7th ed, McGraw-Hill, YorK, pp .3705–3716.

McCance R A, Matheson W J, Gresham G A, et al. (1960). The cerebrooculorenal dystrophies: a new variant. *Arch Dis Child* 35:240–249.

Suchy S F, Nussbaum R L (1998). Subcellular localization of ocr11 by differential centrifugation: comparison of its distribution of Golgi-associated proteins. *Am J Hum Genet* 63 (Suppl): A275, Abstract 1587.

Opitz G/BBB Compound Syndrome

This condition began as two separate disorders, the G syndrome and the BBB syndrome, the senior author of both reports being Opitz (1969 a,b). Subsequent reports suggested the disorders were the same entity. The basic clinical features include hypertelorism, laryngotracheal defects, congenital heart disease, bladder extrophy, and renal defects, along with hypospadias of varying degrees, even to the point of a cleft scrotum, and cryptorchidism in males (Jacobson et al., 1998) Affected females generally show only hypertelorism and no genital anomalies.

Originally, the condition(s) was felt to be X-linked, but male-to-male transmission was subsequently observed, and present evidence supports genetic heterogeneity involving distinct loci on Xp22 and 22q11.2. The two variants are apparently clinically indistinguishable (Robin et al., 1996). The Xp22 locus codes for a RING finger gene that is a transcription regulator and may be important in body axis patterning (Quaderi et al., 1997).

REFERENCES

Jacobson Z, Glickstein J, Hensle T, et al. (1998). Further delineation of the Opitz G/BBB syndrome: report of an infant with complex congenital heart disease and bladder extrophy, and review of the literature. *Am J Med Genet* 78:294–299.

Opitz J M, Frias J L, Gutenberger J E, et al. (1969a). The G syndrome of multiple congenital anomalies. *Birth Defects Orig Art Ser* 5:95–101.

Opitz J M, Summitt R L, Smith D W (1969b). The BBB syndrome: familial telecanthus with associated congenital anomalies. *Birth Defects Orig Art Ser* 5:86–94.

Quaderi N A, Schweiger S, Gaudeuz K, et al. (1997). Opitz G/BBB syndrome, a defect of midline development, is due to mutation in a new RING finger gene on Xp22. *Nat Genet* 17:285–291.

Robin N H, Opitz J M, Münke M (1996). Opitz G/BBB syndrome: clinical comparison of females linked to Xp22 and 22q, and review of the literature. *Am J Med Genet* 62:305–317.

Oto-Facio-Osseous-Gonadal Syndrome

Two brothers described by daSilva and colleagues (1997) had sensorineural deafness, short stature, unusual facies, fusion of carpal bones, Wormian bones, and cryptorchidism. A deceased sister was said to have resembled the boys. The parents were first cousins, further supporting autosomal recessive inheritance.

REFERENCE

daSilva E O, Duarte A R, Lins T S S (1997). Oto-facio-osseous-gonadal syndrome: a new form of syndrome deafness? *Clin Genet* 52:51–55.

Oto-Palatal-Digital Syndrome—Type II

The two oto-palatal-digital syndromes share the features of conductive deafness, cleft palate and short, broad thumbs and great toes. Both also have hypertelorism, prominent forehead, and facial bone hypoplasia. The type II variant is more severe and most patients die early.

Cryptorchidism and hypospadias have been seen in the type II variant (Young et al., 1993). Type I has been mapped to Xq28 (Biancalava et al., 1991). Available evidence points to X-linked inheritance in type II as well, so the two variants may be allelic.

REFERENCES

Biancalava V, Le Marec B, Odent S, et al. (1991). Oto-palatal-digital syndrome type I: further evidence for assignment of the locus to Xq28. *Hum Genet* 88:228–230.

Young K, Barth C K, Moore C, et al. (1993). Otopalatal digital syndrome type II associated with omphalocele: report of three cases. *Am J Med Genet* 45:481–487.

Pallister-Hall Syndrome

Hall and colleagues (1980) described a syndrome consisting of hypothalamic hamartoblastoma, craniofacial defects, postaxial polydactyly, renal and cardiac anomalies, and endocrine dysfunction. The latter undoubtedly results from panhypopituitarism secondary to either mass effect or hypothalamic endocrine dysfunction.

Severely affected males exhibit testicular hypoplasia, cryptorchidism, and micropenis. Milder variants associated with apparently normal genital development and function have since been described, and the suggestion has been made that the syndrome may be a variable autosomal dominant trait (Biesecker and Graham, 1996). As might be expected with CNS hamartomas, precocious puberty has been seen as well (Chapter 12). However, it is quite possible both etiologic and genetic heterogeneity exist. In at least some cases, mutations in GL13 (chromosome 7p13) have been detected (Kang et al., 1997). This is the same gene that is mutated in Grieg's cephalopolysyndactyly and familial postaxial polysyndactyly.

REFERENCES

Biesecker L G, Graham J M (1996). Pallister-Hall syndrome. *J Med Genet* 33:585–589.

Hall J G, Pallister S K, Clarren S K, et al. (1980). Congenital hypothalamic hamartoblastoma, hypopituitarism, imperforate anus, and postaxial polydactyly—a new syndrome? Part I. Clinical, causal and pathogenetic considerations. *Am J Med Genet* 7:47–74.

Kang S, Graham J M, Jr, Olney A H, et al. (1997). GL13 frameshift mutations cause autosomal dominant Pallister-Hall syndrome. *Nat Genet* 15:266–268.

PERLMAN SYNDROME

A syndrome that phenotypically resembles the Beckwith-Wiedemann syndrome was described by Perlman and colleagues (1973) in a male and a female sib who were the products of a consanguineous Yemenite Jewish marriage. The features were those of fetal gigantism, unusual facies, nephroblastomatosis and Wilms tumor in the female sib. A non-Jewish sib pair has been described; the brother had cryptorchidism (Neri et al., 1984), which appears to be a consistent finding in affected males (Greenberg et al., 1986). No genital or gonadal abnormality had been described in affected females. Autosomal recessive inheritance is likely.

REFERENCES

Greenberg F, Stein F, Gresik M V, et al. (1986). The Perlman familial nephroblastomatosis syndrome. *Am J Med Genet* 24:101–110.

Neri G, Martini-Neri M E, Katz B E, et al. (1984): The Perlman syndrome: familial renal dysplasia with Wilms' tumor, fetal gigantism and multiple congenital anomalies. *Am J Med Genet* 19:195–207, 1984.

Perlman M, Goldberg G M, Bar-Ziv J, et al. (1973). Renal hamartomas and nephroblastomatosis with fetal gigantism: a familial syndrome. *J Pediatr* 83:414–418.

PETERS-PLUS SYNDROME

Peters anomaly originally was considered to be a developmental anomaly of the anterior chamber with thinning and opacity of the cornea with iridocorneal adhesions. Family studies of the isolated ocular lesion have broadened the spectrum of the anomaly to include aniridia, and the pedigrees are compatible with autosomal inheritance. In one such family, a PAX 6 mutation was found (Hanson et al., 1994).

Some individuals have the ocular anomaly with other features—pre-and postnatal growth deficiency, short extremities, a high, broad forehead and hypertelorism, cardiac and renal anomalies, mental retardation, and cryptorchidism in males (Hennekam et al., 1993). This more complex condition was described by Van Schooneveld and colleagues (1984), who termed it the Peters-Plus Syndrome. It appears to be an autosomal recessive trait.

REFERENCES
Hanson I M, Seawright A, Hardman K, et al. (1993). PAX6 mutations in aniridia. *Hum Mol Genet* 2:915–920.
Hennekam R C, van Schooneveld M J, Ardinger H H, et al. (1993). The Peters-Plus Syndrome: description of 16 patients and review of the literature. *Clin Dysmorphol* 2:283–300.
Van Schooneveld M J, Delleman J W, Beemer F A, et al. (1984). Peters-Plus: a new syndrome. *Ophthal Paediatr Genet* 4:141–145.

PTERYGIUM SYNDROMES

A number of syndromes have been described that feature striking pterygia variously bridging the popliteal, antecubital, and crural areas (Hall et al., 1982). The popliteal pterygium syndrome is an autosomal dominant trait that also features cleft lip and/or palate and digital hypoplasia (Froster-Iskenius, 1990). One or more autosomal recessive forms with similar pterygia also exist but they are accompanied by a host of other malformations and are lethal (Hall, 1984). A milder autosomal recessive condition is called the multiple pterygium syndrome (Thompson et al., 1987). In this latter condition, pterygia of the neck and digits also occur.

All of the pterygium syndromes variably feature genital abnormalities—for example, penis and scrotal hypoplasia and cryptorchidism in males, and clitoral abnormalities with hypoplasia of the labia majora in females. The uterus may be hypoplastic or bifid as well.

REFERENCES
Froster-Iskenius U G (1990). Popliteal pterygium syndrome. *J Med Genet* 27:320–326.
Hall J G, Reed S D, Rosenbaum, K N, et al. (1982). Limb pterygium syndromes; a review and report of eleven patients. *Am J Med Genet* 12:377–409.
Hall J G (1984). The lethal multiple pterygium syndromes. *Am J Med Genet* 17:803–807.
Thompson E M, Donai D, Baraitser M, et al. (1987). Multiple pterygium syndrome: evolution of the phenotype. *Am J Med Genet* 24:733–749.

RENAL DYSPLASIA-LIMB DEFECTS (RL) SYNDROME

Ulbright and colleagues (1984) reported a male patient with abnormal facies, mesomelia with absence of ulna and severe hypoplasia of the radius with fusion of humerus and radius, absent fibulae, and lethal renal dysplasia. There was a distinct groove around the shaft of the penis, as if it had been constricted by a band. Schradner-Stumpel and colleagues (1990) described a male and a female sib with the condition: the male had an identical penile band as in the initial case and cryptorchidism. The female was said to have prominent labia and a hypertrophic clitoris. Given sibling involvement, autosomal recessive inheritance is possible.

REFERENCES
Schrander-Stumpel C, de Die-Smulders C, Fryns J P, et al. (1990). Limb reduction defects and renal dysplasia: confirmation of a new, apparently lethal, autosomal recessive MCA syndrome. *Am J Med Genet* 37:133–135.

Ulbright C E, Hodes M E, Ulbright T M (1984). New syndrome: renal dysplasia, mesomelia and radiohumeral fusion. *Am J Med Genet* 17:667–668.

RESTRICTIVE DERMOPATHY

The first description of this condition, in sibs, was by Toriello and colleagues (1983) under the rubric of aplasia cutis congenita. Witt and colleagues (1986), noting the multiple joint contractures, due to both abnormal fetal movement and abnormal skin, coined the term restrictive dermopathy. The pregnancy is usually complicated by polyhydramnios. Affected children have absence of facial contours ("porcelain doll") with micrognathia, ankylosis of the temporomandibular joint, thin, fibrotic skin, and other anomalies, including, on occasion, hypospadias (Verloes et al., 1992).

Autosomal recessive inheritance seems assured for this condition, in which the infants are stillborn or die in early neonatal life.

REFERENCES
Toriello H V, Higgins J V, Waterman D F (1983). Autosomal recessive aplasia cutis congenita—report of two affected sibs. *Am J Med Genet* 15:153–156.

Verloes A, Mulliez N, Gonzales M, et al. (1992). Restrictive dermopathy, a lethal form of arthrogryposis multiplex with skin and bone dysplasias: three new cases and review of the literature, *Am J Med Genet* 43:539–47.

Witt D R, Hayden M R, Holbrook K A, et al. (1986). Restrictive dermopathy: a newly recognized autosomal recessive skin dysplasia. *Am J Med Genet* 24:631–648.

RETINITIS PIGMENTOSA AND HYPOGONADISM

Chang and colleagues (1981) described 19-year-old twin girls and their 22-year-old sister, all of whom had primary amenorrhea due to hypogonadotropic hypogonadism, and retinitis pigmentosa. The LH response to repetitive, low-dose GnRH infusion was poor, suggesting that the lesion was basically pituitary in type. Retinitis pigmentosa and hypogonadism are also seen in the Bardet-Biedl syndrome, the Alström syndrome, and the Edwards syndrome (this chapter), but the sisters described by Chang and coworkers had none of the other features consistent with these diagnoses. An autosomal recessive defect seems likely.

REFERENCE
Chang R J, Davidson B J, Carlson H E, et al. (1981). Hypogonadotropic hypogonadism associated with retinitis pigmentosa in a female sibship: evidence for gonadotropin deficiency. *J Clin Endocrinol Metab* 53:1179–1185.

RIEGER SYNDROME (IRIS-DENTAL DYSPLASIA)

The Rieger syndrome (iris-dental dysplasia) consists of malformations of the iris including aniridia and coloboma, pupillary anomalies, and hypoplasia or missing teeth. Associated maxillary hypoplasia gives the patient a prognathic appearance. Hypospadias has been seen on a number of occasions in the absence of any recognized hormonal problem (Jorgenson et al., 1978; Chisholm and Chudley, 1983). Inheritance of the syndrome is autosomal dominant. The gene, located on chromosome 4q25–27, has been cloned (Semina et al., 1996). It is a novel homeobox gene with *Drosophila* and murine homologues.

REFERENCES

Chisholm I A, Chudley A E (1983). Autosomal dominant iridogoniodysgenesis with associated somatic abnormalities: four generation family with Rieger's syndrome. *Br J Ophthalmol* 67:529–534.

Jorgenson R J, Levin L S, Cross H E, et al. (1978). The Rieger syndrome. *Am J Med Genet* 2:
307–318.

Semina E V, Reiter B, Leysens N J, et al. (1996). Cloning and characterization of a novel
bicoid-related homeobox transcription factor gene, RIEG, involved in Rieger syndrome.
Nat Genet 14:392–399.

ROBERTS SYNDROME (PSEUDOTHALIDOMIDE SYNDROME, SC SYNDROME)

Affected individuals exhibit fairly symmetrical tetraphocomelia, craniofacial abnormalities, corneal clouding, cleft lip and palate, cardiac and renal anomalies, and
severe growth retardation (Freeman et al., 1974). Hypospadias and cryptorchidism
have been seen in roughly half the males, although oddly, relative phallic enlargement in both sexes has also been described (VanDenBerg and Franke, 1993). Septate
vagina and bicornate uterus have been seen, but appear to be uncommon (Freeman
et al., 1974). The gonads are not histologically dysgenetic. Whether the female sibs
reported by Schinzel (1990) had this syndrome or not is problematic but possible.
One of these had agenesis of the vagina and uterus. A variety of cellular studies
suggest that the fundamental abnormality in the Roberts syndrome resides in mi-
tosis. The inheritance pattern is that of an autosomal recessive trait.

REFERENCES

Freeman M V, Williams D W, Schimke R N, et al. (1974). The Roberts syndrome. *Clin Genet*
5:1–16.

Schinzel A (1990). Phocomelia and additional anomalies in two sisters. *Hum Genet* 84:539–
541.

VanDenBerg D J, Franke U (1993). Roberts syndrome: a review of 100 cases and a new rating
system for severity. *Am J Med Genet* 47:1104–1123.

ROBINOW SYNDROME

Robinow and colleagues (1969) described an unusual syndrome comprising meso-
melic dwarfism, short digits, hemivertebrae, a peculiar flattened facies with hypertelorism and occasional cleft lip and/or palate, an upturned nose, and genital hypoplasia. The latter is most marked in males, with the phallus often being literally
buried in the scrotum. With time the penis elongates somewhat, so that insemination is possible in some instances as evidenced by the multigeneration occurrence
of the condition including male-to-male transmission (Shprintzen et al., 1982). Some
males may have partial primary hypogonadism as evidenced by mild elevations of
FSH and LH and hyperresponsiveness to GnRH infusion (Lee et al., 1982). A female
with vaginal atresia and hematocolpos has been seen (Balei et al., 1998). Both an
autosomal dominant and recessive form of the syndrome seem to exist.

REFERENCES

Balei S, Beksac S, Haliloglu M, et al. (1998). Robinow syndrome, vaginal atresia, hematocol-
opos, and extra middle finger. *Am J Med Genet* 79:27–29.

Lee P A, Migeon C J, Brown T R, et al. (1982). Robinow's syndrome; partial primary hypo-gonadism in pubertal boys with persistence of micropenis. *Am J Dis Child* 136:327–330.

Robinow M, Silverman F N, Smith H D (1969). A newly recognized dwarfing syndrome. *Am J Dis Child* 117:645–651.

Shprintzen R J, Goldberg, R B, Saenger P, et al. (1982). Male-to-male transmission of Robi-now's syndrome: its occurrence in association with cleft lip and palate. *Am J Dis Child* 136:594–597.

Teebi A S (1990). Autosomal recessive Robinow syndrome. *Am J Med Genet* 35:64–68.

ROTHMUND-THOMPSON SYNDROME

The dermatologic findings are paramount in this disorder and consist of erythema, telangiectasia, atrophy, and irregular pigmentation of the skin along with other dysmorphic features, such as short stature, cataracts, saddle nose, small hands and feet, sparse hair, and mental retardation (Hall et al., 1980). The skin is normal at birth and the various changes begin in the first year of life. Osteosarcoma is a late feature (Drovin et al., 1993). Primary hypogonadism is present in most of the patients and the males are frequently cryptorchid; however, delayed puberty and diminished secondary sex characteristics may occur in both sexes (Starr et al., 1985). The syndrome is inherited as an autosomal recessive trait.

REFERENCES

Drovin C A, Mongrain E, Sasseville D, et al. (1993). Rothmund-Thompson syndrome with osteosarcoma. *J Am Acad Derm* 28:301–305.

Hall J C, Pagon R A, Wilson K M (1980). Rothmund-Thompson syndrome with severe dwarf-ism. *Am J Dis Child* 134:165–169.

Starr O G, McClure J P, Conner J M (1985). Non-dermatologic complications and genetic aspects of the Rothmund-Thompson syndrome. *Clin Genet* 27:102–104.

RUBENSTEIN-TAYBI SYNDROME

The cardinal features of this syndrome are broad thumbs and great toes, mental retardation and peculiar facies (Rubenstein and Taybi, 1963). Cryptorchidism is common in affected males, and both hypospadias and a rather unusual angulation of the phallus have been seen (Rubenstein, 1969). Supernumerary, wide-spaced, or hypoplastic nipples are occasional features. The vast majority of cases are sporadic. Deletions within the chromosome 16p13.3 region have been found in a number of patients, perhaps indicative of a contiguous gene syndrome (Wallerstein et al., 1997). In other instances, autosomal dominant inheritance obtains, presumably due to either a mutation with qualitative effects or haploinsufficiency of a gene for the CREB binding protein (CBP). CBP is known as a transcriptional coregulator: it trans-duces cAMP-regulated gene expression by interacting with a phosphated form of CREB. The latter is a direct transcriptional regulator that binds to a DNA sequence known as the cAMP-regulated enhancer (CRE) (Petrij et al. 1995). Acute leukemia may complicate this disorder, and it is of interest that the breakpoints of the inv(16) and the (16;16) characteristic of the M4 type of acute nonlymphocytic leukemia map within this region (Wessels et al., 1991).

REFERENCES

Petrij F, Giles R H, Dauwerse H G, et al (1995). Rubenstein-Taybi syndrome caused by mu-tations in the transcriptional co-activator CBP. *Nature* 376; 348–351.

Rubenstein J H (1969). The broad thumb syndrome—progress report 1963. *Birth Defects* 5(2): 25–41.

Rubenstein J H, Taybi H (1963). Broad thumbs and toes and facial abnormalities. *Am J Dis Child* 105:588–608.

Wallerstein R, Anderson C E, Hay B E, et al. (1997). Submicroscopic deletions at 16p13.3 in Rubenstein-Taybi syndrome: frequency and clinical manifestations in a North American population. *J Med Genet* 34:203–206.

Wessels J W, Dauwerse J G, Breuning M H, et al. (1991). The inversion 16 and the translocation (16;16) in ANLL M4eo break in the same subregion of the short arm of chromosome 16. *Cancer Genet Cytogenet* 57:225–228.

RÜDIGER SYNDROME

Rüdiger and colleagues (1971) described a male and a female sib with severe developmental failure, unusual coarse facies, bifid uvula, short fingers and toes, and hydronephrosis secondary to distal ureteral stenosis. The female had a bicornuate uterus and bilateral ovarian cysts, whereas her brother had huge inguinal hernias and micropenis. Both died in infancy. Autosomal recessive inheritance seems likely.

REFERENCE

Rüdiger R A, Schmidt W, Loose A, et al. (1971). Severe developmental failure with coarse facial features, distal limb hypoplasia, thickened palmar creases, bifid uvula and ureteral stenosis: a previously unidentified disorder with lethal outcome. *J Pediatr* 79:977–981.

RUVALCABA SYNDROME

Ruvalcaba and colleagues (1971) described male sibs and first cousins with severe mental retardation, short stature, microcephaly, unusual facies, and cryptorchidism with hypoplastic genitalia in males. Other patients have been described under the same rubric who had less dramatic features without mental retardation or hypoplastic genitalia, perhaps indicative of heterogeneity (Sugio and Kajii, 1984). Autosomal dominant inheritance has been suggested, but this mode of inheritance cannot be considered established.

REFERENCES

Ruvalcaba R H A, Reichert A, Smith D W (1971). A new familial syndrome with osseous dysplasia and mental deficiency. *J Pediatr* 79:450–455.

Sugio Y, Kajii T (1984). Ruvalcaba syndrome: autosomal dominant inheritance. *Am J Med Genet* 19:741–753.

SCHINZEL-GIDEON SYNDROME

Midface retraction, frontal bossing, choanal atresia, hirsutism, somatic and mental retardation, and various skeletal anomalies make up this syndrome, which is usually lethal in the first few months of life (Schinzel and Gideon, 1978; Labrune et al., 1994; Elliott et al., 1996). Affected males often have micropenis with or without hypospadias, and a hypoplastic scrotum. Labial hypoplasia, with a deep interlabial sulcus and hymenal atresia, is seen in females (Labrune et al., 1994; Al-Gazali et al., 1990). This condition may be a rare autosomal trait.

REFERENCES

Al-Gazali L I, Farndon P, Burn J, et al. (1990). The Schinzel-Gideon syndrome. *J Med Genet* 27:42–47.

Elliott A M, Meagher-Villemure K, Oudjhave K, et al. (1996). Schinzel-Gideon syndrome: further delineation of the phenotype. *Clin Dysmorphol* 5:135–142.
Labrune P, Lyonnet S, Zupan V, et al. (1994). Three new cases of the Schinzel-Gideon syndrome and review of the literature. *Am J Med Genet* 50:90–93.
Schinzel A, Gideon A (1978). A syndrome of severe midface retraction, multiple skull anomalies, clubfeet and cardiac and renal malformation in sibs. *Am J Med Genet* 1:361–375.

SCHMITT-GILLENWATER-KELLY SYNDROME

Schmitt and colleagues (1982) described a three-generation family in which both males and females had symmetric, nonapposible triphalangeal thumbs and radial hypoplasia along with maxillary diastema. All affected males had first-degree hypospadias. This apparently unique syndrome is inherited as an autosomal dominant trait.

REFERENCE
Schmitt E, Gillenwater J Y, Kelly T E (1982). An autosomal dominant syndrome of radial hypoplasia, triphalangeal thumb, hypospadias, and maxillary diastema. *Am J Med Genet* 13:63–69.

SEPTO-OPTIC DYSPLASIA (DE MORSIER SYNDROME)

This condition, which is likely etiologically heterogeneous, features hypoplastic optic discs with absent septum pellucidum, and often other midline CNS abnormalities such as partial to complete absence of the corpus callosum and changes in the posterior fossa. Various degrees of central endocrine dysfunction are usually also present, including hypogonadotropic hypogonadism with normal genitalia (Willnow et al., 1996). Affected sibs have been recorded (Benner et al., 1990; Dattani et al., 1998). Homozygous mutations in the homeobox gene HESX1 have been identified in two of these sibs, establishing an autosomal recessive form of the disease.

REFERENCES
Benner J D, Preslan M W, Gratz E, et al. (1990). Septo-optic dysplasia in two siblings. *Am J Ophthalmol* 109:632–637.
Dattani M T, Martinez-Barbera J-P, Thomas P Q, et al. (1998). Mutations in the homeobox gene HESX1/Hesx 1 associated with septo-optic dysplasia in human and mouse. *Nat Genet* 19:125–133.
Willnow S, Kiess W, Butenandt O, et al. (1996). Endocrine disorders in septo-optic dysplasia (De Morsier syndrome)—evaluation and follow-up of 18 patients. *Eur J Pediat* 155:179–184.

SHILBACK-ROTT SYNDROME

Shilback and Rott (1988) described a multigeneration family featuring hypotelorism, blepharophimosis with epicanthic folds, and submucous cleft palate. Affected males had variable degrees of hypospadias. As evidenced by the autosomal dominant pedigree pattern, gonadal function in both sexes was normal.

REFERENCE
Shilback U, Rott H-D (1988). Ocular hypotelorism, submucous cleft palate and hypospadias: a new autosomal dominant syndrome. *Am J Med Genet* 31:863–870.

SHORT RIB–POLYDACTYLY SYNDROMES

Several forms of lethal short rib–polydactyly syndromes have been recorded. They are generally differentiated on the basis of the various skeletal radiographic features and the pattern of visceral anomalies, although controversy exists concerning exactly how heterogeneous the category actually is. Some suggest allelism (Beemer at al., 1983), and others that the various syndromes actually represent a single, variably expressed entity (Sillence, 1985; Martinez-Frias et al., 1993).

Four types have been delineated by an international working group (Beighton et al., 1992); type I (Saldino-Noonan), II (Majewski), III (Verma-Naumoff), and IV (Beemer-Langer). All demonstrate variable degrees of genital anomalies to the point of sexual ambiguity and 46,XY sex reversal (Bernstein et al., 1985). This clinical and particularly genital variability is reminiscent of that seen in the Smith-Lemli-Opitz Syndrome (Chapter 13) and with camptomelic dysplasia (Chapter 7). Whether one or multiple entities, the short rib–polydactyly syndrome(s) is inherited as an autosomal recessive trait (s).

REFERENCES

Beemer F A, Langer L O, Klep-dePater, J M, et al. (1983). A new short rib syndrome: report of two cases. *Am J Med Genet* 14:115–123.

Beighton P, Gideon A, Gorlin R, et al. (1992). International classification of osteochondrodysplasias. *Am J Med Genet* 44:223–229.

Bernstein R, Isdale J, Pinto M et al (1985). Short rib-polydactyly syndrome: a single or heterogeneous entity? A re-evaluation prompted by four new cases. *J Med Genet* 22:46–53.

Martinez-Frias M-L, Bermejo E, Urioste M, et al. (1993). Short rib-polydactyly syndrome (SRPS) with anencephaly and other central nervous system anomalies: a new type of SRPS or a more severe expression of a known SRPS entity? *Am J Med Genet* 47:782–787.

Sillence D O (1980). Invited editorial comment: non-Majewski short rib-polydactyly syndrome. *Am J Med Genet* 7:223–229.

SILVER-RUSSELL SYNDROME

Silver and colleagues (1953) and Russell (1954) independently described patients with intrauterine growth retardation, lateral asymmetry, and triangular facies with craniofacial disproportion. Over the years a variety of other anomalies have been added to the clinical spectrum, but they are inconsistent. The facies become more normal with age. Short stature persists into adult life but puberty is usually normal, although sexual precocity has been seen (Silver, 1964). Micropenis, hypospadias and/or cryptorchidism have been reported fairly frequently in males. Although sexual ambiguity also has been recorded (Marks and Bergeson, 1977), the diagnosis of Silver-Russell syndrome was not firm. No definite genital abnormality in females has been identified.

The genetics are unclear and no definite mendelian inheritance pattern has emerged (Patton, 1988). A patient with a chromosome break in 17q25 suggests the possibility of a contiguous gene syndrome (Midro et al., 1993).

Some cases evidently arise on the basis of maternal uniparental disomy of chromosome 7 (Kotzot et al., 1995; Eggerman et al., 1997).

REFERENCES

Eggerman T, Wollmann H A, Kuner R, et al. (1997). Molecular studies in 37 Silver-Russell syndrome patients: frequency and etiology of uniparental disomy. *Hum Genet* 100:415–419.

Kotzot D, Schmitt S, Bernasconi F, et al. (1995). Uniparental disomy 7 in Silver-Russell syndrome and primordial growth retardation. *Hum Mol Genet* 4:583–587.

Marks L J, Bergeson P S (1977). The Russell-Silver syndrome. *Am J Dis Child* 131:447–451.

Midro A T, Debek K, Sawicka A, et al. (1993). Second observation of Silver-Russell syndrome in a carrier of a reciprocal translocation with one breakpoint at site 17q25. *Clin Genet* 44: 53–55.

Patton M A (1988). Russell-Silver syndrome. *J Med Genet* 25:557–560.

Russell A (1954). A syndrome of "intrauterine" dwarfism recognizable at birth with craniofacial dysostosis, disproportionately short arms, and other anomalies (5 examples). *Proc Roy Soc Med* 47:1040–1044.

Silver H K, Kiyasu W, George J, et al. (1953). Syndrome of congenital hemihypertrophy, shortness of stature, and elevated urinary gonadotropins. *Pediatrics* 12:368–376.

Silver H K (1964). Asymmetry, short stature and variations in sexual development: a syndrome of congenital malformations. *Am J Dis Child* 107:498–515.

Simpson-Golabi-Behmel Syndrome

Pre- and postnatal macrosomia with a correspondingly large head, rather coarse facies, postaxial polydactyly, and vertebral segmentation defects in some, mild to moderate mental retardation, cardiac conduction defects, and cystic kidneys are common features of this syndrome (Neri et al., 1988). Either hypospadias or cryptorchidism or both have also been reported. The clinical involvement varies considerably from family to family, and the condition may be lethal in early infancy (Terespolsky et al., 1995). Embryonal tumors such as Wilms tumor and neuroblastoma have been seen prompting comparison of this overgrowth syndrome to the Beckwith-Weidemann syndrome (this chapter). These two disorders may both involve deregulated expression of insulin-like growth factor 2 (IGF 2), considered to be a prime modulator of fetal and perhaps infant growth. The Simpson-Golabi-Behmel syndrome is X-linked and the gene maps to Xq26. The gene itself, termed GPC3, encodes a putative extracellular proteoglycan, glypican 3, that appears to regulate growth in mesoderm by interacting in some fashion with IGF 2 and/or its receptor (Pilia et al., 1996; Weksberg et al., 1996).

REFERENCES

Neri G, Marini R, Cappa M, et al. (1988). Simpson-Golabi-Behmel syndrome: an X-linked encephalo-tropho-schisis syndrome. *Am J Med Genet* 30:287–299.

Pilia G, Hughes-Benzie R M, MacKenzie A, et al. (1996). Mutations in GPC3, a glypican gene, cause the Simpson-Golabi-Behmel syndrome. *Nat Genet* 12:241–247.

Terespolsky D, Farrell S, Siegel-Bartelt J, et al. (1995). Infantile lethal variant of Simpson-Golabi-Behmel syndrome associated with hydrops fetalis. *Am J Med Genet* 59:329–333.

Weksberg R, Squire J A, Templeton D M (1996). Glypicans: a growing trend. *Nat Genet* 12: 225–227.

Sohval-Soffer Syndrome

In 1953, Sohval and Soffer described two male sibs with mental retardation, skeletal anomalies, and small testes with hypogonadism. The testicular histology was identical in the two brothers and quite unlike that seen in other gonadal disorders. All of the seminiferous tubules were involved by either of two distinct processes: true germinal aplasia or complete fibrosis, with no gradations between. In one brother, Leydig cells were sparse, whereas in the other they appeared clumped. No similar cases have been described. Either autosomal or X-linked recessive inheritance is possible.

REFERENCE

Sohval A R, Soffer L J (1953). Congenital familial testicular deficiency. *Am J Med* 14:328–348.

SPASTIC PARAPLEGIA AND SEX REVERSAL

Teebi and colleagues (1998) described two phenotypic female sibs, the offspring of first-cousin Iranian parents, who had microcephaly, normal intelligence, optic atrophy and spastic paraplegia. The elder sib had an XY karyotype, and on further investigation was found to have a normal uterus with fibrotic gonads containing neither ovarian nor testicular tissue. PCR study of SRY along with upstream and downstream sequences revealed no abnormalities and total identity with the father's SRY. The 46,XX sister was not examined further, so her gonadal status is unknown. Autosomal recessive inheritance of this syndrome seems certain.

REFERENCE

Teebi A S, Miller S, Ostrer H, et al. (1998). Spastic paraplegia, optic atrophy, microcephaly with normal intelligence, and XY sex reversal: a new autosomal recessive syndrome? *J Med Genet* 35:759–762.

ULNAR-MAMMARY SYNDROME (SCHINZEL SYNDROME)

Defects of the ulnar rays, often asymmetrical and variable in severity, associated with aplasia or hypoplasia of the breasts and apocrine glands have been described in families as an autosomal dominant trait (Schinzel, 1987; Franceschini et al., 1992). Curiously, affected females have normal external genitalia and apparently normal fertility, whereas affected males frequently have small external genitalia, cryptorchidism, delayed puberty, and reduced fertility. There is no recognized hormonal basis for the differences between the sexes. The gene has been mapped to chromosome 12q23–24.1, a region that also contains the locus for Holt-Oram syndrome, raising the possibility of allelism (Bamshad et al., 1995).

REFERENCES

Bamshad M, Karkowiak P A, Watkins W S, et al. (1995). A gene for ulnar-mammary syndrome maps to 12q23-q24.1. *Hum Mol Genet* 4:1973–1997.

Franceschini P, Varden M P, Dalformo L (1992). Possible relationship between Ulnar-mammary syndrome and split hand with aplasia of the ulnar syndrome. *Am J Med Genet* 44:807–812.

Schinzel A (1987). Ulnar-mammary syndrome. *Am J Med Genet* 24:773–781.

URBAN-ROGERS-MEYER SYNDROME

Urban and colleagues (1979) described two brothers who had mental retardation, genital anomalies, and obesity plus unusual facies, soft tissue contractures of the hands with concomitant atrophy of the intrinsic muscles, mild hypothyroidism, and osteoporosis with frequent fractures. The hypogonadism was mild but was accompanied by cryptorchidism in one of the sibs. HCG therapy was partially successful in initiating testicular descent in this boy. Another unrelated patient had hypospadias (Pagran and Gollop, 1988). Either X-linked or autosomal recessive inheritance is possible.

REFERENCES

Pagnan N A B, Gollop T R (1988). Prader-Willi habitus, osteopenia, and camptodactyly (Urban-Rogers-Meyer syndrome): a probable second report. *Am J Med Genet* 31:787–792.
Urban M D, Rogers J G, Meyers W J III (1979). Familial syndrome of mental retardation, short stature, contractures of the hands and genital anomalies. *J Pediatr* 94:52–55.

URIOSTE SYNDROME

Urioste and colleagues (1993) reported three unrelated 46,XY male patients with persistent müllerian duct derivatives, craniofacial anomalies, and prominent lymphangiectasia of the small intestine and other viscera. Refractory hypoproteinemia was present, most likely due to protein-losing enteropathy. All had cryptorchidism and two had small phalluses. In one instance, the cryptorchid but morphologically normal testes were attached to the Fallopian tubes. Because one of the infants had a brother historically affected, the authors postulated that the syndrome was a rare autosomal recessive or an X-linked trait.

REFERENCE

Urioste M, Rodriguez J I, Barcia J M, et al (1993). Persistence of Müllerian derivatives, lymphangiectasia, hepatic failure, postaxial polydactyly, renal and craniofacial anomalies. *Am J Med Genet* 47:494–503

VAN BENTHEM SYNDROME

Three male sibs have been described with a peculiar constellation of anomalies, including apparent cryptorchidism, severe chest deformities, hypoplasia of the musculature, absence of subcutaneous fatty tissue, and dolichocephaly with severe mental retardation. In the one brother who was autopsied, no remnants of testicular tissue could be found. This may well represent a distinct syndrome inherited as an autosomal or x-linked recessive trait.

REFERENCE

Van Benthem L H, B M, Driessen O, Hanevela G T, et al (1970). Congenital familial testicular deficiency. *Arch Dis Child* 45:590–592.

WALKER-WARBURG SYNDROME (HARD ± E SYNDROME)

This syndrome includes microphthalmia with anterior chamber abnormalities and retinal dysgenesis and lissencephaly with hydrocephalus. Pagon and colleagues (1977) offered the acronym HARD ±E for *h*ydrocephalus, *a*gyria, *r*etinal *d*ysplasia, with or without *e*ncephalocele. Diagnostic criteria were set forth by Dobyns and colleagues (1989). Fukuyama-type congenital muscular dystrophy is probably the same entity (Toda et al., 1995). Affected males may have micropenis and cryptorchidism, likely due to inefficient hypothalamic GnRH. Autosomal recessive inheritance has been established (Rodgers et al., 1994).

REFERENCES

Dobyns W B, Pagon R A, Armstrong D, et al. (1989). Diagnostic criteria for Walker-Warburg syndrome. *Am J Med Genet* 32:195–210.
Pagon R A, Chandler J W, Collie W R, et al (1977). Hydrocephalus, agyria, retinal dysplasia, encephalocele (HARD ± E) syndrome: an autosomal recessive condition. *Birth Defects Orig Art Ser* 14 (6B):233–241.
Rodgers B L, Vanner L V, Pai G S, et al (1994). Walker-Warburg syndrome: report of three affected sibs. *Am J Med Genet* 49:198–201.
Toda T, Yoshioka M, Nakehori Y, et al. (1995). Genetic identity of Fukuyama-type congenital muscular dystrophy and Walker-Warburg syndrome. *Ann Neurol* 37:99–101.

WERNER SYNDROME

The Werner syndrome is characterized by an appearance of premature aging, short stature, cataracts, sclerodermatous skin changes, and mild diabetes (Epstein et al., 1966; Goto et al., 1981). Hypogonadism is a frequent feature in both sexes. Although fertility is definitely reduced, some affected individuals have reproduced. The hypogonadism may be either primary or secondary. The gene for Werner syndrome (WNR) maps to 8p12 and codes for a putative DNA helicase (Yu et al., 1996). Precisely how the defect in DNA metabolism generates premature aging is not immediately clear. The disease seems to be more common in Japan, where 300 are affected per 100 million persons. Werner syndrome is inherited as an autosomal recessive trait.

REFERENCES

Epstein C J, Martin G M, Schultz A I, et al. (1966). Werner's syndrome: a review of its symptomatology, natural history, pathologic features, genetics and relationship to the natural aging process. *Medicine* 45:177–222.
Goto M, Tamimoto K, Horiuci Y, et al. (1981). Family analysis of Werner's syndrome: a survey of 42 Japanese families with a review of the literature. *Clin Genet* 19:8–15.
Yu C-E, Oshima J, Fu Y-H, et al. (1996). Positional cloning of the Werner's syndrome gene. *Science* 272:258–262.

WIEDEMANN SYNDROME

Wiedemann and colleagues (1985, 1989) described male first cousins, related through their mothers, who had postnatal microcephaly, global developmental delay, anomalies of the hands and feet, micropenis with or without scrotal hypoplasia, and cryptorchidism. Two other male patients have been reported, one of whom additionally had unilateral renal agenesis (Nevin et al., 1994); two others had urethral valves (Wieczorek et al., 1996). X-linked inheritance of the syndrome is a good possibility.

REFERENCES

Nevin N C, Stewart F J, Corkey C W B, et al. (1994). Microcephaly with large anterior fontanelle, generalized convulsions, micropenis, and distinct anomalies of the hands and feet. Another example of the Wiedemann syndrome? *Clin Genet* 46:205–208.

Wieczorek D, Gillessen-Kaesbach G, Plewa S, et al. (1996). Microcephaly, seizures, genital hypoplasia, and abnormalities of the hands and feet in a 4 year old boy with possible Wiedemann syndrome. *Clin Genet* 49:106–107.

Wiedemann H-R, Gross K-R, Dibbern H (1985). *An Atlas of Characteristic Syndromes: A Visual Aid to Diagnoses for Clinicians and Practicing Physicians.* London, Wolfe Med Publ Ltd. pp 106–107.

Wiedemann H-R, Kunze J, Dibbern H (1989) *Atlas der Klinischen Syndrome.* Stuttgart Schattauer Verlag. pp. 164–165.

Winter Syndrome

Winter and colleagues (1968) described four sisters who showed varying degrees of renal dysgenesis, deafness due to malformation of the ossicles of the middle ear, and vaginal atresia. Two of the sibs had bilateral renal agenesis, the pathology of these cases having been described in an earlier publication (Schmidt et al., 1952). A second such family was described by Turner (1970). One of the deceased sibs in the latter family had ectopic ovaries and only a small nodule of tissue for a uterus. In a third family (King et al., 1987), one of two affected sibs delivered a normal female infant after vaginal reconstructive surgery. The presence of the characteristic ear defect should distinguish the trait from simple müllerian aplasia. Autosomal recessive inheritance seems likely, although no affected males have been reported as yet.

REFERENCES

King L A, Sanchez-Ramos L, Talledo G E, et al. (1987). Syndrome of genital, renal and middle ear anomalies: a third family and report of a pregnancy. *Obstet Gynecol* 69:491–493.

Schmidt, E C H, Hartley A A, Bower R (1952). Renal aplasia in sisters. *Arch Pathol* 54:403–406.

Turner G (1970). A second family with renal, vaginal and middle ear anomalies. *J Pediatr* 76:641.

Winter J S, Kohn G, Mellman W J, et al. (1968). A familial syndrome of renal, genital and middle ear anomalies. *J Pediatr* 72:88–93.

Xeroderma Pigmentosum

There are a number of types of xeroderma pigmentosum, separable by complementation studies in cultured skin fibroblasts. The latter firmly indicate that the defective DNA repair seen in xeroderma after UV light exposure is due to mutant genes acting at different loci (Cleaver, 1994). One phenotypic form of xeroderma is accompanied by progressive mental retardation, microcephaly, dwarfism, gonadal hypoplasia, and neurologic abnormalities such as ataxia and choreoathetosis, and has been called the De Sanctis–Caccioni syndrome. However, the syndrome has been seen in all complementation types and hence is not specific (Kraemer et al., 1987; Kanda et al., 1990). When present, the hypogonadism appears to be restricted to males and the testes may be cryptorchid. Autosomal recessive inheritance has been established for all complementation types.

REFERENCES

Cleaver J E (1994). It was a very good year for DNA repair. *Cell* 76:1–4.

Kanda T, Oda M, Yonezawa M, et al. (1990). Peripheral neuropathy in xeroderma pigmentosum. *Brain* 113:1025–1044.

Kraemer K H, Lee M M, Scotto J (1987). Xeroderma pigmentosum: cutaneous, ocular, and neurologic abnormalities in 830 published cases. *Arch Dermatol* 123:241–250.

XK APROSENCEPHALY SYNDROME (GARCIA-LURIE SYNDROME)

The phenotype of this condition includes aprosencephaly, congenital heart disease, preaxial limb anomalies, and genital maldevelopment in males—cryptorchidism, micropenis, hypospadias, and even persistent cloaca (Garcia and Duncan, 1977). Lurie and colleagues (1979) suggested X to signify the patient of Garcia and Duncan whose name was not given and the K to denote the initial letter of the last name of the Russian patient described in the paper of Lurie and colleagues.

Most cases are sporadic, but Townes and colleagues (1988) recorded variably affected sibs, suggesting autosomal recessive inheritance. In contrast, virtually the same phenotype can be seen with deletions involving 13q32 (Brown et al., 1995; Guala et al., 1997), suggesting the syndrome might be caused by deletion of contiguous genes. Occasional sib involvement could be due to a cryptic deletion and gonadal mosaicism rather than autosomal recessive inheritance. Molecular studies of all patients with this syndrome will be needed to clarify the issue.

REFERENCES

Brown S, Russo J, Chitayat D, et al. (1995). The 13q-syndrome: the molecular definition of the critical region in band 13q32. *Am J Hum Genet* 57:859–866.

Garcia C A, Duncan C (1977). Atelencephalic microcephaly. *Dev Med Child Neurol* 19:227–232.

Guala A, Dellavecchia C, Mannirino S, et al. (1997). Ring chromosome 13 with loss of the region D13S317-D13S285: phenotypic overlap with XK syndrome. *Am J Med Genet* 72:329–323.

Lurie I W, Nedzved M K, Lazjuk G I, et al. (1979). Brief clinical reports: aprosencephaly and the aprosencephaly (XK) syndrome. *Am J Med Genet* 3:303–309.

Townes P L, Reuter K, Rosquete E E, et al. (1988). XK aprosencephaly and anencephaly in sibs. *Am J Med Genet* 29:523–528.

X-LINKED MENTAL RETARDATION, GYNECOMASTIA, AND HYPOGONADISM

There are a host of syndromes featuring mental retardation, many of which are X-linked. Those with hypogonadism and significant other nongonadal features are discussed specifically in this chapter as well as elsewhere in this volume. Wilson and colleagues (1991) described an X-linked syndrome in which the mental retardation was accompanied by gynecomastia, obesity, and, in some members, obvious hypogonadism, probably on a central basis. The gene was pericentromeric and mapped to the region Xp22.1-q22. Another gene mutation, mapped to Xp11.4-q21, causes a syndrome consisting of spastic paraplegia, microcephaly, neutral retardation, and cryptorchidism (Martinez et al., 1998). Again, the hypogonadism is presumably central.

REFERENCES

Martinez F, Tomás M, Millán J M et al. (1998). Genetic localization of mental retardation with spastic diplegia to the pericentromeric region of the X chromosome: X inactivation in female carriers. *J Med Genet* 35:284–287.

Wilson M, Mulley J, Gideon A, et al. (1991). New X-linked syndrome of mental retardation, gynecomastia and obesity is linked to DXS255. *Am J Med Genet* 40:406–413.

16

Non-Syndromal Abnormalities of Sexual Development in Males and Females

Many of the abnormalities discussed in this chapter as individual entities, such as cryptorchidism or vaginal atresia, can also be part of a variety of other genetic and nongenetic syndromes, and as such are covered elsewhere in this volume. Other conditions are unique defects in development that lead to either simple or complex malformations—for example, bladder exstrophy, sirenomelia. Most are not recognizably heritable, but familial aggregation is seen occasionally. It is possible that some multiplex families are not reported so that genetic factors are underappreciated.

The conditions are divided into those that affect males, those that affect females, and those that involve both sexes. Wherever possible the histologic and functional status of the gonads is described, although in the more complex conditions the anomalies often preclude meaningful survival, so that no relevant information is available.

Abnormalities in Males

CRYPTORCHIDISM

Cryptorchidism is the failure of descent of a testis along its normal path to the scrotum. It must be distinguished from a testis that is retractile, and from one that has strayed outside the normal path of descent (ectopic). Cryptorchidism is unilateral in 90% of cases and is usually sporadic. It occurs in about 0.7% of apparently normal males one year of age or older. About 70% of unilateral cases are right-sided and about 15% are intra-abdominal. An appreciable fraction of the latter represent anorchia or testicular regression (Chapter 8). Isolated cryptorchidism occurs in families but the genetic basis for its recurrence has not been well defined (Rezvani et al., 1976). An empiric risk to sibs of 6% has been suggested (Czeizel et al., 1981). Cryptorchidism in its bilateral form is a frequent sign of any major disturbance in the fetal hypothalamic-pituitary-gonadal axis, and it is a component of many syndromes. Measurement of müllerian inhibiting factor (MIF) may be useful in delineating bilateral cryptorchidism from congenital anorchia (Lee et al., 1997).

Patients with cryptorchidism are less fertile than normal, partly because of associated vasal and epididymal anomalies (Mininberg and Schlossberg, 1983). Medical or surgical means of achieving testis descent increase fertility and permit anticipatory surveillance for neoplasia. The use of GnRH after orchiopexy has been suggested to improve later fertility (Hadźiselimović and Herzog, 1997)

REFERENCES

Czeizel A, Erodi E, Toth J (1981). Genetics of undescended testes. *J Urol* 126:529–539.

Hadźiselimović F, Herzog B (1997). Treatment with a luteinizing hormone-releasing hormone analogue after successful orchiopexy markedly improves the chance of fertility in later life. *J Urol* 158:1193–1195.

Lee M M, Donahoe P K, Silverman B L, et al. (1997). Measurements of serum Müllerian inhibiting substance in the evaluation of children with nonpalpable gonads. *N Engl J Med* 336:1480–1486.

Mininberg D T, Schlossberg S (1983). The role of the epididymis in testicular descent. *J Urol* 128:599–608.

Rezvani I, Rettig K R, DiGeorge A M (1976). Inheritance of cryptorchidism. *Pediatrics* 58:774–775.

TESTICULAR TORSION

This anatomical abnormality may result in infarction of one or both testes. Cunningham (1960) described the condition in three brothers 14, 15, and 21 years of age. Their father and two other brothers were noted to have excessive hypermobility of the gonads without torsion. The condition may appear at any time: one set of sibs was affected in the neonatal period (Castella et al., 1975). It is likely that intrauterine torsion is responsible for some cases of congenital anorchia, the infarcted gonad having been resorbed prior to birth. Only a few families have been reported, but a variably expressed, male-limited autosomal dominant trait seems a plausible explanation for the available family data (Collins and Broecker, 1989).

REFERENCES

Castella E E, Sod R, Anzorena A, et al. (1975). Neonatal testicular torsion in two brothers. *J Med Genet* 12:112–113.
Collins K, Broecker B H (1989). Familial torsion of the spermatic cord. *J Urol* 141:128–129.
Cunningham R F (1960). Familial occurrence of testicular torsion. *JAMA* 174:1330–1331.

Testicular Exstrophy

This is a very rare anomaly in which a normal testis is exposed secondary to a defect in the skin of the scrotum (Gupta et al., 1997). The lesion may be either uni- or bilateral. There are apparently no long-term consequences, and the defect is easily repaired. The condition is not recognizably genetic.

REFERENCE

Gupta D K, Bajpai M, Rattan S (1997). Testicular exstrophy: bilateral presentation in a newborn. *J Urol* 158:599.

Absence of the Vas Deferens

Probably the most common cause of congenital bilateral absence of the vas deferens is cystic fibrosis. However, not all patients with bilateral absence of the vas deferens have mutant CF alleles, indicating genetic heterogeneity and likely different genetic mechanisms (Rave-Harel et al., 1995). Support for the operation of different molecular lesions has been provided by Dumar and colleagues (1996), who found renal anomalies in some men with CBAVD and no mutant CF allele. Study of patients with unilateral vasal aplasia also support genetic heterogeneity (Mickle et al., 1995). These workers divided patients into two groups: group one had an anatomically normal vas on the contralateral side, and no detectable mutant CF allele; the second group had a contralateral occlusion of the vas at either the inguinal or pelvis level, and most had one mutant CF gene. Interestingly, one third of the group-one patients also had ipsilateral renal anomalies (see Urogenital Adysplasia in this chapter).

REFERENCES

Dumar V, Gervais R, Rigot J M, et al. (1996). Congenital bilateral absence of the vas deferens (CBAVD) and cystic fibrosis transmembrane regulator (CFTR): correlation between genotype and phenotype. *Hum Genet* 97:7–10.
Mickle J, Milunsky A, Amos J A, et al. (1995). Congenital unilateral absence of the vas deferens: a heterogeneous disorder with two distinct subpopulations based on aetiology and mutational status of the cystic fibrosis gene. *Hum Reprod* 10:1728–1735.
Rave-Harel N, Madgar I, Goshen R, et al. (1995). CFTR haplotype analysis reveals genetic heterogeneity in the etiology of congenital bilateral aplasia of the vas deferens. *Am J Hum Genet* 56:1359–1366.

Epididymis Defects

Absence of the epididymis usually accompanies ipsilateral absence of the vas deferns. However, Dean and colleagues (1952) found three patients with the defect who had a normal ipsilateral vas deferens. All were cryptorchid.

On occasion, failure of fusion of the epididymis and testis leads to azoospermia. Hamley and Hodges (1959) found various degrees of defective fusion in approximately 1% of a series of 400 azoospermic males.

There is no known genetic basis for these epididymal defects.

REFERENCES

Dean A L Jr, Major J W, Ottenheimer E J (1952). Failure of fusion of the testes and epididymis. *J Urol* 68:754–758.
Hanley H G, Hodges R D (1959). The epididymis in male sterility: a preliminary report of microdissection studies. *J Urol* 82:508–520.

SCROTAL AGENESIS

Agenesis of the scrotum as an isolated anomaly is exceedingly rare (Verga and Avolio, 1996). The penis is in the normal position but the skin at the base is flat and non-rugated. The testes are normally in the inguinal canal. The usual approach is to create a scrotum from penile foreskin, followed by orchiopexy. There is no known genetic basis for the condition.

REFERENCE

Verga C, Avolio L (1996). Agenesis of the scrotum is an extremely rare anomaly. *J Urol* 156: 1467.

HYPOSPADIAS

Hypospadias represents a failure of complete fusion of the genital folds to form a penile urethra. It is a common malformation: estimates of its incidence have ranged from 4.4 per 1000 to 1% (Leung et al., 1985). The extent of fusion failure varies: the urethral meatus may open at the base of the glans (first-degree; coronal), on the shaft (second-degree), or on the perineum (third-degree; perineoscrotal). The fusion process depends on normal dihydrotestosterone production and action.

As in the case of congenital micropenis, isolated hypospadias (especially if it is second- or third-degree) may be a focal presentation of a persistent systemic disorder in androgen production or responsiveness (Alléra et al., 1995). Hence, it is unwise to assume that the patient with hypospadias has the simple "uncomplicated" form that is probably due to a transient delay in androgen production or responsiveness (Allen and Griffin, 1984). Hence, androgen recepter defects, 5 α-reductase deficiency, and partial defects of the final steps in androgen biosynthesis should be excluded.

With the high incidence figure, and assuming polygenic inheritance for uncomplicated hypospadias, a recurrent risk figure of 5% is probably reasonable, although some have suggested sib risks up to 17% (Stoll et al., 1990). In some families the abnormality has been transmitted through three successive generations; male-limited autosomal dominant inheritance may account for a small proportion of such cases (Lowry and Kliman, 1976). Autosomal recessive inheritance has also been advocated (Fryman et al., 1985). Genetic counseling should be predicated on the type of family history, since the malformation is causally heterogenous (Harris and Beatty, 1993).

REFERENCES

Allen T D, Griffin J E (1984). Endocrine studies in patients with advanced hypospadias. *J Urol* 131:310–314.

Alléra A, Herbst M A, Griffen J E, et al. (1995). Mutations in the androgen receptor coding sequence are infrequent in patients with isolated hypospadias. *J Clin Endocrinol Metab* 80: 2697–2699.

Frydman M, Greiber C, Cohen H A (1985). Uncomplicated familial hypospadias: evidence for autosomal recessive inheritance. *Am J Med Genet* 21:51–55.

Harris E L, Beaty T H (1993). Segregation analysis of hypospadias: a reanalysis of published pedigree data. *Am J Med Genet* 45:420–425.

Leung T J, Baird P A, McGillivray B (1985). Hypospadias in British Columbia. *Am J Med Genet* 21:39–48.

Lowry R B, Kliman M R (1976). Hypospadias in successive generations—possible dominant gene inheritance. *Clin Genet* 9:285–288.

Stoll C, Alembik Y, Roth M P et al. (1990). Genetic and environmental factors in hypospadias. *J Med Genet* 27:559–563.

MICROPENIS

Micropenis is defined as a penis whose stretched length is more than 2.5 standard deviations below the mean for age or stage of sexual development (Lee et al., 1980). In its congenital form, one must consider whether the patient has the "simple" form (a local, sometimes transient, disorder of penile growth) or a form that heralds a systemic disorder that will express itself in other ways as development proceeds. These latter disorders include any variety of hypogonadotropic hypogonadism, mild forms of primary testicular failure, or minimal androgen resistance. Importantly, congenital micropenis is sometimes a minimal expression of a familial disorder or syndrome of androgen biosynthesis or responsiveness, in which other relatives suffer from more severe interference with external male genital development. There does not appear to be a reliable short-term biological marker of androgen responsiveness to help predict the outcome of androgen therapy for a male infant with severe, isolated micropenis.

REFERENCE

Lee P A, Mazur T, Danish R, et al. (1980). Micropenis. I. Criteria, etiologies and classification. *Johns Hopkins Med J* 146:156–170.

PENILE TORSION

Congenital torsion of the penis is thought to be caused by differential growth of the two corpora cavernosa. The penis is usually rotated counter-clockwise and hypospadias may be present. When studied, the upper urinary tract has been normal. Paxson and colleagues (1977) observed that three fathers of five affected newborn males also had the anomaly, findings consistent with male-limited autosomal dominant inheritance. The condition is generally benign and requires no therapy unless accompanied by obstructive angulation or urethral stenosis.

REFERENCE

Paxson C L Jr Corriere J N Jr, Morris F H Jr, et al. (1977). Congenital torsion of the penis in father-son pairs. *J Urol* 118:881.

PENOSCROTAL TRANSPOSITION

In this condition, the penis develops caudal to its normal suprascrotal position, with the shaft being within the scrotum or completely separate. Occasionally the scrotum is only hemiectopic (MacKenzie et al., 1994; Parida et al., 1995). The penis may be of normal size or rudimentary, and urethral obstruction occurs frequently. Either uni-or bilateral cryptorchidism may coexist. Hypospadias with or without chordae is common. There may well be a female homologue wherein the clitoris and labia minora are located posterior to the labia majora.

Many affected individuals have other visceral anomalies, especially of the kidneys but also of other systems as well. Penoscrotal transposition may be a component of the caudal regression sequence (p. 335 in this Chapter).

The "shawl scrotum" characteristic of the Aarskog syndrome (Chapter 15) might be considered to be a limited form of the anomaly. The embryogenesis is unclear, but given the frequent occurrence of extragenital anomalies it is likely complex. A critical region on chromosome 13q32-34 has been implicated in some cases (Bartsch et al., 1996). Although male sib cases have been described (Datta et al., 1971; Ghoneim and El Hamadi, 1971), the condition is usually sporadic and may be lethal because of associated renal disease. Given the rarity of the condition, no meaningful genetic statement can be made.

REFERENCES

Bartsch O, Kunle V, Wu L L, et al. (1996). Evidence for a critical region for penoscrotal inversion, hypospadias, imperforate anus with chromosome region 13q32.2-q34. *Am J Med Genet* 65:218–221.

Datta N S, Singh S M, Reddy A V S, et al. (1971). Transposition of the penis and scrotum in two brothers. *J Urol* 105:739–742.

Ghoneim M A, El Hamadi S (1971). Transposition of the penis and testes. *Br J Urol* 43:340–342.

MacKenzie J, Chitayat D, McLorie G, et al. (1994). Penoscrotal transposition: a case report and review. *Am J Med Genet.* 49:103–107.

Parida S K, Hall B D, Barton L, et al. (1995). Penoscrotal transposition and associated anomalies: a report of five new cases. *Am J Med Genet* 59:68–75.

PEYRONIE'S DISEASE

Peyronie's disease is characterized by the formation of thick fibrous plaques on the dorsum of the penis, occasionally in conjunction with fibrous changes elsewhere such as Dupuytren's contracture. Although in most instances the family history is negative, Bias and coworkers (1982) recorded male-limited autosomal dominant inheritance in three kindreds. Affected females appeared to have only Dupuytren's contracture. There was an association of the disease with HLA-B7 but linkage was excluded. Ziegelbaum and colleagues (1987) described affected identical twins whose father was affected. One of the twins had a mildly affected son. Again, all were HLA-B27. Others have found an association with HLA-B27 (Ralph et al., 1997). How many cases of Peyronie's disease might occur on a genetic basis is not known.

REFERENCES

Bias W B, Nybert L M, Hochbert M C, et al. (1982). Peyronie's disease: a newly recognized autosomal dominant disorder. *Am J Med Genet* 12:227–235.

Ralph D J, Schwartz G, Moore W, et al. (1997). The genetic and bacteriologic aspects of Peyronie's disease. *J Urol* 157:291–294.

Ziegelbaum M, Thomas A J, Zachary A A (1987). The association of Peyronie's disease with HLA-B7 cross reactive antigens. A case report of identical twins. *Cleve Clin Quart* 54:427–430.

CHARGE ASSOCIATION

A nonrandom aggregation of anomalies has been proferred as the CHARGE association (coloboma, heart disease, atresia choanae, retarded growth and/or CNS development, genital hypoplasia, ear anomalies or deafness) (Pagon et al., 1981). The genital defects consist of microphallus, poorly developed scrotum, and cryptorchidism in males (Tellier et al., 1998). No female genital anomalies have been described, but hypoplastic breasts and nipples have been seen (Greenberg, 1987). Three males have had hypogonadotropic hypogonadism; this seems logical in view of the rostral location of the other defects. One patient, a 46,XY phenotypic female, was found to have congenital agonadism (Kushnick et al., 1992), but this could have been coincidental. Most cases are sporadic but occasional familial aggregation has been reported, such that the condition, if indeed it is homogeneous (which seems unlikely), is probably multifactorial.

REFERENCES

Greenberg F (1987). Choanal atresia and athelia: methimazole teratogenicity or a new syndrome? *Am J Med Genet* 28:931–934.

Kushnick T, Wiley J E, Palmer S M (1992). Agonadism in a 46, XY patient with the CHARGE association. *Am J Med Genet* 42:96–99.

Pagon R A, Graham Jr J M, Zonana J, et al. (1981). Coloboma, congenital heart disease, and choanal atresia with multiple anomalies: CHARGE association. *J Pediatr* 99:223–227.

Tellier A L, Cormier-Daire V, Abadie V, et al. (1998). CHARGE syndrome: report of 47 cases and review. *Am J Med Genet* 76:402–409.

Abnormalities in Females

CLITOROMEGALY

Clitoromegaly may be the result of intrauterine androgen exposure or be part of a variety of complex syndromes, usually of unknown genesis. It has also been seen with neurofibromatosis (Chapter 15), and in X-linked Alport syndrome with diffuse leiomyomatosis (Cochet et al., 1988), perhaps as a contiguous gene syndrome (Heidet et al., 1995). Isolated cysts of the clitoris that produce enlargement are usually located at the base of the organ and drain spontaneously. Rarely, the location is near the tip of the clitoris, and if drainage is slow, the cyst may be mistaken for a duplicate urethra (Teague and Anglo, 1996). However, there is no communication with the bladder. Clitoral cysts are sporadic.

REFERENCES

Cochet P, Guibaud P, Torres R G, et al. (1988). Diffuse leiomyomatosis in Alport syndrome. *J Pediatr* 113:339–343.

Heidet L, Dehan K, Zhou J, et al. (1995). Deletions of both alpha 5 (IV) and alpha 6 (IV) collagen genes in Alport syndrome associated with smooth muscle tumors. *Hum Mol Genet* 4:99–108.
Teague J L, Anglo L (1996). Clitoral cyst; an unusual cause of clitoromegaly. *J Urol* 156:2057.

LABIAL FUSION

Labial fusion is more often inflammatory rather than a true malformation. However, Sueiro and Pilato (1964) described congenital fusion in four generations. Willman and colleagues (1988) suggested autosomal dominant inheritance with incomplete penetrance. Surgical correction is usually required but fertility is otherwise unimpaired.

REFERENCES

Sueiro M B, Pilato R (1964). Adereneia incompleta dos pequenos labios con caracter familiar. *Arg Anat Antropol* 32:187–192.
Willman S P, Carr B R, Klein V R (1988). Familial fusion of the labia minora. *Proc Greenwood Genet Ctr* 7:140–141.

VAGINAL SEPTA

Vaginal septa are two types, transverse and longitudinal. The transverse type may be complete or incomplete and presumably results from failure of the urogenital sinus and müllerian duct derivatives to fuse or canalize. If the septum is complete, the newborn female may present with a lower abdominal mass secondary to accumulated mucus resulting from maternal estrogen (hydrocolpos). Later, menstrual blood will be evident (hydrometrocolpos). Other pelvic structures are usually normal. Transverse septa have been described in Amish families, and in these instances, a rare autosomal recessive defect is likely (McKusick et al., 1968). When associated with polydactyly, the eponym McKusick-Kaufman syndrome has been applied (Chapter 15).

Longitudinal septa may extend to the introitus or be partial, and fuse with the lower vaginal wall. In this later instance, asymmetric hydrometrocolpos may develop and appear as a bulge in the vaginal wall on pelvic examination. These septa result from either inappropriate mesodermal proliferation or persistent urogenital sinus epithelium. Isolated septa do not appear to be heritable. However, the condition has been described with camptobrachydactyly (Edwards-Gale syndrome, Chapter 15). Importantly, a septate uterus and vagina may be part of the urogenital adysplasia complex (in this chapter).

REFERENCE

McKusick V A, Weilbachber R G, Gregg C W (1968). Recessive inheritance of a congenital malformation syndrome. *JAMA* 204:113–118.

VAGINAL ATRESIA (VAGINAL AGENESIS)

In true vaginal atresia, müllerian elements are intact, but the lower part of the vagina is represented minimally by a fibrous cord. The presentations are the same as those patients with vaginal septae (Togashi et al., 1987). Isolated vaginal atresia does not appear to be heritable, but the malformation has been seen as a component of the Fraser and Winter syndromes (Chapter 15), and the virilizing forms of congenital adrenal hyperplasia (Chapter 13). In otherwise uncomplicated vaginal atresia, reconstructive surgery may allow successful pregnancy.

REFERENCE

Togashi K, Nishimvra K, Itoh K, et al. (1987). Vaginal ageneses: classification by MR imaging. *Radiology* 162:675–680.

MÜLLERIAN APLASIA

Aplasia of the müllerian ducts leads to absence of the entire uterus and upper vagina. Ovarian function is intact so that affected females present with a blind-ending vagina and primary amenorrhea. If a rudimentary uterus is present, the appellation Mayer-Rokitansky-Küstner-Hauser syndrome has been applied, although there is no reason to think complete aplasia differs fundamentally from the remnant variety. Affected sibs have been reported, albeit rarely (Carson et al., 1983). Shokeir (1978) also noted families in which the condition appeared to be inherited as a sex-limited autosomal dominant trait. However, a systematic study of relatives of randomly ascertained patients by Carson and colleagues (1983) revealed no affected sibs or aunts, perhaps indicating the condition usually is polygenic.

It is important to recognize that müllerian aplasia may be associated with renal and vertebral anomalies (MURCS association, urogenital adysplasia, p. 619). Phenotypic female patients with complete androgen insensitivity also have müllerian aplasia; but the absence of sexual hair in those patients should be a clue to the underlying etiology.

REFERENCES

Carson S A, Simpson J L, Malinak L R, et al. (1983). Heritable aspects of uterine anomalies, II. Genetic analysis of Müllerian aplasia. *Fertil Steril* 34:86–90.

Shokier M H K (1978). Aplasia of the Müllerian system: evidence for probable sex-limited autosomal dominant inheritance. *Birth Defects* 14(c):147–165.

MÜLLERIAN FUSION DEFECTS

The paramesonephric or müllerian ducts are originally paired structures that fuse in embryogenesis. Incomplete fusion leads to varying degrees of separation ranging from two distinct hemiuteri to a single uterus with a persistent septum. The term double uterus is occasionally used to describe this condition in its more complete form, but this is a misnomer. Occasionally one müllerian duct is absent, giving rise to a single rudimentary horn. The condition is often detected after recurrent pregnancy loss, although it may be totally asymptomatic.

There are multiple reports of affected sibs as well as mother-daughter pairs, but no mendelian basis for the isolated defect has been established, likely because systematic study would require an invasive procedure (Simpson, 1990). One formal genetic study reported by Elias and colleagues (1984) suggested a sib recurrence risk of roughly 3%, consistent with multifactional inheritance.

Incomplete fusion may be associated with other anomalies, such as in the hand-foot-genital syndrome, and others as described elsewhere in this text and nongenital features should be sought carefully; their presence may change the diagnosis and, therefore, the counseling.

REFERENCES

Elias S, Simpson J L, Carson S A, et al. (1984). Genetic studies in incomplete Müllerian fusion. *Obstet Gynecol* 63:276–279.
Simpson J L (1990). Gynecologic disorders, in King R A, Rotter J I, Histalsky A G (eds.): *The Genetic Basis of Common Disease.* Oxford University Press, Oxford, p. 564.

DOUBLE UTERUS

A true double uterus—two separate uteri, each with two fallopian tubes—is exceedingly rare (Kelso, 1956). Most often, one or both uteri are rudimentary or bicornuate. The condition should be easily distinguishable from impaired müllerian fusion, because in the latter disorder only a single fallopian tube is present on each side. The various anatomic uterine defects have been reviewed (Patton, 1994).

REFERENCES

Kelso J W (1956). Unusual malformation of the uterus. *Am J Obstet Gynecol* 72:922–923.
Patton P E (1994). Anatomic uterine defects. *Clin Obstet Gynecol* 37:705–721.

ABSENCE OF OVARY AND FALLOPIAN TUBE

In Müllerian aplasia, the fallopian tubes are most often intact and the ovaries are in normal position. Isolated absence of one ovary and fallopian tube is generally found incidentally; e.g., during laparascopic sterilization. On occasion, both tubes are absent or present as remnants with either uni-or bilateral absence of the ovaries. The former case would likely present with infertility; in the latter circumstance, primary amenorrhea would be the presenting feature (Eustace, 1992). Unilateral absence could be due to either a primary developmental defect in the rostral Müllerian duct, or secondary to a vascular insult such as torsion, which could also occur in utero or be acquired. There is no known genetic basis for the anomaly.

REFERENCE

Eustace D L (1992). Congenital absence of the fallopian tube and ovary. *Eur J Obstet Gynecol* 46:157–159.

FEMALE PSEUDOHERMAPHRODITISM WITH MULTIPLE CAUDAL ABNORMALITIES

Female pseudohermaphroditism (FPH) is defined as male or ambiguous external genitalia with a normal female karyotype. Following a report by Perloff and colleagues (1953), several additional publications described a distinct form of FPH associated with malformations of the internal genital, urinary, and gastrointestinal tracts (Carpentier and Potter, 1959; Lubinsky, 1980; Hocamp and Muller, 1983; Robinson and Tross, 1984; Seaver et al., 1994). These defects included atresia or duplication of the uterus and vagina, fistulas between the urinary and gastrointestinal and genital tracts, urethral stenosis or atresia, and various skeletal anomalies, including vertebral and radial defects. The urinary tract abnormalities are frequently

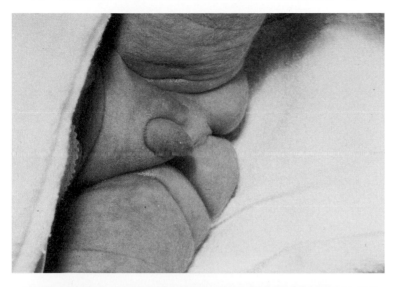

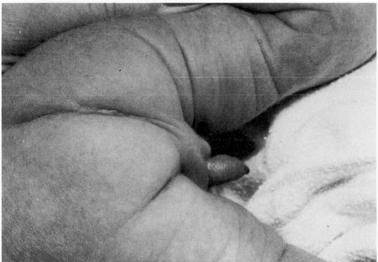

FIGURE 16–1. (A) Note the well-formed phallus; the urethra was penile without hypospadias. (B) Note fused labial/scrotal folds, imperforate anus, and absent raphe. The penile urethra was not probe-patent but leaked small amounts of urine. (From Seaver et al., *Am J Med Genet* 51:16–21, 1994, by permission.)

so severe that oligohydramnios and renal absence/dysplasia is diagnosed by ultrasound *in utero* and elective termination may be performed. The appearance of the external genitalia ranges from ambiguous to that of a normal male (Figs. 16–1 and 16–2). Note the absence of scrotal raphe in Figure 16–1 and its presence in Figure 16–2. The range of malformations routinely seen in four recent cases by Seaver and colleagues (1994) is presented in Table 16–1.

Karyotypes are 46, XX, although one case showed a terminal deletion of 10q [46, XX, del (10) (q25.3 → qter], a region known to be associated with sex reversal

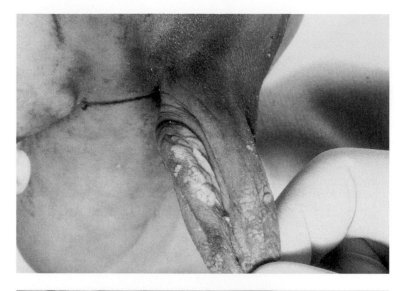

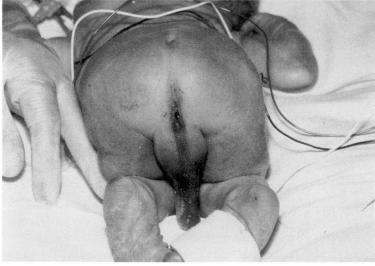

FIGURE 16–2. (A) Sac-like structure found at the normal location of a phallus in a patient. The sac-like structure is under tension. (B) Scrotal raphe seen in this patient. (From Erickson, et al., *Clin Genet* 51:331–337, 1997, by permission)

(Seaver et al., 1994; see also Chapter 2). Autosomal dominant inheritance of multiple caudal anomalies has been postulated by Erickson and colleagues (1990). Y chromosome sequences were not found in those patients so studied (Seaver et al., 1994). In no case has maternal androgen excess been evident. Nonetheless, in a recent case the serum testosterone level in a newborn (2 hours postpartum) was 108 ng/dl—4 times the upper limit of normal (Erickson et al., 1997). No adrenal or gonadal abnormalities were noted on postmortem examination, but the placenta was not examined; hence, placental aromatase deficiency cannot be totally excluded (Chapter 13).

TABLE 16–1. Clinical Summary of Four Cases of Female Pseudohermaphroditism Studied for the Presence of Y-Specific Sequences

Malformation	Case 1	Case 2	Case 3	Case 4
External genitalia	Scrotum Phalus Penile urethra	Scrotum Phallus Penile urethra	Fused labia/scrotal folds No phalus or clitoris	Scrotum Phalus Penile urethra
Gonads	Gonadal agenesis	Apparently normal ovaries	Aparently normal ovaries	Apparently normal ovaries
Internal genitalia	Absence of uterus and vagina	Fallopian tubes and uterus present	Duplicated uterus Duplicated vagina Vesicovaginal fistula Rectovaginal fistula	Fallopian tubes present Dilated uterus present Vesicouterine fistula Vaginal atresia
Urinary	Bilateral renal hypoplasia Megacystis Urethral stenosis	Bilateral renal agenesis Bladder agenesis	Bilateral renal hypoplasia Megacystis Hydroureters	Hydronephrosis Megacystis Hydroureters Urethral stenosis
Gastrointestinal		Imperforate anus	Imperforate anus Omphalocele Meckels diverticulum Tracheo-esophageal fistula	Imperforate anus
Adrenals	Normal[a]	Normal[a]	Normal[a]	Normal[b]
Other	Lax abdominal musculature 13 pairs of ribs Talipes equinovarus Coarctation of aorta	Lax abdominal musculature Vertebral defects Sacral agenesis Talipes equinovarus Truncus arteriosus Ventriculoseptal defect Hydrocephalus Microphthalmia Single umbilical artery	Lax abdominal musculature Vertebral defects Scoliosis	Lax abdominal musculature
Gestational age	19 weeks	22 weeks	28 weeks	30 weeks; monoamniotic twin
Maternal history	32 y/o G2Ab1	17 y/o G2P1	26 y/o G1	29 y/o G1

[a] Gross and histologic examination at autopsy.
[b] Gross appearance at time of surgery.

FPH is likely heterogeneous. Lubinsky (1980) suggested the spectrum of defects could be explained by a disturbance in a specific caudal developmental field with FPH serving as a relatively rare marker of a process that occurs in the absence of testosterone. Robinson and Tross (1984) hypothesized a primary defect in the cloacal membrane, and Escobar and colleagues (1987) proposed a failure of migration of fusion of the urorectal septum with the cloacal membrane.

Some patients likely had the urorectal malformation sequence (see later in this chapter). Cases ascertained because of other defects, such as the prune belly sequence (in this chapter), bladder extrophy (see below), and cloacal extrophy (in this chapter) show a similar pattern of caudal malformations. There is also some clinical overlap with the VATER association and urogenital adysplasia (see later in this chapter).

REFERENCES

Carpentier P J, Potter E L (1959). Nuclear sex and genital malformation in 48 cases of renal agenesis, with special reference to non-specific female pseudohermaphroditism. *Am J Obstet Gynecol* 78:235–258.

Erickson R P, Verga V, Dasouki M (1990). Use of a probe for the putative sex determining gene, Zinc finger Y, in the study of patients with ambiguous genitalia and XY gonadal dysgenesis. *Am J Med Genet* 36:232–236.

Erickson R P, Stone J F, McNoe L A, et al. (1997). Molecular and clinical studies of three cases of female pseudohermaphroditism with caudal dysplasia suggest multiple etiologies. *Clin Genet* 51:331–337.

Escobar L F, Weaver D D, Bixler D, Hodes M R, Mitchell M et al. (1987). Urorectal septum malformation sequence. *Am J Dis Child* 141:1021–1024.

Hokamp H G, Muller K M (1983). Prune belly syndrome and female pseudohermaphroditism. *Path Res Pract* 177:76–83.

Lubinsky M S (1980). Female pseudohermaphroditism and associated anomalies. *Am J Med Genet* 6:123–136.

Perloff W H, Conger K B, Ley L (1953). Female pseudohermaphroditism: description of two unusual cases. *J Clin Endocrinol* 13:783–790.

Robinson Jr. H B, Tross K (1984). Agenesis of the cloacal membrane: a possible teratogenic anomaly. *Perspect Pediatr Pathol* 8:79–96.

Seaver L H, Grimes J, Erickson R P (1994). Female pseudohermaphroditism with multiple caudal anomalies: absence of Y-specific DNA sequences as pathogenetic factors. *Am J Med Genet* 51:16–21.

Abnormalities in Both Sexes

BLADDER EXSTROPHY

In this defect, the bladder wall is exposed, probably because of faulty migration of mesoderm into the cloacal membrane after urorectal septation (Marshall and Muecke, 1962). It occurs in about 1 in 50,000 births, and males outnumber females roughly 4 to 1. Affected males exhibit a short, broad penis with epispadias often extending along the entire penile shaft. Affected females also have epispadias or a bifid clitoris.

The condition is almost always sporadic. When present in more than one family member, transmission appears to be only through affected females, with an empiric recurrence risk of roughly 1% (Ives et al., 1980; Shapiro et al., 1984).

REFERENCES

Ives E, Coffey R, Cartin C O (1980). A family study of bladder exstrophy. *J Med Genet* 17: 139–141.
Marshall V F, Muecke E C (1962). Variations in exstrophy of the bladder. *J Urol* 88:766–796.
Shapiro E, Lepor H, Jeffs R D (1984). The inheritance of the exstrophy, epispadiac complex. *J Urol* 132:303–310.

Caudal Dysplasia (Caudal Regression Sequence)

Broadly defined, this condition consists of varying degrees of agenesis or hypoplasia of the sacrum and lumbar spine (Passarge and Lenz, 1966; Welch and Aterman, 1984). Concomitant with the anatomic defect is disruption of the distal spinal cord with attendant neurologic impairment of the lower extremities and incontinence (Price et al., 1970). The limbs may be short, and both varus and/or valgus deformities along with pterygia are often present as the result of poor movement of the lower extremities. Affected males may have hypospadias, and the external genitalia may be displaced in either sex.

The condition is casually heterogeneous. One accepted teratogenic factor is maternal diabetes. In one series, 16% of affected individuals had a diabetic mother, generally insulin-requiring (Passarge and Lenz, 1966). In one family, sibs of a diabetic mother were affected (Stewart and Stoll, 1979). This could be related to the same teratogen in both pregnancies or be indicative of gene-environment interaction. Finer and colleagues (1978) described sibs with caudal dysplasia along with congenital heart disease and gastrointestinal anomalies. Fullana and colleagues (1986) described caudal deficiency with laterality sequence in sibs, suggesting inheritance of the associated anomalies as an autosomal recessive trait. Although the initial case reports did not note genital anomalies, a later isolated female was described as having a duplication of the uterus and vagina, without further detail. (Rodriguez et al., 1991). In more complex associations, caudal dysplasia could have a single-gene etiology.

The phenotype of caudal dysplasia overlaps to some extent with familial lumbosacral dysgenesis. However, genital anomalies do not occur in the latter condition (Welch and Aterman, 1984). Some have also lumped the sirenomelia sequence with caudal dysplasia because both occur with increased frequency in the offspring of diabetic mothers. Stevenson and colleagues (1986) have offered compelling evidence that sirenomelia has a distinctive and consistent vascular etiology (see later in this Chapter).

REFERENCES

Finer N N, Bowen P, Dunbar L G (1978). Caudal regression anomalies (sacral dysgenesis) in siblings. *Clin Genet* 13:353–358.
Fullana, D, Garcis-Frias E, Martinez-Frias M L, et al (1986). Caudal deficiency and asplenia anomalies in sibs. *Am J Med Genet* (suppl 2):23–29.

Passarge E, Lenz W (1966). Syndrome of caudal regression in infants of diabetic mothers. *Pediatrics* 37:672–675.

Price D L, Dooling E C, Richardson E P (1970). Caudal dysplasia (caudal regression syndrome). *Arch Neurol* 23:212–220.

Rodriguez J I, Palacios J, Omenaca F, et al. (1991). Polysplenia, caudal deficiency and agenesis of the corpus callosum. *Am J Med Genet* 38:99–102

Stevenson R E, Jones K L, Phelan M C, et al. (1986). Vascular steal: the pathogenetic mechanism producing sirenomelia and associated defects of the viscera and soft tissues. *Pediatrics* 78:451–457.

Stewart J M, Stoll S (1979). Familial caudal regression anomalad and maternal diabetes. *J Med Genet* 16:17–20.

Welch J P, Aterman K (1984). The syndrome of caudal dysplasia: a review including considerations and evidence of heterogeneity. *Ped Pathol* 2:313–327.

CAUDAL DUPLICATION

The clinical antithesis of caudal dysplasia is caudal duplication, wherein there is actual duplication of bony structures (sacrum, lumbar vertebrae), anus, various lengths of the large bowel, and the external genitalia (Azmy, 1990; Dominguez et al., 1993). The genital duplication in males includes penis and urethra, scrotum and testes, which may be cryptorchid. The bladder may be septate or duplicated with or without exstrophy. In females, urethra, vagina, cervix, and uterus may be duplicated, often with anomalous drainage. An insult to the developing caudal cell mass and hindgut from the 23rd through the 25th day of gestation has been postulated. This interpretation may be an oversimplification because some patients have had upper gastrointestinal anomalies as well. All cases have been isolated and no common teratogen has been identified.

REFERENCES

Azmy A F (1990). Complete duplication of the hindgut and lower urinary tract with diphallus. *J Pediat Surg* 25:647–649.

Dominguez R, Rott J, Castillo M, et al. (1993). Caudal duplication syndrome. *Am J Dis Child* 147:1048–1052.

CLOACAL EXSTROPHY SEQUENCE

In this rare condition, there is failure of septation of the cloaca into the urogenital sinus and rectum (Jones, 1997). The cloacal membrane subsequently breaks down with resultant exstrophy of the cloaca. This causes failure of fusion of the genital tubercle and pubic rami with subsequent anomalous development of the genitalia in both sexes. Cryptorchidism and severe epispadias are present in affected males. Affected females have unfused müllerian elements with bifid uterine horns and vaginal atresia. Renal anomalies are common in both sexes, and defects in the lumbosacral vertebrae, often with resultant hydromyelia, may be present. Because of the involvement of these various caudal structures, a defect in the development of early mesoderm has been postulated.

There are many overlapping features among cloacal exstrophy, the urorectal malformation sequence (this chapter), and some cases of female pseudohermaphroditism with caudal abnormalities (this chapter). No genetic basis has been identified.

REFERENCE

Jones K L (1997). *Smith's Recognizable Patterns of Human Malformation*, 5th ed. Philadelphia, W B Saunders, pp. 628–629.

DIPHALLUS

Duplication of either the penis or clitoris is almost invariably accompanied by complete urethral duplication and bladder anomalies—for example, either duplication or a separate bladder (Redman and Bissada, 1975; Woodhouse and Williams, 1979). Abortive or Y shaped forms of incomplete urethral duplication may also be associated with bladder anomalies, but not diphallus. A duplicated penis may be contained within a single epithelial covering or be present as two distinct organs.

Bladder exstrophy (p. 611) may simulate diphallus by causing clitoral epispadias or a bifid clitoris (Schey et al., 1980; Feins and Cranley, 1986). Diphallus may be a component of the caudal duplication sequence (613).

REFERENCES

Feins N R, Cranley W (1986). Bladder duplication with one extrophy and one cloaca. *J Pediatr Surg* 21:570–572.

Redman J F, Bissada N K (1975). Complete duplication of the urethra with probable diphallus. *J Pediatr Surg* 10:135–137.

Schey W L, Kandel G, Charles A G (1980). Female epispadias. Report of a case and review of the literature. *Clin Pediatr* 19:212–215.

Woodhouse C R J, William D I (1979). Duplication of the lower urinary tract in children. *B J Urol* 51:481–487.

FETAL AKINESIA SEQUENCE (PENA-SKOKEIR I SYNDROME)

Newborn infants have intrauterine growth retardation, multiple joint contractures, facial abnormalities, and pulmonary hypoplasia (Pena and Shokeir, 1974). Cryptorchidism and hypospadias are often present in males, and clitoral or labial enlargement can be seen in affected females. The phenotype is nonspecific and results from a number of neuromuscular abnormalities that interfere with fetal movement (Hageman et al., 1987). The condition is usually lethal in the first month or so of life. Sibling cases have been described on occasion, but in view of etiologic heterogeneity, a recurrence risk of 10% to 15% has been suggested (Hall, 1986).

REFERENCES

Hageman G, Willemse J, VanKetal B A, et al. (1987). The heterogeneity of the Pena-Shokeir syndrome. *Neuropediatrics* 18:45–50.

Hall J G (1986). Analysis of the Pena-Shokeir phenotype. *Am J Med Genet* 25:99–117.

Pena S D J, Shokeir M H K (1974). Syndrome of camptodactyly, multiple ankyloses, facial anomalies and pulmonary hypoplasia: a lethal condition. *J Pediatr* 85:373–375.

LIMB BODY WALL SEQUENCE

The most common presentation of this disorder is thoracoabdominoschisis usually accompanied by exencephaly or an encephalocele and limb anomalies of various types (Van Allen et al., 1987a). Congenital heart disease, renal and diaphragmatic agenesis, usually unilateral, and genital abnormalities complete the clinical picture. The gonads in both sexes may be absent or dysgenetic, and in females the uterus may be uni-or bicornuate. Rarely, the external genitalia are totally absent (Litwin et al., 1988). The pathogenesis of the sequence is undoubtedly complex and includes vascular disruption, amniotic bands (not mutually exclusive), and perhaps deformation (Van Allen et al., 1987b). The sequence is invariably sporadic. It has been reported as a consequence of maternal cocaine abuse (Viscarello et al., 1992).

REFERENCES

Litwin A, Merlob P, Grunebaum M (1988). Complete absence of external genitalia in limb body wall complex, two cases. *J Med Genet* 25:340–343.

Van Allen M I, Curry C, Gallagher L (1987a). Limb body wall complex: I. Pathogenesis. *Am J Med Genet* 28:529–548.

Van Allen M I Curry C, Walden C E, et al. (1987b). Limb body wall complex: II. Limb and spine defects. *Am J Med Genet* 28:549–565.

Viscarello R R, Ferguson D D, Nores J, et al. (1992). Limb body wall complex associated with cocaine abuse: further evidence of cocaine's teratogenicity. *Obstet Gynecol* 80:523–526.

POLYORCHIDISM

Less than 100 cases of this anomaly have been reported (Shabtal et al., 1991). Roughly half of males have scrotal testes, with the remainder exhibiting various degrees of maldescent of one or more testes. Occasionally all the testes are intraabdominal (Burgers and Gearhart, 1988). In one instance the third testis was discovered only after exploration for failed vasectomy (Hakami and Mosavy, 1975). Females with supernumerary ovaries have also been described (Wharton, 1959), many of which are ectopic—for example, the extra ovary has been found within the kidney (Levy et al., 1997). All these cases are sporadic. Polyorchidism has been found in a child with multiple extragenital malformations and an interstitial deletion of chromosome 21 (Shabtal et al., 1991). Whether the polyorchidism is at all related to the deletion is questionable.

REFERENCES

Burgers J K, Gearhart J P (1988). Abdominal polyorchidism: an unusual variant. *J Urol* 140: 582 528–583.

Hakami M, Mosavy S H (1975). Triorchidism with normal spermatogenesis: an unusual cause for failure of vasectomy. *Br J Surg* 62:632–635.

Levy B, DeFranco J, Parra R, et al. (1997). Intrarenal supernumerary ovary. *J Urol* 157:2240–2241.

Shabtal F, Schwartz A, Hart J, et al. (1991). Chromosomal anomaly and malformation syndrome with abdominal polyorchidism. *J Urol* 146:833–834.

Wharton L R (1959). Two cases of supernumerary ovary and one of accessory ovary with an analysis of previously reported cases. *Am J Obstet Gynecol* 78:1101–1110.

PRUNE BELLY SEQUENCE (EAGLE-BARRETT SYNDROME, TRIAD SYNDROME)

This condition is so named because hypoplastic or absent abdominal muscles cause the abdominal wall to look wrinkled. Some cases are caused by *in utero* lower urinary tract obstruction, with oligohydramnios and pulmonary hypoplasia. Potter facies and clubfoot may be present as in any fetus with oligohydramnios of whatever cause. In other instances, however, no obstructive uropathy has been identified, prompting the suggestion that the condition is actually a developmental field complex related to an early mesodermal defect (Greskovich and Nyberg, 1988). Renal anomalies are common even without obstruction, and congenital defects outside the genitourinary area have been described. Affected males greatly outnumber females, by a ratio of 10 to 1. Cryptorchidism is nearly universal. Even with early orchiopexy, infertility is quite common (Woodhouse and Snyder, 1985). Ambiguous genitalia have been noted in 46,XX females (Rabinowitz and Schellinger, 1977), and vaginal atresia with bicornuate uterus has been seen in females with histologically normal ovaries (Reinberg et al., 1991).

The syndrome is etiologically heterogeneous, hence the recurrence risk must be related to the specific cause. Even when obstructive uropathy is an established etiology, in general the recurrence risk should be considered low because such entities as posterior urethral valves, vesicle neck contractures, or prostatic maldevelopment in themselves have a low heritability.

REFERENCES

Greskovich F J III, Hyberg L M J (1988). The prune belly syndrome: a review of its etiology, defects, treatment and prognosis. *J Urol* 140:707–712.

Rabinowitz R, Schellinger J F (1977). Prune belly syndrome in the female subject. *J Urol* 118: 454–456, 1977.

Reinberg Y, Shapiro E, Manivel J C, et al. (1991). Prune belly syndrome in females: A triad of abdominal muscular deficiency and anomalies of the urinary and genital systems. *J Pediat* 118:395–398.

Woodhouse C R J, Snyder H M III (1985). Testicular and sexual function in adults with prune belly syndrome. *J Urol* 133:607–609, 1985.

SIRENOMELIA SEQUENCE

In the classic form of this disorder, there is only a single central lower limb with or without terminal digital differentiation (Stocker and Heifetz, 1987). Either absence or dysplasia of the kidneys gives rise to the typical lung and facial consequences of oligohydramnios.

Imperforate anus is often accompanied by upper gastrointestinal anomalies, and congenital heart disease is common. The external genitalia in both sexes are absent or rudimentary, and variable degrees of dysgenesis of müllerian structures are present in females. The gonads may be normal, hypoplastic, or absent. Milder forms of the condition have been seen—for example, both legs are present but connected by a soft tissue web. In the less severe forms, the genitalia may be nearly normal. Survival is uncommon and depends largely on the renal status.

Two major theories have been offered to explain this sequence: deficiency of caudal mesoderm and vascular steal. Given the nature and extent of the extracaudal anomalies, the latter theory is more compelling (Stevenson et al. 1986).

Virtually all cases are sporadic. An increased frequency of sirenomelia has been noted in monozygotic twins who are discordant for the abnormality. Rudd and Klimek (1990) have recorded an interesting family in which a man with lumbar spine abnormalities had four children with varying caudal anomalies. Two of the sibs had the sirenomelia sequence, perhaps indicating that on occasion a single variably expressed autosomal dominant gene mutation may be causal.

REFERENCES

Rudd N L, Klimek M L (1990). Familial caudal dysgenesis: evidence for a major dominant gene. *Clin Genet* 38:170–175.
Stevenson R E, Jones K L, Phelan M C, et al. (1986). Vascular steal: the pathogenetic mechanism producing sirenomelia and associated defects of the viscera and soft tissues. *Pediatrics* 78:451–457.
Stocker J T, Heifetz S A (1987). Sirenomelia: a morphologic study of 33 cases and review of the literature. *Perspect Pediat Pathol* 10:7–50.

SPLENOGONADAL FUSION

In this condition, the gonad is either attached to the spleen by a continuous fibrous cord, which usually contains splenic tissue, or ectopic rests of spleen are directly attached to the gonad without any intervening tissue (Walther et al., 1988). When the accessory spleen is fused to the testis, maldescent may result in unilateral cryptorchidism. If the two organs are in the scrotum, the anomaly may be diagnosed as hernia, polyorchidism, or even testicular cancer. If the condition is at all suspected, radionuclide scanning will be diagnostic. One reason to consider accessory splenic tissue in the etiology of a testicular mass is the presence of other anomalies, especially transverse defects of the limbs (Pauli and Greenlaw, 1982). Affected females have been described as well. The defect(s) probably arises when the splenic anlage is in proximity to the urogenital fold, which is why most defects are left-sided.

REFERENCES

Pauli R M, Greenlaw A (1982). Limb deficiency and splenogonadal fusion. *Am J Med Genet* 13:81–90.
Walther M M. Trulock T S, Finnerty D P, et al. (1988). Splenic gonadal fusion. *Urology* 32: 521–524.

UROGENITAL ADYSPLASIA

This term is a construct that refers to varying combinations of uni- or bilateral absence or cystic dysplasia of the kidneys and müllerian fusion abnormalities (Schimke and King, 1980). On occasion vertebral defects (the MURCS association—*mü*llerian aplasia, *r*enal dysplasia, *c*ervico-*t*horacic *s*omite dysplasia) may be seen (Duncan et al., 1979). Opitz (1987) has suggested that the Mayer-Rokitansky-Küster-Hauser (MRKH) anomaly of supposedly isolated vaginal agenesis also belongs in this clinical spectrum, an opinion supported by others (Pavanello et al., 1988). Vaginal agenesis has been associated with the Klippel-Feil anomaly (Baird and Lowry, 1974). Moreover, CNS anomalies have been recorded with the MURCS association (Lin et al., 1996), adding further support to a possible global relationship. Müllerian absence is part of androgen insensitivity, but kidney defects are not, so this condition can easily be excluded in such patients.

Whether all families with müllerian anomalies (Polishuk and Ron, 1974; Carson et al., 1983; Shokeir, 1978) should be included in this category is problematic, but clearly the mother-daughter pair with a double uterus reported by Wiersma and colleagues (1976) should be because the clinical picture included unilateral renal agenesis. Opitz (1987) considers this disorder to be an "iceberg" autosomal dominant trait in that affected families are often not ascertained unless infertility or primary amenorrhea promote evaluation, or an offspring is born with bilateral lethal renal defects. Compounding the problem is the fact that some carrier males may have unilateral absence of the vas deferens with or without other ipsilateral wolffian elements (epididymes, seminal vesicles). Although no supporting evidence exists, males with unilateral absence of the vas with ipsilateral renal agenesis or ectopy may also harbor the same genetic defect. Obviously, genetic heterogeneity is not only possible but likely, as evidenced by the sibs reported by Davee and colleagues (1992) with renal and müllerian duct defects, craniofacial anomalies, and retardation.

McPherson and colleagues (1987) have concluded that in pedigrees showing dominant transmission of unilateral renal adysplasia the empiric risk to offspring of heterozygotes for severe bilateral renal disease is 15% to 20%.

REFERENCES

Baird P A, Lowry R B (1974). Absent vagina and Klippel-Feil anomaly. *Am J Obstet Gynecol* 118:290–291.

Carson S A, Simpson J L, Malinak L R, et al. (1983). Heritable aspects of uterine anomalies II: genetic analysis of uterine aplasia. *Fertil Steril* 34:86–90.

Davee M A, Moore C A, Bull M J, et al. (1992). Familial occurrence of renal and Müllerian duct hypoplasia, craniofacial anomalies, severe growth and developmental delay. *Am J Med Genet* 44:293–296.

Duncan P A, Shapiro L R, Stangel J J, et al. (1979). The MURCS association: Müllerian duct aplasia, renal aplasia, and cervico-thoracic somatic dysplasia. *J Pediatr* 96:399–402.

Lin H J, Cornford M E, Hu B, et al. (1996). Occipital encephalocele and MURCS association: case report and review of central nervous system anomalies in MURCS patients. *Am J Med Genet* 61:59–62.

McPherson E, Carey J, Kramer A, et al. (1987). Dominantly inherited renal adysplasia. *Am J Med Genet* 26:863–872.

Opitz J M (1987). Editorial comment: Vaginal atresia (von Mayer-Robitansky-Küster or MRK anomaly in hereditary renal adysplasia (HRA), *Am J Med Genet* 26:873–876.

Pavancello R d C M, Eigier A, Otto PA (1988). Relationship between Mayer Rokitansky-Küster (MRK) anomaly and hereditary renal adysplasia (HRA). *Am J Med Genet* 29:845–849.

Polishuk W Z, Ron M A (1974). Familial bicornuate and double uterus. *Am J Obstet Gynecol* 119:982–987.

Schimke R N, King C R (1980). Hereditary urogenital adysplasia. *Clin Genet* 18:417–420.

Shokeir MHK (1978). Aplasia of the Müllerian system: evidence for probable sex-limited autosomal dominant inheritance. *Birth Defects* 14(6c):147–165.

Wiersma A F, Peterson L F, Justema E J (1976). Uterine anomalies associated with unilateral renal agenesis. *Obst Gynecol* 47:654–657.

URORECTAL MALFORMATION SEQUENCE

This malformation complex, first reported by Broster (1956), was more fully delineated by Escobar and colleagues (1987). Characteristic features include ambiguous genitalia with a curious phallic-like structure in females, imperforate anus, absent or atretic vaginal and urethral openings, and vesicoureterorectal fistula. Escobar and colleagues (1987) suggested that the defective development was due to failure of the urorectal septum to migrate to or completely fuse with the cloacal membrane so that the latter persists partly or completely. With severe defects, the infants are stillborn or die shortly after birth due to the complications of oligohydramnios. The uterus and vagina are absent or malformed but the ovaries are histologically normal. The initial cases were all 46,XX females and were described as unusual forms of female pseudohermaphroditism (Broster, 1956; Carpentier and Potter, 1959). However, affected males have subsequently been described by Wheeler and colleagues (1997), who also noted a high frequency of associated non-obstructive renal anomalies such as agenesis or cystic dysplasia.

That a possible genetic basis for the condition might exist is supported by a report of a female with an ectopic urethra opening into a septate vagina whose anus and rectum were normal but were separated from the urogenital sinus only by a thin septum (Mills and Pergament, 1997). At age 19, she had an abortion of a 46,XX female fetus with absent urethra, vaginal atresia, and normal anus, bladder, and colon.

REFERENCES

Broster L (1956). A form of intersexuality. *Br Med J* 1:149–151.

Carpentier P, Potter E (1959). Nuclear sex and genital malformation in 48 cases of renal agenesis with special reference to nonspecific female pseudohermorphodi-tism. *Am J Obstet Gynecol* 78:235–258.

Escobar L F, Weaver D D, Bixler D, et al. (1987). Urorectal malformation sequence. *Am J Dis Child* 141:1021–1024.

Mills P L, Pergament E (1997). Urorectal septal defects in a female and her offspring. *Am J Med Genet* 70:250–252.

Wheeler P G, Weaver D D, Obéime M O, et al. (1997). Urorectal septum malformation sequence: report of 13 additional cases and review of the literature. *Am J Med Genet* 73:456–462.

VATER (VACTERL) ASSOCIATION

This acronym refers to *v*ertebral defects, *a*nal atresia, *t*racheo-*e*sophageal atresia, and *r*adial defects. Renal anomalies, other *l*imb defects and congenital *c*ardiovascular anomalies complete the rather broad spectrum of this disorder, which probably has a diverse etiology.

A recent international survey of additional abnormalities in patients with three or more of the main features of the VATER association by Botto and colleagues (1997) revealed occasional examples of cryptorchidism, micropenis, and rarely epispadias in males, and hypoplastic labia in females.

REFERENCE

Botto L D, Khoury M J, Mastroizcovo P, et al. (1997). The spectrum of congenital anomalies of the VATER association: an international study. *Am J Med Genet* 71:8–15.

17

Systemic Disorders of Sexual Development with Gonadal Dysfunction

A number of systemic genetic disorders have been associated with gonadal dysfunction and impaired fertility. The various gene defects do not interfere with male genital differentiation, so there is no sexual ambiguity. But in some instances, such as early-onset lipodystrophic syndromes, the external genitalia, including the clitoris, may be large, perhaps because hyperinsulinism acts as a growth factor.

Maternal exposure to a number of environmental agents also can cause genital defects. Those in which the relationship seems secure are included in this chapter.

Genetic Disorders

CARBOHYDRATE-DEFICIENT GLYCOPROTEIN SYNDROME

There are four types of CDG syndrome. Type 1, the most common, is caused by deficient activity of phosphomannomutase (PMM2), the enzyme that catalyzes the conversion of mannose-6-phosphate to mannose-1-phosphate (Matthijs et al., 1997). This deficit impairs the synthesis of the lipid-linked, mannose-containing oligosaccharide precursor that donates mannose to the asparagine-linked carbohydrate side chains of various secretory glycoproteins, lysosomal enzymes, and, probably, membrane glycoproteins. The deficiency of sialic acid in these side chains causes the affected glycoproteins to migrate more cathodally than normal on isoelectric focusing (IEF). In infancy, the nervous system is most abnormal. There is unprovoked eye movement, axial hypotonia, ataxia, and hyporeflexia. After infancy, retinitis pigmentosa, joint contracture, stroke-like episodes, and epilepsy may appear. Dysmorphisms include large ears and unusual deposition of subcutaneous fat. Later, hepatomegaly, pericardial effusion, or cardiomyopathy may occur. There is a multiplicity of serum metabolite abnormalities, presumably reflecting underglycosylated transport or membrane proteins. A blood clotting disturbance is attributable to factor XI deficiency (Van Geet and Jaeken, 1993).

In adolescence, hypogonadism is frequent, especially among females. Kristiansson and colleagues (1995) studied three women, aged 17 to 25 years. All remained clinically prepubertal, with low serum estradiol levels. Ultrasonography did not reveal any ovaries. However, ovaries without follicular activity have also been observed. Two of three men, aged 20 to 43 years, studied by Kristiansson and colleagues (1995) were fully pubertal; however, one had low testicular volume, and all had relatively low serum testosterone levels, with normal FSH and LH levels. DeZegher and Jaeken (1995) analyzed four adolescent males and four adolescent females. Testicular volume was reduced in all four males, and only one of the girls developed breasts. Serum FSH levels were elevated in both sexes; LH level was increased only in the females, and testosterone was increased in two of them. GnRH provoked hyperresponses of FSH and LH in a pair of 13-year-old monozygotic females. The serum testosterone levels were normal in four male adolescents, but serum estradiol was low in four adolescent girls. Notably, FSH markedly stimulated serum estradiol and increased breast development in one of the 13-year-old twin girls, but only moderately in her co-twin. The serum of these twin girls had low-normal FSH bioactivity and a low-normal FSH bioactivity/immunoreactivity ratio. Most importantly, isoelectric focusing of LH and FSH exposed no change in their charge or median mobility compared to normal. In other words, glycoproteins synthesized in the pituitary are not undersialyated, indicating organ-specific changes. The reason for the primary hypogonadism remains obscure.

As of early 1996, there were about 200 patients with CDG 1 worldwide. Judging from the geographic origin of the patients studied by DeZegher and Jaeken (1995), the distribution of CDG 1 (PMM2) was mapped to 16p13 (Bjursell et al., 1997). Eleven different missense mutations have been found in 16 unrelated CDG 1 patients of diverse geographic origin. A type 1b form results from deficiency of phosphomannose isomerase (Niehues et al., 1998).

CDG 2 results from deficiency of a Golgi-localized form of N-acetyl glucosaminyl transferase II deficiency. The enzyme defects responsible for types 3 and 4 CDG are unknown.

REFERENCES

Bjursell C, Stibler H, Wahlstrom J, Kristiansson B, Skovby F, Stromme P, Blennow G, Martinsson T (1997). Fine mapping of the gene for carbohydrate-deficient glycoprotein syndrome, type 1 (CDG1): linkage disequilibrium and founder effect in Scandinavian families. *Genomics* 39:247–253.

DeZegher F, Jaeken J (1995). Endocrinology of the carbohydrate-deficiency glycoprotein syndrome type 1 from birth through adolescence. *Pediatric Res* 37:395–401.

Kristiansson B, Stibler H, Wide L (1995). Gonadal function and glycoprotein hormones in the carbohydrate-deficient glycoprotein (CDG) syndrome. *Acta Paediatrica* 84:655–660.

Matthijs G, Schollen E, Pardon E, Veiga-Da-Cunha M, Jaeken J, Cassiman J J, Van Schaftingen E (1997). Mutations in PMM2, a phosphomannomutase gene on chromosome 16p13, in carbohydrate-deficient glycoprotein type 1. *Nat Genet* 16:88–92.

Niehues R, Hasilik M, Alton G, et al. (1998). Carbohydrate-deficient glycoprotein syndrome type 1b. *J Clin Invest* 101:1414–1420.

Van Geet G, Jaeken J (1993). A unique pattern of coagulation abnormalities in carbohydrate-deficient glycoprotein syndrome. A unique pattern of coagulation abnormalities in carbohydrate-deficient glycoprotein syndrome. *Pediatr Res* 33:540–541.

Hagberg B A, Blennon G, Kristiansson B, et al. (1993). Carbohydrate-deficient glycoprotein syndromes: peculiar group of new disorders. *Pediatr Neurol* 9:225–262.

Matthijs G, Schollen E, Dardon E, et al. (1997). Mutations in PMM2, a phosphomannomutase gene on chromosome 16p13, in carbohydrate-deficient glycoprotein syndrome (Jaeken Syndrome). *Nat Genet* 16:88–92.

CELIAC DISEASE

Male hypogonadism may be a feature of celiac disease; it is symptomatic in 5% to 10% of untreated patients (Farthing et al., 1983a). Sexual dysfunction may be even more common in the absence of overt signs of gonadal failure. Abnormalities in sperm morphology and motility are not rare but usually revert to normal when the patient is placed on a gluten-free diet (Baker and Read, 1975). Suboptimal nutrition per se can cause male hypogonadism. In one study of 39 men, basal serum FSH was increased in 10 (half treated, the others untreated), but there was no recoguizel oligospermia (Farthing et al., 1983b). Serum LH concentrations were elevated in roughly half the patients with subtotal villous atrophy, but unlike the FSH levels, LH levels returned to normal with treatment. However, exaggerated responses to GnRH were seen even with normal FSH and LH levels. It appears there is a disturbance in pituitary regulation of gonadal function in this disease, but a simultaneous defect in the gonad cannot be excluded (see below).

Celiac disease may be a component of the HLA-related polyendocrine autoimmune syndrome. It is conceivable that gonadal failure associated with the disease could also be primary; in such instances, antigonadal antibodies might be found. As with most autoimmune diseases, the genetic basis is complex and the familial recurrence risk is low.

REFERENCES

Baker P G, Read A B (1975). Reversible infertility in male coeliac patients. *Br Med J* 2:316–317.

Farthing M J G, Edwards C R W, Rees L W, et al. (1983a). Male gonadal function in coeliac disease: 2. sex hormones. *Gut* 24:127–135.

Farthing M J G, Rees L H, Dawson A M (1983b). Male gonadal function in coeliac disease. 3. pituitary regulation. *Clin Endocrinol* 19:661–671.

CONGENITAL PANHYPOPITUITARY DWARFISM (CPHD)

Impaired sexual maturation without genital abnormalities is an integral feature of CPHD. Both autosomal recessive (McArthur et al., 1985) and X-linked (Schimke et al., 1971) varieties have been described. Affected individuals are usually normal at birth, but show progressive loss of anterior pituitary function, most often commencing with deficiency of growth hormone followed by gonadotropins, TSH and ACTH. Congenital absence of the pituitary as described by Steiner and Boggs (1965) may be evident shortly after birth and is probably a separate autosomal recessive disorder.

Deficiency of PIT1, a pituitary specific transcription factor, has been shown to be responsible for some cases of CPHD (Pernasetti et al., 1998). This factor appears to regulate differentiation of growth hormone, prolactin, and thyrotropin cell lineages (Puy and Asa, 1996). Most affected individuals are homozygous, but some are heterozygotes, indicating a dominant negative affect of some mutations (Ohta, 1992).

Another pituitary transcription factor, PROP1 (Prophet of P1T1), appears to regulate *P1T1* (now called *POU1F1*) and also separately control gonadotropin cell specification (Wu et al., 1998). Hence, mutations in *PROP1* result in a hypogonadotropic hypogonadism form of CPHD. Homozygosity or compound heterozygosity for a 301–302 del AG in exon 2 of the PROP1 gene, located on 5q appears to be the most frequent molecular alteration (Cogan et al., 1998).

The Snell and the Ames dwarf mouse strains are the murine equivalents of P1T1 and PROP1 mutations, respectively.

REFERENCES

Cogan J D, Wu W, Phillips J A III, et al. (1998). The PROP1 2-base pair deletion is a common cause of combined pituitary hormone deficiency. *J Clin Endocrinol Metab* 83:3346–3349.

McArthur R G, Morgan K, Phillips J A III, et al. (1985). The natural history of familial hypopituitarism. *Am J Med Genet* 22:553–566.

Ohta K, Nobukuni Y, Mitsubuchi H, et al. (1992). Mutations in the P1T1 gene in children with combined pituitary hormone deficiency. *Biochem Biophys Res Commun* 189:851–855.

Pernasetti F, Milner R D G, Al Ashwal A A Z, et al. (1998). Pro 239 Ser: a novel recessive mutation of the Pit 1 gene in seven Middle Eastern children with growth hormone, prolactin, and thyrotropin deficiency. *J Clin Endocrinol Metab* 83:2079–2083.

Puy L A, Asa S L (1996). The ontogeny of P1T1 expression in the human fetal pituitary gland. *Neuroendocrinology* 63:349–355.

Schimke R N, Spaulding J J, Hollowell J G (1971). X-linked congenital panhypopituitarism. *Birth Defects Org Art Ser* VII (6): 21–23.

Steiner M M, Boggs J D (1965). Absence of pituitary gland, hypothyroidism, hypoadrenalism, and hypogonadism in a 17 year-old dwarf. *J Clin Endocrinol* 25:1591–1598.

Wu W, Cogan J D, Pfaffic R W, et al. (1998) Mutations in PROP1 cause familial combined pituitary hormone deficiency. *Nat Genet* 18:147–149.

CYSTIC FIBROSIS

Infertility and azoospermia are almost constant features of cystic fibrosis (CF). Secondary sexual development and testicular size are usually normal unless malnutrition is severe. Surgical and postmortem specimens have revealed bilateral absence of the vas deferens (see Chapter 15), and often hypoplastic to absent epididymes and seminal vesicles (Chillón et al., 1995). These changes have been noted in the first year of life, perhaps indicating a primary failure of development secondary to some as yet unknown effect of the cystic fibrosis gene on chromosome 7q31, the cystic fibrosis transmembrane conduction regulator (CFTR). Most CF patients are compound heterozygotes. This is especially important because analysis of the CF status should be known prior to microsurgical sperm aspiration from the epididymis for the purpose of *in vitro* fertilization by intracytoplasmic sperm injection (Fitzpatrick et al., 1996). The effect of various CFTR mutations is discussed in Chapter 19. CF mutation frequency may be increased in healthy infertile men with qualitative sperm abnormalities or nonobstructive azoospermia (Van der Ven et al., 1996).

Females with CF can be fertile, providing malnutrition and/or chronic infection have not interfered with hypothalamic-pituitary-gonadal function.

REFERENCES

Chillón M, Casals T, Mercier B, et al. (1995). Mutations in the cystic fibrosis gene in patients with congenital absence of the vas deferens. *N Engl J Med* 332:1475–1480.

Fitzpatrick J L, Hutton E M, Babul R, et al. (1996). Counseling and screening for cystic fibrosis in patients with congenital bilateral absence of the vas deferens: patient perceptions. *J Genet Counseling* 5:1–15.

Van der Ven K, Messer L, Van der Ven H, Jeyendran RS, Ober C (1996). Cystic fibrosis mutation screening in healthy men with reduced sperm quality. *Hum Reprod* 11:513–517.

DEFECTIVE PROHORMONE PROCESSING

Many peptide and glycoprotein hormones are secreted as prohormones and require posttranslational processing. A murine mutation of carboxypeptidase E causes obesity in the fat/fat mouse. An adult female patient studied by O'Rahilly and colleagues (1995) had a history of extreme childhood obesity, successfully treated with diet, who later developed primary amenorrhea. Symptoms of postprandial hypoglycemia led to study of proinsulin levels, which were high, and the physical structure of the impaired cleavage products of both proinsulin and proopiomelanocortin suggested defective processing by the endopeptidase prohormone convertase 1 (PC1). Molecular studies confirmed that the patient was a compound heterozygote for two mutations, the first a Gly $\rightarrow$ Arg^{483} in exon 13, the second an A $\rightarrow$ C^{+4} of the donor splice site of intron 5, leading to deletion of exon 5 and a premature stop codon in the catalytic domain of the enzyme (Jackson et al., 1997).

The serum estradiol level was marginal and both serum FSH and LH levels were low. Pregnancy was induced with gonadotropins, and the patient was delivered of quadruplets, who were shown to segregate for the two PC1 mutations. Presumably the genetic defect in PC1 led to defective processing of either GnRH or the individual gonadotropins and this accounted for the continual amenorrhea; however, these hormones were not formally studied, so the precise reason for the amenorrhea remains uncertain.

REFERENCES

Jackson R S, Creemers J W M, Ohagi S, et al. (1997). Obesity and impaired prohormone processing associated with mutations in the human prohormone convertase 1 gene. *Nat Genet* 16:303–306.

O'Rahilly S, Gray H, Humphreys P J, et al. (1995). Brief report: impaired processing of prohormone associated with abnormalities of glucose homeostasis and adrenal function. *N Engl J Med* 333:1386–1390.

GALACTOSEMIA

The term is genetically nonspecific, for there are three disorders in galactose metabolism that feature galactosemia/galactosuria. Deficiency of the respective enzymes galactokinase, galactose-1-phosphate uridyl transferase, and uridine diphosphate galactose-4-epimerase all result in impaired conversion of galactose to glucose. All are inherited as autosomal recessive traits. Only in the classic form of transferase deficiency (chromosome 9p13) has gonadal function been found to be abnormal, and then only in females. Kaufman and colleagues (1986) first noted hypergonadotropic hypogonadism in 12 of 18 females with presumably adequately treated transferase deficiency. Ultrasonography revealed small to absent ovaries; on laparoscopy, bilateral streak gonads were found in one patient. In one other case the fallopian tubes were also absent (Hoefnagel et al., 1979). Individuals with nonclassic (variant) forms of transferase deficiency typically have normal ovarian function (Kaufman et al., 1988). Nothing is known about gonadal function in either galactokinase or epimerase deficiency, probably because the respective conditions are so rare.

Interestingly, both primary and secondary amenorrhea have been seen, and a normal pregnancy followed by ovarian failure has been reported as well, so ovarian function may fluctuate for some period of time (Aiman and Smentek, 1985; Ginzelman and Steinman, 1984). This latter phenomenon has been termed the "resistant ovary syndrome" (Twigg et al., 1996). However, this term has been used generically to include any form of late-onset hypogonadism, including defective gonadotropin structure or function or receptor abnormalities. The precise reason for the ovarian failure in galactosemia remains obscure.

REFERENCES

Aiman J, Smentek C. (1985). Premature ovarian failure. *Obstet Gynecol* 66:9–14.
Ginzelman R, Steinman B (1984). Galactosemia: how does long term treatment change the outcome? *Enzyme* 32:37–46.
Hoefnagel D, Winston-Hill D, Child E L (1979). Ovarian failure in galactosemia. *Lancet* 2: 1197.
Kaufman F R, Donnell G N, et al. Roe T F, (1986). Gonadal function in patients with galactosemia. *J Inherited Metab Dis* 9:140–146.
Kaufman F R, Xu Y K, Ng W G (1988). Correlation of ovarian function with galactose-1-phosphate uridyl transferase levels in galactosemia. *J Pediat* 112:754–756.
Twigg S, Wallman L, McElduff A (1996). The resistant ovary syndrome in a patient with galactosemia: a clue to the natural history of ovarian failure. *J Clin Endocrinol Metab* 81: 1329–1331.

HEMOCHROMATOSIS

Hypogonadism, testicular atrophy, and loss of libido are well-known complications of the iron storage disorder, hemochromatosis. Although liver involvement may be partially incriminated, most studies suggest the hypogonadism is hypogonadotropic in type and is largely due to iron storage in the pituitary gland (Milman, 1991). Other pituitary hormones are generally normal, but multiple hormone deficiencies have been seen (Oerter et al., 1993). Affected females are protected from the pituitary storage phenomenon until menopause, so that no definite gonadal dysfunction has been seen. The male hypogonadism may be reversible to some extent with phlebotomy (Siemons and Mahler, 1987). The disorder is an autosomal recessive trait. The gene had been termed *HLA-H* (Feder et al., 1996) because of its localization on chromosome 6 within the HLA region and its structural similarity to the MHC class 1 genes; now it is known as *HFE*.

References

Feder J N, Gnirke A, Thomas W, et al. (1996). A novel MHC class 1-like gene is mutated in patients with hereditary hemochromatosis. *Nat Genet* 13:399–400.

Milman N (1991). Heredity hemochromatosis in Denmark 1950–1985: Clinical, biochemical and histologic features in 179 patients and 13 preclinical cases. *Dan Med Bull* 38:385–393.

Oerter K E, Kamp G A, Munson P J (1993). Multiple hormone deficiencies in children with hemochromatosis. *J Clin Endocrinol Metab* 76:357–361.

Siemons L J, Mahler C (1987). Hypogonadotropic hypogonadism in hemochromatosis: recovery of reproductive function after iron depletion. *J Clin Endocrinol Metab* 65:585–587.

Leptin Deficiency and Hypogonadism

Control of energy homeostasis in mammals is complex and incompletely understood. Physiologic studies in mice have revealed at least two genes, mutations in which cause heritable obesity. Homozygosity for the obese (*ob*) and diabetes (*db*) genes on mouse chromosomes 6 and 4, respectively, result in hyperphagic, physically less active animals, who develop early onset obesity and fail to sexually mature. Parabiotic experiments by Coleman (1978) supported the contention that one of these two genes was mutant for a circulating suppressor of food intake, whereas the other was mutant for a receptor for this hormone.

More detailed investigation in mouse and man has proved Coleman correct. The circulating hormone, the product of the murine *ob* gene has been termed leptin (from the greek "lepto," meaning thin) whereas the *db* gene product is the leptin receptor. Later experiments showed that intraperitoneal injection of recombinant leptin to homozygous *ob* mice reversed the phenotype, but had no effect on the *db/db* mouse.

Human leptin (LEP) and the leptin receptor (LEPR) genes share roughly 80% homology at the amino acid level with their respective mouse counterparts. Despite extensive search on the morbidly obese, only two LEP mutations have been identified in man (Montague et al., 1997; Strobel et al., 1998). Both mutations were in sibs who were homozygous. The first sib pair were too young to determine gonadal function, but the second sib pair failed to mature sexually at puberty. Further studies revealed hypothalamic hypogonadism. A single mutation in LEPR, also associated with early onset obesity, has shown the same type of hypogonadism (Clement et al., 1998). It therefore appears that CNS leptin concentration is a signal for the onset of puberty and maintenance of fertility (Ahima et al., 1996).

Whether any other CNS peptides involved in control of body mass also cause hypogonadism is problematic. Two separate frame shift mutations in the melanocortin-4 receptor (MC4R) are responsible for an autosomal dominant form of obesity in man, but do not cause attendant hypogonadism (Vaisse et al. 1998;

Yeo et al. 1998). MC4R and its ligand have been implicated in the central modulation of leptin effects (Seely et al. 1997).

REFERENCES

Ahima R S, Prabakaran D, Mantzoros C, et al (1996). Role of leptin in the neuroendocrine response to fasting. *Nature* 382:250–252.

Clement K, Vaisse C, Lahlou N, et al. (1998). A mutation in the human leptin receptor gene causes obesity and pituitary dysfunction. *Nature* 392:398–401.

Coleman D L (1973). Obese and diabetes: two mutant genes causing diabetes-obesity syndromes in mice. *Diabetologica* 14:141–148.

Montague C T, Faroogi I S, Whitehead J P, et al. (1997). Congenital leptin deficiency associated with severe early-onset obesity in humans. *Nature* 387:903–907.

Seely R J, Yagaloff K A, Fisher S L, et al. (1997). Melanocortin receptors in leptin effects. *Nature* 390:349.

Strobel A, Issal T, Camoin L, et al. (1998). A leptin missense mutation associated with hypogonadism and morbid obesity. *Nat Genet* 18:213–215.

Vaisse C, Clement K, Guy-Grand B, et al. (1998). A frameshift mutation in human MC4R is associated with a dominant form of obesity. *Nat Genet* 20:113–114.

Yeo G S H, Faroogi I S, Aminian S, et al. (1998). A frameshift mutation in MC4R associated with dominantly inherited human obesity. *Nat Genet* 20:111–112.

LIPODYSTROPHY

Lipodystrophy may be genetic or acquired. It may involve the entire body, be asymmetric, or involve only selective areas of the body—for example, face-sparing or limited to the cervicothoracic area. All lipodystrophic syndromes feature insulin resistance with or without overt diabetes mellitus. Patients with congenital total lipodystrophy or the Berardinelli-Seip syndrome have accelerated linear growth, muscle hypertrophy, and genital enlargement (both males and females) as well as hypertrophic cardiomyopathy and occasional CNS defects (Seip and Trygstad, 1996). The condition is an autosomal recessive trait (Gedde-Dahl et al., 1996). No molecular lesion has been defined and the gene is as yet unmapped.

In contrast, mutations in the alpha subunit of the insulin receptor have been identified (O'Rahilly and Moller, 1992) in leprechaunism, which features an unusual facial appearance, growth retardation, hirsutism, enlarged genitalia in both sexes and polycystic ovaries in females, and early death, and a milder variant, the so-called Rabson-Mendenhall syndrome. Patients with Rabson-Mendenhall syndrome have precocious puberty. Patients with either of these two conditions are either homozygous or compound heterozygotes for insulin receptor mutations.

In adult-onset forms of heritable lipodystrophy, mutations in both alpha and beta insulin receptor subunits have been identified in some instances, but in others the structure of the receptor appears to be normal (Desbois-Mouthon et al, 1995). The main gonadal feature of the adult form of the condition is polycystic ovary disease with its clinical consequences of hirsutism, oligomenorrhea, and infertility. Both autosomal dominant and recessive forms have been recorded. In none of these variant forms of lipodystrophy has the relationship between the insulin receptor abnormality and the overall phenotype been adequately explained.

REFERENCES

Desbois-Mouton C, Magré J, Amselem S, et al (1995). Lipotrophic diabetes: genetic exclusion of the insulin receptor gene. *J Clin Endocrinol Metab* 80:314–319.

Gedde-Dahl T J, Trygstad O, VanMaldergem L, et al. (1996). Genetics of Beradinelli-Seip Syndrome (congenital generalized lipodystrophy) in Norway: epidemiology and gene mapping. *Acta Paediatr Suppl* 413:52–58.
O'Rahilly S, Moller D E (1992). Mutant insulin receptors in syndromes of insulin resistance. *Clin Endocrinol* 36:121–132.
Seip M, Trygstad O (1996). Generalized lipodystrophy, congenital and acquired (lipoatrophy). *Acta Paediatr Suppl* 413:2–28.

POLYCYSTIC OVARY DISEASE (STEIN-LEVENTHAL SYNDROME)

Hirsutism accompanied by amenorrhea or more often oligomenorrhea and polycystic ovaries classically make up this syndrome. However, the condition varies considerably even within the same family, as the ovaries may be small or enlarged and significant cystic alteration is not always evident by ultrasound. Varying degrees of hyperthecosis, nests of luteinized cells within the ovarian stroma, are also seen. The biochemical hallmarks are elevated serum androgens (DHEA, androstenedione and/or testosterone), low or normal FSH, and elevated LH (McKenna, 1988). Many patients exhibit insulin resistance as well.

The syndrome commonly appears in families: in sibs, in multiple generations, or in monozygotic twins (Givens, 1988). Sex-limited autosomal dominant inheritance has been suggested. However, male relatives of such patients may have premature baldness (Lunde et al., 1989). In fact, there is an excess of affected female relatives in some families, perhaps indicating the presence of phenocopies.

Some families exhibiting apparent dominant inheritance of PCOD show both linkage to and/or associations with regulatory polymorphisms of the VNTR region of the insulin gene (Waterworth et al., 1997). However, the syndrome is genetically heterogeneous. For example, ovarian 17-ketosteroid reductase deficiency, late-onset 21-hydroxylase deficiency, and even enhanced hepatic 5-alpha reductase activity have been found in some families (Chapter 13), and in those insurances, autosomal recessive inheritance would be expected. PCOD occurs in some patients with lipodystrophy and insulin resistance (see above). Targeted overexpression of LH in transgenic mice produced infertility and polycystic ovaries, suggesting a possible hypothalamic causation (Risma et al., 1995). It is quite likely that other patients have still different etiologies.

REFERENCES

Givens J R (1988). Familial polycystic ovary disease. *Endocrin Metab Clin North Am* 17:771–783.
McKenna T J (1988). Pathogenesis and treatment of polycystic ovary syndrome. *N Engl J Med* 318:588–562.
Lunde O, Magnus P, Sandvik L, et al. (1989). Familial clustering in the polycystic ovary syndrome. *Gynecol Obstet Invest* 28:23–30.
Risma K A, Clay C M, Nett T M, et al (1995). Targeted overexpression of luteinizing hormone in transgenic mice leads to infertility, polycystic ovaries and ovarian tumors. *Proc Nat Acad Sci USA* 92:1322–1326.
Waterworth D M, Bennett S T, Gharani N, et al. (1997). Linkage and association of insulin gene VNTR regulating polymorphisms with polycystic ovary disease. *Lancet* 349:986–990.

POLYGLANDULAR AUTOIMMUNE SYNDROMES AND HYPOGONADISM

Immune-mediated failure of more than one endocrine gland has been described in families on a number of occasions. At least two forms exist, one with childhood onset that additionally features mucocutaneous candidiasis and is inherited as an autosomal recessive trait (Type I or APECD, Ahonen, 1985) and another that is more likely multifactorial, showing a strong association with alleles at the HLA B and D loci (Type II). Circulating endocrine gland autoantibodies are found in both forms. Hypogonadism is not a common component of these syndromes, but it does occur. Shapiro and colleagues (1987) have suggested that a further form exists based on the findings of hypogonadism in five Persian Jews. The gonadal failure is usually primary—that is, the autoantibodies are directed against gonadal steroidogenic enzymes (Chen et al., 1996); on occasion gonadal failure may be secondary to gonadotropin failure (Barkan et al., 1985). The diagnosis of these complex syndromes should be considered in any patient with symptoms of hypogonadism who has (or has had) one or more of the more common forms of autoimmune endocrine dysfunction, such as diabetes mellitus, Hashimoto's thyroiditis, or even idiopathic Addison's disease.

The type I disease, previously linked to 21q22.3, has been found to be due to mutations in a novel gene AIRE, expressed in thymus, pancreas and adrenal cortex, that appears to be a transcription regulator (Björses et al., 1998).

REFERENCES

Ahonen P (1985). Autoimmune polyendocrinopathy-candidiasis-ectodermal dystrophy: autosomal recessive inheritance. *Clin Genet* 27:535–542.

Ahonen P, Myllärniemi, Sipilä I, et al. (1990). Clinical variation of autoimmune polyendocrinopathy-candidiasis-ectodermal dystrophy (APECED) in a series of 68 patients. *N Engl J Med* 322:1829–1836.

Barkan A L, Kelch R P, Marshall J C (1985). Isolated gonadotrope failure in the polyglandular autoimmune syndrome. *N Engl J Med* 312:1535–1540.

Björses P, Aaltonen J, Horelli-Kuitunen N, et al. (1998). Gene defect behind APECD: a new clue to autoimmunity. *Hum Mol Genet* 7:1547–1553.

Chen S, Sawicka J, Betterle C, et al., (1996). Antiantibodies to steroidogenic enzymes in autoimmune polyglandular syndrome, Addison's disease, and premature ovarian failure. *J Clin Endocrinol Metab* 81:1871–1876.

Shapiro M S, Zamir R, Weiss E, et al. (1987). The polyglandular deficiency syndrome: a new variant in Persian Jews. *J Endocrinol Invest* 10:1–7.

WILSON DISEASE

This condition is a copper storage disorder chiefly characterized by progressive liver damage and basal ganglia dysfunction (Danks, 1995). However, deposition occurs in other places: the cornea (Kayser-Fleisher rings), renal tubule, bones, joints, heart, and parathyroid glands.

Liver dysfunction, if it occurs early enough, can lead to delayed puberty and gynecomastia in males, and either primary or secondary amenorrhea in females. It has been suggested that the ovulatory disturbance in women is due to copper-induced decrease in follicular aromatase (Kaushausky et al., 1987).

Wilson disease is treated with chelating agents, which are effective if the condition is detected before irreversible liver failure develops. The inheritance is autosomal recessive and the gene, located on chromosome 13, has been cloned. The protein product is a copper-binding ATPase (ATP7B), highly homologous to the gene product identified in another copper-transport disorder, Menkes syndrome (Tümer and Horn, 1997).

REFERENCES

Danks D M (1995). Disorders of copper transport. *The Metabolic and Molecular Basis of Inherited Disease*, Scrivner C R, et al (eds.), McGraw-Hill, New York, 7th ed., pp. 2211–2235.

Kaushamskry A, Frydman M, Kaufman H, et al. (1987). Endocrine studies of the ovulatory disturbance in Wilson's disease (hepatolenticular degeneration). *Fertil Steril* 47:270–273.

Tümer Z, Horn N (1997). Menkes disease: recent advances and new aspects. *J Med Genet* 34: 265–274.

Teratogenic Causes of Sexual Maldevelopment

One of the most extensively studied drugs shown to have a teratogenic effect on genital development is *diethylstilbestrol* (DES). This compound is a synthetic estrogen-like substance used extensively from 1940 to 1970 for regularizing menses and preventing abortion. It was subsequently discovered that female fetuses exposed to this drug developed a significantly increased incidence of clear cell adenomas and, less commonly, adenocarcinomas of the cervix and vagina. Somewhat later it was recognized that upper genital tract anomalies were also fairly common. Kaufman and colleagues (1980) performed hysterosalpingography on 267 DES-exposed women, and found nearly 70% to have some abnormality, including T-shaped and small uteri, constrictions, diverticula, and filling defects. The cervix was frequently also abnormal, and there was a good correlation between these anatomical changes and both vaginal epithelial changes and pregnancy wastage (Giusti et al., 1995).

Less commonly recognized is the fact that males exposed to DES *in utero* also may have anomalies, among which are varicoceles, epididymal cysts, hypoplastic and cryptorchid testes, small penis, and hypospadias (Whitehead and Leiter, 1981). Even in the absence of recognized anatomical abnormalities, results of semen analysis are frequently not normal. Surprisingly, however, DES-exposed men do not seem to have any impairment of sexual function or fertility.

A variety of other environmental agents—drugs, infections, physical factors, and so on, also can have adverse effects on the developing fetus. However, in comparatively few instances have sufficient numbers of fetuses been exposed so that distinctive patterns of maldevelopment have emerged. Genital abnormalities are not a prominent feature of these conditions, save for those associated with maternal diabetes (caudal regression, Chapter 16; see also Becerra et al. (1980), or androgen ingestion by a mother of a female fetus, with consequent masculinization. Of the other agents, probably the best known are the *effects of fetal alcohol*, in which hypospadias and cryptorchidism in males and hypoplastic labia majora in females have been seen (Clarren and Smith, 1978). In the *fetal hydantoin syndrome*, male genital abnormalities range from micropenis to genital ambiguity (Hanson et al., 1976). Another anticonvulsant, *trimethadione*, has also been associated with a syndrome that includes genital anomalies similar to those seen in males exposed to hydantoin *in utero* (Zachai et al., 1975). Hypospadias, micropenis, bifid scrotum, and cryptorchidism are frequent in males with *valproate embryopathy*, and fusion defects of müllerian structures have been noted in females (Ardinger et al., 1988). *Maternal cocaine abuse* may result in hypospadias and cryptorchidism in males, with less predictable effects in females (Chasnoff et al., 1988; Chavez et al., 1989). Aplasia of müllerian derivatives and bicornuate uterus have been recorded as part of *thalidomide embryopathy* (Hoffman et al., 1976).

Any teratogen that interferes with CNS growth and development could give rise to early gonadotropin failure in a male, with resultant defective androgen secretion. *Maternal hyperthermia* due to febrile illness or prolonged sauna bathing has been implicated in CNS malformations (Pleet et al., 1981). Some male infants delivered after these high-temperature exposed pregnancies have had micropenis, implying that the hypothalamic-pituitary-gonadal axis malfunctioned. This implication requires further study.

Extensive fetal damage can follow maternal infection with *rubella* virus (Menser et al., 1967). Paramount involvement occurs in the eye, ear, CNS, and cardiovascular systems, but on occasion hypospadias and cryptorchidism will be found in affected males. Large-scale use of a attenuated rubella vaccine in adolescent females has substantially decreased the incidence of the condition.

REFERENCES

Ardinger H H, Atkins J F, Blackston R D, et al. (1988). Verification of the fetal valproate syndrome phenotype. *Am J Med Genet* 29:171–185.

Becerra J E, Koury M J, Cordero J F, et al. (1990). Diabetes mellitus during pregnancy and the risks for the specific birth defects: a population-based case control study. *Pediatrics* 85:1–9.

Chasnoff I J, Chisum G M, Kaplan W E (1988). Maternal cocaine use and genitourinary tract malformation. *Teratology* 37:201–204.

Chavez G F, Mulinare J, Cordero J F (1989). Maternal cocaine use during early pregnancy as a risk factor for congenital urogenital anomalies. *JAMA* 263:795–798.

Clarren S K, Smith D W (1978). The fetal alcohol syndrome. *N Engl J Med* 298:1063–1067.

Giusti R M, Iwamoto K, Hatch E E (1995). Diethylstilbestrol revisited: a review of the long-term health effects. *Ann Intern Med* 122:778–788.

Hanson J W, Myrianthopoulos N C, Harvey M A S, et al. (1976). Risks to the offspring of women treated with hydantoin anticonvulsants, with emphasis on fetal hydantoin syndrome. *J Pediatr* 89:662–668.

Hoffman W, Grospiecth G, Kuhn W (1976). Thalidomide and female genital malformation. *Lancet* 2:794.

Kaufman R H, Adam E, Binder G L, et al. (1980). Upper genital tract changes and pregnancy outcome in offspring exposed *in utero* to diethylstilbestrol. *Am J Obstet Gynecol* 137:299–308.

Menser M A, Dods L, Harley J D (1967). A twenty-five-year follow-up of congenital rubella. *Lancet* 2:1347–1350.

Pleet H, Graham J M Jr, Smith D W (1981). Central nervous system and facial defects associate with maternal hyperthermia at 4 to 14 weeks gestation. *Pediatrics* 67:785–789.

Whitehead E D, Leiter E A (1981). Genital abnormalities and abnormal semen analysis in male patients exposed to diethylstilbestrol *in utero*. *J Urol* 125:47–50.

Wilcox A J, Baird D D, Weinberg C R, et al. (1995). Fertility in men exposed prenatally to diethylstilbestrol. *N Engl J Med* 332:1411–1416.

Zachai E H, Mellman W J, Neiderer B, et al. (1975). The fetal trimethadione syndrome. *J Pediatr* 87:280–284.

18

Autosomal Aneusomy and Sexual Maldevelopment

CLINICAL BIOLOGY OF AUTOSOMAL ANEUSOMY

Although defective genital and/or gonadal development is commonplace and can be expected when there are visible or molecular alterations of the X or Y chromosome, it is noteworthy that the same physical features occur with autosomal chromosome defects as well. This chapter treats a variety of chromosome "syndromes" involving partial or complete trisomy as well as partial or complete monosomy for a number of different chromosomes. Usually it is the external genitalia that are abnormal, and little or nothing is known about gonadal status, for most reported cases are in children. Moreover, the spectrum of defects in sexual development recorded herein must be considered in proper perspective because many case studies, especially those reporting partial or segmental trisomy or monosomy, are derived from patients with various translocations—the implication being that the phenotype may be variable to some extent, depending on the reciprocal chromosome(s) involved. For this reason, absolute or even relative incidence figures for the genital involvement are virtually impossible to obtain. The nongenital features of the syndromes are presented only briefly in this chapter; detailed accounts can be obtained from the original references. It must be emphasized that the chapter includes only those chromosomal syndromes in which genital/gonadal involvement has been reliably ascertained. Other chromosome aneusomic states with genital changes but no other definitive features, such as occasional genital hypoplasia with partial trisomy 10p (Clement et al., 1996) or even sex reversal with partial trisomy 1p (Wieacker et al., 1996), are not described, mainly because of the scarcity of clinical material. For simplicity's sake, a brief discussion of polyploid states is given.

REFERENCES

Clement S J, Leppig K A, Jarvik G P, et al. (1996). Trisomy 10p: report of an unusual mechanism of formation and critical evaluation of the clinical phenotype. *Am J Med Genet* 65: 197–204.
Wieacker P, Missbach D, Jakubiazka, S, et al. (1996). Sex reversal in a child with the karyotype 46,XY,dup (1) (p 22.3, p 32.3). *Clin Genet* 49:271–273.

Complete Autosomal Trisomies

TRISOMY 7

This lethal trisomy has been fully described in two unrelated females who had cystic kidneys and the oligohydramnios tetrad. One infant also had marked clitoromegaly (Pflueger et al., 1984), whereas the other had a blind-ending vagina and no evident uterus (Yunis et al., 1980). Mosaicism was not specifically sought.

REFERENCES

Pflueger S M, Scott C I, Moore C M (1984). Trisomy 7 and Potter syndrome. *Clin Genet* 25: 543–548.
Yunis E, Ramirez E, Uribe J G (1980). Full trisomy 7 and Potter syndrome. *Hum Genet* 54:13–18.

TRISOMY 8

Viable trisomy 8 is likely always mosaic. As would be expected with mosaicism, features are variable but usually include mental retardation, abnormal facies, absent or dysplastic patella, rather unusual furrowing of palms and soles, joint contractures, hallucal anomalies, vertebral defects, and heart and renal anomalies.

The various anomalies overlap those seen in patients with partial duplication of both 8p and 8q; in fact, the three conditions are probably not separable on clinical grounds alone (Riccardi and Crandall, 1978). Spinner and colleagues (1995) described an affected patient who was mosaic for only an extra small centromeric fragment of chromosome 8.

With mosaic or partial 8 trisomies, cryptorchidism and hypoplastic genitalia are common in males (Walker and Bocian, 1987). Female genital anomalies have not been described. Some patients are fertile (Habecker-Green et al., 1998)

REFERENCES

Habecker-Green J, Naeem R, Goh W, et al. (1998). Reproduction in a patient with trisomy 8 mosaicism: case report and literature review. *Am J Med Genet* 75:382–385.

Riccardi V M, Crandall B F (1978). Karyotype-phenotype correlations: mosaic trisomy 8 and partial trisomies of different segments of chromosome 8. *Hum Genet* 41:363–368.

Spinner N B, Grace K R, Owens N L, et al. (1995). Mosaicism for a chromosome 8–derived minute marker chromosome in a patient with manifestations of trisomy 8 mosaicism *Am J Med Genet* 56:22–24.

Walker A P, Bocian M (1987). Partial duplication 8q12 → q21.2 in two sibs with maternally derived insertional and reciprocal translocations: case reports and review of partial duplications of chromosome 8. *Am J Med Genet* 27:3–22.

TRISOMY 9 (INCLUDES MOSAIC TRISOMY 9)

There is no appreciable phenotypic difference between mosaic and non-mosaic trisomy 9, probably indicating that the former is underdiagnosed (Cantú et al., 1996). Children are of low birth weight and exhibit developmental delay, microcephaly, and a variety of different CV, skeletal, and CNS defects.

Hypoplastic genitalia, including micropenis and cryptorchidism in males and hypoplastic labia in females, are present in roughly half the reported patients (Arnold et al., 1995).

REFERENCES

Arnold G L, Kirby R S, Stern T P, et al. (1995). Trisomy 9: review and report of two new cases. *Am J Med Genet* 56:252–259.

Cantú E S, Eicher D J, Pai G S, et al. (1996). Mosaic vs. non-mosaic trisomy 9: a report of a liveborn infant evaluated by fluorescence in situ hybridization and review of the literature. *Am J Med Genet* 62:330–335.

TRISOMY 13

The range of malformations in trisomy 13 is well known and has been repeatedly documented (Gorlin et al., 1990).

Affected males commonly have cryptorchidism with or without scrotal anomalies. Hypospadias is less common. Affected females may have clitoral hypertrophy and septate vagina and uterus; ovarian dysgenesis is almost universal (Cunniff et al., 1991).

Partial trisomy of the long arm, particularly q22 → qter has many of the features of the full trisomic state, including cryptorchidism (Rao et al., 1995).

REFERENCES

Cunniff C, Jones K L, Benirschke K (1991). Ovarian dysgenesis in individuals with chromosome abnormalities. *Hum Genet* 86:552–556.

Gorlin R J, Cohen M M Jr, Levin L S (1990). *Syndromes of the Head and Neck*. Oxford University Press, New York, pp 40–43.

Rao V V, Carpenter N J, Gucsavas M, et al. (1995). Partial trisomy 13q identified by sequential fluorescence in situ hybridization. *Am J Med Genet* 58:50–53.

TRISOMY 14

Viable examples of this condition probably exist only in mosaic form. Birth weight may be near normal but postnatal growth and psychomotor development are severely impaired (Johnson et al., 1979). The head is small, the nose is broad and prominent, the mouth is large, but there is micrognathia. Congenital heart disease is common.

Undescended testes and micropenis occur commonly in affected males. Some of the features overlap those of patients with dup 14q (Kaplan et al., 1986). Interestingly, maternal uniparental disomy may give rise to short stature and precocious puberty (Antonarakis et al., 1993).

REFERENCES

Antonarakis S E, Blovin J-L, Maher J, et al. (1993). Maternal uniparental disomy for human chromosome 14, due to loss of 2 chromosome 14 from somatic cells with t (13;14) trisomy 14. *Am J Hum Genet* 52:1145–1152.
Kaplan L C, Wayne A, Crowell S, et al. (1986). Trisomy 14 mosaicism in a liveborn male: clinical report and review of the literature. *Am J Med Genet* 23:925–930.
Johnson V P, Aceto T, Likness C (1979). Trisomy 14 mosaicism: case report and review. *Am J Med Genet* 3:331–339.

TRISOMY 18

Taylor (1968) and Hodes and colleagues (1978) have reviewed the various features of trisomy 18, and Matsuoka and colleagues (1983) have summarized autopsy findings.

Cryptorchidism is probably universal in males and most females have gonadal dysgenesis. Otherwise, the gross appearance of the genitalia in both sexes is normal. Secondary amenorrhea has been reported with mosaicism (Uehara et al., 1996).

Hypoplastic genitalia and cryptorchidism have been inconsistently noted with tetrasomy 18p (due to an extra marker isochromosome for 18p) (Callen et al., 1990).

REFERENCES

Callen D F, Freemantle C J, Ringenbergs M L, et al. (1990). The isochromosome 18p syndrome: confirmation of cytogenetic diagnosis by in situ hybridization. *Am J Med Genet* 47:493–498.
Hodes M E, Cole J, Palmer C G, et al. (1978). Clinical experience with trisomies 18 and 13. *J Med Genet* 15:48–60, 1978.
Matsuoka R, Misugi K, Goto A, et al. (1983). Congenital heart anomalies in the trisomy 18 syndrome with reference to congenital polyvalvular disease. *Am J Med Genet* 14:657–668.
Taylor A I (1968). Autosomal trisomy syndromes. *J Med Genet* 5:227–252.
Uehara S, Obara Y, Obara T, et al. (1996). Trisomy 18 mosaicism associated with secondary amenorrhea: ratios of mosaicism in different samples and complications. *Clin Genet* 49: 91–94.

TRISOMY 21

The various clinical manifestations of this, the most common autosomal trisomy, have been extensively recorded and reviews are readily available to the interested reader.

Hypogonadism is likely always present in males, but gonadal function is variable in females (Cunniff et al., 1991). A small phallus, occasionally with cryptorchidism, can be seen in affected males, but the appearance of the external genitalia in either sex is usually normal.

REFERENCE
Cunniff C, Jones K L, Benirschke K (1991). Ovarian dysgenesis in individuals with chromosome abnormalities. *Hum Genet* 86:552–556.

TRISOMY 22

Bacino and colleagues (1995) pointed out that trisomy 22 is common in spontaneous abortuses, but occasional survival to term may occur, perhaps on the basis of mosaicism (Robinson and Kalousek, 1996). Affected infants exhibit intrauterine growth retardation, microcephaly, facial dysmorphism, microtia, commonly a cleft palate, a high frequency of congenital heart disease, renal anomalies, and distal digital hypoplasia.

Affected males frequently have micropenis, hypospadias, and/or cryptorchidism.

REFERENCES
Bacino C A, Schreck R, Fishel-Ghodsian N, et al. (1995). Clinical and molecular studies in full trisomy 22: further delineation of the phenotype and review of the literature. *Am J Med Genet* 56:359–365.
Robinson W P, Kalousek D K (1996). Mosaicism most likely accounts for extended survival of trisomy 22. *Am J Med Genet* 62:100.

Partial Autosomal Trisomies (Segmental Duplications)

DUP 2P

All patients described have severe mental and growth retardation with microcephaly, high forehead, midface hypoplasia, wide-spaced toes, and thin, hyperextensible fingers (Francke and Jones, 1976). The presence or absence of additional visceral anomalies likely depends on the extent of the partial trisomy (Pueschel et al., 1987). Most of the salient features are seen with interstitial duplications (p13 → p25) (Mégarbané et al., 1997).

Micropenis with or without hypospadias, shawl scrotum, and cryptorchidism are common in males. No definite female genital abnormality has been identified.

REFERENCES
Francke U, Jones K L (1976). The 2p partial trisomy syndrome. *Am J Med Genet* 130:1244–1249.
Mégarbané A, Souraty N, Prieur M, et al. (1997). Interstitial duplication of the short arm of chromosome 2: report of a new case and review. *J Med Genet* 34:783–786.
Pueschel S M, Scola P S, Mendoza T (1987). Partial trisomy 2p. *J Ment Def Res* 31:293–298.

DUP 3P

A square face with brachycephaly, hypertelorism, and occasional cleft lip are the facial features of this syndrome (Reiss et al., 1986). Congenital heart disease is common and various degrees of holoprosencephaly have been seen with more proximal duplications (Kurtzman et al., 1987). Affected males frequently have micropenis, with or without hypospadias, and cryptorchidism. Hypoplasia of female external genitalia occur, but less commonly (Conte et al., 1995). The association of these various defects suggests that genes controlling a hypothetical midline developmental field might be in this region.

REFERENCES

Conte P A, Pitter J H, Verma R S (1995). Molecular characterization of trisomic segment 3p24.1 → 3pter: a case with review of the literature. *Clin Genet* 48:49–53.

Kurtzman D N, vanDyke D L, Rich C A, et al. (1987). Brief clinical report: duplication of 3p21-3pter and cyclopia. *Am J Med Genet* 37:33–37.

Reiss J A, Sheffield, L J, Sutherland G R (1986). Partial trisomy 3p syndrome. *Clin Genet* 30: 50–58.

DUP 3Q

The facial features of patients with dup 3q resemble those in the de Lange syndrome (Chapter 15) largely because of hypertrichosis and synophrys. However, those with dup 3q lack the extreme extremity abnormalities and the low birth weight of the deLange syndrome; instead they are more likely to have craniosynostosis, cleft palate, and eye, cardiac, and renal defects (van Essen et al., 1991).

The critical chromosome region for the full syndrome appears to be q26.31q27.3 (Aqua et al., 1995). Interestingly, Ireland and colleagues (1991) reported a *de novo* translocation in a patient with the deLange syndrome where the breakpoint on chromosome 3 was at q26.3, perhaps indicating that the two phenotypically related syndromes involve a common gene(s).

Genital anomalies are common in males and include micropenis, hypospadias, cryptorchidism, and scrotal hypoplasia (Wilson et al., 1985).

REFERENCES

Aqua M S, Rizzo P, Lindsay E A, et al. (1995). Duplication 3q syndrome: molecular delineation of the critical region. *Am J Med Genet* 55:33–37.

Ireland M, English C, Cross I, et al. (1991). A *de novo* translocation t (3;17) (q26.3;q23.1) in a child with Cornelia de Lange syndrome. *J Med Genet* 28:639–640.

van Essen A J, Kok K, van der Berg A, et al. (1991). Partial 3q duplication syndrome and assignment of D3S5 to 3q25-3q28. *Hum Genet* 87:151–154.

Wilson G N, Dasouki M, Barr M J (1985). Further delineation of the dup (3q) syndrome. *Am J Med Genet* 22:117–123.

DUP 4P

Patel and colleagues (1995) have summarized the clinical features of this condition, which when present seems to involve trisomy of most of the short arm of chromosome 4. The facies are characterized by a prominent glabella and/or supraorbital ridge with a bulbous nose. The chin is prominent, and the neck is short with a low hairline. Long fingers, frequently with camptodactyly, are common and the feet have a "rocker-bottom" configuration.

Micropenis, hypospadias, cryptorchidism, and a hypoplastic scrotum are common in males. No specific female genital anomaly has been identified. At least some degree of sexual maturation generally occurs in both sexes, but puberty is often delayed.

REFERENCE
Patel S V, Dagnew H, Parekk A, et al. (1995). Clinical manifestations of trisomy 4p. *Eur J Pediatr* 154:425–431.

Dup 4Q

Microcephaly, severe psychomotor retardation, and unusual but not diagnostic facies are seen in this partial trisomy (Cervenka et al., 1976; Andrle et al., 1979). Complex cardiac lesions often lead to neonatal death, and urinary tract anomalies are common.

Hypoplastic external genitalia are regularly seen in both sexes, and the males generally have cryptorchidism.

REFERENCES
Andrle M, Erlach A, Rett A (1979). Partial trisomy 4q in two unrelated cases. *Hum Genet* 49: 179–183.

Cervenka J, Djavadi G R, Gorlin R J (1976). Partial trisomy 4q syndrome: case report and review. *Hum Genet* 34:1–7.

Dup 6Q

More severe phenotype effects result from more proximal duplications within 6q2.3 → 6qter. Mental and somatic retardation are universal. The head is small and often misshapen, and a variety of other craniofacial alterations may be present (Conrad et al., 1998)

The genitalia in both sexes are usually hypoplastic and males may have hypospadias and cryptorchidism (Stamberg et al., 1981). In two sisters, whose partial trisomy arose from a maternal 6;11 translocation, Clark and colleagues (1980) found histologically normal ovaries.

REFERENCES
Clark C E, Cowell H R, Telfer M A, et al. (1980). Trisomy 6q25 → qter in two sisters resulting from a maternal 6;11 translocation. *Am J Med Genet* 5:171–175.

Conrad B A, Higgins R R, Pierpoint M E (1998). Duplication 6q22 → qtr: definition of the phenotype. *Am J Med Genet* 78:123–126.

Stamberg J, Shapiro J, Valle D, et al. (1981). Partial trisomy 6q due to a balanced maternal translocation (6;22) (q21;p13) or (q21∂er). *Clin Genet* 19:122–125.

Dup 7P

There seems to be little difference in phenotype whether the entire short arm is duplicated or simply the segment from 7p15 → pter—the critical region seems to be 7p15 (Reish et al., 1996). Affected infants have hypertelorism, often accompanied by hydrocephalus, Dandy-Walker malformation, or other CNS defects, largely septal defects of the heart, hyperextensible joints with dislocation, and severe retardation. The condition is often lethal in early infancy.

Hypoplastic external genitalia have been described in both sexes, along with cryptorchidism in males and vaginal and uterine septae in females.

REFERENCE

Reish O, Berry S A, Dewald G, et al. (1996). Duplication of 7p: further delineation of the phenotype and restriction of critical region to distal part of short arm. *Am J Med Genet* 61:21–25.

DUP 9P (INCLUDES BOTH TRISOMY AND TETRASOMY 9P)

The difference between the presence of trisomy and tetrasomy 9p (the latter usually due to an isochromosome) are of degree, because the same general features are found in both (reviewed by Wilson et al., 1985, and Tonk, 1997). The craniofacies are abnormal but nondiagnostic; growth and mental retardation are almost invariable, and visceral defects are common.

Hypoplastic external genitalia are present in both sexes, and males may have additional cryptorchidism and hypospadias.

REFERENCES

Tonk V S (1997). Moving towards a syndrome: a review of 20 cases and a new case of non-mosaic tetrasomy 9p with long-term survival. *Clin Genet* 52:23–29.
Wilson G N, Raj A, Baker D (1985). The phenotype spectrum of partial trisomy 9. *Am J Med Genet* 20:277–282.

DUP 10Q

Partial trisomy of the distal long arm of chromosome 10-10q25 → qter-gives rise to a reasonably consistent phenotype with a recognizable facies (Yunis and Sanchez, 1974; Klep-dePater et al., 1979). The children are severely retarded and often succumb early from the effects of complex cardiovascular, pulmonary, and renal malformations.

Males commonly have cryptorchidism, and streak gonads in females have been described.

REFERENCES

Klep-dePater J, Bijlsma J B, deFrance H F, et al. (1979). Partial trisomy 10q: a recognizable syndrome. *Hum Genet* 46:29–40.
Yunis J J, Sanchez O (1974). A new syndrome resulting from partial trisomy for the distal third of the long arm of chromosome 10. *J Pediatr* 84:567–570.

TETRASOMY 12P (ISOCHROMOSOME 12P, PALLISTER-KILLIAN SYNDROME)

This condition exists only in mosaic form. If the diagnosis is suspected on clinical grounds, cytogenetic studies should be done on cultured skin fibroblasts or on direct bone marrow examination because peripheral blood lymphocytes may show a normal karyotype (Hunter et al., 1985). In infancy, noteworthy features are sparse frontal and temporal hair with hypopigmented areas on the scalp and forehead, which tends to be high. The nose is upturned, the upper lip is thin, and the mandible is small. The infants are deaf and mentally retarded, and seizures are frequent. The facies tends to coarsen with age.

Genital or gonadal abnormalities are not common. However, Reynolds and colleagues (1987) described one female fetus with a persistent cloaca. The overall gonadal status in surviving individuals with mosaic tetrasomy 12p has not been assessed.

REFERENCES

Hunter A G W, Clifford B, Cox D M (1985). The characteristic physiognomy and tissue specific karyotype distribution—the Pallister-Killian syndrome. *Clin Genet* 28:47–53.

Reynolds J F, Daniel A, Kelly T E, et al. (1987). Isochromosome 12p mosaicism (Pallister mosaic aneuploidy or Pallister-Killian syndrome): report of 11 cases. *Am J Med Genet* 27: 257–274.

DUP 15Q

Partial trisomy of 15q, particularly 15q22 → qter gives rise to microcephaly, unusual facies, postnatal growth deficiency, mental retardation, arachnodactyly, and cardiovascular anomalies. Cryptorchidism has been seen in males and hypoplastic labia have been noted in females (Lacro et al., 1987).

REFERENCE

Lacro R V, Jones K L, Masacarelba J T, et al. (1987). Duplication of distal 15q. *Am J Med Genet* 26:719–728.

DUP 16Q

Trisomy 16 is the most common cytogenetic finding among spontaneous abortuses. Surviving infants usually have partial trisomy of part or all of the respective long or short arms. Long arm duplication leads to low birth weight, severe retardation, dysmorphic facies with a high forehead, flat nasal bridge, hypertelorism, occasional cleft palate, hypertrichosis, flexion contracture of the extremities, and various visceral anomalies.

Genital ambiguity has been noted, with males having micropenis, bifid scrotum, and cryptorchidism; both sexes have been seen with what appears to be at least partial persistence of the cloaca (Ridler and McKeown, 1979; Garau et al., 1980).

REFERENCES

Garau A, Crisponi G, Peretti D, et al. (1980). Trisomy 16q21-qter. *Hum Genet* 53:165–167.

Ridler M A C, McKeown J A (1979). Trisomy 16q arising from a maternal 15p;16q translocation. *J Med Genet* 16:317–319.

DUP 17P

Common features include severe developmental delay, microcephaly, low-set ears, micrognathia, flexion deformity of the fingers, and occasional cardiovascular and renal anomalies.

Cryptorchidism in males and hypoplastic genitalia in females have been seen (Feldman et al., 1987).

REFERENCE

Feldman G M, Baumer J G, Sparks R S (1982). Brief clinical report: the dup (17p) syndrome. *Am J Med Genet* 11:299–304.

DUP 17Q

The phenotype includes short stature; growth and mental retardation; microcephaly, often with associated anomalous CNS development; dysmorphic facies; and frequent severe cardiac and renal malformations. Lax joints and postaxial polydactyly have been recorded (Bridge et al., 1985; Naccacha et al., 1984).

Cryptorchidism is common.

REFERENCES

Bridge J, Sanger W, Mosher G, et al. (1985). Partial duplication of distal 17q. *Am J Med Genet* 22:229–235.
Naccacha N F, Vianna-Morgante A M, Richieri-Costa A (1984). Duplication of distal 17q: report of a familial observation. *Am J Med Genet* 17:633–639.

DUP 22P (INCLUDES TRISOMY AND TETRASOMY 22P, CAT-EYE SYNDROME)

The syndrome received its name because the initial patients had rather striking colobomas of the iris that may extend to the retina and choroid. However, these features may be missing in up to half the patients. Other hallmarks of this chromosome-excess syndrome include frequent anal atresia, congenital heart disease, and usually mild retardation.

The syndrome usually results from an extra dicentric marker chromosome consisting of a duplication of 22pter → q11; this segment is present in quadruplicate. However, an interstitial duplication of 22q11 gives rise to most of the features so that trisomy of this critical region appears to be sufficient for the syndrome (Liehr et al., 1992).

Occasional features include male hypospadias (Schinzel et al., 1981) and müllerian agenesis (Jones 1997).

REFERENCES

Jones K L (1997). *Smith's Recognizable Patterns of Human Malformation.* Saunders, Philadelphia, 5th ed. pp. 68–69.
Liehr T, Pfeiffer R A, Trautmann U (1992). Typical and partial cat eye syndrome: identification of a marker chromosome by FISH. *Clin Genet* 42:91–96.
Schinzel A, Schmid W, Fraccaro M, et al. (1981). The "cat eye syndrome": dicentric small marker chromosome probably derived from a No. 22 (tetrasomy 22 pter → q11) associated with a characteristic phenotype. *Hum Genet* 57:148–158.

Autosomal Monosomy

Complete monosomy of most autosomes appears to be lethal unless the individual is mosaic. The other exception is perhaps represented by monosomy of the two smallest chromosomes, 21 and 22, but even here, monosomy of certain parts of the respective chromosomes provide evidence for critical region loss that may account, in large part, for the phenotypic effects. Also included within the discussion of these partial monosomies are well-defined syndromes that are likely the result of loss of contiguous genes; however, it must be recognized that some of these presumed contiguous gene syndromes may turn out to be single-gene defects, with allelism accounting for phenotypic variability.

DEL 1P36

Shapiro and colleagues (1997) have recently summarized the clinical features of this newly recognized condition. The most salient findings are postnatal growth delay with mental retardation and facial dysmorphism.

Affected females exhibited what was felt to be later catch-up growth due to "precocious" puberty, but menses commencing at 10 years does not really constitute isosexual precocity (Chapter 12). Scrotal hypoplasia and cryptorchidism have been seen in affected males, whose gonadal status is otherwise unknown (Reish et al., 1995)

REFERENCES

Reish O, Berry S A, Hirsch B (1995). Partial monosomy of chromosome 1p36.3: characterization of the critical region and delineation of the syndromes. *Am J Med Genet* 59:467–475.
Shapiro S K, McCaskill C, Northrup H, et al. (1997). Chromosome 1p36 deletions: the clinical phenotype and molecular characterization of a common newly delineated syndrome. *Am J Hum Genet* 61:642–650.

DEL 1Q42

The clinical consequences of deletions of the terminal part of the long arm of chromosome 1 (q42 → qter) were first described by Mankinen and colleagues (1976). Other reports have corroborated and extended the initial case report such that the condition should be considered a valid entity (Johnson et al., 1985; Meinecke and Vögtal, 1987). Affected children usually show growth and psychomotor retardation, microbrachycephaly, a round face with a thin upper vermillion border in a "cupids bow" configuration, a short, broad nose, and a small jaw. Absence of the corpus callosum and neural tube closure defects are also relatively common.

Affected males commonly have various degrees of hypospadias, shawl or bifid scrotum, and cryptorchidism. The original female patient had vaginal stenosis. Prominent labia have been reported in others. Functional status of the gonads in either sex is unknown.

REFERENCES

Johnson V P, Hack L J, Carter G A, et al. (1985). Deletion of the distal long arm of chromosome 1: a definable syndrome. *Am J Med Genet* 22:685–694.
Mankinen C B, Sears J W, Alverez V R (1976). Terminal (1) (q43) deletion of chromosome 1 in a three-year-old female. *Birth Defects OAS* 11(5): 132–136.
Meinecke P, Vögtal D (1987). A specific syndrome due to deletion of the distal long arm of chromosome 1. *Am J Med Genet* 28:371–376.

DEL 2Q

With long arm deletions of chromosome 2, the extent of the deletion seems to determine the phenotype. Patients with terminal loss of 2q37 have most of the salient features—developmental delay, macrocephaly with frontal bossing, depressed nasal bridge, and congenital heart disease (Conrad et al., 1995).

Hypospadias has been recorded in males, and hypoplasia of the labia has been noted in females (Jansen et al., 1982). Viot-Szoboszlai and colleagues (1998) reported an 18-month-old female with gonadal dysgenesis, bifid uterus and Wilms' tumor whose karyotype was [46,XX,del(2)(q37.1 → qter).

REFERENCES

Conrad B, Dewald G, Christensen E, et al. (1995). Clinical phenotype associated with terminal 2q37 deletion. *Clin Genet* 48:134–135.
Jansen M, Beemer F A, van der Heiden C, et al. (1982). Ring chromosome 2: clinical, chromosomal and biochemical aspects. *Hum Genet* 60:91–95.
Viot-Szoboszlai G, Amiel J, Doz F, et al. (1998). Wilms' tumor and gonadal dysgenesis in a child with the 2q37.1 deletion syndrome. *Clin Genet* 53:278–280.

DEL 4P (INCLUDES WOLF-HIRSCHHORN SYNDROME AND OTHERS)

Children with 4p deletions are usually small for gestational dates and fail to thrive. They have microcephaly with hypertelorism and a broad-based nose, along with poorly differentiated external ears. Growth and mental retardation are constant. Cleft palate and micrognathia may be present, congenital heart lesions are common, and a variety of renal anomalies may be evident as well (Gorlin et al., 1990).

The deletion may be submicroscopic. The critical region appears to be within 4p16.3 (Altherr et al., 1991). HOX7 (MSX1) is on chromosome 4p, and deletion of this locus could conceivably contribute to the phenotype.

Cryptorchidism and hypospadias are common in males, and absent uterus and streak gonads have been recorded in females (Johnson et al., 1976).

It is controversial whether the Pitt-Rogers-Danks (PRD) syndrome is a variant of the Wolf-Hirschhorn syndrome or is a separate entity also contained within 4p16.3 ("syndrome within a syndrome"). Interestingly, Partington and colleagues (1997) described three families in which translocations giving rise to deletions and duplications within 4p16.3 contained individuals with deletions and the PRD syndrome and others with duplications and a distinctive overgrowth syndrome. These authors postulated deficiency and excess of the fibroblast growth factor receptor gene 3 located in the 4p16.3 region, respectively, as being partially responsible for the phenotypic differences. Neither type of patient had recorded genital anomalies or hypogonadism.

A more proximal deletion involving 4p12p15 produced a different phenotype, also without recognized genital involvement (White et al., 1995)

REFERENCES

Altherr M R, Gusella J F, Wasmuth J J, et al. (1991). Molecular confirmation of Wolf-Hirschhorn syndrome with a subtle translocation of chromosome 4. *Am J Hum Genet* 49:1235–1242.

Gorlin R J, Cohen M M, Jr, Levin L S (1990). *Syndromes of the Head and Neck*, Oxford, New York, 3rd ed. pp 46–48.

Johnson V P, Mulder R D, Hosen R (1976). The Wolf-Hirschhorn (4p-) syndrome. *Clin Genet* 10:104–112.

Partington M W, Fagan K, Soubjaki V, et al. (1997). Translocations involving 4p16.3 in three families: deletion causing the Pitt-Rogers-Danks syndrome and duplication resulting in a new overgrowth syndrome. *J Med Genet* 34:719–728.

White D M, Pellers D M, Reiss J A, et al. (1995). Interstitial deletions of the short arm of chromosome 4 in patients with a similar combination of multiple congenital anomalies and mental retardation. *Am J Med Genet* 57:588–597.

DEL 7P

Nearly half the patients with partial monosomy 7p have craniosynostosis with variably shaped skulls depending on the suture(s) prematurely closed (Schömig-Spingler et al., 1986). Facial dysmorphism is generally related to the cranial asymmetry. Two of the patients recorded by Bianchi and colleagues (1981) had terminal duplication of the phalanx of the great toe. This finding is common in the Grieg syndrome, in which there is deletion or mutation of GL13 located in 7p.

Clitoral hypertrophy in females and hypospadias in males have been recorded (Bianchi et al., 1981; Crawfurd et al., 1979).

REFERENCES

Bianchi D, Cirillo Silengo M, Luzzatti L, et al. (1981). Interstitial deletion of the short arm of chromosome 7 without craniosynostosis. *Clin Genet* 10:456–461.

Crawfurd M, Kessel I, Liberman et al. (1979). Partial monosomy 7 with interstitial deletions in two infants with differing congenital anomalies. *J Med Genet* 16:453–460.

Schömig-Spingler M, Schmid M, Brosi W, et al. (1986). Chromosome 7 short arm deletion, 7p21 → pter. *Hum Genet* 74:323–325.

DEL 7Q (INCLUDES WILLIAMS-BEUREN SYNDROME AND OTHERS)

Terminal deletions of 7q (7q32 → qter) result in a recognizable syndrome, which includes occasional male patients with micropenis and hypospadias (Young et al., 1984), whereas the clinical findings in deletions involving more proximal bands (7q2 → 32) are nonspecific.

Visible or molecular deletions involving genes within 7q11.23 give rise to the Williams-Beuren syndrome comprising characteristic facies, developmental delay, ebullient personality, short stature, cardiovascular anomalies (mainly supravalvular aortic stenosis), and transient infantile hypercalcemia (Budarf and Emmanuel, 1997). Micropenis is common in males. Gonadal status in both sexes is probably normal, but reports of autosomal dominant transmission of the syndrome are not convincing. The 7q11.23 region includes the elastin (ELN) gene, which is quite likely responsible for the cardiovascular lesion of the Williams syndrome.

REFERENCES

Budarf M L, Emanuel B S (1997). Progress in the autosomal segmental aneusomy syndromes (SAS): single or multilocus disorders. *Hum Mol Genet* 6:1657–1665.

Young R S, Weaver D D, Kukolich M K, et al. (1984). Terminal and interstitial deletions of the long arm of chromosome 7: a review with five new cases. *Am J Med Genet* 17:437–440.

DEL 8P

Postnatal growth retardation, mental retardation, a wide, flat face, and congenital heart disease are the prominent features of 8p-, and these seem to be largely, if not solely, related to loss of the more distal segment 8p21.1 → pter (Dobyns et al., 1985; Digilio et al., 1998).

Genital anomalies in males include cryptorchidism and hypospadias. Hypogonadism has been established and it appears to be primary: elevated serum FSH levels were detected in those patients so studied (Taillemite et al., 1975).

REFERENCES

Digilio M C, Marino B, Guccione P, et al. (1998). Deletion 8p syndrome. *Am J Med Genet* 75: 534–536.

Dobyns W B, Dewald G W, Carlson R O, et al. (1985) Deficiency of chromosome 8p21.1 → 8 pter: case report and review of the literature. *Am J Med Genet* 22:125–134.

Taillemite L, Channarond J, Tinel H, et al. (1975). Délétion partiale du bras court du chromosome 8. *Ann Genet (Paris)* 20:13–17.

DEL 8Q (INCLUDES BRANCHIO-OTO-RENAL, TRICHORHINOPHALANGEAL SYNDROMES AND OTHERS

Branchio-oto-renal syndrome (BOR) is an autosomal dominant syndrome, the locus for which is located within 8q12.1-q21.2. Microdeletions in proximal 8q that are more extensive give rise to the BOR syndrome plus hydrocephalus, Duane syndrome, and perhaps other features, thereby producing a contiguous gene syndrome (Vincent et al., 1994). Genital anomalies have not been described.

Trichorhinophalangeal (TRP) syndrome type I is another autosomal dominant trait that maps to 8q. Deletion in 8q24.11 → q24.13 removes this gene and gives rise to TRP along with multiple exostoses (due to deletion of a bone growth control gene, EXT1), or so-called TRP type II, or the Langer-Giedion syndrome. Depending on the size of the deletion, mental retardation may or may not be a feature of TRP type II. Fryns (1997) described three patients with TRP type II who had hydrometrocolpos as an additional anomaly.

REFERENCES

Fryns J P (1997). Syndromic forms of hydrometrocolpos. *Prenatal Diag* 17:87.

Vincent C, Kalatzis V, Compain S, et al. (1994). A proposed new contiguous gene syndrome in 8q consists of branchio-oto-renal syndrome, Duane syndrome, a dominant form of hydrocephalus, and trapeze aplasia: implications for the mapping of the BOR gene. *Hum Mol Genet* 3:1859–1866.

DEL 9P

The dominant facial features of this syndrome are trigonocephaly and pronounced upslanting palpebral fissures, flat and elongated philtrum, and abnormal pinnae. Cardiac septal defects are common, and growth and mental retardation are probably universal.

Hypoplastic external genitalia in males with or without hypospadias occurs in roughly 40% (Huret, 1988). Sex reversal has been seen in XY males with deletions including 9p24 (reviewed in McDonald et al., 1997; see Chapters 2 and 7 for more details about this feature). The critical region for sex reversal appears to be at or distal to masker D9S1799 (Guioli et al., 1998). Gonadoblastoma has also been seen.

REFERENCES

Guioli S, Schmitt K, Critcher R, et al. (1998). Molecular analysis of 9p deletions associated with XY sex reversal: refining the localization of a sex-determining gene to the tip of the chromosome. *Am J Hum Genet* 63:905–909.

Huret J L, Leonard C, Forestier B, et al. (1988). Eleven new cases of del (9p) and features from 80 cases. *J Med Genet* 25:741–749.

McDonald M T, Flejter W, Sheldon S, et al. (1997). XY sex reversal and gonadal dysgenesis due to 9p24 monosomy. *Am J Med Genet* 73:321–326.

DEL 10P

The physical findings are not uniform because the case reports include variably deleted segments. Generally patients have microcephaly, short palpebral fissures, epicanthus, a short upturned nose, and a small jaw. If the deletion involves 10p13, hypoparathyroidism, conotruncal cardiac malformations, and T cell defects are evident (Greenberg et al., 1986)—deletion of this segment gives rise to the phenotype of DiGeorge syndrome (Schuffenhauer et al., 1995).

Hypoplastic external genitalia and cryptorchidism have been described, along with absent or hypoplastic olfactory bulbs (Hon et al., 1995), raising the possibility that the hypogenitalism is central, and might affect female gonadal function as well.

REFERENCES

Greenberg F. Valdes C, Rosenblatt H, et al. (1986). Hypoparathyroidism and T-cell immune defect in a patient with 10p deletion syndrome. *J Pediatr* 109:489–492.

Hon E, Chapman C, Gunn T R (1995). Family with partial monosomy 10p and trisomy 10p. *Am J Med Genet* 56:136–140.

Schuffenhauer S, Seidel H, Oechsler H, et al. (1995). DiGeorge syndrome and partial monosomy 10p: case report and review. *Ann Genet* 38:162–167.

DEL 10Q

Severe mental retardation, microcephaly, a prominent beaked nose, large and/or malformed ears, and cardiovascular anomalies characterize this aneusomy (Wulfsberg et al., 1989). Affected males frequently have undescended testes and micropenis, and frank sex reversal has been seen with terminal deletions from 10q26 on (Wilkie et al., 1993—see also Chapter 2 for a fuller discussion of a possible sex determination gene on 10q).

REFERENCES

Wilkie A O, Campbell F M, Danbeney P, et al. (1993). Complete and partial sex reversal associated with terminal deletion of 10q: report of 2 cases and literature review. *Am J Med Genet* 46:597–600.

Wulfsberg E A, Weaver R P, Cunniff C M, et al. (1989). Chromosome 10qter deletion syndrome: a review and report of three new cases. *Am J Med Genet* 32:364–367.

DEL 11P (INCLUDES WAGR SYNDROME)

Loss of sequences from 11p11-p13 gives rise to a contiguous gene syndrome consisting of multiple exostoses, enlarged parietal foramina, craniofacial dysostosis with brachycephaly, mental retardation, and often seizures (Bartsch et al., 1996). The region contains one of the two loci for multiple exostoses (EXT 2); the other is on chromosome 8.

Micropenis is common in males. If the deletion encompasses the WTI and PAX6 genes, some or all of the components of the WAGR syndrome would also be evident, which includes genital ambiguity in males (see Chapters 2 and 7).

REFERENCE

Bartsch O, Wuyts W, van Hul W, et al. (1996). Delineation of a continuous gene syndrome with multiple exostoses, enlarged parietal foramina, craniofacial dysostosis, and mental retardation caused by a deletion of the short arm of chromosome 11. *Am J Hum Genet* 58: 734–742.

DEL 11Q (JACOBSEN SYNDROME)

Jacobsen and colleagues (1973) described the most reproducible phenotype in a family with multiple individuals having deletion of 11q23 → qter. Trigonocephaly with either micro-or macrocephaly, mental retardation, eye anomalies (hypertelorism, strabismus, ptosis, colobomas), a carp-shaped mouth, micrognathia, cardiac anomalies, and deformities of the extremities characterize this disorder, which has many features of the C syndrome (see Chapter 15 (Wardinsky et al., 1990). The critical region for the phenotype appears to be 11q24.1 (Fryns et al., 1986).

Hypospadias and/or cryptorchidism occur in roughly half the males—who are relatively few in number, for most reported cases are female. The latter occasionally exhibit hypoplastic external genitalia.

REFERENCES

Fryns J, Kleezkowska A, Buttiene M, et al. (1986). Distal 11q monosomy. *Clin Genet* 30:255–260.

Jacobsen P, Hauge M, Henningsen K, et al. (1973). A (11;21) translocation in four generations with chromosome 11 abnormalities in the offspring. *Hum Hered* 23:568–585.

Wardinsky T D, Weinberger E, Pagon R A, et al. (1990). Partial deletion of chromosome 11 [del(11)(q23.3 → qter)] with abnormal white matter. *Am J Med Genet* 35:60–62.

DEL 13Q

Terminal deletions of 13q have been extensively analyzed by Brown and colleagues (1993,1995). Patients whose interstitial deletions are proximal to q32 exhibit mild to moderate mental retardation, growth failure, and mild facial dysmorphism. They may or may not have retinoblastoma but are at risk if the deletion includes q14. With deletions that include q32, brain, digital, ocular, and genitourinary anomalies, along with imperforate anus, occur, whereas terminal deletions of q33-34 cause severe mental retardation only. The brain malformations may be due to haploinsufficiency in ZIC2 in 13q32 (Brown et al., 1998), in which mutations cause holoprosencephaly usually with microcephaly.

While hypoplastic to frankly ambiguous genitalia are most often associated with deletions of the q32 region, penoscrotal transposition has been seen with loss of 13q33 (Gershoni-Baruch, 1996). Males with loss of the 13q32 sequence commonly have bifid or shawl scrotum, micropenis, and hypospadias; females may have a septate uterus. Urorectal septal defects/persistent cloaca have been recorded (Vittu et al., 1989; Urioste et al., 1995; Bartsch et al., 1996). Ovarian dysgenesis has been seen with a ring 13 chromosome (Cunniff et al., 1991).

The phenotype associated with terminal 13q deletions so strongly resembles that of the XK aprosencephaly syndrome that it seems quite possible that XK aprosencephaly is a microdeletion syndrome (Guala et al., 1997; see also Chapter 15).

REFERENCES

Bartsch O, Kunhle V, Wu L L, et al. (1996). Evidence for a critical region for penoscrotal inversion, hypospadias, and imperforate anus within chromosome region 13q32.2q34. *Am J Med Genet* 65:218–222.

Brown S, Gerson S, Anyane-Yaboa K, et al. (1993). Preliminary definition of a "critical region" of chromosome 13 in q32: report of 14 cases with 13q deletions and review of the literature. *Am J Med Genet* 45:52–59.

Brown S, Russo J, Chitayat D, et al. (1995). The 13q- syndrome: the molecular definition of a critical deletion region in band 13q32. *Am J Hum Genet* 57:859–866.

Brown S A, Warburton D, Brown L Y, et al. (1998). Holoprosencephaly due to mutations in ZIC2, a homologue of Drosophila odd-paired. *Nat Genet* 20:180–183.

Cunniff C, Jones K L, Benirschke K (1991). Ovarian dysgenesis in individuals with chromosome abnormalities. *Hum Genet* 86:552–556.

Gershoni-Baruch R, Zekaries D (1996). Deletion (13)(q22) with multiple congenital anomalies, hydranencephaly and penoscrotal transposition. *Clin Dysmophol* 5:289–294.

Guala A, Dellavecchia C, Mannarino S, et al. (1997). Ring chromosome 13 with loss of the region D135317-D135285: phenotypic overlap with XK syndrome. *Am J Med Genet* 72:319–323.

Urioste M, Arroyo I, Villa A, et al. (1995). Distal deletion of chromosome 13 in a child with the "Opitz" GBBB syndrome. *Am J Med Genet* 59:114–122.

Vittu G, Croquette M F, Donney A, et al. (1989). Syndrome polymorformatif léthal avec délétion 13q secondaire à une translocation maternelle X;13. *J Génét Hum* 37:141–147.

DEL 15Q (INCLUDES PRADER-WILLI SYNDROME AND OTHERS)

Loss of terminal sequences on the long arm of chromosome 15 generally give rise to a ring chromosome. Affected individuals exhibit mental and growth retardation, microcephaly, a triangular face, short fingers, and congenital heart defects.

Males may have cryptorchidism and hypospadias, and infertility has been documented in adult males with otherwise normal genitalia (Moreau and Teyssier, 1982; Butler et al., 1988).

If the interstitial deletion includes 15q11 → q13 and the involved chromosome is paternally derived, the Prader-Willi syndrome may result, in which affected individuals have hypotonia, mental retardation, characteristic facies, small hands and feet, and potentially life-threatening hyperphagia (Holm et al., 1993). In this syndrome the vast majority of males have hypogonadism with small testes, scrotal hypoplasia, and occasionally cryptorchidism. Females may have hypoplasia of the labia and clitoris, with absent or delayed menses. The available evidence suggests that the syndrome results from deletion of contiguous genes, at least some of which are imprinted, because some patients who do not have these deletions have maternal disomy (Mascari et al., 1992). The hypogonadism is likely central. Oddly enough, both precocious adrenarche and true precocious puberty have been seen (Kauli et al., 1978; Vanelli et al., 1984). Not all deletions of this region produce the typical phenotype (Schwartz et al., 1985).

One gene that is deleted in the Prader-Willi syndrome and is also paternally imprinted is the necdin-encoding gene (NDM), the murine counterpart of which apparently regulates neuron cell growth (MacDonald and Wevrick, 1997). Loss of this gene function by deletion or maternal disomy could be at least partly responsible for the CNS findings in the Prader-Willi syndrome.

REFERENCES

Butler M G, Fogo A P, Fuchs D A, et al. (1988). Two patients with ring chromosome 15 syndrome. *Am J Med Genet* 29:149–154.
Holm V A, Cassidy S B, Butler M G, et al. (1993). Prader-Willi syndrome: consensus diagnostic criteria. *Pediatrics* 91:398–402.
Kauli R, Prager-Lewin R, Laron Z (1978). Pubertal development in the Prader-Labbart-Willi syndrome. *Acta Paediatr Scand* 67:763–767.
MacDonald H R, Wevrick R (1997). The necdin gene is deleted in Prader-Willi syndrome and is imprinted in human and mouse. *Hum Mol Genet* 6:1873–1878.
Mascari M J, Gottlieb W, Rogan P K, et al. (1992). The frequency of uniparental disomy in Prader-Willi syndrome. *N Engl J Med* 326:1599–1607.
Moreau N, Teyssier M (1982). Ring chromosome 15: report of a case in an infertile man. *Clin Genet* 21:273–279.
Schwartz S, Max S R, Panny S R, et al. (1985). Deletions of proximal 15q and non-classical Prader-Willi syndrome phenotype. *Am J Med Genet* 20:255–263.
Vanelli M, Bernasconi S, Caronna N, et al. (1984). Precocious puberty in a male with Prader-Labbart-Willi syndrome. *Helv Paediatr Acta* 39:373–377.

Del 18p

As with most partial monosomic states, there is considerable phenotype variability, and no features are diagnostic. Affected children are mentally retarded and may have microcephaly. Some have holoprosencephaly with the critical region defined within 18p13 (Overhauser et al., 1995). Others have ptosis with or without epicanthal folds; hypertelorism; wide mouth; protruding, often misshapen, ears; and cardiac defects.

Underdeveloped external genitalia are often seen in both sexes (Zumel et al., 1989). Gonadal dysgenesis has been demonstrated by ultrasound in one female patient who had elevated serum gonadotropins (Telvi et al., 1995), whereas a central cause of amenorrhea has been documented in another (Stoffer et al., 1989).

REFERENCES

Overhauser J, Mitchell H F, Zachai E H, et al. (1995). Physical mapping of the holoprosencephaly critical region in 18p13. *Am J Hum Genet* 57:1080–1085.
Stoffer S S, Koen A L, Abbasi A A, et al. (1989). 46,XX, del(18p) with amenorrhea, hypothyroidism and ptosis. *Am J Med Genet* 9:285–290.
Telvi L, Bernheim A, Ion A, et al. (1995). Gonadal dysgenesis in del(18p) syndrome. *Am J Med Genet* 57:598–600.

Zumel R M, Darmanda M T, Delicado A, et al. (1989). The 18p- syndrome. Report of five cases. *Am Genet* 32:160–163.

Del 18q

The phenotype includes short stature, microcephaly with midface hypoplasia, a broad mouth, and a prominent anthelix. In general, patients are significantly mentally retarded, although there are exceptions.

Labial hypoplasia is common in females, and micropenis, scrotal hypoplasia, cryptorchidism, and hypospadias have all been seen in males (Kline et al., 1993). The gene(s) that cause the genital malformations probably lie within q22.1 → qter (Frizell et al., 1998).

REFERENCES

Frizell E R, Sutphen R, Diamond F B Jr., et al. (1998). Short report: t(1;18)(q32.1;q22.1) associated with genitourinary malformations. *Clin Genet* 34:330–333.

Kline A D, White M E, Wapner R, et al. (1993). Molecular analysis of the 18q- syndrome and correlation with phenotype. *Am J Hum Genet* 52:895–906.

Del 21q (includes monosomy 21)

Huret and colleagues (1995) have compared the physical features of patients having 21q deletions with those with apparent monosomy 21 and concluded that the two conditions cannot be reliably differentiated. The critical region for the overall phenotype appears to be in 21q22 → qter (Theodoropoulos et al., 1995), but the clinical features are not specific. Affected infants tend to be small, with down-slanting palpebral fissures, broad nose with a broad base, low-set enlarged ears, cleft palate, and, less commonly, cardiac and renal anomalies.

Micropenis, cryptorchidism, clitoromegaly, and frank genital ambiguity have also been described (Huret et al., 1995; Phillip et al., 1984).

REFERENCES

Huret J L, Léonard C, Chery M, et al. (1995). Monosomy 21q: two cases of del(21q) and review of the literature. *Clin Genet* 48:140–147.

Phillip N, Baetman M A, Mattei M G, et al. (1984). Three new cases of partial monosomy 21 resulting from one ring 21 chromosome and two unbalanced reciprocal translocations. *Eur J Pediatr* 142:61–64.

Theodoropoulos D S, Cowan J M, Elias E, et al. (1995). Physical findings in 21q22 deletions suggest critical region for 21q- phenotype in q22. *Am J Med Genet* 59:161–163.

Del 22q (DiGeorge syndrome and others)

Deletions of variable length gives rise to a spectrum of malformations. Classically, the DiGeorge syndrome involves the craniofacies, the heart, thymus, and parathyroid glands, but other organs can be affected as well (Ryan et al., 1997). Hence, contained within this chromosome region may be a gene or genes responsible for the velocardiofacial (Shprintzen) syndrome, for familial conotruncal defects, familial hypoparathyroidism, the Opitz G/BBB syndrome (Chapter 15), and so forth. The smallest chromosome region that can produce the entire clinical picture is loss of

22q11 (Kurahashi et al., 1996). A number of candidate genes are present within the region, but specific mutations have not been identified (Budarf and Emanuel, 1997).

A recent collaborative European study reported renal anomalies in more than a third of 136 patients. There was an 8% incidence of undescended testes. Present but less common were micropenis, hypospadias, and shawl scrotum.

REFERENCES

Budarf M L, Emanuel B S (1997). Progress in the autosomal aneusomy syndromes (SASs): single or multilocus disorders. *Hum Mol Genet* 6:1657–1665.

Kurahashi H, Nakayama T, Osugi Y, et al. (1996). Deletion mapping of 22q11 in CATCH syndrome: identification of a second critical region. *Am J Hum Genet* 58:1377–1381.

Ryan A K, Goodship J A, Wilson D I, et al. (1997). Spectrum of clinical features associated with interstitial chromosome 22q11 deletions: a European collaborative study. *J Med Genet* 34:798–804.

POLYPLOIDY

There are numerous case reports of fetuses and occasionally viable infants with triploidy or tetraploidy; most of the surviving individuals are mosaic for a diploid cell line (mixoploidy). Blackburn and colleagues (1982) and Wilson and colleagues (1988) have reviewed the phenotypes.

Affected males generally exhibit abnormal genitalia—micropenis, cryptorchidism, hypoplastic scrotum—even to the point of sexual ambiguity. The external genital features in females are less consistent. They usually include hypoplasia, but occasionally clitoral enlargement is sufficient to cause diagnostic uncertainty. Both trisomy 13 and 18 are associated with ovarian dysgenesis, so similar findings in trisomic/tetrasomic states are not surprising. Hence, although sex chromosome imbalance might be causally inferred in sexual maldevelopment in these cases, autosomal imbalance is more likely to be responsible, as in cases in which the karyotype has been further expanded by supernumerary X or Y chromosomes (e.g., 70,XXYY) (Meisner et al., 1987). However, there are possible exceptions—for example, the 71, XXXXY female reported by Maaswinkel-Mooij and colleagues (1992).

REFERENCES

Blackburn W R, Miller W P, Superneau D W, et al. (1982). Comparative studies in infants with mosaic and complete triploidy: an analysis of 55 cases. *Birth Defects (OAS)* 18(3B): 251–274.

Maaswinkel-Mooij P D, van Zwieten P, Mollervanger P, et al. (1992). A girl with 71,XXXXY karyotype. *Clin Genet* 41:96–99.

Meisner L F, Lorie L R, Aryas S, et al. (1987). Triploidy with an extra sex chromosome (70,XXYY) and increased alpha fetoprotein. *Birth Defects (OAS)* 23:333–339.

Wilson G N, Vekemans M J J, Kaplan P (1988). MCA/MR syndrome in a female infant with tetraploidy mosaicism: review of the human polyploid phenotype. *Am J Med Genet* 30: 953–965.

V

GENETIC FORMS OF GAMETE FAILURE

19

Genetic Disorders of Gamete Delivery

One can envision "gamete failure" as a progression of possible abnormal events beginning with impaired migration of primordial germ cells to the gonadal ridge and ending with impaired function of the egg or sperm at, and just after, fertilization. Intermediate defects could include impaired gametogenesis, impaired storage of gametes, and impaired delivery of gametes to the location of fertilization.

Impaired spermatogenesis with Yq alterations was discussed in Chapter 5 as a form of testicular maldevelopment and accelerated oocyte attrition was discussed in Chapter 6 as one consequence of X chromosome aberrations leading to ovarian maldevelopment. In Chapter 16, we dealt with several overlapping disorders of gamete delivery affecting females, under the terms vaginal septa, vaginal atresia, and müllerian aplasia.

In this chapter, we deal with two discrete disorders of gamete delivery that affect males. In the following chapter, we present autosomal genomic and chromosomal disorders associated with impaired gametogenesis. This is followed by a survey of mutations in the mouse that impair male fertility, female fertility, or both.

As researchers exploit orthologous and syntenic relations between the human and mouse genomes, it is likely that much will soon be learned about the genetics of human infertility from these mutations.

Kartagener Syndrome with Dysfunctional Sperm

Kartagener first described a hereditary disease consisting of situs inversus, bronchiectasis, and chronic sinusitis (Kartagener, 1933). The "immotile-cilia syndrome" was the term designed for hereditary disease with ultrastructural abnormalities of the ciliary dynein arms resulting in bronchiectasis and sinusitis (Afzelius, 1976). The association with male sterility was soon recognized (Eliasson et al., 1977) but the realization that situs inversus only occurred in about half of the patients with immotile cilia took longer (Afzelius, 1981). It has been postulated that ciliary movement is involved in the normal rotations of viscera and that with ciliary abnormalities, a right-sided or left-sided heart occurs with fifty-fifty probability. Thus, one eighth of the children of carrier parents have situs inversus plus chronic sinusitis and bronchiectasis and another one eighth have only the chronic sinusitis and bronchiectasis; males in both groups are usually sterile because of defective sperm.

Clinical and Imaging Presentation. Recurrent episodes of sinusitis, bronchiectases, and otitis media may lead to an early diagnosis. This is especially true if x-rays performed to study bronchitis reveal dextrocardia. In some cases, the patient's chronic infections have not led to the diagnosis of Kartagener syndrome, and male sterility leads to evaluations. Polysplenia, another aspect of laterality defects (along with asplenia) has sometimes been found (Schidlow et al., 1982).

Laboratory Features. Studies of tracheobronchial mucociliary clearance will confirm a defect in ciliary motility. Scrapings of nasal mucosa may be examined under the microscope to observe ciliary motion. Frequently the cilia are dysmotile rather than immotile (Rossman et al., 1980). Electron microscopy of biopsies of ciliated tissues may disclose a variety of abnormalities: (1) dynein arms that are short or absent or spokes that are shorter or absent; (2) random orientation of cilia, or (3) a high proportion of cilia with extra or absent microtubules (Sturgess et al., 1979, 1980; Afzelius, 1981; Antonelli et al., 1981). Semen analysis usually shows immotile sperm, but some individuals with Kartagener syndrome have been infertile despite motile sperm (Jonsson et al., 1982).

Genotyping. Most families have shown a pattern of inheritance highly consistent with autosomal recessive inheritance for the bronchiectasis and chronic sinusitis, whereas situs inversus is present in only about 50% of these affected individuals (Moreno and Murphy, 1981). One pedigree has been strongly consistent with X-linked inheritance (Narayan et al., 1994, and another has shown linkage to microsatellites mapping to Xq24-q27.1 (Casey et al., 1993). To our knowledge, linkage for the usual autosomal recessive forms has not yet been found. This may well be due to the expected extent of locus heterogeneity. Over 100 components of the cilia are known (Afzelius, 1981) and the multiplicity of likely defective genes is exposed by the variety of pathological pictures seen by electron microscopy. Several mouse mutations affect situs laterality (Klar, 1994), which, again, suggests heterogeneity and provides candidate regions using the mouse-human synteny map while human dynein genes preferentially expressed in testes provide other candidates (Kastury, et al, 1997). Mapping recessive diseases is, of course, much more difficult than mapping dominant ones; the probable great locus heterogeneity causing this syndrome will make the task all the greater.

Discussion. Kartagener syndrome usually presents as a chronic respiratory illness, but the immotile spermatozoa often result in infertility and a semen analysis may be the first clue to the ciliary dyskinesis problem. Although genetic analysis of these disorders has been slow, the cloning of sperm-specific ciliary proteins (Gastmann et al., 1993; Milisav et al., 1996) indicates that there ought to be a class of patients with immotile spermatozoa but without the chronic respiratory problems. Undoubtedly, such cases will soon come to light.

REFERENCES

Afzelius B A (1976). A human syndrome caused by immotile cilia. *Science* 193:317–319.

Afzelius B A (1981). Genetical and ultrastructural aspects of the immotile-cilia syndrome. *Am J Hum Genet* 33:852–864.

Antonelli M, Modesti A, De Angelis M, Marcolini P, Lucarelli N, Crifo S (1981). Immotile cilia syndrome: radial spokes deficiency in a patient with Kartagener's triad. *Acta Paediatr Scand* 70P:571–573.

Casey B, Devoto M, Jones K L, Ballabio A (1993). Mapping a gene for familial situs abnormalities to human chromosome Xq24-q27.1. *Nat Genet* 5:403–407.

Eliasson R, Mossberg B, Camner P, Afzelius B A (1977). The immotile-cilia syndrome: a congenital ciliary abnormality as an etiologic factor in chronic airway infections and male sterility. *N Engl J Med* 297:1–6.

Gastmann O, Burfeind P, Gunther E, Hameister H, Szpirer C, Hoyer-Fender S (1993). Sequence, expression, and chromosomal assignment of a human sperm outer dense fiber gene. *Mol Reprod Dev* 36:407–418.

Jonsson M S, McCormick J R, Gillies C G, Gondos B (1982). Kartagener syndrome with motile spermatozoa. *N Engl J Med* 307:1131–1133.

Kartagener M (1933). Zur Pathogenese der Bronchiektasien: Bronchiektasien bei situs viscerum inversus. *Beitr Klin Tuberk* 83:489–501.

Kastury K, Taylor W E, Shen R, Arver S, Gutierrez M, Fisher C E, Coucke P J, Van Hauwe P, Van Camp G, Bhasin S (1997). Complementary deoxyribonucleic acid cloning and characterization of a putative human axonemal dynein light chain gene. *J Clin Endocrinol Metab* 82:3047–3053.

Klar A J S (1994). A model for specification of the left-right axis in vertebrates. *Trends Genet* 10:392–396.

Milisav I, Jones M H, Affara N A (1996). characterization of a novel human dynein-related gene that is specifically expressed in testis. *Mamm Genome* 7:667–672.

Moreno A, Murphy E A. (1981). Inheritance of Kartagener syndrome. *Am J Med Genet* 8:305–313.

Narayan D, Krishnan S N, Upender M, Ravikumar T S, Mahoney M J, Dolan Jr, T F, Teebi A S, Haddad G G (1994). Unusual inheritance of primary ciliary dyskinesia (Kartagener's syndrome). *J Med Genet* 31:493–496.

Rossman C, Forrest J, Newhouse M (1980). Motile cilia in "immotile cilia" syndrome. *Lancet* 1:1360.

Schidlow D V, Cats S M, Turtz M G, Donner R M, Capasso S (1982). Polysplenia and Kartagener's syndrome in a sibship: association with abnormal respiratory cilia. *J Pediatr* 100: 401–403.

Sturgess J M, Chao J, Wong J, Aspin N, Turner J A P (1979). Cilia with defective radial spokes: a cause of human respiratory disease. *N Engl J Med* 300:53–56.

Sturgess J M, Chao J, Turner J A P (1980). Transposition of ciliary microtubules. *N Engl J Med* 303:318–322.

OBSTRUCTIVE AZOOSPERMIA AND MUTATIONS IN THE CYSTIC FIBROSIS TRANSMEMBRANE CONDUCTANCE REGULATOR

Congenital absence of the vas deferens is a rare cogenital malformation but one that may explain infertility in 1.3% of infertile men (Jequier et al., 1985; Goldstein and Schlossberg, 1988); the condition may occur in siblings (Budde et al., 1984). It has long been known that almost all males affected with cystic fibrosis have congenital bilateral absence of the vas deferens (CBAVD; Kaplan et al., 1968; Olson and Weaver, 1969). (It is probable that the vas deferens develops and is then reabsorbed because of blockage.) Thus, when the gene for cystic fibrosis, the cystic fibrosis transmembrane conductance regulator gene (*CFTR*), was cloned, it became possible to study individuals with congenital absence of the vas deferens for mutations in this gene. It was quickly found that nearly 50% of men with CBAVD were heterozygous for the ΔF508 mutation of the *CFTR* gene (Rigot et al., 1991). This represents a frequency of about 10 times that expected. Thus, many mutations in the *CFTR* were sought in men with CBAVD. These studies are the subject of this section.

Clinical and Imaging Presentation. Most cases are ascertained because of infertility and the demonstration of azoospermia on semen analysis. The scrotal vas deferens is usually not palpable on physical examination and its absence can be confirmed by vasography or transrectal ultrasonography (Kuligowska and Fenlon, 1998). The latter will reveal that nearly all those with bilateral vasal agenesis also have absent ejaculatory ducts and abnormal seminal vesicles.

Laboratory Features. Semen analysis shows azoospermia. Although the frequency of detecting serum anti-sperm antibodies has varied greatly in different studies (Amelar et al., 1975; Girgis et al., 1982; Patrizio et al., 1992), about 50 % of men with congenital absence of the vas deferens will have circulating IgG or IgA antibody to sperm.

Genotyping. Early studies suggested certain mutant alleles were particularly associated with congenital absence of the vas deferens. For instance, the R117H mutation was found to be strongly associated with CBAVD, both in the heterozygous (Gervais et al., 1993) and homozygous (Bienvenu et al., 1993) condition. As studies of CFTR continued, the percentage of men with CBAVD and documented mutations in the gene has increased (up to 82%; Oates and Amos, 1994) and the classes of mutations extended. There is a polypyrimidine tract in intron 8, and individuals vary in the number of pyrimidines on one strand in this tract; there are 5T, 7T, and 9T variants. The 5T variant is believed to result in less efficient splicing of exon 9 and reduced CFTR expression (Kiesewetter et al., 1993). It appears that there is a stronger influence of the 5T variant on decreased splicing in vasa tissue than in nasal epithelium, suggesting a mechanism for the absence of pulmonary pathology (Mak et al., 1997). The frequency of this variant is found to be markedly increased when it is located trans to *CFTR* mutations in CBAVD (Jarvi et al., 1995; Chillón et al., 1995). Thus, decreased expression of functional CFTR, due to either mild mutations or compound heterozygosity for more severe mutations with the intronic variant, are found in a high frequency of CBAVD patients. Presumably, this decreased expression of the CFTR results in abnormal development of the vas deferens. The altered status for CFTR in these patients can also be detected by studies of nasal epithelial chloride ion transport (Osborne et al., 1993). CBAVD is sometimes associated with renal anomalies. This association reflects a shared developmental ancestry in the wolffian duct. These individuals are rarely found to have *CFTR* mutations (Schlegel et al., 1996).

Management. Sperm aspiration with subsequent *in vitro* fertilization allows conception for some individuals with CBAVD (Silber et al., 1990). Of course, because most of these individuals are carriers for *CFTR* mutations with propensity for serious disease if found in homozygous or compound heterozygous states with other severe alleles, it is important for the egg donor to be tested for *CFTR* status.

Discussion. Perhaps one of the most intriguing aspects of *CFTR* mutations and congenital bilateral absence of the vas deferens is the phenotypic heterogeneity found with the same mutations (which is also true of classic cystic fibrosis). R117H compound heterozygotes with ΔF508 sometimes present with mild cystic fibrosis and sometimes only with CBAVD (Williams et al., 1993). An individual with ΔF508 on one chromosome, and a F508C polymorphism on the other chromosome, had CBAVD (Meschede et al., 1993); in another case, this same genotype with an additional polymorphism (M470C) resulted in a perfectly normal male (Desgeorges et al., 1994). Other examples of both fertility and sterility from the same combination of *CFTR* alleles in families are reported by both Mercier and colleagues (1995) and Rave-Harel and colleagues (1995). Modifying genes outside the *CFTR* region, and/ or stochastic factors, must be implicated in this phenotypic heterogeneity, for the same *CFTR* alleles were being inherited in these families.

REFERENCES

Amelar R D, Dubin L, Schoenfeld C (1975). Circulating sperm-agglutinating antibodies in azoospermic men with congenital biateral absence of the vasa deferentia. *Fertil Steril* 26: 228–231.

Bienvenu T, Beldjord C, Adjiman M, Kaplan J C (1993). Male infertility as the only presenting sign of cystic fibrosis when homozygous for the mild mutation R117H. *J Med Genet* 30: 797.

Budde W J A M, Verjaal M, Hamerlynck J V T H, Borrow M (1984). Familial occurrence of azoospermia and extreme oligozoospermia. *Clin Genet* 26:555–562.

Chillón M, Casals T, Mercier B, Bassas, L, Lissens W, Silber S, Romey M C, Ruiz-Romero J, Verlingue C, Claustres M, Nunes V, Férec C, Estivill X (1995). Mutations in the cystic fibrosis gene in patients with congenital absence of the vas deferens. *N Engl J Med* 332: 1475–1480.

Desgeorges M, Kjellberg P E, Demaille J, Claustres M (1994). A healthy male with compound and double heterozygosities for ΔF508, F508C, and M47OV in exon 10 of the cystic fibrosis gene. *Am J Hum Genet* 54:384–385.

Gervais R, Dumur V, Rigot J-M, Lafitte J-J, Roussel P, Claustres M, Demaille J (1993). High frequency of the R117H cystic fibrosis mutation in patients with congenital absence of the vas deferens. *N Engl J Med* 328:446–447.

Girgis S M, Ekladious E M, Iskander R, El-Dakhly R, Girgis F N (1982). Sperm antibodies in serum and semen in men with bilateral congenital absence of the vas deferens. *Arch Androl* 8:301–305.

Goldstein M, Schlossberg S (1988). Men with congenital absence of the vas deferens often have seminal vesicles. *J Urol* 140:85–86.

Jarvi K, Zielenski J, Wilschanski M, Durie P, Buckspan M, Tullis E, Markiewicz D, Tsui L-C (1995). Cystic fibrosis transmembrane conductance regulator and obstructive azoospermia. *Lancet* 345:1578.

Jequier A M, Ansell I D, Bullimore N J (1985). Congenital absence of the vasa deferentia presenting with infertility. *J Androl* 6:15–19.

Kaplan E, Swachman H, Perlmutter A D, Rule A, Khaw K-T, Holsclaw D S (1968). Reproductive failure in males with cystic fibrosis. *N Engl J Med* 279:65–69.

Kiesewetter S, Macek M Jr, Davis C, Curristin S M, Chu C-S, Graham C, Shrimpton A E (1993). A mutation in CFTR produces different phenotypes depending on chromosomal background. *Nat Genet* 5:274–278.

Kuligowska E, Fenlon H M (1998). Transrectal US in male infertility: spectrum of findings and role in patient care. *Radiology* 207:173–181.

Macek M Jr, Ladanyi L, Bürger J, Reis A. Missense variations in the cystic fibrosis gene: heteroduplex formation in the F508C mutation. (1992) *Am J Hum Genet* 51:1173–1174.

Mak V, Jarvi K A, Zielenski J, Durie P, Tsui L-C (1997). Higher proportion of intact exon 9 CFTR mRNA in nasal epithelium compared with vas deferens. *Hum Mol Genet* 6:2099–2107.

Mercier B, Verlingue C, Lissens W, Silber S J, Novelli G, Bonduelle M, Audrézet M P, Férec C (1995). Is congenital bilateral absence of vas deferens a primary form of cystic fibrosis? Analyses of the *CFTR* gene in 67 patients. *Am J Hum Genet* 56:272–277.

Meschede D, Eigel A, Horst J, Nieschlag E (1993). Compound heterozygosity for the ΔF508 and F508C cystic fibrosis transmembrane conductance regulator (*CFTR*) mutations in a patient with congenital bilateral aplasia of the vas deferens. *Am J Hum Genet* 53:292–293.

Oates R D, Amos J A (1994). The genetic basis of congenital bilateral absence of the vas deferens and cystic fibrosis. *J Androl* 15:1–8.

Olson J R, Weaver D K (1969) Congenital mesonephric defects in male infants with mucoviscidosis. *J Clin Pathol* 22:725–730.

Osborne L R, Lynch M, Middleton P G, Alton E W F W, Geddes D M, Pryor J P, Hodson M E, Santis G K (1993). Nasal epithelial ion transport and genetic analysis of infertile men with congenital bilateral absence of the vas deferens. *Hum Mol Genet* 2:1605–1609.

Patrizio P, Silber S J, Ord T, Moretti-Rojas I, Asch R H (1992). Relationship of epididymal sperm antibodies to their *in vitro* fertilization capacity in men with congenital absence of the vas deferens. *Fertil Steril* 58:1006–1010.

Rave-Harel N, Madgar I, Goshen R, Nissim-Rafinia M, Ziadni A, Rahat A, Chiba O, Kalman Y M, Brautbar C, Levinson D, Augarten A, Kerem E, Kerem B (1995). CFTR haplotype analysis reveals genetic heterogeneity in the etiology of congenital bilateral aplasia of the vas deferens. *Am J Hum Genet* 56:1359–1366.

Rigot J M, Lafitte J J, Dumur V, Gervais R, Manouvrier S, Biserte J, Mazeman E, Roussel P (1991). Cystic fibrosis and congenital absence of the vas deferens. *N Engl J Med* 325:64–65.

Schlegel P N, Shin D, Goldstein M (1996). Urogenital anomalies in men with congenital absence of the vas deferens. *J Urol* 155:1644–1648.

Silber S J, Ord T, Balmaceda J, Patrizio P, Asch R H (1990). Congenital absence of the vas deferens: the fertility capacity of human epididymal sperm. *N Engl J Med* 323:1788–1792.

Williams C, Mayall E S, Williamson R (1993). A report on CF carrier frequency among men with infertility owing to congenital absence of the vas deferens. *J Med Genet* 30:973.

20

Autosomal Genomic and Chromosomal Disorders with Meiotic Abnormalities Causing Impaired Gametogenesis

Autosomal Imbalance and Infertility

Changes in the number and configuration of the autosomes are well known to be associated more frequently with male infertility than with female infertility. This fact is well exemplified by the situation in Down syndrome: fertile, apparently non-mosaic males are so rare as to be reportable (Sheridan, et al., 1989); in contrast, women with Down syndrome have normal menstrual cycles (Goldstein, 1988), and a number of them have had pregnancies (Sheridan, et al., 1989). The same sex difference occurs in mice, where a number of chromosomal changes affecting male fertility but not female fertility are known (Searle, 1974). Basic differences in meiosis between the two sexes are reflected in their timing (prenatal in females and post-pubertal in males) and in recombination frequencies (genome-wide average in females nearly twice that in males). A number of cytogenetic surveys on infertile males have documented a relatively high frequency of abnormalities of number or association of autosomes paired with male infertility (Table 20-1). These surveys

TABLE 20-1. Autosomal Genomic and Chromosomal Abnormalities Associated with Male Infertility

Condition	Incidence among Infertile Men	References
Reciprocal autosomal translocations	0.4%–0.7%	Chandley, 1979; Testart et al., 1996
X-autosomal translocations	rare	Madan, 1983; Chandley, 1979
Robertsonian translocations	0.16%–2.3%	Chandley, 1979; Testart et al., 1996
Pericentric inversions	rare–0.7%	Chandley, et al., 1987; Testart et al., 1996
Marker chromosomes	0.16%–0.4%	Chandley, 1979; Testart et al., 1996
Trisomy 21	0.06%	Hsiang et al., 1987

have revealed that autosomal abnormalities are more frequently associated with oligospermia, while sex chromosome abnormalities are more frequently associated with azoospermia (Van Assche et al., 1996). On the other hand, similar surveys on females did not expose a higher frequency of cytogenetic abnormalities among infertile females than in control populations, and one survey, at least, was discontinued because of the very low yield of chromosomal abnormalities (Chandley, 1979).

REFERENCES

Chandley AC (1979). The chromosomal basis of human infertility. *Brit Med Bull* 35: 181–186.

Chandley AC, McBeath S, Speed RM (1987). Pericentric inversion in human chromosome 1 and the risk for male sterility. *J Med Genet* 24: 325–334.

Goldstein H (1988). Menarche, menstruation, sexual relations and contraception of adolescent females with Down syndrome. *Eur J Obstet Gynecol Reprod Biol* 27: 343–349.

Hsiang Y-HH, Berkovitz GD, Bland GL, Migeon CJ, Warren AC (1987). Gonadal function in patients with Down syndrome. *Am J Med Genet* 27: 449–458.

Madan K (1983). Balanced structural changes involving the human X: effect on sexual phenotype. *Hum Genet* 63: 216–221.

Searle AG (1974). Nature and consequences of induced chromosome damage in mammals. *Genetics* 78: 173–186.

Sheridan R, Llerene J Jr, Matkins S, Debenham P, Cawood A, Bobrow M (1989). Fertility in a male with trisomy 21. *J Med Genet* 26: 294–298.

Testart J, Gautier E, Brami C, Rolet F, Sedbon E (1996). Intracytoplasmic sperm injection in infertile patients with structural chromosome abnormalities. *Hum Reprod* 11: 2609–2612.

Van Assche E, Bonduelle M, Tournaye H, Joris H, Verheyen G, Devroey P, Van Steirteghem A, Liebaers I (1996). Cytogenetics of infertile men. *Hum Reprod* 11:1–24; discussion 25–26.

AUTOSOMAL CHROMOSOME ABNORMALITIES WITH MALE INFERTILITY

There are a number of karyotypic changes that have been found in infertile men (Table 20-1). Although relatively rare, they are common enough that approximate incidence figures can be given for the different varieties. The frequency is high enough that men with idiopathic infertility usually have karyotypes performed during examination and evaluation for infertility. In any event, it is strongly recommended that karyotypes be performed before intracytoplasmic sperm injection (ICSI) is used in the treatment of male infertility due to severe oligospermia or azoospermia (Johnson, 1998). Many of these chromosomal changes could result in

TABLE 20-2. Autosomal Genomic and Chromosomal Abnormalities Associated with Ovarian Dysgenesis

Condition	Oocyte Abundance	References
Trisomy 21	decreased	Hojager et al., 1978
Trisomy 18	markedly decreased	Russell and Altshuler, 1975; Cunniff et al., 1991
Trisomy 13	rare	Cunniff et al., 1991
Lethal translocations	rare or decreased	Cunniff et al., 1991

offspring with severely imbalanced chromosomes (Gianaroli, et al, 1997). Knowledge of their presence allows detection of such abnormalities after ICSI, either before implantation or after amniocentesis.

REFERENCES

Gianaroli L, Munn S, Magli MC, Ferraretti AP (1997). Preimplantation genetic diagnosis of aneuploidy and male infertility. *Intl J Androl* 20: 31–34.

Goldstein H (1988). Menarche, menstruation, sexual relations and contraception fo adolescent females with Down syndrome. *Eur J Obstet Gynecol Reprod Biol* 27: 343–349.

Johnson MD (1998). Genetic risks of intracytoplasmic sperm injection in the treatment of male infertility: recommendations for genetic counseling and screening. *Fertility and Sterility* 70: 397–411.

AUTOSOMAL CHROMOSOME ABNORMALITIES ASSOCIATED WITH OVARIAN DYSGENESIS

Except for trisomy 21, most of the genomic mutations known to be associated with oogenic failure, presumably due to meiotic arrest, are lethal. Therefore, the information in Table 20-2 had to be obtained from autopsy specimens. Female meiosis seems to be very insensitive to meiotic arrest caused by autosomal chromosome imbalance. This may reflect a different sensitivity to abnormal pairing of the unpaired autosomal segment with the X chromosomes (Lyon and Meredith, 1966). In females, this pairing will not interfere with X-inactivation (since both Xs are active at this time), while in males such pairing may interfere with the obligatory X-inactivation during spermatogenesis (Forejt, 1982; see Klinefelter syndrome Chapter 6).

REFERENCES

Cunniff C, Jones KY, Benirschke K (1991). Ovarian dysgenesis in individuals with chromosomal abnormalities. *Hum Genet* 86: 552–556.

Forejt J (1972). X-Y involvement in male sterility caused by autosome translocations: a hypotheses. *In:* Genetic control of gamete production and function. (Proc Serono Clinical Colloquia on Reproducton No. 3) Crosignani PG, Rubin BL, Fraccaro M (eds), Academic Press, New York, 261–273.

Hojager B, Peters H, Byskov AG, Faber M (1978). Follicular development in ovaries of children with Down's syndrome. *Acta Paediatr Scand* 67: 637–643.

Lyon MF, Meredith R (1966). Autosomal translocations causing male sterility and viable aneuploidy in the mouse. *Cytogenetics* 5: 335–354.

Russell P, Altshuler G (1975). The ovarian dysgenesis of trisomy 18. *Pathology* 7: 149–155.

21

Mouse Models of Infertility

MUTATIONS WITH EFFECTS ON MALE FERTILITY

Many mutations are known to affect male fertility in inbred strains of mice and a number of these are presented in Table 21–1. They have been subdivided according to whether they affect germ cell migration, germ cell–Sertoli cell interaction, meiosis, or sperm differentiation. This is not a complete classification of the possibilities, for instance, hormonal influences on gonad function were discussed in Chapters 10–14. Nonetheless, several generalizations can be made. The first is that a number of mutations affect germ cell migration and, because of the deficiency of germ cells in the resultant gonad, cause decreased fertility or sterility. In the case of *Steel* and *White-spotting*, the molecular mechanism has been elucidated. *White-spotting* codes for the *c-kit* tyrosine kinase receptor on germ cells (Flanagan and Leder, 1990). *Steel* codes for the stem cell factor that is the ligand for this *c-kit* receptor (Zsebo et al., 1990). Thus, this pair of mutations forms a complementary pair defined by a receptor and its ligand. Their defective interaction seems to prevent proper homing

TABLE 21–1. Mutations with Effects on Male Fertility

Gene	Phenotype	Female Effect	Reference
Germ Cell Migration			
at (atrichosis)	Sertoli cell only	Yes	Hummell, 1966 Handell and Eppig, 1979
gcd (germ cell deficient)	Sertoli cell only	Yes	Duncan et al., 1995
Steel	Deficient germ cells	Yes	Bennet 1956
ter	Teratomas & Sertoli cell only	No	Noguchi and Noguchi, 1985
White-spotting	Sertoli cell only	Yes	Mintz and Russell, 1957
Germ Cell/Sertoli Cell Interaction			
jsd (juvenile spermatogonial cell depletion)	Early loss of germ cells	No	Beamer et al., 1988
mshi (male sterility and histoincompatibility)	Disorganized spermatogenesis suggesting abnormal Sertoli cell function	No	Ward-Bailey et al., 1996
Meiosis			
sks (skeletal fusions with sterility)	Spermatogonial arrest	Yes	Handel et al., 1988
Sperm Differentiation			
lvs (lacking vigorous sperm)	Abnormally shaped nuclei	No	Magram and Bishop, 1991
bs (blind-sterile)	Arrest of post-spermatid differentiation	No	Varnum, 1983
hop (hop sterile)	Sperm tails absent or highly modified	No	Johnson and Hunt, 1971
hpy (hydrocephalic-polydactyly)	Partially assembled sperm structure	No	Bryan, 1977
azh (abnormal spermatozoon headshape)	Abnormal manchette structure but fertile	No	Cole et al., 1988
ps (pink-eyed, sterile)	Giant sperm with abnormal heads and multiple tails	No	Hunt and Johnson, 1971
pcd (purkinje cell degeneration)	Sperm with abnormally shaped heads and tails	No	Handel and Dawson, 1981
qk (quaking)	Abnormal sperm heads and flagella	No	Sidman et al., 1964
wr (wobbler)	Defects in sperm tail structure	Yes	Leestma and Sepsenwol, 1980

of the germ cells to the gonadal ridge. Piebaldism is a human homologue of *White-spotting* (Giebel and Spritz, 1991; Fleischman et al., 1991); the dominantly inherited human mutations are obviously not associated with sterility. A second class of mutation involves germ cell–Sertoli cell interactions. In this case, it is presumed that a defect in trophic factors from the Sertoli cells leads to an early loss of germ cells (*jsd*) or disorganized spermatogenesis (*mshi*). It is not surprising that genes affecting meiosis (more vividly illustrated by several knockouts—see next section) affect gamete development. Some human pedigrees suggest autosomal recessive (Chaganti et al., 1980) or sex-linked (Chaganti et al., 1979) inheritance of meiotic abnormalities. The more complete genetic analyses in mice indicate that multiple autosomal (Blecher et al., 1981; Biddle et al., 1985) and sex-linked loci (Biddle et al., 1985) are involved. Finally, there are many mutations of sperm differentiation that illustrate that it is not only the Y chromosome that contains many genes requisite for normal male gametogenesis.

KNOCKOUTS WITH EFFECTS ON MALE FERTILITY

An interesting finding from many knockout studies is the frequency with which male fertility has been affected. Some of these knockouts were designed to affect genes with suspected roles in spermatogenesis. These knockouts are summarized in Table 21–2 (if an official gene symbol for the gene encoding the protein is not available, the name of the protein is used). The knockout of acrosin, a sperm tryptic-like enzyme thought to be essential for zona pellucida penetration, is still fertile but shows delayed *in vitro* fertilization (Adham et al., 1997). Defects in a number of genes whose roles in meiosis were known or suspected have caused male sterility. This is not surprising given the crucial role of meiosis in forming gametes. Perhaps more surprising has been the finding of male sterility with a number of knockouts whose genes were not suspected to have an affect on gamete formation. For instance, in the apo-B (apolipoprotein B) knockout, males are mostly sterile despite normal-appearing sperm (Huang et al., 1995). Given the blood-testes barrier, apo-B would not have been thought to be important in the metabolism of cells within the spermatogenic tubule. Perhaps the effect relates to malfunction of structures important for sperm after they leave the testes, the epididymides and/or vas deferens.

MUTATIONS AFFECTING FEMALE FERTILITY

Very few mutations are known that specifically affect female fertility. This may be a reflection of the fact that an oocyte is not as highly differentiated a structure as a spermatozoan. Not surprisingly, mutations that affect germ cell migration (Table 21–1) usually affect female gametogenesis as well as male. Also, some mutations affecting meiosis also affect oogenesis. The fact that other mutations (knockouts) affect only male meiosis, and not female, points out important differences in male and female meiosis that are also reflected in different frequencies of recombination. There is one example of a knockout affecting female fertility and not male—p27^{kip1}-deficient mice show female, but not male, sterility (Fero et al., 1996).

TABLE 21–2. Knockouts with Effects on Male Fertility (in homozygotes unless otherwise indicated)

Gene or Protein	Phenotype	Reference
Gene Function Known/Predicted to Affect Male Fertility		
acrosin	Delayed *in vitro* fertilization (but still fertile)	Adham et al., 1997
Bmp8b (bone morphogenetic protein 8)	Variable germ-cell deficiency and infertility	Zhao et al., 1996
calmegin (calnexin-like endo-plasmic reticulum chaperone)	Nearly sterile, sperm do not adhere to egg matrix	Ikawa et al., 1997
ACEt (angiotensin converting enzyme, testicular)	Markedly reduced fertility	Krege et al., 1995
Sprm-1 (male germ cell POU transcription factor)	Subfertility	Pearse II et al., 1997
Genes Affecting Meiosis		
mHR6B (ubiquitin-conjugating enzyme)	Post-meiotic condensation of chromatids defective	Roest et al., 1996
Mlh1 (mismatch-repair related gene)	Prematurely separated chromosomes, arrest in meiosis I	Baker et al., 1996 Edelmann et al., 1996
pms2 (mismatch-repair related gene)	Only abnormal spermatozoa found	Baker et al., 1995
Genes with Unknown Relationship to Male Fertility		
apo B (apolipoprotein B)	Male heterozygotes predominantly sterile despite normal-appearing sperm	Huang et al., 1995
ATM	Meiotic chromosomal fragmentation	Xu et al., 1996
CREM (cAMP) response element modulator)	Defective spermiogenesis	Nantel et al., 1996 Blendy et al., 1996
dhh (desert hedgehog)	Arrested spermatogenesis	Bitgood et al., 1996
γ-glutamyl transpeptidase	Hypoplastic testes, seminal vesicles, and epididymides	Lieberman et al., 1996
Hsp70-2 (spermatocyte heat shock protein)	Germ cell apoptosis and meiotic arrest	Dix et al., 1996
RXR beta (retinoic acid X receptor)	Surviving homozygotes oligo-azoospermic	Kastner et al., 1996

REFERENCES

Adham I M, Nayernia K, Engel W (1997). Spermatozoa lacking acrosin protein show delayed fertilization. *Mol Reprod Dev* 46:370–376.

Baker S M, Bronner C E, Zhang L, Plug A W, Robatzek M, Warren G, Elliott E A, Yu J, Ashley T, Arnheim N, Flavell R A, Liskay R M (1995). Male mice defective in the DNA mismatch repair gene *PMS2* exhibit abnormal chromosome synapsis in meiosis. *Cell* 82:309–319.

Baker S M, Plug A W, Prolla T A, Bronner C E, Harris A C, Yao X, Christie D-M, Monell C, Arnheim N, Bradley A, Ashley T, Liskay R M (1996). Involvement of mouse *Mlh1* in DNA mismatch repair and meiotic crossing over. *Nat Genet* 13:336–342.

Barton D E, Yangfeng T L, Mason A J, Seeburg P H, Francke U (1989). Mapping of genes for inhibin subunit-alpha, subunit-β-a, and subunit-β-b on human and mouse chromosomes and studies of *jsd* mice. *Genomics* 5:91–99.

Beamer W G, Cunliffebeamer T L, Shultz K L, Langley S H, Roderick T H (1988). *Juvenile spermatogonial depletion (jsd)*—a genetic defect of germ-cell proliferation of male mice. *Biol Reprod* 38:899–908.

Bennett D (1956). Developmental analysis of a mutation with pleiotropic effects in the mouse. *J Morphol* 98:199–234.

Biddle F G, MacDonald B G, Eales B A (1985). Genetic control of sex-chromosomal univalency in the spermatocytes of C57BL/6J and DBA/2J mice. *Can J Genet Cytol* 27:741–750.

Bitgood M J, Shen L Y, McMahon A P (1996). Sertoli-cell signaling by desert hedgehog regulates the male germline. *Curr Biol* 6:298–304.

Blecher S R, Gollapudi B B, Kamra O P (1981). Preliminary evidence of genetic control of sex chromosomal synapsis in the mouse. *Can J Genet Cytol* 23:155–157.

Blendy J A, Kaestner K H, Weinbauer G F, Nieschlag E, Schutz G (1996). Severe impairment of spermatogenesis in mice lacking the CREM gene. *Nature* 380:162–165.

Bryan J H D (1977). Spermatogenesis revisited. IV. Abnormal spermiogenesis in mice homozygous for another male-sterility-inducing mutation, *hpy* (Hydrocephalic-Polydactyl). *Cell Tissue Res* 180:187–201.

Chaganti R S K, German J (1979). Human male infertility, probably genetically determined, due to defective meiosis and spermatogenic arrest. *Am J Hum Genet* 31:634–641.

Chaganti R S K, Jhanwar S C, Ehrenbard L T, Kourides I A, Williams J J (1980). Genetically determined asynapsis, spermatogenic degeneration, and infertility in men. *Am J Hum Genet* 32:833–848.

Cole A, Meistrich M L, Cherry L M, Trostle-Weige P K (1988). Nuclear and manchette development in spermatids of normal and *azh/azh* mutant mice. *Biol Reprod* 38:385–401.

Dix D J, Allen J W, Collins B W, Mori C, Nakamura N, Poorman-Allen P, Goulding E H, Eddy E M (1996). Targeted gene disruption of Hsp70-2 results in failed meiosis, germ cell apoptosis, and male infertility. *Proc Natl Acad Sci USA* 93:3264–3268.

Duncan M K, Lieman J, Chada K K (1995). The germ-cell deficient locus maps to mouse chromosome 11A2-3. *Mamm Genome* 6:697–699.

Edelmann W, Cohen P E, Kane M, Lau K, Morrow B, Bennett S, Umar A, Kunkel T, Cattoretti G, Chaganti R, Pollard J W, Kolodner R D, Kucherlapati R (1996). Meiotic pachytene arrest in *MLH1*-deficient mice. *Cell* 85:1125–1134.

Fero M L, Rivkin M, Tasch M, Porter P, Carow C E, Firpo E, Polyak K, Tsai L H, Broudy V, Perlmutter R M, Kaushansky K, Roberts J M (1996). A syndrome of multiorgan hyperplasia with features of gigantism, tumorigenesis, and female sterility in p27[kip1]-deficient mice. *Cell* 85:733–744.

Flanagan J G, Leder P (1990). The *kit* ligand—a cell-surface molecule altered in *steel* mutant fibroblasts. *Cell* 63:185–194.

Fleischman R A, Slatman D L, Stastny V, Zneimer S (1991). Deletion of the *c-kit* protooncogene in the human developmental defect piebald trait. *Proc Natl Acad Sci USA* 88:10885–10889.

Giebel L B, Spritz R A (1991). Mutation of the *KIT* (mast/stem cell growth factor receptor) protooncogene in human piebaldism. *Proc Natl Acad Sci USA* 88:8696–8699.

Handel M A, Dawson M (1981). Effects on spermiogenesis in the mouse of a male sterile neurological mutation, Purkinje cell degeneration. *Gamete Res* 4:185–192.

Handel M A, Eppig J J (1979). Sertoli cell differentiation in the testes of mice genetically deficient in germ cells. *Biol Reprod* 20:1031–1038.

Handel M A, Lane P W, Schroeder A C, Davisson M T (1988). New mutation causing sterility in the mouse. *Gamete Res* 21:409–423.

Hummel K P (1966). Atrichosis. *Mouse News Lett* 34:31.

Huang L S, Voyiaziakis E, Markenson D F, Sokol K A, Hayek T, Breslow J L (1995). apo-B gene knockout in mice results in embryonic lethality in homozygotes and neural tube defects, male infertility, and reduced HDL cholesterol ester and apo A-I transport rates in heterozygotes. *J Clin Invest* 96:2152–2161.

Hunt D M, Johnson D R (1971). Abnormal spermiogenesis in two pink-eyed sterile mutants in the mouse. *J Embryol Exp Morph* 26:111–121.

Ikawa M, Wada I, Kominami K, Watanabe D, Toshimori K, Nishimune Y, Okabe M (1997). The putative chaperone calmegin is required for sperm fertility. *Nature* 387:607–611.

Johnson D R, Hunt D M (1971). Hop-sterile, a mutant gene affecting sperm tail development in the mouse. *J Embryol Exp Morph* 25:223–236.

Kastner P, Mark M, Leid M, Gansmuller A, Chin W, Grondona J M, Decimo D, Krezel W, Dierich A, Chambon P (1996). Abnormal spermatogenesis in RXR beta mutant mice. *Genes Dev* 10:80–92.

Krege J H, John S W M, Langenbach L L, Hodgin J B, Hagaman J R, Bachman E S, Jennette J C, O'Brienc D A, Smithies O (1995). Male-female differences in fertility and blood pressure in ACE-deficient mice. *Nature* 375:146–148.

Leestma J E, Sepsenwol S (1980). Sperm tail axoneme alterations in the Wobbler mouse. *J Reprod Fertil* 58:267–270.

Liberman M W, Wiseman A L, Shi Z-Z, Carter B Z, Barries R, Ou C-N, Chévez-Barrios P, Wang Y, Habib G-M, Goodman J C, Huang S L, Lebovitz R M, Matzuk M M (1996). Growth retardation and cysteine deficiency in γ-glutamyl transpeptidase-deficient mice. *Proc Natl Acad Sci USA* 93:7923–7926.

Magram J, Bishop J M (1991). Dominant male sterility in mice caused by insertion of a transgene. *Proc Natl Acad Sci USA* 88:10327–10331.

Mintz B, Russell E S (1957). Gene-induced embryological modifications of primordial germ cells in the mouse. *J Exp Zool* 134:207–230.

Nantel F, Monaco L, Foulkes N S, Masquilier D, LeMeur M, Henriksen K, Dierich A, Parvinen M, Sassone-Corsi P (1996). Spermiogenesis deficiency and germ-cell apoptosis in CREM-mutant mice. *Nature* 380:159–162.

Noguchi T, Noguchi M (1985). A recessive mutation (ter) causing germ-cell deficiency and a high incidence of congenital testicular teratomas in 129/sv-ter mice. *J Natl Cancer Inst* 75:385–391.

Pearse R V II, Drolet D W, Kalla K A, Hooshmand F, Bermingham J R Jr, Rosenfeld M G (1997). Reduced fertility in mice deficient for the POU protein sperm-1. *Proc Natl Acad Sci USA* 94:7555–7560.

Roest H P, van Klaveren J, de Wit J, van Gurp C G, Koken M H, Vermey M, van Roijen J H, Hoogerbrugge J W, Vreeburg J T, Baarends W M, Bootsma D, Grootegoed J A, Hoeijmakers J H (1996). Inactivation of the HR6B ubiquitin-conjugating DNA-repair enzyme in mice causes male sterility associated with chromatin modification. *Cell* 86:799–810.

Sidman R L, Dickie M M, Appel S H. (1964). Mutant mice (Quaking and Jimpy) with deficient myelination in the central nervous system. *Science* 144:309–311.

Swanger W J, Robert J M (1983) p57[kip2] targeted disruption and Beckwith-Wiedemann syndrome: is the inhibitor just a contributor? *Bioessays* 19:839–842, 1997.

Varnum D S. Blind-sterile: a new mutation on chromosome 2 of the house mouse. *J Hered* 74:206–207.

Ward-Bailey P F, Johnson K R, Handel M A, Harris B S, Davisson M T (1996). A new mouse mutation causing male sterility and histoincompatibility. *Mamm Genome* 7:793–797.

Xu Y, Ashley T, Brainerd E E, Bronson R T, Meyn M S, Baltimore D (1996). Targeted disruption of *ATM* leads to growth retardation, chromosomal fragmentation during meiosis, immune defects, and thymic lymphoma. *Genes Dev* 10:2411–2422.

Zhao G-Q, Deng K, Labosky P A, Kiaw L, Hogan B L M (1996). The gene encoding bone morphogenetic protein 8B is required for the initiation and maintenance of spermatogenesis in the mouse. *Genes Dev* 10:1657–1669.

Zsebo K M, Williams D A, Geissler E N, Broudy V C, Martin F H, Atkins H L, Hsu R Y, Birkett N C, Okino K H, Murdock D C (1990). Stem-cell factor is encoded at the S I locus of the mouse and is the ligand for the *c-kit* tyrosine kinase receptor. *Cell* 63:213–224.

Appendix

Selected Features of Various Genetic and Other Disorders of Human Sexual Development and the Chapters in Which They Are Discussed

Clitoral/Labial Hypertrophy

aromatase deficiency	13
Beckwith-Wiedemann syndrome	15
Beemer lethal malformation syndrome	15
bird-headed dwarfism	15
C syndrome	15
cerebrohepatorenal syndrome	15
craniosynostosis syndromes	15
cryptophthalmos (Fraser) syndrome	15
del 1q42	18
del 7p	18
del 21q	18
fetal akinesia sequence	16
3β-hydroxysteroid dehydrogenase deficiency	13
17β-hydroxysteroid dehydrogenase type 1	13
17β-hydroxysteroid dehydrogenase type 3	13
21-hydroxylase deficiency	13
Johanson-Blizzard syndrome	15
lipodystrophy	17
neurofibromatosis type 1	15
polyploidy	18
renal dysplasia-limb defects (RL)	15
SRY alteration	5
trisomy 13	18

cloacal extrophy sequence	16
craniosynostosis syndromes	15
cryptophthalmos (Fraser) syndrome	15
de Lange syndrome	15
dup 7p	18
del 8q	18
female pseudohermaphroditism	16
Fryns syndrome	15
Halal syndrome	15
hand-foot-genital syndrome	15
hydrolethalus syndrome	15
17β-hydroxysteroid dehydrogenase type 3	13
Johanson-Blizzard syndrome	15
Laurence-Moon syndrome	15
McKusick-Kaufman syndrome	15
Meckel syndrome	15
prune belly sequence	16
5α-reductase type 2 deficiency	13
Roberts syndrome (pseudothalidomide syndrome, SC syndrome)	15
Schinzel-Giedeon syndrome	15
trisomy 7	18
urogenital adyplasia	16
urorectal malformation sequence	16
Winter syndrome	15

Vaginal Anomalies

acro-renal-mandibular syndrome	15
alterations of the androgen receptor	14
Bardet-Biedl syndrome	15
camptobrachydactyly	15
cardio-pulmonary-genital syndrome	15

Uterine Anomalies

acro-renal-mandibular syndrome	15
alterations of AMH and its receptor	9
alterations of the androgen receptor	14
Bardet-Biedl syndrome	15

Hypoplastic (undervirilized) Male or Female Genitalia: Cryptorchidism

Gonadal Dysgenesis

Index

Page references followed by the letter 'f' are for figures.
Page references followed by the letter 't' are for tables.